The French Invention of Menopa
the Medicalisation of Women's

The French Invention of Menopause and the Medicalisation of Women's Ageing

A History

ALISON M. DOWNHAM MOORE

OXFORD
UNIVERSITY PRESS

OXFORD
UNIVERSITY PRESS

Great Clarendon Street, Oxford, OX2 6DP,
United Kingdom

Oxford University Press is a department of the University of Oxford.
It furthers the University's objective of excellence in research, scholarship, and education by publishing worldwide. Oxford is a registered trade mark of Oxford University Press in the UK and in certain other countries

First Edition published in 2022

Impression: 1

Published in the United States of America by Oxford University Press
198 Madison Avenue, New York, NY 10016, United States of America

British Library Cataloguing in Publication Data
Data available

Library of Congress Control Number: 2022937049

ISBN 978–0–19–284291–6

DOI: 10.1093/oso/9780192842916.001.0001

Printed and bound by
CPI Group (UK) Ltd, Croydon, CR0 4YY

Acknowledgements

While the writing of a historical monograph is mostly a solitary affair, it is also patently indebted to countless others.

The writing of such a huge book would never have been possible without substantial research-focused time, which was enabled between 2019 and 2021 by several institutional entities. The flexibility and consideration provided by all these entities faced with the challenges of the Covid-19 pandemic, during which most of the work on this book occurred, was crucial to its completion. Western Sydney University supported the initial development of the project by providing a Women's Fellowship in 2016, sabbatical leave in 2017, as well as substantial research support and collegiality continuously since I began working there in 2012, and permitting my absence during the visiting fellowships in Germany in 2019–2021. Special thanks at Western go to Professors Peter Hutchings, Robert Mailhammer, Anna Pertierra, and Simon Burrows, as well as to Jenny Purcell, Manager of the School of Humanities and Communication Arts. My WSU colleagues Jennifer Mensch, Chris Fleming, Asha Chand, Margarite Poulos, Mark Kelly, Diego Bubbio, Rashmi Pithavadian and Tinashe Dune also inspired my hope and courage through the volatile and uncertain times in Australian higher eduction of 2020–2021.

The Australian Research Council (ARC) awarded me a Discovery grant for the larger project *Sexual Ageing in the History of Medicine* from 2019–2022 of which this book is the primary outcome.

Eleven months were spent on this book on a research fellowship at the Hanse Wissenschaftskolleg (HWK) in Germany, permitting me copious writing time, multidisciplinary feedback, and outstanding collegial support. The unique arrangement of the HWK where fellows are housed within the leafy and spacious Institute grounds itself turned out to be especially robust in absorbing the shock that was the Covid-19 pandemic lockdowns. All the staff of the HWK, especially the Rector, Professor Kerstin Schill, Professor Dorothe Poggel, Wolfgang Stenzel, and Christine Thiel, and all the wonderful scholars, writers, artists, and scientists who were fellows there in 2019–2020, especially Dr Harmen Gudde, Lida Sherafatmand, Dr Caj Neubauer, Professor Ward Keenan, Christoph Delory, Associate Professor Carsten Levisen, Ulrike Syha, Associate Professor Amy Hasinoff, Associate Professor Marci Cottingham, Dr Monika Turk, Dr Eva Fischer, Dr Sarah Coehlo, Dr Chrissy Kolya and Professor Brooke Miller, have left me with many fond memories of this time.

I warmly thank the Freiburg Institute for Advanced Studies (FRIAS), where I spent 4.5 months enjoying the multidisciplinary rigour and inspiration of that remarkable institute, first as a Marie Skłodowska-Curie Senior Fellow, and secondly as an Alumni Fellow when Australian border restrictions made my return to Sydney impossible. Special thanks for this time go to Professors Bernd Kortmann and Jürgen Osterhammel, to Petra Fischer and Niklaus Binder, and to concurrent humanities fellows Professor Janet E. Johnson (Brooklyn College) and Dr Adam Szymanski (University of Chicago).

The Chateau du Fëy commune in Burgundy (France) provided an invigorating and nurturing haven of sociability in the final month of my stay in Europe in 2021 while intensive work on the manuscript continued. Thank you Jessica Flore Angel and thankyou all Fëytopians.

Much of the research on which this book relied was enabled by both in-person visits and digital scanning services provided by the Bibliothèque Interuniversitaire de Santé (BIUS) and by the Bibliothèque Nationale de France (BNF).

Early work on the initial development of the idea for this book was enabled by a small Society for the Study of French History travel grant in 2017, by the London Critical Sexologies seminar series, by Birkbeck University of London's School of History and Archaeology, and by the Institute for Historical Studies (UK), where I first presented my initial findings from the project in 2017–2018. Special thanks go to Professor Joanna Bourke at Birkbeck, University of London who supported me in numerous ways throughout this time. The George Rudé Society for French history in Australasia also provided immense support and opportunity for feedback on my work throughout my career, and particularly during the development of this book.

I am grateful to the anonymous reviewers of my first paper published in the journal *French History* in 2018, another related paper published in *French History & Civilisation* in 2019, and to the reviewers of my initial book proposal and final monograph at Oxford University Press, who all provided significant advice toward improvement of the book concept and manuscript. Oxford UP editor Cathryn Steele was a beacon of personable professionalism and a constant support and guide throughout this process, with Bhavani Govindasamy overseeing with excellence the final copy-edit and proof stage.

I am most grateful to those who proof-read, edited, provided research assistance, and gave collegial feedback on versions of all the chapters, especially Dr Paul Reeve, whose careful multi-lingual eye on my prose and translations was particularly valuable; Dr Lucia Pozzi, who helped me to verify my understanding of Latin sources consulted in the early chapters; and Dr Antje Kühnast, who helped me to establish how much German scholarship on menopause was occurring during the emergence of the French concept and set up the website for my ARC project.

Dr Russell Downham patiently and kindly heard me rant on about, puzzle over, and worry about the manuscript at every stage of its development, ever believing in my capacities and cheering for my flourishing. Special thanks go also to Ed Cooke of Memrise for his hospitality and constant incitement to mischief in welcoming Russel and I, first in London at the start of my travel to work on this book and in Burgundy towards the end.

I want to thank all the idiosyncratic and delightful older (than me) people, both family and friends, who were part of my life during the writing of this book, especially Dr André Blum in Romainmôtier (Switzerland), Astara Henderson, Pele Sadler, and Ruth Levy (Northern NSW), my beautiful sister Catherine Kirkman and her husband Dr Ross Kirkman (Tasmania), my mother Dr Helen Cameron (South Australia) and my father Dennis Aubrey Moore (Tasmania).

I also want to thank the fearless and inspiring strength athletes and trainers of all ages I met, trained alongside, and learnt from throughout the time I was writing this book and who I observed always to be nothing but encouraging of older women pursuing their own strength and athleticism: Paul Con, Ricky and Sarah Gulyamov (Sydney), the Bethnal Green Weightlifting Club (London), Berlin Strength (Berlin), and the Société Athlétique Montmartroise (Paris).

Finally, I want to thank the medical clinicians Dr Lyndal Tendek (Sydney), Dr Erlich Sem (Goldcoast) and Associate Professor Marcelo Nascimento (Goldcoast) who all provided personable and respectful patient-centred care to me in managing my own health challenges during the years I spent working on this book, and so helped me to feel incredibly grateful not to have been seeking medical treatment in a nineteenth-century hospital.

Contents

List of Images

Introduction

The Layering of Medical Concepts

It may surprise many readers to learn that this book resulted not from a narrowly focused single-culture historical investigation, but from a wide-ranging, global, diachronic, intercultural, multi-lingual, and interdisciplinary reading of biomedical accounts of sex-differentiated ageing across time and place. And yet this is a book largely about French medical concepts, mostly those of the long nineteenth century and specifically about women's ageing and its reduction to the concept of menopause. Over a five-year period of global research, it became increasingly clear that from the late eighteenth to early twentieth centuries, there was a massively disproportionate magnitude of different European cultures' preoccupation with women's final cessation of menses and its implication for their ageing as a matter of medical concern. French doctors, vastly more than any others throughout the long nineteenth century (*c.*1790–*c.*1930), produced a vast corpus of works about women's final cessation of menses and the special forms of self-care and medical surveillance it was thought to require, which was unparalleled in any other contemporaneous culture, even if a few specialist works of a similar nature occasionally appeared in both English and German.[1] This book is about why that was so.

Nonetheless, medical concepts never spring forth from nowhere and have never been bounded within nation-states. Chapter 1 discusses relevant precedent English, Latin and German ideas to that of menopause in the long history of medicine since the late sixteenth century, and other chapters mention those German and English works published on women's critical age or climacteric during the long nineteenth century—some of which were read and discussed in

[1] The major German and English/American works were: Enoch Heinrich Kisch, *Das klimaterische Alter der Frauen: Physiologischer und pathologischer Beziehung* (Erlangen: Ferdinand Enke, 1874); Ernst Börner, *Die Wecheseljahre der Frau* (Stuttgart: Ferdinand Enke, 1886); John Fothergill, 'On the Management Proper at the Cessation of the Menses', *Medical Observations and Inquiries* vol. 5 (London: Cadell, 1776): 160–186; Edward John Tilt, *The Change of Life in Health and Disease: A Practical Treatise on the Nervous and Other Affections Incidental to Women at the Decline of Life* [1857], 3rd ed. (London: J. Churchill, 1870); Andrew Fay Currier, *The Menopause* (New York: D. Appleton & Co.: 1897). On the history of German gynaecological writing that occasionally referred to the cessation of menses, see Birgit Panke-Kochinke, *Die Wechseljahre der Frau: Aktualität und Geschichte 1772–1996* (Opladen: Leske & Budrich, 1998). On English menopause writing see Ornella Moscucci, 'Medicine, Age and Gender: The Menopause in History', *British Menopause Society*, 5/4 (1999): 149–153.

The French Invention of Menopause and the Medicalisation of Women's Ageing: A History. Alison M. Downham Moore, Oxford University Press. © Alison M. Downham Moore 2022. DOI: 10.1093/oso/9780192842916.003.0001

France, just as several of the major French works on the topic were influential elsewhere. However, all these non-French sources, as well as those French and other sources published before 1790 which mentioned the final cessation of menses, taken together constitute merely a drop in the ocean of the major topic which menopause became in French medicine between 1790 and 1920. General French medical textbooks and surveys of women's health in this period also assimilated the specialist topic far more than was the case in either German or English general medicine. This striking disparity demands explanation. It has been overlooked in most previous attempts to historicise menopause substantially, which have either tended to sample selective French and other sources as if they were representative of a broad European trend in modern biomedicine; or have skimmed the surface of several different cultures' medical concepts of menstruation, or cultural attitudes to older women, which are then conflated with menopause; or have given equal importance to all western cultures from medieval times to the present in the production of a handful of texts ambiguously referring to menstrual stoppage which is not clearly that relating to ageing, and not recognising that for France, the selected sources were barely a fraction of what was actually written on the topic.[2] French medical scholars not only invented the word menopause and generated the first truly specialist works (hundreds of them) on the topic; they frankly *owned* the concept for over 100 years, making it a central topic of modern biomedical pedagogic induction.

The period between 1790 and 1821 saw the publication of the first of many subsequent works to champion a radical new interpretation of women's reproductive ageing, including that of the inventor of the word *la ménopause*, Charles-Pierre-Louis de Gardanne between 1812 and 1821.[3] Throughout the nineteenth century, menopause became a common thesis topic for doctoral students at both the Montpellier and Paris medical faculties, with over 170 specialist theses written on it—a phenomenon unparalleled in any other contemporaneous culture. Indeed, much of the work of fleshing-out the concept surrounding women's final cessation of menses as a category of disease was done by doctoral students. While theses were not available to French readerships outside the academy, they were both extremely important in the internal development of medical concepts, and a crucial vector of international dissemination, since from the early nineteenth century, medical journals in other countries frequently listed all the recent medical theses produced in major universities globally, and French thesis titles on

[2] Ruth Formanek, ed., *The Meanings of Menopause: Historical, Medical and Clinical Perspectives* (Hillsdale, NJ: The Analytic Press, 1990); Jessica E. Godfrey, *Attitudes to Post-Menopausal Women in the High and Late Middle Ages, 1100–1400* (Jessica E. Godfrey, self-published, 2011); Michael Stolberg, 'A Woman's Hell? Medical Perceptions of Menopause in Preindustrial Europe', *Bulletin of the History of Medicine*, 73/3 (1999): 404–428.

[3] Charles-Pierre-Louis de Gardanne, *Dissertation sur les avis à donner aux femmes qui entrent dans l'âge critique*. Thèse (Paris: Didot Jeune, 1812); Charles-Pierre-Louis de Gardanne, *De la ménopause ou de l'âge critique des femmes* (Paris: Méquignon-Marvis, 1821).

menopause were commonly reported in the English, American, German, and Italian journals. But also, the established medical scholars who began generating popularised books about menopause or women's critical age after the 1830s, following Gardanne's successful 1821 publication, evidently drew heavily from the work of doctoral students, translating their specialist ideas for a wider elite public readership. Indeed, it seems apparent that the topic of women's final cessation of menses was identified as important by several eminent late eighteenth- and early nineteenth-century medical figures, such as Paul-Joseph Barthez, Philippe Pinel, and Joseph-Marie-Joachim Vigarous, but was viewed as too narrowly specific or uninteresting for established scholars to bother with themselves, which is why the professors of Montpellier and Paris assigned it to their students instead. By the 1830s, that perception had begun to shift and increasing numbers of established clinicians thereafter produced their own specialist works on women's health with reference to the 'critical' times of uterine change, such as the final cessation of menses.[4] The revolutionary character of the neologism lay less in its radical content relative to previous medical ideas from which it inherited and repurposed many central themes, but rather in the historical and materialist self-consciousness of French doctors in this period, who saw themselves as cleaving a new era of scientific reasoning about women's health and ageing.[5] That identity was crucial to the invention and elaboration of menopause as a crisis of women's ageing health, without which many important later developments, such as the most common surgical practices of modern gynaecology, and the development of the

[4] Gardanne, *De la ménopause*; Sébastien Guyétant, *Le Médecin de l'âge de retour et la vieillesse: conseils aux gens du monde, qui ont passé l'âge de quarante-cinq ans* (Paris: Dufey, 1836); Charles Menville, *De l'Âge critique chez les femmes, des maladies qui peuvent survenir à cette époque de la vie et des moyens de les combattre et de les prévenir* (Paris: Imprimerie de Bourgogne et Martinet, 1840); Alexandre. F. Brierre de Boismont, *De la menstruation, considérée dans ses rapports physiologiques et pathologiques* (Paris: Germer Baillière, 1842); Adam Raciborski, *De la puberté et de l'âge critique chez la femme, au point de vue physiologique, hygiénique et médical* (Paris: J. B. Baillière 1844); Virginie Messager, *Guide pratique de l'âge critique, ou Conseils aux femmes sur les maladies qui peuvent les attaquer à cette époque de leur vie; suivis de Réflexions et d'observations sur les maladies laiteuses* (Paris: chez l'auteur, 1859); Émile Bertin, *De la ménopause considérée principalement au point de vue de l'hygiène* (Montpellier: C. Coulet/Paris: Adrien Delahaye, 1866); Adam Raciborski, *Traité de la menstruation, ses rapports avec l'ovulation, la fécondation, l'hygiène de la puberté et de l'âge critique* (Paris: J. B. Baillière, 1868); Sébastien Guyétant, *L'Âge de retour et la vieillesse: Conseils au gens du monde* (Paris: L. Brunet, 1870); Alex Mayer, *Conseils aux femmes sur l'âge de retour; médecine et hygiène* (Paris: J. B. Baillière et Fils, 1875); Dr Hayès, *Hygiène de l'âge critique* (Paris: Librairie des publications modernes, 1891); Dr Charles Barbaud & Dr A. Rouillard, *Histoire clinico-thermale de la femme aux trois grandes périodes de sa vie: puberté, union sexuelle, ménopause. Troubles et accidents de la ménopause (âge critique de la femme), traitement thermal aux eaux de Luxeuil* (Paris: Jouvet, 1895); André Castan, *Hygiène de l'âge de retour* (Paris: J. B. Baillière et Fils, 1901); Ernest Barié, *Étude sur la ménopause* (Paris: V. Adrien Delahaye, 1877); Charles Vinay, *La Ménopause* (Paris: Masson, 1908); Louis Genest, *Comment prévenir et guérir les maladies du retour d'âge: Hygiène préventive; les soins spéciaux; les meilleurs remèdes* (Paris: M. Drouin, *c.*1920).

[5] Alison M. Moore, 'Conceptual Layers in the Invention of Menopause in Nineteenth-Century France', *French History*, 32/2 (2018): 226–248.

multi-billion-dollar global pharmaceutical hormone replacement therapy industry in the twentieth century, would have been unimaginable.

Several of the most influential figures who helped to make the subject of menopause a substantial theme in French medicine throughout the long nineteenth century also elaborated a unique vision of what they described as the 'hygienic' management of women's ageing, which became a major sub-genre of its own throughout the long nineteenth century.[6] Menopause, in fact, appears to have been one of the central examples through which medical scholars of both the Paris and Montpellier medical faculties developed the concept of *hygiène*, which fused ideas about humoral constitutions, vitalism, dietetics, moral psychology, and preventive medicine, with an emphasis on personalised treatment, drawing attention to the distinctions between patients on the basis of age, sex, class,

[6] Jacques Louis Moreau (de la Sarthe), *Histoire naturelle de la femme, suivie d'un traité d'hygiène appliqué à son régime physiques et moral aux différentes époques de la vie*, 3 vols (Paris: Duprat, 1803); Jean-Antoine Poussié, *Réflexions sur l'hygiène qui convient aux femmes arrivées à l'âge de retour.* Thèse (Montpellier: Jean Martel aîné, 1813); Louis Gubian, *Considérations générales sur l'état physiologique de la femme parvenue à l'âge critique, et sur les moyens hygiéniques qui lui conviennent.* Thèse (Paris: Didot Jeune, 1816); Antoine-Alexandre Olive, *Dissertation inaugurale sur la première menstruation, l'âge critique et les soins hygiéniques que réclament les femmes à ces deux époques.* Thèse (Paris: Didot Jeune, 1819); Joseph-François Garnier, *Considérations sur l'âge critique, et sur l'hygiène des femmes à cette époque.* Thèse (Paris: Didot Jeune, 1820); Gardanne, *De la ménopause ou de l'âge critique des femmes*; Albert Assegond, *De la Femme, considérée à l'âge critique: Changements physiologiques qui s'opèrent dans on état physiques et moral, et de l'application des règles de l'hygiène à cette principale époque de la vie.* Thèse (Paris: Didot Jeune, 1821); Pierre-Jean-Baptiste Bertrand, *Dissertation sur l'aménorrhée définitive ou âge critique des femmes sur les accidents auxquels elles sont exposées à cette époque, et sur les moyens thérapeutiques, hygiéniques et prophylactiques les plus appropriés à leur situation* (Paris: Didot le Jeune, 1824); Claude Lachaise, *Hygiène physiologique de la femme ou de la femme considérée dans son système physique et moral* (Paris: Mequignon Marvis, 1825); S. G. Chazal, *De l'Hygiène des femmes à l'époque de la cessation des menstrues.* Thèse (Paris: Didot Jeune, 1826); Jacques-Philippe Labarraque, *Aperçu physiologico-pathologique sur la menstruation en général, et quelques conseils d'hygiène pour l'âge critique en particulier.* Thèse (Montpellier: Jean Martel aîné, 1827); E. Duplessis, *De l'âge critique et des soins hygiéniques que réclament les femmes à cette époque.* Thèse (Paris: Didot Le Jeune, 1828); Louis-Marie-André Jeannin, *Considérations physiologiques, pathologiques et hygiéniques sur l'âge de retour des femmes.* Thèse (Strasbourg: F. G. Levrault, 1830); Lucien-Hector Docé, *Dissertation sur la cessation des menstrues vulgairement appelée âge critique, et sur les moyens hygiéniques que réclame la santé de la femme à cette époque.* Thèse (Paris: Didot Jeune, 1831); Louis-Marie Lafontaine-Margariteau, *Conseils hygiéniques aux femmes depuis leur naissance jusqu'à l'âge critique, ayant pour but principal de les préserver de la leucorrhée flueurs blanches), ou de la diminuer si elle existe.* Thèse (Paris: Didot le Jeune, 1835); Menville, *De l'âge critique chez les femmes*; Joseph-Hortense Houlès, *De la ménopause considérée au point de vue de l'hygiène.* Thèse (Montpellier: Isadore Tournel, 1843); Marie-Gustave Léopold Chéneaux, *De la menstruation et de la ménopause, au point de vue de la physiologie et de l'hygiène.* Thèse (Paris: Rignoux, 1859); Charles Van Leynseele, *Hygiène de la femme, ou l'art de conserver la santé et de prolonger la vie, depuis la naissance jusqu'à l'extrême vieillesse*, 2 vols (Gand: H. Hoste, 1860); Théophile-Charles-Emmanuel-Édouard Auber, *Hygiène des femmes nerveuses ou Conseils aux femmes pour les époques critiques de leur vie* (Paris: Germer Baillière, 1864); Émile Bertin, *De la ménopause considérée principalement au point de vue de l'hygiène* (Montpellier: C. Coulet/Paris: Adrien Delahaye, 1866); Raciborski, *Traité de la menstruation*; Mayer, *Conseils aux femmes sur l'âge de retour*; Hayès, *Hygiène de l'âge critique*; Marie de Thilo, *L'Hygiène intime: Conseils aux femmes pour tous les âges de la vie* (Paris: Fischbacher, 1892); Castan, *Hygiène de l'âge de retour*; Genest, *Comment prévenir et guérir les maladies du retour d'âge.*

temperament, and other forms of typology.[7] Hygienic medicine claimed to be providing a necessary clinical service to ageing women that was particular to them, even if they had no diseases and sought no treatments. This was the beginning of something recognisable to us today in the pharmacological targeting of women 'in menopause' with hormone replacement therapies, herbal supplements, and prophylactic surgeries: French menopause hygiene of the long nineteenth century marked the beginning of modern biomedical practices of differentiating ageing women from men as the sex in greater need of care by medical professionals. It was also the beginning of the ongoing generation of health advice to women to actively manage post-reproductive life, rather than simply living it—or indeed rather than using it to achieve some purpose beyond themselves and beyond their roles within family, as indeed the American doctor Emma Drake alternatively proposed in her 1901 work which appeared in French translation in 1908.[8]

From the above account it may seem as if this book itself means to imply that the incorporation of menopause into modern biomedicine was an entirely unnecessary or unwelcome historical development and that the final cessation of menses should be simply treated as a natural life stage without much more to be said of it—a valid normative argument sometimes made by older women themselves and by different kinds of scholars.[9] But this is not the argument made in this book, which refrains entirely from the activity of menopause advice, of which there is already a dazzling abundance. The word 'medicalisation' has different meanings in the humanities and social sciences, which can lend themselves to misunderstandings. It is often thought to imply criticism of the medical treatment of natural human conditions, which biomedicine is seen as both negatively characterising and unnecessarily subjecting to therapeutic regimes and practices that may bring new forms of illness in themselves.[10] But among medical historians, the term is also used to describe the growth of medical research and writing on specific themes, the increased scientific attention given to particular facets of human physiology, the growth of new medical specialisms, the increased number

[7] Elizabeth A. Williams, *A Cultural History of Medical Vitalism in Enlightenment Montpellier* (London: Routledge, 2003), 102–104; 215; Gérard Seignan, 'L'Hygiène sociale au XIXe siècle: Une physiologie morale', *Revue d'histoire du XIXe siècle*, 40 (2010), 113–130; Erwin H. Ackernecht, 'Hygiene in France, 1815–1848', *Bulletin of the History of Medicine*, 22/2 (1948): 117–155.

[8] Emma Angell Drake, *What a Woman of Forty-Five Ought to Know* (Philadelphia: Vir Publishing, 1901); Emma Angell Drake, *Ce que toute femme de 45 ans devrait savoir (l'âge critique)* (Geneva: J. H. Jeheber, 1908).

[9] Germaine Greer, *The Change: Women, Ageing and the Menopause* (London: Bloomsbury, 2018).

[10] Ivan Illich, *Medical Nemesis* (London: Calder & Boyars, 1974).); Peter Conrad, *The Medicalization of Society: On the Transformation of Human Conditions into Treatable Disorders* (Baltimore: Johns Hopkins University Press, 2007); Robert A. Nye, 'The Evolution of the Concept of Medicalization in the Late Twentieth Century', *Journal of the History of the Behavioural Sciences*, 39/2 (2003): 115–129; Ilana Löwy & Jean-Paul Gaudillière, 'Médicalisation de la ménopause, mouvements pour la santé des femmes et controverses sur les thérapies hormonales', *Nouvelles Questions féministes*, 25/2 (2006): 48–65.

of doctors per inhabitants of a town, and the proliferation of clinical services and pharmaceutical products directed at specific populations; as well as encompassing the growth of traditional and alternative forms of medical and health practices, not merely biomedicine.[11] Medicalisation is not necessarily an inherently critical term; it is also a descriptive one which characterises the modern era as a unique time in human history, in which medicine has become increasingly enmeshed in our lives as never before.[12] Medicalisation has clearly brought enormous benefits both for lifespan preservation and for the treatment of many serious diseases. Nonetheless, the case of menopause is a clear example of how the specific conceptual content of medicalisation—its ever densifying discursive weft and weave throughout the long nineteenth century—has profoundly shaped the kinds of clinical norms and research questions that continue to inform current therapeutic practices relating to the health of older women.

In the period where this book begins (at the end of the seventeenth century), doctors were rarely encountered by most French people, and even in the nineteenth century, it was only in large towns and cities that such official practitioners could be found. They were outnumbered, by a factor of at least three or four to one, by a vast array of folk and empiric practitioners of different kinds, *charlatans*, *empiriques*, *guérisseurs*, and *commères*, as well as surgeons and pharmacists who remained on the edges of legal medicine until the late nineteenth century;[13] most women gave birth not in hospitals but at home; and most medicaments were based on herbal and animal products that were harvested, dried, ground, and packaged by the individual pharmacy workers who sold them; all abdominal surgeries were almost invariably lethal; and women themselves were barred from being doctors, even in the growing specialist area of the treatment of the diseases of women.[14] Over the course of the nineteenth century, during the time of the formation and elaboration of the concept of women's critical age or menopause in the university faculties of Paris and Montpellier, all these important contexts underwent dramatic change, with important implications for how women's

[11] Matthew Ramsey, *Professional and Popular Medicine in France, 1779–1830* (Cambridge: Cambridge University Press, 1988); Ann La Berge & Mordechai Feingold, eds, *French Medical Culture in the Nineteenth Century* (Amsterdam: Rodopi, 1994); Martin Dinges, Kay Peter Jankrift, Sabine Schlegelmilch, & Michael Stohlberg, *Medical Practice 1600–1900*, trans. Margot Saar (Leiden/Boston: Brill/Rodopi, 2016); Lise Dumasy-Queffélec & Hélène Spengler, eds, *Médecine, sciences de la vie et littérature en France et en Europe de la Révolutioin à nos jours: Le Médecin entre savoirs et pouvoirs*, vol. 3 (Geneva: Librairie Droz, 2014).

[12] W. R. Albury, 'Heart of Darkness: J. N. Corvisart and the Medicalization of Life', in Jean-Pierre Goubert, ed., *La Médicalisation de la société française, 1770–1830* (Waterloo: Historical Reflections Press, 1982), 17–31.

[13] Ramsey, *Professional and Popular Medicine in France*, 129–246.

[14] Ibid., 50, 79; June K. Burton, *Napoleon and the Woman Question: Discourses of the Other Sex in French Education, Medicine, and Medical Law 1799-1815* (Lubbock: Texas Tech University Press, 2007), 103–106.

ageing became medically treated.[15] The rise of menopause medicine in France was greeted by a wide array of responses among physicians, hygienists, medical pedagogues, chemists, surgeons, midwives, health writers, as well as women novelists and epistolary writers who are discussed in Chapter 9. Rather than mounting a case for or against the medicalisation of menopause, this book primarily explores how the reduction of women's ageing to the cessation of menses was assimilated, contested, complicated, and transcended by different minds of the long nineteenth century. Whatever values we, as historians and readers, may bring to the past described here, the people who lived it had their own ideas about what was important, what was dangerous, what needed to be questioned, and what could be done better. If this book indeed appears at times critical of specific trends, practices, or individuals of the past, it is because their own contemporaries showed that it was indeed possible to think otherwise.

Furthermore, medicalisation is even more central to this book than simply describing its broad object. The critique of medicalisation was in fact itself central to the discourse surrounding the invention of the neologism, *la ménopause*, which referred simply to the cessation of menses, in contrast to alternative terms, such as *l'âge critique* or *climatérique*, and *le retour d'âge*, which, it was thought, all variously implied something worrying about the dramatic nature of the change. Doctors writing on this topic throughout the nineteenth century championed their own anti-pathological stance, arguing that they were the first medical scholars in history not to see 'it' as a disease that required medicating. In fact, they were the first scholars in history to see 'it' as a specific thing at all. The critique of medicalisation was actually part of the very process through which menopause was itself made into a topic of substantial medical description. While doctors repeatedly insisted that menopause was a normal and natural process which was not to be feared or medicated, they also, just as commonly, invoked the frightening spectre of uncomfortable illnesses and dangerous diseases that would occur if a woman failed to observe the elaborate set of prescriptions and proscriptions with which hygienic advice for them was filled. Paradoxically, doctors sought to manage menopause medically as never before, while also arguing against its pathologisation. The paradox is succinctly contained in the following 1846 sentences from the work of the Paris hygienist Antonin Bossu (1809–1897):

> The disappearance of the menses, or the turn of age (critical age) is generally considered to create a dangerous environment in a woman's body. These fears are exaggerated: the cessation of the menstrual flux is physiological fact, a normal function . . . In general, however, the critical time modifies the vitality of the

[15] Jacques Léonard, *La France médicale: Médecins et malades au XIXe Siècle* (Paris: Aubier, 1978); Jean-Pierre Goubert, ed., *La Médicalisation de la société française, 1770–1830* (Waterloo: Historical Reflections Press, 1982).

womb and the entire economy, in such a way as to facilitate the development of diseases to which a woman is already predisposed, or which the disturbance or lack of precautions has allowed to breed.[16]

In a sense then, French doctors actively medicalised something which they clearly understood to be a universal natural process, both elaborating specific clinical principles for the treatment of menopausal women, while insisting nonetheless that the cessation of menses was 'not a disease', and criticising (often unnamed) others whom they blamed for catastrophising it. The twentieth-century critical meaning of 'medicalisation', then, has an older lineage in nineteenth-century French medicine, where it was instrumentalised precisely to do the very work of medicalisation it claimed to critique.

It was only in France of the long nineteenth century that the topic of menopause, or women's critical age, became central to medical pedagogy and to the development of clinical hygiene. Nonetheless, global pressures played an important role in the unique French manifestation of ideas about women's ageing, both through the intercultural demographic revolution occurring during the eighteenth century, which converged on the view that women naturally lived longer; and through the ethnographic description of diverse cultures which naturalised the functional end of menses in women as a universal biological fact. Strikingly, the concept of women suffering a sex-specific crisis of ageing resulting from the end of menses emerged in French medicine precisely in the context of the wider European demographic revelation of women's greater life expectancy. The first French thinkers to discuss women's longer lifespans in relation to medicine, the mathematician-demographers Antoine Deparcieux and Louis-François Benoiston de Châteauneuf, referred specifically to statistical mortality data as evidence against the view of the end of menses as dangerous to women's health, or as something that required specific medical attention.[17] The longevity advantage of women was indeed so great that at the beginning of the nineteenth century, the adult female population outnumbered men by two to one, with more women living past their reproductive years than ever previously before.[18] But this also made older women the most important demographic for doctors' economic need for patients. Thus, rather than the fact of women's longevity deterring French doctors from developing the concept of a menopause symptomology and hygiene, on the contrary, it provided the stimulus for a novel scientific identity which

[16] Antonin Bossu, *Anthropologie, ou Étude des organes, fonctions et maladies de l'homme et de la femme, comprenant l'anatomie, la physiologie, l'hygiène, la pathologie et la thérapeutique*, 2 vols (Paris: Comon, 1846), vol. 1, 450.

[17] Antoine Deparcieux, *Essai sur les probabilités de la durée de la vie humaine, d'où l'on déduit la manière de déterminer les rentes viagères, tant simples qu'en Tontines* (Paris: Frères Guerin, 1746); Louis-François Benoiston de Châteauneuf, *Mémoire sur la mortalité des femmes de l'âge de quarante à cinquante ans, lu à l'Académie des Sciences, dans la séance du 13 mai 1818* (Paris: Martinet, 1822).

[18] Ramsey, *Professional and Popular Medicine in France*, 226.

championed what they claimed was a revolutionary new approach to medically treating women's ageing morbidity. In fact, menopause was an important case example for the development of theories of ageing and longevity in both the Paris and Montpellier faculties, resulting in the shift from a vitalist conception of life as a force of finite quantity that produced health, longevity, and fertility in equal measure, towards a new bifurcation of morbidity from mortality. Women, long considered the sicker sex on account of the sacrifice of vital force that their bodies made to create new humans, were thought to age more poorly and yet live longer. The cessation of menses was made the focus of explanation for this apparently paradoxical situation.

Menopause was not suddenly invented at the moment of its nominal scientific designation; rather it was composed of multiple embedded conceptual layers, each bearing their own temporally specific inheritances relating to ageing, lifespan, women, and disease. Some of these layers were clearly partially carried over into later forms of the concept, such as the eighteenth-century concept of sanguinary plethora, which remained part of ideas about menopause physiology throughout the nineteenth century;[19] while others were put into a long recess until a later resurgence, like the astrological concept of the seventh septenary climacteric which French doctors of the nineteenth century largely eschewed due its unacceptably metaphysical underpinnings but which has occasionally been referenced in the twentieth century.[20] From one perspective, the modern French medicalisation of women's ageing was consistent with a much larger and older trend towards the view of women as inherently more diseased. 'From antiquity to the classical age, women's bodies were the paradigm of the sick body,' remarks Elsa Dorlin in her 2006 study of medical views of women's reproductive health in the history of French national and colonial regimes.[21] Nonetheless, it was only in the final decades of the eighteenth century that post-reproductive women became reclassified as more prone to disease, even as their greater longevity relative to men was widely recognised, referring to the splitting of morbidity from mortality (Chapter 3).

The oldest conceptual current that began the long historical layering of modern menopause derived from Ptolemaic astrology which referred to the seven-year cycles of the lifespan as 'climacteric' years of special portent, in which one either died or entered a new phase of being.[22] Early modern engagements with

[19] The esteem of plethora theory was nonetheless less than in the nineteenth than in the eighteenth century and was subject to repeated criticisms, summarised in Ernest Perthuisot, *De la crise médicale: Pléthore, discrédit, concurrence, imposition* (Lyon: A. Storck & Cie, 1898).

[20] Colette, *La Naissance du jour* [1928] (Paris: Flammarion, 1984), 48; Michel Ducet, *L'Âge climatérique de l'homme et de la femme, retour d'âge et crise sexuelle* (Soissons: Aubenas, 1964).

[21] Elsa Dorlin, *La Matrice de la race: Généologie sexuelle et coloniale de la nation française* [2006] (Paris: La Découverte/Poche, 2009), 109.

[22] Max Engammare, *Soixante-trois: La Peur de la grande année climactérique à la Renaissance* (Genève: Droz, 2013); Jean-Christophe Sanchez, 'Observations des météores et médecine aux temps

Ptolemy interpreted the seventh septenary—age 49—as a particularly important climacteric year in which ageing properly began in both men and women; and this idea collided with the emergence of a growing medical interest in the diseases of women from the end of the sixteenth century to produce the very first questions raised by doctors about women's final cessation of menses which had often been observed to occur in women around the turn of their 49th year.[23] However, the end of menstruation was barely considered significant by scholars before the eighteenth century, and ideas about it initially emerged as a subset of the larger medical concern with suppressed menstruation in women of reproductive age, which was often taken as a proxy of conceptive capacity.[24] Suppressed menses, ageing in general, and a wide range of other diseases in eighteenth-century medicine were reconceived according to the doctrine of sanguinary plethora, for which the most common remedy was phlebotomy, but also, sometimes, purgative medications. It was in this context the women's final cessation of menses first came to be treated medically, not as a significant matter of its own, but as one of the many forms of plethora with which women and men, old and young, were diagnosed (Chapter 1).

On the other hand, a significant and crucial part of the conceptual work towards the nineteenth-century development of both menopause hygiene and menopause psychiatry was in fact worked out in an entirely separate branch of medical writing of the eighteenth century, which referred to the vapours, hysteria, and hypochondria—a connection which Jocelyne Livi suggested in her 1984 book *Vapeurs de femmes*.[25] Livi's evocative and generative account nonetheless evaded the precise relationship between eighteenth-century vapours and nineteenth-century menopause, for perfectly understandable reasons: vapours and hysteria scholars of the eighteenth century rarely had much to say about older women, and largely characterised such nervous diseases as specific to young women; but a few of them did identify the final cessation of menses as one of the critical times of uterine change that were thought to trigger women's nervous disorders.[26] On the other hand, there was an obscure lateral relationship between these two

modernes', *Histoire, médecine et santé*, 1 (2012): 95–113; Rutkin, H. Darrel, 'The Use and Abuse of Ptolemy's *Tetrabiblos* in Renaissance and Early-Modern Europe: Two Case Studies (Giovanni Pico Mirandola and Filippo Fantoni)', in Alexander Jones (ed.), *Ptolemy in Perspective: Use and Criticism of his Work from Antiquity to the Nineteenth Century* (New York: Springer, 2010), 135–150.

[23] Daniel Schäfer, *Old Age and Disease in Early Modern Medicine*, trans. Patrick Baker (London: Routledge, 2015).

[24] Cathy McClive, *Menstruation and Procreation in Early-Modern France* (London/New York: Routledge, 2015).

[25] Jocelyne Livi, *Vapeurs de femmes: Essai historique sur quelques fantasmes médicaux et philosophiques* (Paris: Navarin, 1984).

[26] Robert Whytt, *Les Vapeurs et maladies nerveuses, hypocondriaques ou hystériques reconnues & traitées dans les deux sexes* [1765], 2 vols (Paris: Vincent, 1767); Edme-Pierre Chauvot de Beauchêne, *De l'influence des affections de l'âme dans les maladies nerveuses des femmes, avec le traitement qui convient à ces maladies* [1781], 2nd ed. (Montpellier & Paris: Méquignon, 1783).

distinct discursive currents relating to women. The earlier vapours and hysteria writers crucially developed the mechanistic explanation which remained the basis of most nineteenth-century alienist and psychiatric writing about menopausal madness, erotomania, and hypochondria. Nineteenth-century menopause hygiene too was able simply to attach a complete therapeutic apparatus to its structure using the recycled parts of ideas about women's hygiene as the pursuit of an ideal peasant model, and which were elaborated extensively in eighteenth-century vapours scholarship.[27]

The final conceptual layer which helped to cohere the emerging interest in older women's cessation of menses came from Montpellier vitalist approaches which placed tremendous emphasis both on the personalisation of patient care according to sex, age, humoral temperament, and individual character; on the healthful properties of bodily excretions and exudations;[28] and on the positive view of physiological 'crises' which defined these as the passage of bodies from one state to another which medicine should abstain from trying to treat (Chapter 3).[29] But Montpellier also generated some of the most influential thinkers to theorise about the nature of women's vital force and its decline with ageing, namely the medically trained Paris journalist Pierre Roussel (1742–1802) whom numerous historians have identified as a crucial figure in the emergence of modern medical ideas about what was often called 'the natural history of women'.[30] Roussel was certainly the most influential, but far from the only late eighteenth-century French scholar to insist on a radical dimorphism of the sexes in matters of culture, society, politics, and medicine. In the medical elaboration of such arguments about women's nature, other Montpellier-trained scholars such as Samuel Tissot, Théophile de Bordeu, and Philippe Pinel played a particularly prominent role. As Elizabeth Williams observes, vitalist scholars' views of women tended to see sex and child-rearing as 'the only activities consonant with the

[27] Joseph Raulin, *Traité des affections vaporeuses du sexe, avec l'exposition de leurs symptômes, de leurs différentes causes, et la méthode de les guérir* (Paris: Jean-Thomas Hérissant, 1758); Jean-Baptiste Pressavin, *Nouveau Traité des vapeurs, ou traité des maladies des nerfs, dans lequel on développe les vrais principes des vapeurs* (Paris: La Veuve Reguilliat, 1770); Edme-Pierre Chauvot de Beauchêne, *De l'influence des affections de l'âme dans les maladies nerveuses des femmes, avec le traitement qui convient à ces maladies* [1781], 2nd ed. (Montpellier & Paris: Méquignon, 1783).

[28] Elizabeth A. Williams, 'Eating after the Climacteric: Food, Gender and Aging in the Long Eighteenth Century', in James Kennaway & Rina Knoeff, eds, *Lifestyle and Medicine in the Enlightenment: The Six Non-Naturals in the Long Eighteenth Century* (London: Routledge, 2020), unpaginated.

[29] Théophile Bordeu, *Recherches sur le pouls, par rapport aux crises* (Paris: De Bure l'aîné, 1756); Dominique Raymond, *Traité des maladies qu'il est dangereux de guérir*, 2 vols (Avignon: F. B. Merande, 1757).

[30] Pierre Roussel, *Système physique et moral de la femme* (Paris: Chez Vincent, 1775); Anne C. Vila, 'Sex and Sensibility: Pierre Rousseau's *Système physique et moral de la femme*', *Représentations*, 52 (1995): 76–93; Kathleen Anne Wellman, 'Physicians and Philosophes: Physiology and Sexual Morality in the French Enlightenment', *Eighteenth-Century Studies*, 35/2 (2002): 267–277; Sean M. Quinlan, *Morbid Undercurrents: Medical Subcultures in Postrevolutionary France* (Ithaca, NY: Cornell University Press, 2021), 68–94.

character of the female vital force',[31] with important implications for their conceptualisation of the end of fertility and menstruation. When these currents encountered the growing materialist and mechanistic strands of post-revolutionary Paris science with its strident claims to rupture from past medical error and reformulations of the ideal of Hippocratic medicine, the modern concept of menopause was finally formed (Chapter 6).

The new concept was rapidly made an exemplary topic in scientific medical pedagogy of the first years of the nineteenth century, where it became entangled in the inter-faculty rivalries between Montpellier and Paris and assimilated to the larger struggle of biomedicine against rival health practitioners. Importantly, it was a concept formed in the context of women's exclusion from practising as doctors and their relegation as official medical practitioners only to the care of birthing mothers (discussed in Chapter 8).[32] The concept of menopause did not come from women themselves but rather from medical men for whom it was a tremendously useful and generative case example: as a tool for biomedical reformulations of treatment practices and of the conceptual separation of morbidity from mortality; as a teaching tool for inducting medical students into the new mechanistic approach to women's medicine; as a weapon with which to fight folk healers, other doctors, rival medical faculties, and competing treatment practices; as well as a pathway for new medical disciplines such as hygiene (Chapter 5), psychiatry (Chapter 7), as well as gynaecological surgery and emergent endocrinology (Chapter 10), to expand their patient markets, develop their theoretical precepts and test their clinical techniques.

A further consideration which supports the view of menopause as a concept grounded in new French biomedical identities, industries and pedagogies is that most doctors writing on women's ageing at this time denigrated what they considered 'popular myths' about menopause, in some cases specifically blaming women folk-healers and empirics for the erroneous view that the cessation of menses was a disease-state that required medication.[33] Numerous doctors of women's health warned against alternative pharmacological remedies in which, they claimed, too many women put their faith.[34] French hygienic medicine of the nineteenth century made increasingly strident claims about its unique authority to treat women in menopause, in opposition to these other kinds of healers. There is very little indication that unofficial health practitioners of any kind provided

[31] Williams, *A Cultural History of Medical Vitalism*, 229.

[32] Ramsey, *Professional and Popular Medicine in France*, 50, 79.

[33] Marc Colombat de l'Isère, *Traité des maladies des femmes et de l'hygiène spéciale de leur sexe*, 2 vols (Paris: Librairie médicale de Labé, 1838–1843), vol. 2, 658–659.

[34] Gardanne, *Avis aux femmes qui entrent dans l'âge critique*, 96; Sebastien Guyétant, *Conseils aux femmes, ou Moyens de se préserver et de se guérir de la leucorrhée* (Paris, chez l'auteur, 1836), v; Prosper-Louis Sauvé, *Réflexions dur l'âge critique, et particulièrement sur le régime le plus convenable pour préserver les femmes des accidens qui ont coutume de survenir cette époque de leur vie.* Thèse (Strasbourg: F. G. Levrault, 1826), 8.

any specific remedies to menopausal women until long after the nineteenth-century medical concept had been elaborated, and an exhaustive survey of midwifery sources conducted in the early stages of this project yielded no substantial examples in this corpus of ideas about the final cessation of menses being viewed as symptomatic before the 1850s (discussed in Chapters 1, 6, and 8).

In part this fixation by doctors on the competing remedies available to women around the final cessation of menses reflected a much larger struggle in the history of medicine between chemical, mechanical, and vitalist approaches to disease.[35] Purgative remedies, which many doctors claimed were widely abused both by patients and by empirics hawking them, had been criticised by major figures of French medicine since the early eighteenth century,[36] seen as reflecting the Galenic humoral view of physiology focused on pharmacology, rather than the iatro-mechanist strands which emphasised such practices as phlebotomy, leeches, cauterisation, cupping, and surgery, but also dietary, exercise, and lifestyle advice of the kind that became increasingly categorised and elaborated under the new medical discipline of *hygiène*; as well as redefinition of all those many illnesses that presented without lesions as 'nervous' disorders. Purgatives were particularly singled out for attack by doctors writing on menopause, both as a shorthand for the discrediting of competing empirics and charlatans, and as a shorthand for the refocusing of medical science on the new mechanistic approaches to physiology.[37]

The matter played out in complicated ways too in relation to the rivalry between France's two largest medical faculties of Paris and Montpellier since the University of Montpellier remained both more Galenic in its orientation towards constitution-specific pharmacy, and was the highest producer of French medical graduates at the end of the eighteenth century.[38] As Colin Jones has remarked, the University of Montpellier's students constituted the very figures through whom the process of medicalisation most unfolded prior to the dissolution of medical institutions during the French Revolution.[39] Nonetheless, in the transformation of medicine after 1794, the establishment in Paris in 1803 of the École de Pharmacie, and the assimilation of both surgery and pharmacy into the new

[35] Michael Stolberg, 'Menstruation and Sexual Difference in Early Modern Medicine', in Andrew Shail & Gillian Howed, eds, *Menstruation: A Cultural History* (New York: Palgrave, 2005), 90–101; Charles T. Wolfe, 'Models of Organic Organization in Montpellier Vitalism', *Early Science & Medicine*, 22 (2017): 1–24.

[36] Philippe Hecquet, *De Purgandâ medicinâ a curarum sordibus* (Paris: Chavelier, 1714).

[37] Matthew Ramsey, 'Academic Medicine and Medical Industrialism: The Regulation of Secret Remedies in Nineteenth-Century France', in Ann La Berge and Mordechai Feingold, eds, *French Medical Culture in the Nineteenth Century* (Amsterdam: Rodopi, 1994), 25–78; L. W. B. Brockliss, 'Before the Clinic: French Medical Teaching in the Eighteenth Century', in Caroline Hannaway & Ann la Berge, eds, *Constructing Paris Medicine* (Amsterdam: Rodopi, 1998), 71–115.

[38] Williams, *A Cultural History of Medical Vitalism*, 24, 117.

[39] Colin Jones, 'Montpellier Medical Students and the "Medicalisation" of Eighteenth-Century France', in R. Porter & A. Wear, eds, *Problems and Methods in the History of Medicine* (London: Croom Helm, 1987), 59 [57–80].

national curriculum of medical pedagogy, all reinforced the role of Paris as the French centre of the new modern biomedicine throughout the nineteenth century,[40] rapidly relocating the pedagogic fascination with women's reproductive ageing throughout the early nineteenth century (Chapters 5 and 6).

In the mid-nineteenth century, menopause also became assimilated into the specialist emergent psychiatric scholarship on hysteria and other nervous and mental pathologies, never as a central theme, but as one of the many vulnerable times, when susceptible women might succumb to hysterical symptoms or manifest the signs of their inherited degenerate traits (Chapter 7). The association of menopause with hysteria was consistent with the widespread view that nervous or mental derangement in general was more likely to occur in a woman's life during periods of uterine change: puberty, menstruation, pregnancy, lactation, and the final cessation of menses.[41] However, the association of madness with menopause persisted even long after the uterine-atrophy model was overturned in the 1840s in the growing recognition that the ovaries were the primary organ of internal chemical secretion.[42] A marked divergence about menopause and hysteria emerged after this time, with many doctors insisting that women were actually less prone to hysteria at this time of life due to the atrophy of the genital organs, while others argued instead that menopausal women suffered their own unique form of hypochondria which manifested in sexual perversion and erotomania. Sexuality was a central focus of these concerns and numerous doctors considered that 'perversion of the sexual appetite' was one of the central symptoms of menopause.[43] French medical writers of the early twentieth century inherited ideas about women's reproductive ageing that had emerged in French alienism of the nineteenth century, reiterating the claims of the discipline in treating women after menopause. Even after the hysteria movement had peaked in the 1890s, the visions of women's midlife madness prevailed well into the late twentieth century.[44]

[40] La Berge & Hannaway, 'Paris Medicine', 5.

[41] Étienne-Jean Georget, *De la physiologie du système nerveux et spécialement du cerveau, recherches sur les maladies nerveuses en général et en particulier sur le siège, la nature et le traitement de l'hystérie, de l'hypochondrie, de l'épilepsie et de l'asthme convulsif*, 2 vols (Paris: J.-B. Baillière, 1821); Alexandre F. Brierre de Boismont, *De la menstruation, considérée dans ses rapports physiologiques et pathologiques* (Paris: Germer Baillière, 1842); Henri-Eugène Rocque, *Essai sur la physiologie et la pathologie de la ménopause*. Thèse (Paris: Rignoux, 1858); Pierre Berthier, *Des névroses menstruelles, ou La Menstruation dans ses rapports avec les maladies nerveuses et mentales* (Paris: Delahaye, 1874); Henri Guimbail, *De la folie à la ménopause*. Thèse (Paris: A. Delahaye, 1884); Valentin Magnan & Paul Maurice Legrain, *Les Dégénérés: État et syndromes épisodiques* (Paris: Rueff, 1895).

[42] Victor C. Medvei, *A History of Endocrinology* (Lancaster: MTP Press, 1982), 215.

[43] Alexandre F. Brierre de Boismont, 'Recherches bibliographiques et cliniques sur la folie puerpérale, précédées d'un aperçu sur les rapports de la menstruation et de l'aliénation mentale', *Annales médico-psychologiques* (1851): 574–610; Noël Guéneau de Mussy, 'Érotisme de la ménopause', *Gazette hebdomadaire de médecine et de chirurgie*, 37 (13 October 1871): 591–595; Berthier, *Des névroses menstruelles*; Henri Guimbail, *De la folie à la ménopause*. Thèse (Paris: A. Delahaye, 1884).

[44] Alexandre-Jacques-Bernard Gerdessus, *La Ménopause et son rôle en psychiatrie* (Toulouse: Dirion, 1910); Antoine Rémond & Paul Voivenel 'Essai sur le rôle de la ménopause en pathologie mentale', *L'Encéphale: Revue de psychiatrie clinique, biologique et thérapeutique*, 6/2 (1911): 133–126.

Women-authored general medical works which mentioned menopause appeared from the late nineteenth century onwards, often taking a markedly different tone from the specialist works on the topic written by men (Chapter 8). From the 1880s onwards, a small number of women became successful doctors in France, most often publishing theses on matters of women's reproductive medicine, and midwives too wrote medical manuals of women's health throughout the lifespan. These works often had strikingly little to say about the final cessation of menses requiring any special hygienic management or medical care, directing the bulk of their concerns to the ongoing dangers of childbirth given the persistently high maternal and infant mortality, as well as to the novel challenges of marital relations and parenting in the industrial age.[45] Pharmacists on the other hand, were another competing provider of health services only partially aligned to the emergent official biomedical culture. Indeed, it was in apothecaries and mail-order pharmacy enterprises of the eighteenth century where the earliest general pharmacological remedies for the complaints and comforts of ageing bodies could be found, targeting women only towards the end of the nineteenth century in response to the now substantial medical discourse about menopause.[46]

Why France?

The growing medical interest in the diseases of women between the late sixteenth and mid-nineteenth centuries, and the accompanying view that women were so

See Daniel Delanoë, 'Les Troubles psychique attribués à la ménopause et le regard des hommes', in Pascale Bélot-Foucarde & Diane Winaver, eds, *La Ménopause: Regards croisés entre gynécologues et psychanalystes* (Toulouse: Érès, 2004), 151–170.

[45] Virginie Messager, *Guide pratique de l'âge critique, ou Conseils aux femmes sur les maladies qui peuvent les attaquer à cette époque de leur vie; suivis de réflexions et d'observations sur les maladies laiteuses* (Paris: chez l'auteur, 1859); Amélie Wion Pigalle, *Le Conseiller secret des femmes, ou Conseils sur les moyens de se préserver des maladies qui atteignent spécialement les femmes* [1858], 3rd ed. (Paris: Georges Kugelmann, 1861); Mme Delestrée, *Le Conseiller secret des femmes, ou Conseils sur les moyens de se préserver des maladies qui atteignent spécialement les femmes*, septième édition entièrement refondue (Paris: Chez l'auteur, 1875); Angélina Guillarmou, *Kinésithérapie gynécologique: Valeur hémostatique de certains mouvements musculaires contre les méno et métrorrhagies chroniques (système de Brandt). Etude pratique.* Thèse (Paris: Steinheil, 1896); Mme A. Gensse, *Les Quatre Âges de la femme au point de vue physiologique* [1894], 5th ed. (Corbeil: E. Crété, 1899); Marie Schultz, *Hygiène générale de la femme, alimentation, vêtements, soins corporels, d'après l'enseignement et la pratique du Dr Auvard* (Paris: O. Doin, 1903); Anne Darcanne-Mouroux, *Contribution à l'étude clinique de la ménopause précoce.* Thèse (Paris: H. Jouve, 1904); Madeleine Tessier, *Établissement de la ménopause.* Thèse (Paris: Ollier-Henry, 1911); Isabelle Gaboriau, *Contribution à l'étude des métrorragies dites essentielles de la ménopause.* Thèse (Paris: Jouve, 1919); Hélina Gaboriau, *Les Trois Âges de la femme: Puberté, maternité, ménopause* (Paris: Larousse, 1923).

[46] Pharmacie Moride, *Accidents du retour d'âge et maladies du système veineux: Varices et ulcères variqueux, hémorroîdes, varicocèles, phlebites, oedèmes chronique, congestions, hémorragies, etc. leur traitement par l'exilir de Virginie* (Paris: Pharmacie Moride, c.1897); M. S. Gomès, *De l'opothérapie ovarienne, contribution à l'étude physiologique et thérapeutique de l'ovarine.* Thèse (Paris: Georges Carré & C. Naud, 1898); J. Noé, *La Nicine Rol dans le traitement des hémorroïdes, varices, phlébites, artériosclérose, emphysème, asthme, bronchites, métrites, accidents de l'âge critique, cirrhoses, affections cardiaques et vasculaires, etc.* (Paris: Nicine Rol, 1908).

distinct from men as to require their own medical specialism, were certainly not confined to France.[47] So why was France the vastly dominant culture in medicalising menopause throughout the long nineteenth century? There were several unique tendencies of eighteenth-century French politics, culture, and scientific thought relating to questions of sexual difference which, in turn, stimulated the radical bifurcation of ageing along gender lines and with reference to women's end of menses. Some scholars have suggested that French gender questions have been broadly characterised by a 'Gallic singularity' impacting representations of women since the Middle Ages and which have tended to imagine the sexes in particularly dimorphic ways.[48] Such claims might be considered a fruitful line of inquiry for asking how ageing came be to sexually bifurcated in French medicine with reference to menstruation and women's declining conceptive capacity. Karen Offen's work has highlighted the centrality of French debates about the place of women and the proper roles of each sex, as well as the 'strategic importance accorded to biomedical thinking in French society' throughout the eighteenth and nineteenth centuries in relation to anti-clericalist and republican challenges to the authority of the Church. Offen thus suggests, in a footnote of her renowned 2017 book on French gender history, that the sudden medical interest in menopause in the final years of the eighteenth century was another manifestation of the unique propensity to fixate on 'the woman question' in French Enlightenment and nationalist values, particularly emphasising women's roles as wives and mothers, serving both their husbands and the nation.[49] These roles, certainly, were officialised both in the Napoleonic Code which made women legally the property of their husbands in 1804, and in the criminalisation of abortion in 1810.[50] The revolutionary *Déclaration des droits de l'homme et du citoyen* of 1789 had excluded women from the entire polity, and the new rights accorded them (to divorce and inheritance) were quickly eroded under the reign of Napoléon Bonaparte and during the Bourbon restoration after 1816. The marked turn throughout the first half of the nineteenth century towards an emphasis on women's subordinate and childbearing capacity cast non-reproductive and rebellious women of all kinds—prostitutes, libertines, revolutionaries, and menopausal women—in a sombre light. As Karen Offen notes, the population issue and its impact on ideas about women's roles was a particularly French obsession throughout the nineteenth and early twentieth centuries.[51] Given that the significant

[47] Helen King has charted the trans-cultural growth of early modern gynaecology in: Helen King, *Midwifery, Obstetrics and the Rise of Gynaecology* (London: Routledge, 2007).

[48] Jean Elisabeth Pedersen, 'Representations of Women in the French Imaginary: Historicizing the Gallic Singularity', *French Politics, Culture & Society*, 38/1 (2020): 1–20).

[49] Karen Offen, *The Woman Question in France, 1400–1870* (Cambridge: Cambridge University Press, 2017), 1–9, 110.

[50] Jack R. Censer & Lynn Hunt, *Liberty, Equality, Fraternity: Exploring the French Revolution* (University Park, Pa: Pennsylvania State University Press, 2001), 147.

[51] Offen, *The Woman Question in France*, 113–114.

French political obsession with population decline began long before the marked downturn in births of at the end of the nineteenth century, it may also have set the tone for the generation of ideas of menopause as a kind of general negative phenomenon.[52]

Was the menopausal woman now appearing in medical scholarship at the cusp of the nineteenth century because she was simply a misfit of the new conservative and pro-natal social order, and hence a viable medical target for pathologisation? Certainly, many of the medical works discussing menopause addressed the question of older women's fitness for sexual relations and denigrated their changing physiology, taking the 'crisis' of the end of menstruation and conception to signal yet another moment (of many in the female life cycle) in which women were negatively influenced by their unruly uterus or ovaries. Some doctors railed against the modern freedoms elite women enjoyed for sociability, gourmandise, drunkenness, gambling, debauchery, and copious leisure, once they were free of child-rearing responsibilities; others used the spectre of a later symptomatic menopause as a threat for younger women should they 'deny the wish of nature' and fail to bear children, as their 'nature' dictated. On the other hand, many doctors insisted that menopause passed without consequence for most women if they were in general good health. Others viewed the loss of reproductive capacity as making older women more like men, thus qualifying them for new forms of inclusion and authority denied to those younger, while others insisted upon the unique charms of post-reproductive life or argued that conception could even sometimes still occur after menstruation ceased, or even that men too suffered a 'critical age'. Medical thought was no simple or homogeneous mirror of broader cultural and political concerns, and doctors' ideas about menopause were also influenced by their patients, their wives, and by women writers who responded to the medicalisation of menopause after the 1870s. Clearly too, the assemblage of many of the layers of meaning that the medical concept of menopause contained had begun to cohere well before either the French Revolution or the demographic worry about births that became so insistent in the nineteenth century. This assemblage began in German vitalist medicine of the Halle school around 1700, in mid-eighteenth-century French medical evocations of 'the vapours', in Encyclopedist descriptions of human life cycles across world cultures between 1751 and 1772, and in French responses of 1746 to 1850 to pan-European scientific discussions of sex-differentiated population mortality statistics which indicated women's greater longevity. So, while the 'woman question' in political culture after the French Revolution may have helped to fuel the growing

[52] On early discourses of declining population growth, see Lynn Salkin Sbiroli, 'Generation and Regeneration: Reflections on the Biological and Ideological Role of Women in France (1786–96)', in M. M. Roberts & Roy Porter, eds, *Literature and Medicine during the Eighteenth Century* (London: Routledge, 1993), 266–285.

importance of menopause as a topic of medical concern, it does little to explain how the concept cohered in the first instance.

Other cultural developments relating to the place of older women in changing social custom and to the new scientific discourse of women's 'nature' are more suggestive for understanding how menopause came to matter for France more than for other cultures of the late eighteenth century. The vitalist view of women's nature espoused by a range of scholars, especially those in the Montpellier medical faculty, had far reaching effects in wider public discourses about gender throughout France, as Elizabeth Williams has shown: vitalist physicians were influential in the Paris salons both of Paul Thiry d'Holbach in the 1750s and of Anne Catherine Helvétius in the 1780s where they asserted naturalistic arguments about the necessity for women to stay away from intellectual and public life, through the view that the only activities aligned to the vital nature of the 'sensitive sex' were those relating to reproduction and child-rearing.[53] Williams remarks on the irony of vitalist physicians using the French *salon* as the very locale for the espousal of arguments against women's public and intellectual activities, given they were precisely the one cultural milieu that permitted elite women, particularly older women, to flourish in precisely such ways.[54] The important late eighteenth-century genre of writing on the 'natural history of women' about which Anne Vila, Karen Offen, Sean Quinlan, and others have all written,[55] and with which many of the major menopause doctors also engaged, was another significant gender discourse that helped to fuel the growing medical emphasis placed upon the particular pathologies of women's reproductive physiology and which was not present in other cultures of this time. It reflected the uniquely French insistence, in multiple facets of medical and philosophical thought, upon the radical differentiation of the sexes and the particular character of women's life cycles and vital essence.

French medicine at the end of the eighteenth century, even more than other domains of French society and culture, was also subject to a marked rupture provoked by the French Revolution of 1789–1795, which impacted the tone and fervour with which the topic of menopause was greeted in both medical pedagogy and clinical practice thereafter. The relatively stable universities of Paris, Montpellier, and others that had functioned since the thirteenth century, with a three- or four-year degree costing as much as 6,000 livres—more than one year of a doctor's salary once qualified—were dissolved in 1793;[56] the result was a period

[53] Elizabeth A. Williams, 'Physicians, Vitalism, and Gender in the Salon', *Studies in Eighteenth-Century Culture*, 29 (Baltimore: Johns Hopkins University Press, 2000), 1–21; Williams, *A Cultural History of Medical Vitalism*, 229.

[54] Williams, 'Physicians, Vitalism, and Gender in the Salon', 4–5.

[55] Vila, 'Sex and Sensibility', 76–93; Offen, *The Woman Question in France*, 109–110; Quinlan, *Morbid Undercurrents*, 68–94.

[56] Charles Coury, 'The Teaching of Medicine in France from the Beginning of the Seventeenth Century', in Charles Donald O'Malley, ed., *The History of Medical Education* (Berkeley: University of California Press, 1970), 123–124 [121–172].

of free, unregulated, and disorganised medical reality in which all the many kinds of health practitioners, charlatans, empirics, drug merchants, and folk healers were permitted the same licence to practice as university-trained doctors.[57] While the new École de Santé in Paris was created in 1795, the system that replaced the medical faculties of the *ancien régime*—the work of the anatomist Félix Vicq d'Azyr (1748–1794) and the chemist Antoine-François de Fourcroy, informed by the physician Philippe Pinel (1745–1826), the physiologists Pierre Jean Georges Cabanis (1757–1808), and others—emerged only between 1795 and 1808, instituting the new medical underclass of *officiers de santé* who operated until 1892.[58] Medical pedagogy thereafter massively expanded: the number of students at the Paris faculty more than doubled between 1797 and 1830, and by the 1840s, the supply of French doctors outstripped demand.[59] But the training of doctors was also now based on a radically different university curriculum that combined medical, pharmacy, and surgical training, with much higher exposure of students to clinical practice during their studies—the revolutionary change that Michel Foucault referred to in his 1964 *The Birth of the Clinic* and which John Lesch described with great nuance in his 1984 *Science and Medicine in France.*[60]

The political transformation of the French Revolution had set the stage for the revolution of medical concepts towards what Phillippe Pinel in 1797 (who had been a student at Montpellier in the 1770s) most famously called nosography—referring to the new modern classification of distinct diseases,[61] and what the great Montpellier professor of medicine François de Boissier de Sauvages (de Lacroix) in 1771 had called nosology.[62] It was precisely in the revolutionary period of crisis, chaos, competition, renewal, and the collapse of tradition in French medicine that the first specialist French medical theses were written on women's final cessation of menses, depicting it as a 'critical time' in the female life cycle—perhaps projecting onto women's ageing the very perturbation of French medicine itself in this period. Medical specialisation was also coming to be seen as the more sophisticated and scientific form of clinical practice, while generalism was increasingly associated with charlatans and empirics.[63] This too was a

[57] Colin Jones, 'Montpellier Medical Students and the "Medicalisation" of Eighteenth-Century France', in R. Porter & A. Wear, eds, *Problems and Methods in the History of Medicine* (London: Croom Helm, 1987), 74 [57–80]; Ramsey, *Professional and Popular Medicine in France*, 71–77.

[58] Coury, 'The Teaching of Medicine in France', 149–153.

[59] Ibid., 159; George D. Sussman, 'The Glut of Doctors in Mid-Nineteenth-Century France', *Comparative Studies in Society and History*, 19/3 (1977): 289–290 [287–304].

[60] Michel Foucault, *La Naissance de la clinique* [1963] (Paris: Presses Universitaire de France, 2015); John E. Lesch, *Science and Medicine in France: The Emergence of Experimental Physiology, 1790–1855* (Cambridge, Mass.: Harvard University Press, 1984).

[61] Philippe Pinel, *Nosographie philosophique, ou la méthode de l'analyse appliquée à la médecine*, 2 vols (Paris: Maradon, 1797).

[62] François de Boissier de Sauvages, *Nosologie méthodique, dans laquelle les maladies sont rangées par classes, suivant le système de Sydenham, & l'ordre des botanistes*, 10 vols (Paris: Hérissant le fils, 1771).

[63] Ramsey, *Professional and Popular Medicine in France*, 243.

transnational trend by the end of the nineteenth century, but as George Weisz's comparison of France with other medical cultures in Europe has shown, French medicine was far advanced over others in these modern tendencies in the first half of the nineteenth century.[64] The modern shift towards clinical pedagogy and nosography of disease were also occurring in other medical cultures in Europe too, but in France they were hurriedly installed as official curricula far more abruptly on account of the revolutionary changes to institutional structures.[65] Napoleon Bonaparte's own personal physician, Jean-Nicholas Corvisart-Demarets (1755–1821), was a powerful advocate of the new approach, according to which patients could have diseases without lesions, requiring 'the continual monitoring of apparently health bodies', as W. R. Albury has described it.[66] From this time on, as Ann La Berge and Caroline Hannaway have remarked, 'clinicians no longer simply saw sick individuals, they saw diseases'.[67] In fact, French doctors and doctoral students became so excited about classifying diseases that they even began treating phenomena that everyone agreed were natural and normal as if they were diseases—including menopause. This was the context in which French medicine of the early nineteenth century elaborated a new vision of women as the sicker sex, their physiology punctuated by a constant series of perturbations from puberty to menstruation to pregnancy, to childbirth, to lactation, and finally to menopause. Although women's mortality was often found to be lower than men's at every age, and their lifespans were widely acknowledged as longer, their ageing was seen as more morbid, requiring greater surveillance and management both by women themselves and by medical clinicians.

Importantly too, the new French medical education system actively excluded women, except as midwives whose roles were also increasingly formalised. Prior to the Revolution, many widows had managed their deceased husbands' pharmacy practices, but an 1803 law forbade this.[68] Women had been excluded from practising as physicians by a 1755 Paris parliamentary law.[69] This is important because women were patently not involved in the elaboration of the concept of menopause which took place in the pedagogic and scholarly context of an entirely male-dominated medical system. Women continued to practice as folk healers, especially outside major cities, often called *commères* (godmothers), but were increasingly denigrated as ill-informed and dangerous menaces to society by official medical scholars, including those writing about menopause and claiming

[64] George Weisz, 'The Emergence of Specialism in the Nineteenth Century', *Bulletin of the History of Medicine*, 77 (2003): 536–575.

[65] Jean-Charles Sournia, *Histoire de la médecine* (Paris: Éditions la Découverte, 1992), 219.

[66] Jean-Nicholas Corvisart, *Essai sur les maladies et les lésions organiques du cœur et des gros vaisseaux* (Paris: Imprimerie Migneret, 1806); Albury, 'Heart of Darkness', 30.

[67] Ann La Berge & Caroline Hannaway, 'Paris Medicine: Perspectives Past and Present', in Caroline Hannaway & Ann La Berge, *Constructing Paris Medicine* (Amsterdam: Rodopi, 1998), 5 [1–70].

[68] Ramsey, *Professional and Popular Medicine in France*, 79–80.

[69] Ibid., 50.

themselves as the only legitimate clinicians qualified to treat it (considered in Chapter 6). Midwives did not generally address women's health needs beyond those relating to pregnancy, childbirth, and lactation. Only in the second half of the nineteenth century were there a handful of women medical writers who considered the final cessation of menses, but mostly still only to dismiss it as of little importance relative to the dangers that threatened nineteenth-century women in childbirth (considered in Chapter 8).

The competition among doctors for patients was particularly fierce in the revolutionary period of 1793–1805, during which time France lacked a regulatory system for privileging university medical graduates as it had under the *ancien régime*, and which was restored under the Directorate. Even after the restored system was substantially installed by 1808, the new class of *officiers de santé* provided legitimation to a novel category of semi-qualified health practitioner with whom doctors competed for patients, and despite the new pressure placed on other kinds of popular practitioners, charlatans, folk healers, drug merchants, and empirics who continued to outnumber doctors massively throughout the first half of the nineteenth century.[70] The revolutionised French university schools after 1805, especially those of Paris, pumped out graduates as never before, resulting in what some historians have described as a 'glut' of doctors relative to demand throughout much of the nineteenth century.[71] Women numbered more than double the population of men on account of their greater survival into the older ages, and with the need for healthcare generally increasing with ageing, older women clearly constituted a crucial demographic for medical services.[72] The description of women as the sicker sex in ageing, with their ageing also widely recognised as longer than men's—which were both observations commonly made in medical writings on menopause—meant that older women were implicitly identified as an important cohort for the maintenance of doctors' livelihoods in this exceptionally competitive market. French hygiene, with its emphasis on healthy living, longevity, and regimes of self-care, clearly had an interest in singling older women out for special attention. *Fin-de-siècle* gynaecological surgery particularly needed older women to perform the role of patients, since the benign uterine and ovarian masses that were common among them were far more likely than cancer to result in a successful surgery that would both permit the technical development of the experimental field of laparotomy and build the super-star careers of individual surgeon-doctors such as Jules Péan (1830–1898) and Samuel Pozzi (1846–1918) (discussed in Chapter 10). Like most inventions, the French invention of menopause was enabled by precedent conceptual developments,

[70] Albury, 'Heart of Darkness', 25.

[71] Ramsey, *Professional and Popular Medicine in France*, 113; Sussman, 'The Glut of Doctors in Mid-Nineteenth-Century France', 287–304.

[72] Ramsey, *Professional and Popular Medicine in France*, 226.

fuelled by prevailing cultural beliefs and contextual pressures, and was not the product of a single brilliant mind; but it was the work of medical men and its appearance as a complete concept was both strikingly sudden and very much a product of the rupture in French medicine following the French Revolution. Once in place though, the concept of menopause was instrumentalised for a wide range of professional and pedagogic purposes in French medicine throughout the nineteenth century.

Methodological Questions

The methodologies of this book are grounded in the conceptual and intellectual history of medicine, but are also informed by biomedical, anthropological, sociological, philosophical, and feminist scholarship, without adhering to any specific models derived from these fields. It is not a social constructionist account of contemporary French menopause, which can be found in the excellent work of the sociologist Cécile Charlap.[73] In fact much sociological scholarship on medicalisation has treated it as a matter of social construction, an approach which is even often erroneously attributed to Michel Foucault, both by those critical of Foucault's influence and by those referencing it towards a constructionist critical perspective.[74] It is important here to distinguish the characterisations of Foucault's approach in the anglophone humanities and social sciences, from Foucault's own account, as exemplified in his historical scholarship in the four volumes of the epic *Histoire de la sexualité* on which he worked intently between *c.*1972 and his death in 1984, and as he explained it in his lectures in relation to the biosciences.[75] What Foucault called 'history of the present' certainly entailed an element of critique, but it had distinctly different objectives from the anglophone social constructionist agenda aimed at discrediting biologistic assumptions. Foucault sought instead to disentangle present concepts and practices from their past origins with a view to engendering greater freedom for understanding ourselves.[76]

[73] Cécile Charlap, *La Fabrique de la ménopause.* Thèse de sociologie (Strasbourg: Université de Strasbourg, 2015).

[74] A point well made in both Peter Conrad, *The Medicalization of Society: On the Transformation of Human Conditions into Treatable Disorders* (Baltimore: Johns Hopkins University Press, 2007), 8 and Deborah Lupton, 'Foucault and the Medicalisation Critique', in Alan Peterson & Alan Bunton, eds, *Foucault, Health and Medicine* (London/New York: Routledge, 1997), 94–110. See also Alison M. Downham Moore & Stuart Elden, 'Foucault's 1960s Lectures on Sexuality', *Theory, Culture and Society*, Special Issue on Foucault Before the Collège de France (2021): 1–15.

[75] Michel Foucault, *Histoire de la sexualité*, 4 vols (Paris: Gallimard, 1976–2018); Michel Foucault, *La Sexualité: Cours donné à l'université de Clermont-Ferrand (1964), suivi de Le Discours de la sexualité: Cours donné à l'université de Vincennes (1969)*, ed. Claude-Olivier Doron (Paris: Gallimard/Seuil, 2018).

[76] Michel Foucault, *'Il faut défendre la société': Cours au Collège de France (1975–1976)*, ed. François Ewald & Alessandro Fontana (Paris: l'Association pour le Centre Michel Foucault, 2012). See Martina Tazzioli, Sophie Fuggle, & Yari Lanic, 'Introduction', in Sophie Fuggle, Yari Lanic, & Martina Tazzioli,

Here the medical past is problematised, not with a view to debunking and rejecting it per se, but rather with a view to reconstructing how our current perspectives have formed historically and gained their legitimacy. The point is to open new possibilities for thought both with and beyond these past legacies, rather than creating yet another closed reactive system—such as one in which there is an assumed holistic or 'natural' way of experiencing menopause which biomedical categories are construed as disrupting.

In the second volume of the *History of Sexuality*, Foucault referred to his larger historical project as located 'at the apex of an archaeology of problematisation and a genealogy of practices of the self',[77] whereas social constructionist scholarship on medicine has largely focused uniquely on the negative impacts of medicine on people and their self-understandings.[78] Foucault's work has thus been instructive for the present study, not in the sense of providing a radical critical frame, but rather in focusing its epistemology as an inquiry into how our present medical conceptions of women's reproductive ageing came into being. Similarly, while the title of this book playfully invokes the notion of resisting an assumed universal biological fact of women's menses definitively ending, reframed instead as something that was suddenly 'invented' at a specific historical moment in French medical history, it also attends to the older antecedents of the neologism in European medical thought, and to the changing bodily lifeways of French women in the context of nineteenth-century urbanisation, industrialisation, and the massively expanding reach of biomedicine.

In theorising 'history of the present', Foucault identified the spaces of opening for the beginning of historical questions about concepts in the contested fields of the historian's own discursive context. In the time of this book's writing, menopause has indeed been such a contested field: a vast medical commercial interest—that of surgeons, prescribing physicians, and pharmaceutical companies—underlies its widespread clinical treatment; while a growing critique of biomedical approaches flourishes from feminist sociological perspectives, from within the minimally invasive surgery current, and from the edges of medicine in the competing commercial interest of compounding pharmacy producers of 'bio-identical' hormone alternatives. Researchers attempting to study contemporary menopause complain of it being shrouded in secrecy,[79] characterising it as a matter of shame and 'taboo' about which women are reluctant to speak,[80] while journalists claim

eds, *Foucault and the History of our Present* (Basingstoke: Palgrave, 2015), 1–12; and Alison M. Downham Moore, 'Foucault's Scholarly Virtues and Sexuality Historiography', *History: The Journal of the Historical Association*, 105/366 (July 2020): 446–469.

[77] Michel Foucault, *Histoire de la sexualité 2: L'Usage des plaisirs* (Paris: Éditions Gallimard, 1984), 19.

[78] Lupton, 'Foucault and the Medicalisation Critique'.

[79] Charlap, *La Fabrique de la ménopause*, 19.

[80] Maria Kathryn Tomlinson, *From Menstruation to Menopause: The Female Fertility Cycle in Contemporary Women's Writing in French* (Liverpool: Liverpool University Press, 2021), 14, 53, 55;

that medicine is still withholding proper hormonal treatment from those menopausal women who need it, informed by outdated fears of cancer generated by flawed but highly publicised safety studies of the early 2000s.[81] Nonetheless, a vast literature of recent advice books for menopausal women both in French and in English now runs for more than ten pages of a search through Googlebooks, as Cécile Charlap has considered.[82] Conflicting claims about the status of contemporary menopause are so common, and women's reported experiences of it so diverse, that it seems unlikely for greater clarity to emerge in humanistic and social scientific inquiry on the matter simply via further critical contestation. And while several scholarly books have already historicised menopause through different methodologies of popular cultural history, anthropological or sociological history, or broad western world history, none has previously traced precisely how the medical concept emerged and cohered in the one spectacularly dominant culture, France, where medical ideas about it were most intensively elaborated throughout the long nineteenth century;[83] though there have also been a number of excellent small scholarly studies on aspects of menopause in French medical history, with which it has been a pleasure to engage in the writing of this book.[84]

In considering historical inheritances—both our own in relation to the nineteenth century, as well as the nineteenth century's in relation to early modern and ancient medicine—this book has also been informed by the work of the German historian Reinhart Koselleck, who referred to 'temporal layers' embedded in the

Paul Komesaroff, Philipa Rothfield, & Jeanne Daly, eds, *Reinterpreting the Menopause: Cultural and Philosophical Issues* (New York: Routledge, 1997).

[81] Kate Muir, 'Women have struggled to get help with the menopause for decades but its about to change', *The Guardian*, 6 October 6 2021. <https://www.theguardian.com/commentisfree/2021/oct/06/women-menopause-change-hormone-replacement-therapy>; Kate Muir, 'Mission Menopause: My hormones went off a cliff—and I'm not going to be ashamed', *The Guardian*, 9 May 2021: <https://www.theguardian.com/society/2021/may/09/mission-menopause-my-hormones-went-off-a-cliff-and-im-not-going-to-be-ashamed>.

[82] Charlap, *La Fabrique de le ménopause*, 76–96.

[83] Susan P. Matterns, *The Slow Moon Climbs: The Science, History and Meaning of Menopause* (Princeton: Princeton University Press, 2019); Jeannette King, *Discourses of Ageing in Fiction and Feminism: The Invisible Woman* (London: Palgrave, 2013); Louise Foxcroft, *Hot Flushes, Cold Science: A History of the Modern Menopause* (London: Granta Books, 2011); Judith A. Houck, *Hot and Bothered: Women, Medicine, and Menopause in Modern America* (Cambridge, Mass.: Harvard University Press, 2008); Charlap, *La Fabrique de la menopause.*

[84] Joel Wilbush, 'La Ménespausie: The Birth of a Syndrome', *Maturitas*, 1 (1979): 145–151; Joel Wilbush, 'What's in a Name? Some Linguistic Aspects of the Climacteric', *Maturitas*, 3 (1981): 1–9; Jocelyne Livi, *Vapeurs de femmes: Essai historique sur quelques fantasmes médicaux et philosophiques* (Paris: Navarin, 1984); Joel Wilbush, 'Menorraghia and Menopause: A Historical Review', *Maturitas*, 10 (1988): 5–26; Annick Tillier, 'Un Âge critique: La Ménopause sous le regard des médecins des XVIIIe et XIXe siècles', *CLIO: Femmes, genre, histoire*, 21 (2005): 268–280; Nicoletta Diasio, '"Habillée de temps": La Femme à l'âge critique dans le discours médical au tournant du XIXe siècle', in Virginie Vinel, ed., *Féminin/masculin: Approches anthropologiques des catégories et des pratiques médicales* (Strasbourg: Cahiers du portiQue, 2007), 101–129; Véronique Moulinié, 'Andropause et ménopause: La Sexualité sur ordonnance', *CLIO: Histoire, femmes et sociétés*, 37 (2013): 105–121; Christine Théré, 'Âge de retour et retour d'âge: L'Asymétrie entre les sexes dans les discours médicaux en France (1770–1836)', *CLIO: Femmes, genre, histoire*, 42 (2015): 54–75.

history of concepts.[85] Conceptual history has been located as between intellectual and cultural history, closer to the former through its attention to the nuances of ideas expressed by past thinkers located within distinct intellectual traditions, and closer to the latter in its non-doctrinaire account of what counts as a relevant source, hence considering both the works published within scholarly genres, as well as those outside them or beneath them (low-brow works), attending as much to the ideas expressed as to emotive aspects of expression.[86] Koselleck's frame was less precisely theorised than evocative, but it provides an important perspective through which to accommodate historical continuities and discontinuities by referring to concepts via a spatial, geological metaphor. Recent scholarship on Koselleck's language draws attention to this aspect of his thought, which permits concepts to be understood as cultural artefacts of the past in which multiple temporal layers are sedimented, some making themselves known in the rich evocations of everyday or technical language; others lying dormant until they are exhumed by historical inquiry.[87] Foucault too used spatial metaphors in his historical epistemology, referring to 'archaeology', 'architecture', 'structure', and 'panopticon', while his use of 'genealogy' evoked both the visual image of the family tree as well as the biological notion of genetic inheritance.[88] Foucault's archaeology, like Koselleck's temporal layering, implied that the task of historiography may be one of excavation to find the buried sediments of the past over which our current concepts are fashioned.[89] While there are two different digging disciplines referenced here (for Foucault archaeology, for Koselleck geology), in both cases, there is an idea of past layers as once buried, hidden but present, embedded in concepts and retrievable through historical probing.

Koselleck also described the long nineteenth century as a *Sattelzeit* (saddle time), referring to troughs in geological formations where sedimented layers become particularly densely compacted, bringing deeply buried past layers closer

[85] Reinhart Koselleck, '"Neuzeit": Zur Semantik moderner Bewegungsbegriffe', *Vergangene Zukunft: Zur Semantik geschichtlicher Zeiten* (Frankfurt am Main: Suhrkamp, 1979), 260–277; 'Wie neu is die Neuzeit?' *Historische Zeitschrift*, 251 (1990): 539–554; see also Alison M. Downham Moore, 'Temporal Layering in the Long Conceptual History of Sexual Medicine: Reading Koselleck with Foucault', *Journal of the Philosophy of History*, 15 (2019): 5–27; For more general introductions to conceptual history as an approach see Niklas Olsen, *History in the Plural: An Introduction to the Work of Reinhart Koselleck* (New York: Berghahn, 2012); and Jan-Werner Müller, 'On Conceptual History', in Darrin M. McMahon & Samuel Moyn, eds, *Rethinking Modern European Intellectual History* (New York: Oxford University Press, 2014), 74–93.

[86] Margrit Pernau & Dominic Sachsenmaier, eds, *Global Conceptual History: A Reader* (London: Bloomsbury, 2016).

[87] Sean Franzel & Stefan-Ludwig Hoffman, *Sediments of Time: On Possible Histories*, ed. Hent de Vries (Stanford, Calif.: Stanford University Press, 2018); Carsten Dutt & Reinhard Laube, eds, *Zwischen Sprache und Geschichte: Zum Werk Reinhart Kosellecks* (Göttingen: Wallstein, 2013).

[88] Nikolas Rose, 'Medicine, History and the Present', in Colin Jones & Roy Porter, eds, *Reassessing Foucault: Power, Medicine and the Body* (London: Routledge, 1994), 48–72.

[89] Peter Cryle, 'Words and Things: The Uncertain Place of Philology in Intellectual History', *Journal of Languages, Literatures and Culture*, 65 (2018): 65–80 [71]; Stuart Elden, *Mapping the Present: Heidegger, Foucault and Project of a Spatial History* (London: Continuum, 2001).

to the surface, where they can be more readily incorporated in current concepts; but also where rupture can occur by bringing contradictory elements into relation with one another, producing dynamic conflicts relating to concepts, between the voices of different temporal layers.[90] Foucault's work clearly oscillated between emphasis on long historical continuities of concepts and the description of important ruptures which separated one era of medical treatment practices from another, at times explicitly defending this inconsistency as a matter of principle.[91] The *Sattelzeit* too was marked by a distinctive historicity by virtue of the multiple temporal layers available to those thinking about their relationship to the past.[92] This finds a parallel too in Foucault's 1966 work *Les Mots et les choses* (The Order of Things) where he described a similar nineteenth-century historicity reshaping the European human sciences.[93] French medical sciences in the nineteenth century were no less exquisitely historically self-consciousness, and there is little doubt that the formation of the concept of menopause relied heavily on doctors' stories about the medical past through which they invested their novel developments with traditionalist authority.[94] Chapter 6 focuses on the most important of these historical stories, in which doctors invented their very own 'Hippocratic' aphorism that reduced women's nature to the functions of the uterus, helping to justify a vast medical fascination with the cessation of menses which was framed as a process of uterine atrophy.

The long nineteenth-century elaboration of menopause appears on the surface to confirm the Berkeley historian Thomas W. Laqueur's famed account of modern medicine radically differentiating the biology of the sexes, in contrast to early modern and ancient views that described male and female as structurally homologous.[95] Certainly, the medical scholarship on menopause throughout this time was insistent upon the idea of women having completely different organs, internal secretions, patterns of ageing, and needs for medical care from men—an idea particularly upheld by the Montpellier vitalist view of women's physiology as

[90] Koselleck, '"Neuzeit", 260–277.

[91] Michel Foucault, *Histoire de la Sexualité*, vol. 2: *L'Usage des plaisirs* (Paris: Gallimard, 1984), 10; Colin Jones & Roy Porter, 'Introduction', in Colin Jones & Roy Porter, eds, *Reassessing Foucault: Power, Medicine and the Body* (London: Routledge, 1994), 1–16.

[92] Reinhart Koselleck, 'Wie neu ist die Neuzeit?', in Reinhart Koselleck, *Zeitschichten: Studien sur Historik*, mit einem Beitrag von Hans-Georg Gadamer (Frankfurt am Main: Suhrkamp Verlag, 2000), 225–239. See also Reinhart Koselleck, *The Practice of Conceptual History: Timing History, Spacing Concepts*, trans. Todd Presner (Stanford, Calif.: Stanford University Press, 2002), 138–139.

[93] Michel Foucault, *Les Mots et les choses: Une archéologie des sciences humaines* (Paris: Éditions Gallimard, 1966).

[94] See also See Kate Fisher & Rebecca Langlands, eds, *Sex, Knowledge and Receptions of the Past* (Oxford: Oxford University Press, 2015); Alison M. Downham Moore, 'The Historicity of Sexuality: Knowledge of the Past in the Emergence of Modern Sexual Science', *Modern Intellectual History*, 18/2 (2021): 1–24.

[95] Thomas W. Laqueur, *Making Sex from the Greeks to Freud* (Cambridge, Mass.: Harvard University Press, 1990); Cécile Charlap, *La Fabrique de la ménopause* (Paris: CNRS, 2019), 55–56.

highly determined by motherhood.[96] Nonetheless, even though the concept of menopause referred to menstruation, making it applicable uniquely to women, in fact many French medical scholars writing about menopause referred repeatedly to the idea that men too suffered a critical age, or what later came to be known as andropause. So, while menopause appeared to separate women from men in ageing, it was also commonly leveraged precisely to argue for an androgynous view of what it meant to grow old. The theme of women losing their femininity in ageing was a recurrent motif in many of the medical theses and works of mature clinicians writing about the critical age or menopause. Consequently, despite menopause being described as a natural process and 'not a disease', menopausal bodies were also sometimes depicted as tragic and monstrous because they were considered no longer entirely female but also not fully male.

Readers of specialist medical and psychiatric history have also become accustomed to close studies of clinical practices, not merely medical concepts, with many excellent works of recent scholarship demonstrating that past doctors' publications on diseases and how they actually treated live human patients show important disparities.[97] The focus of this book is on medical publication, pedagogy, and professional identity, and on the relationship of women intellectuals to medical discourses about their ageing. As such, it is grounded more in the history of medical concepts and their public reception, rather than in the social history of medicine, focused on the lived experience of medical subjects. The reason for this focus is because via published works, scholars influenced one another and exchanged ideas, producing distinct intellectual genealogies which were also available to non-medical literate publics. Unpublished clinical case notes, on the other, were rarely read by anyone at all in their own time, nor were they commonly used for pedagogic purposes until the late twentieth century. There is indeed substantial discussion in this book of clinical case-observations which help to illustrate how medical concepts were applied in practice and the kinds of people who were treated through them as patients. But the focus here is on those clinical case notes that were cited in published works and so did indeed become part of the public discourse. Here it is worth bearing in mind that in its more recent history, menopause treatment has been subject to a generalised universal advice to women, based on the needs of the minority of women who experience severe symptoms. Nineteenth-century doctors' case notes invariably only reflected the tiny cohort of elite women who sought medical care for symptoms severe enough to warrant a doctor's visit, while the voices of most women who either noticed nothing in particular following the cessation of menses, or who

[96] Williams, *A Cultural History of Medical Vitalism*, 229.

[97] Alannah Tomkins, 'Case Notes and Madness', in Mark Jackson, ed., *The Routledge History of Disease* (London: Routledge, 2016), 529–546; Monika Class, 'Medical Case Histories as Genre: New Approaches', *Literature and Medicine*, 32/1 (2014): 12–26.

had no access to doctors and so managed their experience of ageing in other ways, are nowhere reflected in this archive. Published works, including medical theses, on the other hand, frequently considered the larger question of whether all women generally should expect symptoms associated with the cessation of menses, and made sharp distinctions along class lines and in relation to constitutional types, corpulence, and lifestyle habits such as alcohol consumption, diet, sleep patterns, and physical activity. They were particularly acute observers of the new sedentary and dietary changes in the bodily lifeways of elite women.

From the 1930s onwards, French medicine no longer owned menopause, as globalised medical research on both prophylactic surgeries and hormone replacement therapies proliferated. Nonetheless, it had left an indelible mark on the shape of the modern concept with many of its legacies enduring still today. The nineteenth-century French invention of menopause viewed it as something that must be made the object of medical attentions because although it was not itself a disease, it was assumed to make one susceptible to disease. This novel idea, which was not to be found in any substantial form in earlier medical concepts, is still clearly enduring into our own time in the widespread modern biomedical approach both to treating menopausal women with prophylactic gynaecological surgeries and pharmaceutical hormone replacement therapies; but also in the ever-expanding market of popular health books, websites, weight-loss and health programmes, online videos and podcasts, special diets, exercise regimes, sleep hygiene, stress management, as well as herbal medicine and organotherapy interventions specific for women's ageing and menopause, which have become increasingly globalised in the twenty-first century. The most important continuity in the legacy of nineteenth-century French medical concepts of menopause into our own time is in the fact of directing midlife women's attention inwards towards themselves in the pursuit of anti-ageing products, identity crisis-management, cosmetic beautification or modification, and health-conscious self-care interventions, rather than outward, at the very moment, perhaps, when they are more than ever able to influence the world around them wisely and confidently. A simple constructionist critique of medicalisation would not be adequate for understanding this phenomenon, either in the sense of whom it benefits, or from whence it came.

1

Amenorrhea, Plethora, and the Final Cessation of Menses in Early Modern Medicine

One might be forgiven for expecting that a complete concept of menopause (albeit without a name) would have appeared already in the source corpus of Latin works published from the end of the sixteenth century, since this was when specialist medical writing on the diseases of women's reproductive system first began to flourish. Indeed, several scholars have made such a claim, albeit on rather thin evidential ground. This chapter evaluates such claims, presenting an alternative perspective based on the reading of a wide variety of Latin and French early modern medical sources focused on women. Through this tracing of the first medical discussions of the cessation of menses, mentions were only found as very minor subclauses in works predominantly focused on menstrual disorders in women of reproductive age. There was an emerging consensus about the age of the final cessation of menses appearing in this time largely without reference to any specific symptomatology. Early modern physicians were often concerned about suppressed menses in women of reproductive age (what later gynaecology called *amenorrhea*), and a large corpus of works elaborated a detailed symptomatology of this phenomenon which was increasingly considered nefarious to the health of young women—though even this remained subject to considerable debate.[1] However, the first substantial discussions of the final cessation of menses in older women appeared only during the eighteenth century, as a subclause of these wider medical concerns with suppressed menses in young women. Doctors of women's health in the sixteenth and seventeenth centuries paid scant attention to the cessation of menses in older women (what later medicine called *menopause*). Where they did refer to the normal age-related cessation of menses, it was mostly in terms of it being one of the exceptions to the rule that the lack of menses should be considered a sign of pathology: both pregnancy and being older than 45–50 years were commonly cited as 'natural' causes of the menses ceasing, with little more to be said about the matter. Only a few physicians in this time referred to the final cessation of menses as a time of potential difficulty in the

[1] Cathy McClive, *Menstruation and Procreation in Early Modern France* (Farnham: Ashgate, 2015), chapter 3, unpaginated.

The French Invention of Menopause and the Medicalisation of Women's Ageing: A History. Alison M. Downham Moore, Oxford University Press. © Alison M. Downham Moore 2022. DOI: 10.1093/oso/9780192842916.003.0002

same way as suppressed menses was for young women. But in referring to older women, they also typically acknowledged that such troubled experiences were not the universal norm and were largely only to be expected in a tiny minority of physically inactive, elite women.

Several scholars writing about the long history of menopause have sought examples of symptoms associated with the final cessation of menses in the canon of ancient medicine, namely in the work of Aristotle, Hippocrates, Galen, Soranus of Ephesus, Rufus of Ephesus, and Pliny the Elder.[2] Certainly, numerous Hippocratic aphorisms referred to diseases relating to suppression or absence of menses.[3] However, none of them specifically referred to the cessation of menses with ageing. There was no substantial concept of anything like a menopause symptomatology in ancient medicine, a matter not further discussed hereafter, as it has already been substantially treated by other medical historians.[4] Historians of Islamicate sexual and reproductive medicine have also mentioned discussion of suppressed menses in women of reproductive age in the medieval Arabic and Persian corpus, but similarly do not appear to have found any specific pathological accounts of the end of menses in older women.[5] The pathological view of menopause was a novel, mostly French confection of the long nineteenth century which has too often been assumed to derive from ancient and early modern lineages. This is an easy mistake to make if we believe past medical scholars' own insistence of their ancient pedigree, overlooking the extent to which they wished to be thought of as inheriting the wisdom of the ancient Greeks. Nineteenth-century doctors often implied that Hippocratic medicine had been passed down to them through a continuous lineage since the Renaissance, both ignoring the medieval Arabic mediation of ancient medicine, and denying the influence of medieval Latin traditions on early modern European thought.

[2] Louise Foxcroft, *Hot Flushes, Cold Science: A History of the Modern Menopause* (London: Granta, 2011); Ruth Formanek, 'Continuity and Change and the "Change of Life": Premodern Views of the Menopause', in Ruth Formanek, ed., *The Meanings of Menopause: Historical, Medical, and Cultural Perspectives* (Hillsdale, NJ: The Analytic Press, 1990), 3–42. A good contexualisation of the minimal focus on older women in ancient Greek medicine can be found in Helen King, *Hippocrates' Woman: Reading the Female Body in Ancient Greece* (London: Routledge, 1998). On women's ageing in Roman medicine, see Karen Cokayne, *Experiencing Old Age in Ancient Rome* (London: Routledge, 2003), 144.

[3] For example, aphorisms V, 33; V, 40; V, 57; see Christine Bonnet-Cadilhac, 'Les Aménorrhées dans le "Corpus hippocratique": La Vision du médecin actuel', in Antoine Thivel & Arnaud Zucker, eds, *Le Normal et le pathologique dans la collection hippocratique*, Actes du xe colloque international hippocratique (Nice: Publications de la Faculté des Lettres, Arts et Sciences humaines, 2002), 575–589; also Helen King, *Hippocrates' Woman: Reading the Female Body in Ancient Greece* (London/New York: Routledge, 1998).

[4] Susan P. Matterns, *The Slow Moon Climbs: The Science, History and Meaning of Menopause* (Princeton: Princeton University Press, 2019), 265–268.

[5] Pernilla Myrne, *Female Sexuality in the Early Medieval Islamic World: Gender and Sex in Arabic Literature* (London: Bloomsbury, 2019), 25–36; Avner Giladi, *Muslim Midwives: The Craft of Birthing in the Premodern Middle East* (New York: Cambridge University Press, 2015), 20–22; Emily Selove & Rosalind Batten, 'Making Men and Women: Arabic Commentaries on the Gynaecological Hippocratic Aphorisms in Context', *Annales islamologiques*, 48/1 (2014): 239–262.

Nineteenth-century doctors in general made great mileage of their supposed inheritance from ancient medicine, even as they radically displaced many of its central presuppositions. However, ancient medicine of women's health was innovatively reimagined between the sixteenth and nineteenth centuries in ways that neither Hippocrates nor Galen would have recognised.[6] Chapter 6 considers the nineteenth-century appeals to ancient inheritance, noting the significant liberties French doctors often took in their generalisations about the medical past relative to ideas about women's reproductive physiology. But as far as ideas about the medical description of the end of menses which appeared in the late eighteenth century are concerned, there was very little inheritance from premodern medical traditions, despite physicians' own frequent pretensions to a continuous ancient fidelity.

By overlooking those sources which specifically referred to the final cessation of menses as natural and unremarkable, and by conflating early modern medical accounts of menstrual disorders and plethora with the later construction of menopause, it is possible to imagine the modern pathologising view of menopause as already fully formed in accounts of women's ageing in early modern medicine.[7] Michael Stolberg acknowledges that 'medical writing before 1650 does not abound in discussions of menopausal disorders', though in clustering medical ideas about women's ageing of the seventeenth and early eighteenth centuries under the category of 'menopause', he projects the nineteenth-century category back onto the past before this concept had formed.[8] Cathy McClive considers early modern sources as replete with negative views of what she too calls 'menopause' in her 2015 monograph on the history of menstruation and procreation, even finding Stolberg too dismissive of early modern pathological accounts of it in the history of medicine.[9] However, the evidence provided for her claim is unconvincing.[10] McClive's fascinating work demonstrates an important divergence of French medical opinion of the meaning of menstruation—the central focus of her monograph. But the ambiguous examples of what she takes to be 'menopause' are far less distinctive as such, and incomparably less elaborated than the medical accounts of women's reproductive ageing in nineteenth-century France.

[6] Helen King, *Midwifery, Obstetrics and the Rise of Gynaecology* (London: Routledge, 2007), 83–98; 155–163; Monica H. Green, *Making Women's Medicine Masculine: The Rise of Male Authority in Pre-Modern Gynaecology* (Oxford: Oxford University Press, 2008). On general early modern uses of Hippocrates see: David Cantor, ed., *Reinventing Hippocrates* (Abingdon: Palgrave, 2016).

[7] In particular Michael Stolberg, '"A Woman's Hell"? Medical Perceptions of Menopause in Preindustrial Europe', *Bulletin of the History of Medicine*, 73/3 (1999): 404–428; Ruth Formanek & Valerie Ann McKeon, 'Dispelling Menopause Myths', *Journal of Gerontological Nursing*, 14/8 (1988): 26–29.

[8] Stolberg, '"A Woman's Hell"?'

[9] McClive, *Menstruation and Procreation in Early Modern France*, 111, 120–122.

[10] Ibid., 158–160.

The problem stems in part from the power of the current medical concept of menopause in our own time, which historians thus expect to find everywhere and so read it back onto sources where it was not present in the description of older women—a problem which McClive herself acknowledged in an earlier paper.[11] Susannah Ottaway too identifies this problem in relation to scholarly readings of early modern English sources where the concept of menopause had not in fact yet formed.[12] Lynn Botelho's study of seventeenth-century Suffolk archives found negative descriptions of older women which she described with reference to their presumed 'menopause'.[13] Jessica Godfrey's 2011 book *Attitudes to Post-Menopausal Women in the High and Late Middle Ages* used the term 'postmenopausal' loosely to refer to older women in general, reflecting twentieth-century, not medieval categories. Godfrey importantly shows that medieval medical works between 1200 and 1500 developed a distinct interest in the idea of life cycles and the question of when the ageing process began, torn between the three life stages in the Aristotelian tradition, and the seven stages in the Ptolemaic mathematical tradition, with estimates of ageing beginning somewhere between 40 or 60 years.[14] The popular 1186 work *De amore* (Art of Courtly Love) of Andreas Capellanus, produced for the royalty of Aquitaine, defined old age in women as beginning at 50, while for men it began at 60, and considered that while people over these ages could still have sex, they could not experience love.[15] Nonetheless, neither Capellanus nor any other medieval scholar who attempted to define life cycles referred specifically to the end of menses as medically significant. Medieval and early modern Catholic theologians typically considered all sexual acts that could not lead to conception as sinful (though the Church became far less concerned with this from the eighteenth century onwards). Consequently, insofar as it was understood that women were no longer fertile after their menses ended, sexual activity after this time might be considered implicitly sinful.[16] Nonetheless, medieval accounts lacked a concept of menopause altogether and provided no elaboration of how menstruation mattered in anything like a sex-specific account of the stages of ageing.

[11] Cathy McClive, '"Quand les fleurs s'arrêtent": La Ménopause et l'imaginaire médical', in Cathy McClive, ed., *Femmes en fleurs, femme en corps: Sang, santé, sexualité du Moyen Âge aux Lumières* (Saint-Étienne: L'École du genre, 2010), 277–299 [281].

[12] Susannah R. Ottaway, *The Decline of Life: Old Age in Eighteenth-Century England* (Cambridge: Cambridge University Press, 2004), 35.

[13] Lynn Botehlo, 'Old Age and Menopause in Rural Women of Early Modern Suffolk', in Lynn Botelho & Pat Thane, eds, *Women and Ageing in British Society since 1500* (London: Pearson Educational, 2001), 43–65.

[14] Jessica E. Godfrey, *Attitudes to Post-Menopausal Women in the High and Late Middle Ages, 1100–1400* (Jessica E. Godfrey, 2011), 9–11.

[15] Andreas Capellanus, *The Art of Courtly Love*, trans. John Jay Parry (New York: W. W. Norton & Co, 1969), 32.

[16] Godfrey, *Attitudes to Post-Menopausal Women*, 30–32.

Certainly, there were important medieval books, such as the *c.*1500 *De secretis mulierum* attributed to the Dominican bishop of Cologne, Albertus Magnus and his German followers, which denigrated older women and described them as both sexually undesirable and dangerous to have around children, referring to suspicions of them in relation to witchcraft.[17] However, the authors of this work also considered young menstruating women dangerous, based on the Pentateuch view of menstrual blood as poisonous.[18] Both old men and old women were sometimes viewed in abject terms and were the objects of comic mockery in Old English literary sources and in Old French vernacular proverbs.[19] The French physician François de Fougerolles in 1610 also evoked the concept of women ageing faster than men, but only in cold climate zones.[20] Through the view of broad cultural histories of ageing, some scholars then have attributed modern medical forms of medicalisation of menopause to ancient and medieval antecedents in the cultural denigration of older women throughout history.[21] But this is frankly not menopause. It is perhaps of interest that several medieval medical scholars viewed women's ageing as beginning earlier than men's (without proposing any specific mechanism for this difference). However, given they generally saw women as weaker and inferior, and given the poor survival chances of medieval and early modern women into old age due to high deaths in childbirth, it probably seemed intuitive to many scholars to assume that women simply aged faster too. Nonetheless, this was a far cry from the nineteenth-century French establishment of an entire specialist genre of medical writing dedicated to the newly named symptomatic category of 'menopause', its hygienic and psychiatric management, and finally its surgical and pharmacological treatment.

Several scholars have dated medical descriptions of women suffering illness around the time of menses ceasing as far back as the 1563 work of the Italian physician Giovanni Marinello, though notably in a recent study of the history and science of menopause, Susan Matterns attributes this more to the French physician Jean Liébault's plagiarised translation of Marinello published in 1598.[22] How

[17] Albertus Magnus, *Women's Secrets: A Translation of Pseudo Albertus Magnus's De Secretis Mulierum with Commentaries*, trans. Helen Rodnite Lemay (New York: State University of New York Press, 1992), 129–134.

[18] Magnus, *Women's Secrets*, 131.

[19] McClive, '"Quand les fleurs s'arrêtent"', 277–299; Sarah Toulalan, '"Elderly Years Cause a Total Dispaire of Conception": Old Age, Sex and Infertility in Early Modern England', *Social History of Medicine*, 29/2 (2016): 333–359.

[20] François de Fougerolles, *De senum affectibus prœcavendis, nonnullisque curandis enarratio* (Lyon: J. de Gabiano et L. Durand, 1610), 29–30.

[21] Godfrey, *Attitudes to Post-Menopausal Women*; McClive, '"Quand les fleurs s'arrêtent"'; Houck, *Hot and Bothered*; Ruth Formanek, 'Continuity and Change and the "Change of Life": Premodern Views of the Menopause', in Ruth Formanek, ed., *The Meanings of Menopause: Historical, Medical, and Clinical Perspectives* (Hillsdale, NJ: Analytic Press, 1990), 3–41.

[22] Stolberg, '"A Woman's Hell"?', 406; Louise Foxcroft, *Hot Flushes, Cold Science: A History of the Modern Menopause* (London: Granta, 2011), 76; Matterns, *The Slow Moon Climbs*, 269–271; Giovanni Marinello, *Le medicine partenenti alle infermita delle donne* [1563] (Venetia: Giovanni Valgrisio,

extensive was Marinello's description then, and does it warrant the periodisation of modern menopause as a concept dating from the late sixteenth century, rather than from the long nineteenth when it was named and developed into an entire branch of medical specialisation? The 1574 printed edition of Marinello's 730-page Italian work provides both a table of contents and a detailed index of the significant topics contained within it, none of which refers to older women's cessation of menses.[23] Buried amidst Marinello's discussion of sterility, frigidity, and suppressed menses in women of reproductive age and how to treat these problems (for the most part, with suppositories, purgative medicaments, herbal teas, and baths), there is a passage which describes symptoms of suppressed menses in young women, including abdominal pains, fever, vomiting, sore eyes, breathing difficulties, and intensified sexual desires. And this single sentence includes a sub-clause mentioning that women who have recently permanently ceased menstruating may also exhibit similar effects.[24] As Matterns notes, Marinelli's lengthy book was overwhelmingly concerned with matters of fertility and pregnancy in women of reproductive age and his short description of physical symptoms associated with suppressed menses was not even specific to older women.[25] His barely detectable reference to the final cessation of menses in ageing as symptomatic is hardly equivalent to the several hundred works—specifically focused uniquely on the symptomology and management of a distinct condition now with its very own name—menopause—elaborated in France during the nineteenth century. Liébault, for his part, was also considerably ambivalent in his discussion of the cessation of menses in older women and can little more than Marinello be taken to represent an early modern pathologisation of menopause, as we consider further in this chapter.

An important turning point occurred between 1712 and 1750, when there were increasingly more works on the general diseases of women which similarly contained a few lines, or more rarely in a single chapter, referring to a 'change of life, 'decline of life', a 'critical age', or a 'climacteric' thought to produce negative symptoms in some women, while also often naturalising the cessation of menses and providing positive accounts of its benefits. Importantly, a handful of Latin theses written by German medical students, mostly at the University of Halle, in the first half of the eighteenth century made the cessation of menses in women of all ages a minor topic of disease description with reference to the larger non-sex-specific concept of plethora.[26] These theses were rarely subsequently cited by other medical scholars writing on the topic thereafter. It is worth recalling here

1574); Jean Liébault, *Trois livres appartenans aux infirmitez et maladies des femmes* [Giovanni Marinelli] (Lyon: J. Veyrat, 1598).

[23] Marinello, *Le medicine partenenti*, 688–729.

[24] Ibid., 96.

[25] Matterns, *The Slow Moon Climbs*, 270.

[26] Daniel Schäfer, *Old Age and Disease in Early Modern Medicine*, trans. Patrick Baker (London: Routledge, 2015), 161–166.

too that in the eighteenth century, Latin was an elite language known only to scholars and clergy. On the other hand, many of the most renowned early modern doctors, writing in both Latin and in vernacular languages, frankly naturalised the final cessation of menses and were widely cited by other scholars. If they did mention any symptoms associated with it, they also distinguished between the vast majority who were peasant women and who reported no symptoms at all, and a tiny minority of urban elite women living sedentary, indoor, gluttonous lifestyles who they claimed more commonly experienced temporary health problems in adjusting to the loss of menses as the body's means of relieving the plethora that menstruation entailed.[27]

Plethora was an important piece in the assemblage of the modern concept of menopause, though it was not itself such a concept. Plethora (from the Greek *plēthōrē*, meaning 'fullness') referred to a mechanistic theory espoused by medical scholars in numerous western European cultures from the end of the sixteenth century which modified the strictly humoralist view of disease of the kind associated with Galenic medicine, proposing a novel physics-based account of ageing in which excess healthy fluids created pressure in the venous system, resulting in a gradual solidification of the tissues.[28] Importantly, the plethora concept of ageing was not sex differentiated and was applied just as much to men's ageing, although menstruation and its cessation did become assimilated to the theory in eighteenth-century German, Dutch, French, and English medicine.[29] Other conditions that were ascribed to plethora included gout (a disease most common in men), arthritic pain, epilepsy, tumours, stroke, as well as menstrual disorders in women of all ages. The most common treatment for plethora, since it was assumed to be a problem of excess fluids, was phlebotomy (blood-letting), which was a widespread prescription for a vast range of medical conditions in early modern medicine.[30] This was an ancient therapeutic practice, most often associated with the ancient Greek physician Erasistratus (*c.*310–250 BCE), and was described both in medieval European and Arabic texts, as well as in Chinese medicine, but it underwent a considerable revival from the end of the fifteenth

[27] Elizabeth Williams, 'Eating after the Climacteric: Food, Gender and Ageing in the Long Eighteenth Century', in James Kennaway & Rina Knoeff, eds, *Lifestyle and Medicine in the Enlightenment: The Six Non-Naturals in the Long Eighteenth Century* (London: Routledge, 2020), unpaginated; Alison M. Moore, 'Conceptual Layers in the Invention of Menopause in Nineteenth-Century France', *French History*, 32/2 (2018): 226–248.

[28] Schäfer, *Old Age and Disease in Early Modern Medicine*, 160–161; Colin Jones & Laurence Brockliss, *The Medical World of Early Modern France* (Oxford: Oxford University Press, 1997), 156–157.

[29] Daniel Schäfer, 'Alte Frau = Alter Mann? Die Wahrnehmung von Matronen in der medizinischen Fachprosa des 18. Jahrhunderts', in Heike Hartun, ed., *Alter und Geschlecht: Repräsentationen, Geschichten und Theorien des Alter(n)s* (Beilefeld: Transcript Verlag, 2005), 135–154; also Michael Stolberg, 'Menstruation and Sexual Difference in Early Modern Medicine (1500–1800)', in A. Shail & G. Howie, eds, *Menstruation: A Cultural History* (Basingstoke: Palgrave, 2005), 90–101; McClive, *Menstruation and Procreation*, 109–111.

[30] Jones & Brockliss, *The Medical World of Early Modern France*, 146–159.

century in Europe, enduring through to the end of the nineteenth century.[31] If one goes looking for early modern equivalents of the later modern pathologisation of menopause, it is easy to mistake the practice of blood-letting among older women for an indication that their absent menses was assumed to have accumulated in the body, requiring mechanical release. Cathy McClive, for instance, looking for evidence of menopause symptoms in seventeenth-century women's writing, cites a 1679 letter from Mme de Sévigné to her daughter which describes the monthly use of blood-letting to maintain her health in old age.[32] But in fact, blood-letting once per month from the feet was an extremely common prescription in the seventeenth century, given to men and women alike in the view that it could alleviate all the diseases of ageing—without specific reference to menstruation or its cessation—and a considerable Latin, French, and English medical corpus was devoted to this singular therapeutic method and its theory.[33]

This chapter hereafter considers a range of late sixteenth-, seventeenth-, and early eighteenth-century medical descriptions of women's specific ageing, selecting major works from the Latin, French, and English corpus of the late fifteenth to early eighteenth centuries, considering both those sources which have been recently cited by other scholars in support of a pathological view of early modern menopause, as well as other influential medical works which can be taken to indicate significant currents of medical opinion since they were published in numerous editions, translated into other languages, or cited by many other scholars.

The Early Modern Naturalisation of the Final Cessation of Menses

We begin with the French royal surgeon under Henri II, Ambroise Paré (1510–1590), who was undoubtedly one of the most widely read and cited French medical scholars of the late sixteenth century. He devoted much consideration in his *De la génération* of 1573 to the questions of sterility in women and of suppressed menses, listing a variety of reasons why this might occur, including because of sadness, fear, hunger, excessive work, sleep loss, being pregnant, being

[31] Lois N. Magner, *A History of Medicine* (New York: Marcel Dekker, 1992), 79, 203; Charles Green Cumston, *An Introduction to the History of Medicine: From the Time of the Pharaohs to the End of the XVIIIth Century* (New York: Routledge, 2018), chapters VII and XVII, unpaginated.

[32] McClive, '"Quand les fleurs s'arrêtent"', 297. See *Lettres de Madame de Sévigné*, 2 vols, ed. Roger Duchene (Paris: Gallimard, 1977), vol. 2, 700.

[33] See e.g., Michael Alberti, *De venae sectione* (Halle: Hendel, 1725); Andreas-Elias Büchner, *De plethora senum ejusque rationali therapeutica tractatione per venaesectionem speciatim suscipienda* (Halle: Hendel, 1749); Georg Ernst Stahl, *De senum affectibus* (Halle: Henckel, 1710), 27–30; Pierre Calemare de La Fayette, *Essai sur la pléthore ou polyémie* (Paris: Faculté de Médecine, 1809); John Scudder, *A Dissertation on the Diseases of Old Age as Connected with a Plethoric State of System* (New York: Van Winkle & Wiley, 1815).

ill, eating too much raw fruit, because of an ulcer, from using too many astringent douches, because of blood loss from other parts of the body, because of extended fever, 'par âge, comme vieillesse' (because of age, such as old age), during lactation, and other reasons.[34] Sterility (still with menses) could also result from tumours, from a blockage of the uterus, or from having a uterus that is too hot, cold, dry, or moist, from drinking too much cold water, eating too much raw fruit, being too thin or too fat, or from working too hard.[35] Paré worried about the border between the sexes in a range of ways, as Valerie Traub has demonstrated.[36] He thought that retaining the menses in general could turn women into men, citing the example of Phaëtusa in the work of Hippocrates, who was a married woman who lost her menses after her husband went away to war, and who grew a beard and became a man thereafter.[37] 'Such women are naturally stronger and of hotter and drier temperature, such that they can easily dissipate, by imperceptible perspiration, the superfluities of their nourishment in the manner of men: They are, moreover, sterile.'[38] Paré did not appear to consider older women more prone to this slide into masculinity, as indicated by his specification that this could happen to any women 'or girls' who were too uppity. He considered that suppression of menses could be a sign of vapours or of 'suffocation of the uterus', but made no mention of older women in this discussion either, and indeed proposed that those most vulnerable to the condition were young married women who had not yet conceived, or whose husbands were absent.[39] The remainder of his discussion of suppressed menses and sterility and how to treat them also made no mention of older women, whereas he noted elsewhere in passing that women were generally only capable of conceiving between the ages of 14 and 50 years.[40] There was here neither an explicit naturalisation of the cessation of menses such as we will see in the work of Jean Liébault shortly afterwards, but nor was there any apparent suspicion of this time in a woman's life as one of greater disease.

One reason for the absence of any discussion of the final cessation of menses here is that Paré did not consider menstruation necessarily required for fertility, though it could generally be taken as a proxy for conceptive capacity.[41] He emphasised variability between types of individuals, citing unusual cases of women conceiving without menstruation and claiming that young brunette women always had heavier periods. He certainly made distinctions between the menstruation of

[34] Ambroise Paré, *De la génération de l'homme, recveilli des anciens et modernes* [1573], in *Œuvres complètes d'Ambroise Paré*, ed. J. F. Malgaigne, vol. 2 (Paris: J. B. Baillière, 1840), 18e Livre, 633–799 [764].

[35] Paré, *De la génération de l'homme*, 733–735.

[36] Valerie Traub, *The Renaissance of Lesbianism in Early Modern England* (Cambridge: Cambridge University Press, 2002), 94–110.

[37] See Helen King, *The One-Sex Body on Trial: The Classical and Early Modern Evidence* (London & New York: Routledge, 2013), 80–123.

[38] Paré, *De la génération de l'homme*, 765. [39] Ibid., 751–761. [40] Ibid., 738.

[41] On French medical debates about this matter see McClive, *Menstruation and Procreation*, 99–136.

younger and older women: he considered the process of ageing in general to be one of solidification, remarking that the bones of young people are easier to break than those in the 'virile' age.[42] He cited Aristotle's claim, in *De generatione animalium*, that younger women 'who have a lot of blood and are stronger and cheerful', menstruate on the new moon, while older women menstruate on the full moon since they have less blood and 'require a stronger, more vigorous moon' to invoke their menses—an idea evoked by Marinello as well.[43] But he also recounted nothing pathological that was thought to be specific to women after the final cessation of their menstrual cycles.

Certainly, if a woman wished to continue conceiving into her fifties or beyond, following Paré's advice on how to treat the suppression of menses in younger women (with vomiting, leeches placed around the cervix, with purgative herbal remedies, baths, pessaries), she might adopt such measures in the hope of avoiding the final cessation of menses. But Paré himself made no recommendation of this kind, and it seems likely, given the many pregnancies to which most women were subjected in the early modern period, that few women would have wished to undergo further pregnancies later in life, unless they had lost all their children to infectious diseases (which certainly happened sometimes). Comparative recent anthropological studies of the menstrual lifespan, which are discussed at length by Susan Matterns, indicate that most women in cultures where pregnancies are high in number typically have their final pregnancies long before their final menstruation, and welcome the end of their reproductive capacity as providing relief from the burdens of childbearing.[44] Of course, there are exceptions—there usually are in everything.

At least part of the reason that early modern medical scholars did not all agree on the significance of the cessation of menses is that it was widely observed that some women, rarely, conceived long after ceasing to menstruate. Numerous scholars, in generalising the age of the change as occurring around 45, 49, or 50 years, also cited exceptions in which women of 60, or even as old as 80 became pregnant.[45] Often, these observations did not specify if the pregnancies were brought to term in live infant births, but in some cases they did: Louis de Serres in 1625 noted that women rarely conceived after 50 or 55 years, but cited the historical exception of the 56-year-old wife of the German emperor Henry (probably II), who bore a son to him after being sterile for many years, giving birth in public so that no one could doubt the veracity of her delivery.[46] Exceptions in the other direction were noted too, with women as young as 30 years ceasing to menstruate and never resuming. In the larger conversation about the meaning of menstruation

[42] Ibid., 714. [43] Ibid., 762; Marinello, *Le medicine partenenti*, 96.

[44] Matterns, *The Slow Moon Climbs*, 302–328.

[45] McClive, *Menstruation and Procreation*, 105–112.

[46] Louis de Serres, *Discours de la nature, causes, signes et curation des empeschemens de la conception et de la stérilité des femmes* (Paris: Antoine Chard, 1625), 293.

as a proxy for fertility, doctors also noted that some women conceived even when they had not been menstruating, while other women with regular menstrual cycles could still be infertile. While most medical scholars concerned with women's health naturalised the cessation of menses in ageing to some degree and took it to be an approximate indication of the loss of conceptive capacity, it made little sense to them to tightly connect conceptive capacity to the continuance of menstruation in the manner that occurred later in the French fascination with 'menopause'.

In this period there was substantial transmission of medical concepts across different cultures sharing the scholarly Latin lingua franca, and also across different vernacular languages, in regard to reproductive health and ageing, stimulated by the proto-biological frames of mechanism, solidism, vitalism, organicism, and materialism in their displacement of the humoral model associated both with Galen and Hippocrates, and with medieval Arabic medicine.[47] Certainly, as Michael Stolberg notes, in this period, the different models of the purpose of menstruation all rejected the simple 'cathartic' account of Galenism in favour of either an iatromechanical view of menstruation as plethora, or an iatrochemical view of it as fermentation—which similarly was thought to create pressure on the venous system, requiring release.[48] Nonetheless, there is also no doubt that doctors of the seventeenth and eighteenth centuries increasingly viewed matters of medical generalisation informed by ethnographic accounts produced in the colonial contexts of French, Dutch, Spanish, Portuguese, and English imperial endeavours in South America, South Asia, and North Africa, as well as the internal colonisations of indigenous lands in the northern and eastern extremities of the European continent and Mediterranean islands. The work of the sixteenth-century French Protestant minister Jean de Léry appears to have had an important intercultural impact on the emergence of medical ideas about the meaning of the end of menses. Léry worked in the Guanabara Bay Calvinist colony in Rio de Janeiro in 1574, and spent several months afterwards living among the Tupinambá Indians on the east coast of Brazil. He claimed to have observed that most Tupinambá women did not regularly menstruate and speculated that they must have had other means of expelling blood and enabling conception, pointing to various skin-cutting rituals practised among them.[49] The idea, derived from Léry, that indigenous women in different parts of the world did not require menstruation for conception appeared in numerous other French medical texts thereafter, notably cited by the highly influential early eighteenth-century Montpellier-trained physician Jean Astruc (1684–1766), and by the renowned

[47] Schäfer, *Old Age and Disease*, 108–112.
[48] Stolberg, 'Menstruation and Sexual Difference', 93–96.
[49] Jean de Léry, *Histoire d'un voyage fait en Brésil, autrement dite Amérique* (Geneva: Pour Antoine Chuppin, 1578), 302.

late eighteenth-century medical scholar Pierre Roussel (1742–1802), whom we consider in Chapter 3.[50]

Very much in the iatrochemical tradition of medicine, the 1585 *Treasury of Secret Remedies for the Diseases of Women* by the Dijonnais physician Jean Liébault, published in both Latin and French, had mostly worried about the 'vapours' that suppressed menses could induce as a result of 'vicious humours' from the uterus infiltrating the venous system.[51] Liébault thought this suppression made women become stupid, irrational, and cry all the time, or else made them think that the Devil was trying to strangle them. But in this work, he discussed the problem without any reference to older women.[52] He undoubtedly realised that the menses ended at a certain age—elsewhere in the book, he proposed that young girls do not menstruate because they are holding on to their blood as long as possible in order to grow their own bodies, and that similarly, once a woman ceased to menstruate 'around the end of the seventh septenary' (on the cusp of 49–50 years), her blood would be reabsorbed and distributed to those parts of the body that needed it most.[53] Here an astrological climacteric concept appears to have informed the estimation of women's age of change.[54] Liébault rejected the view, which he attributed to both Aristotle and Pliny the Elder, that menstrual blood is morbid or 'venomous', but he did consider it 'excremental' if it accumulated for too long, and hence it was necessary to expel it periodically, which is why 'unnatural' causes of suppressed menstruation were generally of concern. Importantly though, Liébault made a sharp distinction between causes for the suppression of menses that were 'natural' and those that were 'against nature' ('contre la nature'): natural causes were firstly pregnancy, in which the woman's blood nourished the growing foetus and so did not need to be expelled; secondly, frequent exercise such as occurred among 'rustic women', and among 'les sauterelles' (very thin women) and 'chanteresses' (singers) which could result in diminished or suppressed menses; the third *natural* example was among 'les vieilles' (old women).[55]

Liébault devoted a whole chapter (XXVII) to the problem of 'suppressed or diminished monthlies' but it focused entirely on those causes which he considered 'contre la nature' among women who were mature (beyond adolescence) but neither pregnant *nor old*.[56] He had nothing here to say about illnesses associated with the final cessation of menses nor about this fact of women's physiology implying anything specific in relation to their ageing. This is an important

[50] Jean Astruc, *Traité des maladies des femmes* [1737], vol. 5 (Paris: P. Guillaume Cavelier, 1765), 85.

[51] Jean Liébault, *Trésor des remèdes secrèts pour les maladies des femmes*. Pris du Latin, fait français par Jean Liébault (Paris: Jacques du Puys à la Samaritaine, 1585), 23.

[52] Ibid., 329–330. [53] Ibid., 332.

[54] Elizabeth Sears, *The Ages of Man: Medieval Interpretations of the Life Cycle* (Princeton: Princeton University Press, 1986), 38–53.

[55] Liébault, *Trésor des remèdes secrèts pour les maladies des femmes*, 337. [56] Ibid., 341–346.

distinction which has been commonly overlooked by historians writing on the early modern medical description, some of whom have even cited Liébault's ideas about menstruation in support of the view that early modern medicine considered 'menopause' to be universally symptomatic, ignoring this doctor's important statements which specifically naturalised the age-related cessation of menses. Michael Stolberg, seeking to debunk what he takes to be a Foucaldian dogma of 'medicalisation' critique plaguing medical historians in the English-speaking world, remarks that early modern menopause 'could have been portrayed as a perfectly natural, innocuous process.... But few writers allowed that possibility.'[57] However Liébault, like many others, in fact made precisely this claim, explicitly naturalising the end of menses. Additionally, Stolberg footnotes (though does not discuss) several other naturalising exceptions to his own historical interpretation, including the Spanish royal physician Luis de Mercado (1525–1611) who in 1587 stated simply that most women ceased menstruating at 45 or 50 years, after which they were no longer fertile. Mercado appeared to consider menstruation itself so fraught with disease that its cessation could only be a good thing.[58] Further, the Dutch physician Pieter van Foreest (1521–1597) in 1589, in similar terms to Liébault, naturalised the end of menses after the age of 40 years, categorically dismissing it from the concerns of doctors.[59] The 1590 *Archidoxis magica*, an alchemical treatise attributed to Paracelsus, proposed pharmacological remedies to return menses and fertility in young women but made no mention whatsoever of such treatments being advisable for older women.[60] The Swiss anatomist Felix Platter (1536–1614), in the highly successful 1604 *Quaestionum medicarum* which was published in multiple editions throughout the seventeenth century, claimed that women's reproductive capacity ending around the age of 50 was designed deliberately by God;[61] and the English physician John Freind (1675–1728) in 1703 explicitly (discussed further in this chapter) denied that the end of menses was problematic.[62] While it is not possible to treat all the many naturalising sources in detail, a number of them are discussed here with close textual attention in order to show that a non-pathological view of the cessation of menses was indeed significant in early modern medical works, if they discussed the matter at all. Numerous highly influential medical scholars writing on the

[57] Stolberg, '"A Woman's Hell"?' 408.

[58] Luis de Mercado, *Gynaeciorum siue De mulierum affectibus commentarii Graecorum, Latinorum, Barbarorum iam olim & nunc recens editorum: in quatuor tomos digesti, et necessariis passim imaginibus illustrate* (Venice: Conrad Vualdkirch, 1587), vol. 4, 17.

[59] Peter van Foreest, *Observationum et curationum medicinalium liber vigesimus-octavus, de mulierum morbis. Unà cum scholiis* (Leiden: Raphelengium Christophorum, 1589), 8–9.

[60] Archidoxis magic, lib. V, in Johannes Huser, ed., *Zehender Theil Der Bücher und Schriften Adiunctus est Index rerum et verborum accuratiß et copiosissimus* (Basel: Conrad Waldkirch, 1590), vol. 4, 51–52.

[61] Felix Platter, *Quaestionum medicarum paradoxarum et endoxarum, juxta partes medidnae dispositarum centuria posthuma* [1604] (Basel: Impensis Ludovici Regis, 1625), 107–110.

[62] John Freind, *Emmenologia* [1703] trans. Thomas Dale, MD (London: T. Cox, 1729), 61–62.

disease of women or on menstruation made scant reference to the incidence of women experiencing negative symptoms in the age-related final cessation of menses. This was in marked contrast to nineteenth-century French medical sources discussed throughout the rest of this book, in which doctors wrote hundreds of entire specialist works devoted to the 'critical age' or 'menopause'—now named as a distinct epoque in women's lives, and elaborated with reference to both a specific symptomatology and a hygienic programme of treatment.

Numerous medical works devoted to questions of the diseases of women and the description of sexed difference flourished in the late sixteenth and early seventeenth centuries, first in Latin and then in French, English, and German, inspired by the new studies of women's anatomy produced since the late fifteenth century.[63] There is no doubt that in many such works, the problem of suppressed menstruation became more commonly viewed as indicating pathology in women of reproductive age—what modern medicine calls *amenorrhea*, not menopause. It most likely preoccupied doctors in this time because both women's deaths in childbirth and infant mortality were extremely common, making concerns to optimise conception a central topic of medicine focused on women. From the beginning of the eighteenth century, there were some doctors in Germany who described women among the aristocracy and bourgeoisie suffering a wide range of general plethoric diseases whenever their menses was suppressed, including around the time of its final cessation, as well as other doctors who explicitly naturalised the cessation of menses in ageing and claimed it to pass normally without symptoms.

Luis de Mercado was the personal physician to Phillip II and III of Spain and one of the most influential scholars in the early history of gynaecology, who began writing about the reproductive physiology of women in his 1579 *De communibus mulierum*, before embarking on the four-volume *Gynaeciorum siue De mulierum affectibus* (Gynaecology, or the Afflictions of Women) published 1587. These were among the first major studies in the subject area which made full use of the new translations of Hippocrates derived from Arabic sources only recently

[63] In addition to those already named above, see Giovanni Battista da Monte, *De affectibus uterinis libellus, cum decem consiliis muliebribus* (Basel: no publisher named, 1554); Abucasis (Abū al-Qāsim Khalaf ibn 'Abbās al-Zahrāwī), *Gynaeciorum, hoc est, de mulierum tum aliis, tum gravidarum, parientium & puerperarum affectibus & morbis, libri veterum ac recentiorum aliquot, partim nunc primum editi, partim multo quam antea castigatiores* (Basel: Thomam Guarinum, 1566); Maurice de la Corde, *Commentarii in librum priorem Hippocratis de muliebribus* (Paris: Dionysium Duvallium, 1585); Girolamo Mercuriale, *De morbis muliebribus prælectiones* [1584] (Venice: Juntas, 1591); Martin Akakia, *De morbis muliebribus libridus* (Strasbourg: Lazari Zetzneri, 1597); Rodrigo de Castro, *De universa mulierum medicina* (Hamburg: Frobeniana, 1603). See King, *The One-Sex Body on Trial*; Londa Schiebinger, *Nature's Body: Gender in the Making of Modern Science* (Boston: Beacon, 1993); Ian McLean, *The Renaissance Notion of Woman: A Study in the Fortunes of Scholasticism* (Cambridge: Cambridge University Press, 1980); Thomas W. Laqueur, *Making Sex: Body and Gender from the Greeks to Freud* (Cambridge, Mass.: Harvard University Press, 1990); Michael Stolberg, 'A Woman Down to her Bones: The Anatomy of Sexual Difference in the Sixteenth and Early Seventeenth Centuries', *Isis*, 94/2 (June 2003): 274–299.

available in Latin after 1525, as well as the popular manual of women's health known as the *Trotula* which had circulated throughout medieval Europe.[64] Scholars who wish to evoke the ancient origins of a medical view of the cessation of menses as pathological would do well to read Mercado—he appears to have scoured the ancient sources for everything they had to say about menstruation and its absence, and as far as statements about ageing women were concerned, he appears to have found... *nihil.* Intriguingly too, in the opening pages of this major work of early modern gynaecology, Mercado referred to the astrological traditions which ascribed meaning to particular years in a person's life as bearing dangerous portent, explicitly dismissing these as grounds for explaining anything about women's menstrual cycles, health risks, or fertility windows.[65] The fusion of Chaldean astrology with plethora theory which appeared ambivalently only in early eighteenth-century German medicine, is not only absent from Mercado's late sixteenth-century Spanish perspective, but is even emphatically denied as a possible pathway for rational conceptualisation of reproductive medicine.

General medical works of the early seventeenth century, written in Latin for other doctors and scholars, also touched upon the matter of the temporality of women's fertility, often naturalising the age-related end of menses without reference to pathologies specific to this time in a woman's life. The Swiss physician Felix Platter's 1604 *Quaestionum medicarum* (Medical Questions) considered several matters relating to menstruation, such as why women were the only animals to menstruate (he countered that he had seen dogs do it too),[66] and why women, but not men, were only able to conceive for a finite period of their lives. He said that this was because women have a fixed number of menstrual cycles which occur monthly (so long as they are healthy and not pregnant or breastfeeding) until the age of somewhere between 40 and 50 years, after which they can neither conceive nor continue to menstruate.[67] He sharply distinguished between men and women in relation to their conceptive capacity in old age: 'Verum tempus, quo ad generandum non amplius idonei sunt, non utriusque aeque contingit' ('that time, when they are no longer able to generate, actually does not affect equally both'), remarking that his own father had remarried at the age of 70 after he was widowed, and with his new (presumably much younger) wife, begat a daughter when he was 86 years old.[68] As Stolberg acknowledges, Platter here also explained the sex difference in ageing reproductive capacity as part of God's deliberate design in order to prevent the earth from becoming overpopulated.[69] While Platter did not use the modern language of 'nature' or 'biology' to invoke

[64] Helen King, *Midwifery, Obstetrics and the Rise of Gynecology: The Uses of a Sixteenth-Century Compendium* (Aldershot: Ashgate, 2007), 31.

[65] Mercado, *Gynaeciorum*, vol. 1, 2–3.

[66] Felix Platter, *Quaestionum medicarum paradoxarum et endoxarum, juxta partes medidnae dispositarum centuria posthuma* (Basel: Impensis Ludovici Regis, 1625), 107.

[67] Ibid., 109. [68] Ibid., 109–110. [69] Stolberg, '"A Woman's Hell"?', 410, footnote 25.

this explanation, his description of the cessation of menses as something intended by God for a rational purpose served a similar function to the naturalising statements of the kind Stolberg claims were not a significant part of early modern medical description. Other doctors, such as Liébault, did indeed explicitly evoke the natural/against nature distinction to situate the cessation of menses in ageing as outside the scope of medical concerns which generally applied to matters of missing menstruation.

Hydraulic and mechanistic explanations of women's physiology became more insistent in Latin and English medical works from the beginning of the eighteenth century, including consideration of the physiology of menstruation and the meaning of its suppression. Commonly, the mechanism of menstruation was now described as plethora—the abundance of healthy fluid—which in the case of the menses, must be released, not because the blood was toxic, but simply because it was in excess.[70] However, this alone was not sufficient to produce a pathological view of the final cessation of menses. The 1703 Latin *Emmenologia* of the Cornish physician and chemist John Freind was an important and widely read work as indicated by the multiple English and Latin editions of it that appeared throughout the eighteenth century following its translation in 1729.[71] It was also translated into French in 1738, and into Swedish in 1786.[72] Freind devoted a whole chapter of the *Emmenologia* to the causes of suppressed menses,[73] and another to the methods for treating the problem, which included blood-letting and induced vomiting, as well as cathartic and emmenagogic medicaments.[74] However Freind made no mention of such treatments being advisable for women over 45 years old and in fact specifically devoted another short passage to the question of women's natural end of menses which did not require medication.[75] As John Rowlinson has shown, Freind employed Newtonian physics of hydraulics to describe the mechanics of menstruation.[76] He referred to the notion of numerically regular life cycles producing the prediction that menstruation should cease most commonly around the 49th year, since this was seven times seven years, as in the earlier description of the French physician Liébault.[77] The 'seventh septenary' was

[70] Schäfer, *Old Age and Disease*, 68–72.

[71] John Freind, *Emmenologia: in qua fluxus muliebris menstrui phaenomena, periodi, vitia cum medendi methodo, ad rationes mechanicas exiguntur* (Oxford: Thomas Bennet, 1703). Freind, *Emmenologia* (1729); Freind, *Emmenologia*, 2nd ed. (London: T. Cox, 1752).

[72] John Freind, *Emménologie, ou traité de l'évacuation ordinaire aux femmes: Où l'on explique les phénomènes, les retours, les vices, et la méthode curative, qui la concernent selon les loix de la méchanique* (Paris: Jacques Clouzier, 1738); John Freind, *Underrättelse om månads-reningen: til des natur, orsaker, tid, tilfälligheter, fel och botemedel, jämte sättet huru en stor del sjukdomar, härrörande af blodets elaka beskaffenhet, framalstras, såsom ock wissa läkemedels kraft och wärkan* (Stockholm: Nordström, 1786).

[73] Freind, *Emmenologia* (1729), 77–110. [74] Ibid., 111–128. [75] Ibid., 60–62.

[76] J. S. Rowlinson, 'John Freind: Physician, Chemist, Jacobite and Friend of Voltaire's', *Notes & Records of the Royal Society*, 61 (2007): 109–127.

[77] Liébault, *Trésor des remèdes secrèts pour les maladies des femmes*, 332.

the natural moment for menses to end because by this time the vessels of the uterus had rigidified, preventing blood from entering them. Therefore, there was no blood banking up in the uterus of the older woman, because no blood was able to enter it in the first place. Nature had 'wisely ordered' that the menses gradually diminish so that it would not need to force its way into the more rigid vessels of the ageing uterus. Even if some blood did manage to squeeze though, Freind reasoned, 'other secretory vessels will by custom be brought to that pass, as to be able to receive and discharge that plethora which heaped up every month. Therefore no very bad symptoms happen in elderly woman, although the menses should be wanting.'[78]

Daniel Schäfer has argued that the early eighteenth-century plethora theory of ageing to emerge from iatromechanical medicine (challenging Galenic humour theory) might have allowed the cessation of menses to be assimilated into a pathogenetic view of sex-specific ageing, creating the potential conditions for the description of menopause as disease-ridden; at the same time, the emerging evidence of women's greater longevity created a counter-pressure against this trend.[79] Convincing as this interpretation is for the early eighteenth century, in fact both kinds of arguments that variously naturalised or catastrophised the final cessation of menses were soon to be made on both iatrochemical and iatromechanical grounds with reference either to plethora or to the nervous disorders (the focus of our Chapter 4). Moreover, as we shall see in Chapter 2, the intercultural demographic revolution which converged on a consensus about women's greater longevity during the seventeenth and eighteenth centuries, was also specifically assimilated into the early nineteenth-century French elaboration of medical ideas about menopause. There it performed as a touchstone for doctors' anti-pathological insistences which appeared, surprisingly, within a new menopause symptomatology substantiating the need for older women's medical surveillance. How this curious and rather counter-intuitive paradox was richly elaborated in the context of the contest for new patient markets and scholarly esteem between the medical faculties of both Montpellier and Paris universities is the focus of Chapters 3, 4, and 5.

Menstruation and Its End from Iatrochemical to Iatromechanical Perspectives

Both iatrochemical accounts of ageing, associated with the Swiss polymath Paracelsus, and iatromechanical approaches to physiology developed by the German physicians Friederich Hoffmann and Herman Boerhaave, emphasised the

[78] Freind, *Emmenologia*, 61–62. [79] Schäfer, *Old Age and Disease*, 186–187.

physical and chemical properties of fluids in the body with reference to pressure, motion, alkalinity, and acidity, thereby displacing Galenic approaches focused on the balancing of humours, with reference to cold, heat, dampness, and dryness. The Montpellier scholar and royal physician Jean de Varanda (1564–1617) exemplified an iatrochemical account of menstruation in his 1666 *Traité des maladies des femmes*, defining it as a 'concoction' or 'benign excretion' of the uterus that 'discharges itself every month' among those women who were 'of age without being pregnant' ('en aage sans estre grosses'), taking it as a reliable sign of fertility since the purpose of menstrual blood was to nourish a foetus.[80] He recognised that women ceased menstruating after the age of 50 or 55, at which point they could no longer conceive.[81] He took this fact to resolve the much debated matter of whether menstruation indicated fertility, since neither girls too young nor women too old menstruated and both also rarely ever conceived.[82] The cessation of menses 'without any other vice than age' was 'when the vigour of age and strength is lacking': this meant there was no longer sufficient heat and what little of it remained became dedicated to 'nourishing and conserving the self', freed from the ardour of childbearing.[83] In all his subsequent remarks, there is no mention of older women. Varanda too referred to the ethnographic account of Amazonian women barely menstruating.[84] He described numerous symptoms of the suppression of menses in women who were of the age to menstruate, including diarrhoea, vomiting, constant sweating and urination, nose-bleeds, and haemorrhoids, which were caused especially by excess consumption of salt, aromatics, or pepper. The failure to menstruate made the blood rise up to more sensitive parts, becoming corrupted, cold, and putrefied, and after three months of not menstruating, women could experience 'suffocations, lumbar pains, heaviness and even fever'.[85] But this did not always occur since menses could also be suppressed by 'too violent exercise', which was why Amazonian women, dancers, and peasant women all barely menstruated at all or not very often.[86] Tumours of the uterus could also suppress menstruation and resemble pregnancy he noted, and advised that if such occurred then a competent *sage-femme* should be called to inspect the interior orifice, since tumours could be distinguished from foetuses by their hardness and the pain they caused when touched.[87] Importantly, Varanda defined as 'against nature' ('contre la nature') and per se in need of medication only those stoppages of menses which were due to 'bad disposition' ('par une mauvaise disposition'), causing 'an infinity of ill effects' ('une infinite de maux') and were neither due to 'age, nor pregnancy, nor the nourishing of an infant' ('sans que l'âge, ny la grossesse, ny la nourriture d'un enfant en soient la cause').[88]

[80] Jean de Varanda, *Traité des maladies des femmes* (Paris: Robert de Ninville, 1666), 30–31.
[81] Ibid., 31, 302. [82] Ibid., 309. [83] Ibid., 31.
[84] Ibid., 32. [85] Ibid., 56–57.
[86] Ibid., 56. [87] Ibid., 60. [88] Ibid., 62.

The late seventeenth-century Montpellier medical scholar Daniel Duncan (1649–1735) provided an iatrochemical model of how suppressed menses in women could be interpreted as pathological. Consequently his work has been widely cited by scholars writing on the pre-history of 'menopause' symptomatology.[89] The early Montpellier vitalist current was certainly a key element in the formation of medical ideas about periods of physiological change as moments of crisis, with associated health risks seen as peculiar to specific age groups.[90] However, the idea that the end of menses represented a type of 'critical age' or life-cycle turning point particularly flourished in France only towards the close of the eighteenth century and was still notably absent from both Varanda's and Duncan's work on women's physiology. The 1687 second and third parts of Duncan's larger *Chimie naturelle* provided one of the first detailed iatrochemical medical accounts of women's reproductive function, including a short passage devoted to the hydraulics of menstruation, its cleansing role in women's physiology, and the meaning of its final cessation. He claimed that women's blood was generally less pure than men's, hence they needed to expel it through menstruation. Reflecting on the Old Testament view of menstruation, he remarked that this impurity was not as God had made it, but rather was part of Eve's punishment for the Fall.[91] In ageing then, women must suffer again for the Fall: 'Old women are even often made sick by the cessation of their monthlies, even though they only stop at the time marked by nature', he remarked. The reason was that the menses were trapped inside them and the impurities of their blood were now unable to exit the body, the 'door closed by which they were accustomed to discharge'. These impurities must therefore extrude by other means, producing symptoms of discomfort elsewhere in the body, though Duncan claimed the most common ailments related to the belly, without detailing anything specific.[92]

Duncan's account provided a target for many later Parisian medical claims of overturning past religious views of menstruation which implied its cessation to be inherently pathological, though he was rarely correctly identified as the singular exceptional individual responsible for this view. Certainly though, purely iatrochemical accounts of menstruation were widely discredited within the Montpellier faculty after Théophile Bordeu (1722–1776), and references to the Bible were rarely found in medical works after the mid-eighteenth century. However, even Duncan's work had very little to say about any specific symptoms of the end of menses, or about its ending as a meaningful moment in the

[89] Daniel Duncan, *Seconde et troisième partie de la chimie naturelle, ou L'Explication chimique et mécanique de l'évacuation particulière aux femmes et de la génération* (Paris: L. d'Houry, 1687). See Evelyne Berriot-Salvadore, *Un corps, un destin: La Femme dans la médecine de la Renaissance* (Paris: Champion, 1993); Ruth Formanek, 'Continuity and Change and "the Change of Life": Premodern Views of the Menopause', in Formanek, *Meanings of Menopause*, n. 2:3–41; Patricia Crawford, 'Attitudes to Menstruation in Seventeenth-Century England', *Past & Present*, 91 (1981): 47–73.

[90] Stolberg, '"A Woman's Hell"?'

[91] Duncan, *Seconde et troisième partie de la chimie naturelle*, 4–8.

[92] Ibid., 182.

progression of women's ageing. And while he referenced the Pentateuch touchstone of menstruation as Eve's impure curse, generalising it to the experience of the end of menses, he also qualified what this meant for medical practice—explicitly rejecting the possibility of remedying or reversing the process by pharmacological or other interventions. The troubles of the end of menses, he claimed, only endured for a few years, after which the blood became accustomed to not being able to exit in its usual way and the fermentation which produced its impurities thereafter diminished.[93] He devoted the bulk of his discussion to matters of whether it was possible to resume the menses of an older woman with the use of blood-thinning medicaments, or by balancing the alkalinity of the blood: a snake, after all, was able to shed its skin. But he concluded that while volatile salts were sometimes able to resume suppressed menses, in the event that such occurred, it invariably meant that the suppression was not due to age but to some other cause. He insisted that once the menses had finally ceased, nothing could bring them back because the 'fermentation spirit' which animated them had been extinguished—only Jesus could return from the dead.[94] This combination of a lack of symptomology, the designation of older women's suffering as Eve's curse, and the dismissal of the idea of trying to stimulate the resumption of menses in ageing, amounted to a categorical denial of the final cessation of menses as a suitable object for medical treatment of any kind.

The matter of whether stoppages of menses in women of reproductive age were even abnormal or unhealthy was subject to a broad disagreement after the end of the seventeenth century, with those most focused on obstetrics (and therefore on fertility questions) tending towards the insistence that women should menstruate regularly to be fertile, while those more aware of comparative ethnography considered that regular menstruation was not necessarily a universal human norm. Some, like the renowned Parisian obstetrician François Mauriceau (1637–1709) considered that if a woman was not menstruating, she was not well, but he clearly was thinking about women of an age to become pregnant, not even considering if the principle would apply to women whose cessation of menses was due to age.[95] In his 1668 work on the diseases of pregnant women, Mauriceau, like his Montpellier contemporary Varanda, defined the term of menstruation and of women's reproductive capacity as ordinarily between the ages of 13 and 50 or 55 years.[96] Menstruation was 'a natural evacuation' to be expected in all women who were not pregnant and 'who were of an age to be able to become so'.[97] He described

[93] Ibid., 183. [94] Ibid., 184–190.

[95] François Mauriceau, *Aphorismes touchant la grossesse, l'accouchement, les maladies, et autres dispositions des femmes* (Paris: L. d'Houry, 1694), 14–16.

[96] François Mauriceau, *Des maladies des femmes grosses et accouchées, avec la véritable et bonne méthode de les bien aider dans leurs accouchements naturels, et les moyens de remédier à tous ceux qui sont contre nature, et aux indispositions des enfans nouveau-nés* (Paris: J. Hénault, 1668), 45.

[97] Ibid., 46.

a woman trader (*une marchande*) from the wooded quarter (*bois quarré*) of Paris, who had never borne children 'though she had strange passions for it', and who was still menstruating at the age of 50 when she developed an inflated belly (*le ventre enflé*) coinciding with suppression of her menses. This led her to believe for ten months that she was pregnant, of which several midwives reassured her. The error only became clear when the woman voided a large quantity of 'waters and some gases'.[98] This anecdote is intriguing in that served to mock libidinous older women as well as the authority and expertise of midwives, but it clearly evoked nothing resembling the later medicalisation of menopause. Even as late as 1754, the Paris military doctor Pierre Hurtaut, describing a version of the iatromechanical plethora model in his treatise on menstruation (which was translated from Latin into French by the Montpellier-trained English scholar Emmett), provided no mention of negative symptoms associated with the final cessation of menses.[99] Hurtaut said women menstruated up to the age of 52 years, stopping because the uterine vessels became less susceptible to pressure differentials caused by the atmosphere changes related to the lunar cycle.[100] Menstruation itself, on the other hand, caused headaches, apoplexy, mania, and epilepsy.[101] Hurtaut thought that menstrual suppression caused women pains in the back and heart that endured for as long as the period would normally last if it were present, as well as acute fevers, headaches, and general lassitude. But he said nothing of women who no longer menstruated at all due to age.[102]

Statements defining the age of natural cessation of menses without any associated symptomatology were also the pattern in major contemporaneous English works on the diseases of women: the 1696 treatise of the English physician John Pechey, on the *Diseases of Maids, Big-Bellied Women, Child-Bed Women, and Widows*, only briefly mentioned the disappearance of women's 'courses' on account of age, like others, viewing this as one of the exceptions to the rule that suppressed menses was generally a medical concern.[103] Pechey was a tremendous intermediary of different medical traditions from around the world, promoting botanical medicaments from South America, the Middle East, Africa, and India, but in none of his diverse prescriptions can we find anything specific for ageing women or the final cessation of menses.[104] As Wendy Churchill notes, while Pechey offered many remedies for the restoration of suppressed menses in young

[98] Ibid., 67–68.

[99] Pierre-Thomas-Nicolas Hurtaut, *Essais de médecine sur le flux menstruel et la curation des maladies de la tête, ou Par rapport à la première partie on donne une théorie nouvelle sur le flux périodique des femmes: & par rapport à la seconde, on propose un remède nouveau contre les maladies céphaliques*, trans. Robert Emett (Paris: J. B Despilly, Jac. Ch. Chardon & S. Severin, 1754).

[100] Ibid., xxii, xxxvii. [101] Ibid., xiii. [102] Ibid., 39, 47.

[103] John Pechey, *General Treatise on the Diseases of Maids, Big-Bellied Women, Child-Bed Women, and Widows* (1696), 24.

[104] John Pechey, *The Compleat Midwife's Practice Enlarged in the Most Weighty and High Concernments of the Birth of Man Containing a Perfect Directory or Rules for Midwives and Nurses* (London: J. Philips, J. Taylor & K. Bentley, 1698).

women, he recommended to older women only that they apply remedies in the event of developing gout, for which the solution (as for men) was regular phlebotomy and dietary restriction.[105] In contrast to the views of several other scholars in characterising seventeenth-century medical sources in several cultures as replete with views of 'menopause' as symptomatic, Churchill too finds early modern English sources to treat the age-related cessation of menses largely as a 'natural life stage for women', noting that medical practitioners were certainly aware of age as a factor that could explain loss of menses, but also mostly considered it to require no particular medical treatment.[106]

The Influence of the Halle School?

The first whispers of an important shift towards medicalisation of the age-related cessation of menses in women began in the first decades of the eighteenth century in Germany and Holland, where an important body of work integrating the plethora view of disease into the concept of climacteric ages occurred among doctoral candidates mostly at the University of Halle, and later too at Helmstadt and Leiden. In his 1704 work *De annorum climactericorum*, the Halle scholar Friederich Hoffmann considered the validity of the ancient view of climacteric ages in the lifespan which followed the movement of the planets.[107] He frankly doubted this was so, but he noted that there clearly were temporal consistencies in human bodies, all which corresponded to sex-specific experiences—citing the nine months of pregnancy, the pubertal development of girls around 14 years and the growth of men's beards around the age of 21.[108] He proposed that when men reached their seventh septenary, they would be challenged by 'violent forces of order' which if they survived, would resolve into an age of wisdom, strength, and excellence—an idea he thought implicit in a popular German verse about the decades of life: 'Fünffzig Jahre stille Stan' (fifty years standing steady). Women, on the other hand, around 49 simply became deficient in their capacity to reproduce as signalled by the cessation of menstruation, corresponding to 'a great turbulent disturbance in the movement of the blood'; thereafter was simply a descent into wrinkles, despair, and debility.[109] Medieval scholars before Hoffmann had similarly claimed that women aged faster and more poorly than men, as we saw, but here suddenly women's ageing was catastrophised specifically in relation to the cessation of menses.

[105] Wendy D. Churchill, *Female Patients in Early Modern Britain: Gender, Diagnosis and Treatment* (London & New York: Routledge, 2012), 114.

[106] Ibid., 113–115.

[107] Friedrich Hoffmann, *De annorum climactericorum rationali & medica explicatione. Opera Omnia Physico, Tomus Quintus* (Geneva: Fratres de Tournes, 1704).

[108] Ibid., 8–11. [109] Ibid., 15.

The other Halle luminary Georg Stahl (1659–1734) was also interested in the temporal matters of physiology. In his 1707 *Theoria medica vera* he discussed the critical days theory of Galen and Hippocrates, according to which the seventh day and fourteenth days of an illness were thought to be turning points, which Stahl credited with some validity.[110] He did not appear to engage with the astrological climacteric-age concept in the manner of Hoffmann but he nonetheless gave a temporal frame to women's generative capacity and menstruation of up to the seventh septenary (age 49), after which there would be plethora with copious haemorrhages and mental afflictions.[111] The reason for the significance of the forty-ninth year was not anything to do with the planets, though, which Stahl considered science had not satisfactorily demonstrated had any influence on human health, despite the persistence of popular beliefs of this kind.[112] Elsewhere in his magnum opus he took pains to reject the notion that the moon governed epileptic fits, describing such beliefs as vulgar, fantastical, and frankly embarrassing ('tanquam per somnium fabulari, non piget solum, sed pudet etiam').[113] He also expressed contempt for the mystical belief that menstruation corrupted women's bodies, which he related to the emotional perturbations women themselves experience during their periods, producing a tendency to attribute their distress to nefarious forces in their bodies.[114] Nonetheless, he appeared to take as self-evident that there would be illnesses associated with the suppression of menses in young women, because perturbations of any kind of change within the body produced disease states: any variation of a tranquil state resulted in disturbances of both the humours and of the mind.[115] Further in his 1711 work on women's fertility, Stahl proposed an iatromechanical explanation for the final cessation of menstruation in women, emphasising the weakened excretory and vital power of the uterus in the process of ageing, resulting in plethora, hysteria, and abdominal (*hypochondriacos*) pains.[116]

It was Stahl's student David Titius who appears to have been the first doctoral candidate in medicine instructed to write his entire dissertation on the cessation of menses in women both young and old, effectively sweeping up a new inclusion of age-related cessation of menses into the larger topic of menstrual suppression in younger women.[117] His 1710 dissertation entitled *Fine mensium initiis morborum variorum opportune* (The End of Menses Initiating Various Diseases) used the Latin word *fine* (suggesting something ended and not to return) rather than *cesantibus* (cessation or stoppage, suggesting something that could resume).

[110] Georg Ernst Stahl, *Theoria medica vera: Physiologiam & pathologiam* (Halle: Literis Orphanotrophei, 1707), 386.
[111] Ibid., 1099–1100. [112] Ibid., 900. [113] Ibid., 1344–1345.
[114] Ibid., 390–391. [115] Ibid., 1100.
[116] Georg Ernst Stahl, *De sterilitate foeminarum: Dissertatio inauguralis medica* (Halle: Henckel, 1711), 13–15.
[117] David Titius *De fine mensium initiis morborum variorum opportune: Dissertatio inauguralis medica* (Halle: Henckelii, 1710).

Nonetheless, while he included older women in his definition of menstrual plethora, he still focused largely on what later medical language would call amenorrhea—menstrual stoppage in women who might be expected to menstruate, rather than older women's menopause. He situated this topic in relation to the widely known practice of treating suppressed menses in young women as a gynaecological disorder, adding that while this was generally a good practice, there was one kind of stoppage of the menses that could not be avoided—that which occurred in ageing.[118] He leaned on the iatrochemical authorities Paracelsus and Van Helmont, as well as on Hippocrates,[119] referring to the plethora concept of suppressed menses in young women causing stagnant humours and congestion, and he described associated symptoms as arthritis, fevers and itching, hypochondria entailing shortness of breath, hiccups, abdominal pain, and digestive problems. He considered the symptoms to be worse the younger and more suddenly the menses ceased, and also described women engaging in sexual pleasures after the final cessation of menses as a sign of hysteria—a theme that was to become a topic of French alienist fascination after the mid-nineteenth century as we shall see in Chapter 7.[120] He recommended a variety of medicaments, to be used according to constitutional type, such as cinnamon, aloe, olive, sage, and balsamic pills, as well as clysters and vomiting, though he warned against the abuse of narcotics (opium).[121] This text, which several scholars have assumed to be primarily about menopause, did not in fact focus at length on older women. Rather, it is significant in illustrating how the medicalisation of the age-related cessation of menses first emerged as a subtopic from within the eighteenth-century medical theorisation of suppressed menses as a plethoric disorder.

Titius' dissertation represented an important connectionist juncture which implicitly drew two distinct intellectual traditions together for the first time in medical history, though both Stahl and Hoffmann had hinted at an emergent new model of sex-differentiated ageing around the same time.[122] Up until now, those evoking climacteric crises had rarely thought to wonder if these would be the same for women as for men, while those writing about the diseases of women who had begun to consider those over 50 as prone to plethora symptoms rarely made the larger claim about this as a crisis of ageing. The separate components were now in place for the assemblage of menopause, though there was still much to be fleshed out about how the cessation of menses constituted a climacteric or critical age. The theme hardly caught on fast though: it would be another twenty-seven years before the Dutch medical student Johann Regemann produced his

[118] Ibid., 5. [119] Ibid., 8, 22. [120] Ibid., 14–23. [121] Ibid., 32–33.

[122] Georg Ernst Stahl, *Theoria medica vera: Physiologiam & pathologiam* (Halle: Literis Orphanotrophei, 1707); Friedrich Hoffmann, *De annorum climactericorum rationali & medica explicatione. Opera Omnia Physico, Tomus Quintus* (Geneva: Fratres de Tournes, 1704).

thesis on the diseases of the cessation of menses at the University of Leiden in 1737, which also focused largely on women of reproductive age.[123]

By this time important French medical works discussing both the suppression of menses in women of reproductive age, and how it related to the natural cessation that occurred in ageing, had reached a new level of elaboration. The Montpellier-trained Paris professor of medicine Jean Astruc (1684–1766), in his six-volume 1737 *Traité des maladies des femmes*, reviewed all the existing major works relevant to the diseases of women produced in Latin, French, German, English, Italian, and Spanish, including those of John Leake, John Freind, Herman Boerhaave, Friederich Hoffmann, John Sydenham, Gerald Fitzgerald, François Mauriceau, Jean Varanda, Giovanni Marinello, Jean Liébault, Luis de Mercado, Ambroise Paré, Felix Platter, Jacob Rueff, the medieval Persian physician el-Rhazi, the medieval Trotula, as well as all the major ancient authors (Aristotle, Hippocrates, Galen, Soranus, Rufus, Pliny the Elder, and others), reflecting either explicitly or implicitly upon many of these differing accounts of menstruation and the questions of its suppression or absence. Astruc's work was published in six editions between 1737 and 1785 and was widely cited by many of the French doctors who later elaborated on the concept of menopause, who mostly found it frustratingly dismissive of the age-related cessation of menses as a matter of medical concern. Astruc was very much of the same generation as the first German scholars to describe the age-relation cessation as a new addendum to the description of menstrual suppression in young women, with its broad symptomatology of plethora. Astruc had completed his own doctoral dissertation in Latin at Montpellier in 1702, a *Tract on the Causes of Fermentative Movement, Containing a New Mechanical Hypothesis*, which like Stahl's work sought a synthesis of iatrochemical and iatromechanical principles.[124] He appears to have read many of the relevant doctoral dissertations from the Halle school, as indicated by the annotated bibliography he provided in the fourth volume of his 1737 *Traité des maladies des femmes*. Here, in referring to the dissertations relating to the disease of women over which Stahl had presided between 1702 and 1711, he said simply that Stahl's esteem obliged him to mention them, 'though I have no design to report upon any of them'.[125] It seems likely that, in so abruptly dismissing these dissertations, he was indicating his low estimation of them, despite their eminent supervisor, rather than that he simply had not inspected them, since elsewhere in

[123] Johann L. Regemann, *De morbis ex menstruis per aetatem cessantibus* (Leiden: Conrad Wishoff, 1737).

[124] Jean Astruc, *Tractatus de motus fermentativi causa, novam et mechanicam hypothesim continens* (Montpellier: H. Pech, 1702).

[125] Jean Astruc, *Traité des maladies des femmes* [1737], vol. 4 (Paris: P. Guillaume Cavelier, 1761), 318.

this bibliography he explicitly indicated when he knew of works only by their title but not by their contents.[126]

The fifth volume of Astruc's five-volume *Traité* is where he elaborated primarily on matters of menstruation and its absence, as well as the physiological causes of sterility—he counted thirteen of these, not including several incidental forms, including that which comes 'not from the husband but from the age of the woman'.[127] Astruc prescribed numerous emetic, emmenagogic, and purgative medications to treat suppressed menses and sterility in women of reproductive age, as well as an extract of horse testicle to stimulate fertility (Image 1.1)—an opotherapy practice remarkably prefiguring, by several hundred years, the later emergence of gonadal and hormone replacement treatments, appearing also in Jean de Renou's *Œuvres pharmaceutiques* of 1626 which listed a rooster's testicle extract used for this same purpose.[128] Despite such products being quite common in early modern apothecary lists, they do not ever seem to have been prescribed for health complaints of women after the final cessation of menses, as Astruc's mention of them indicates. He recommended blood-letting and the use of purgatives as treatments for suppressed menses, gastric complaints, abdominal pains, and cancers of the uterus in women under 55 years old, but for women after this age, he recommended reduced blood-letting and warned against the use of purgative medications.[129]

In the second volume of his massive treatise, Astruc briefly described how the menses comes to its natural end in ageing, generally between the ages of 45 and 50 years, sometimes by ending abruptly, but usually by becoming gradually lighter, sometimes disappearing periodically, then returning again, until eventually ceasing altogether. He said that in some women 'the periods cease without any incident, or with such light incident that it does not merit attention'. In some women the cessation 'attracts very strong, very vivid hysterical vapours'—pathologies about which Astruc generally wrote a great deal relative to younger women. In other women, the cessation produced dangerously large blood loss, while yet other women suffered white discharge that was 'difficult to cure'.[130] He emphasised the wide variability of different women's experiences of the final cessation of menses, which was in part explained by the different temperaments: sanguine and phlegmatic women had the easiest cessation of menses since theirs tended to dwindle over a period of between six months to two years, allowing a longer span of time for their bodies to adapt to the change; whereas melancholic

[126] Ibid., 302. [127] Astruc, *Traité des maladies des femmes*, vol. 5, 143.

[128] Ibid., 187; Jean de Renou, *Œuvres pharmaceutiques* [1626], 2nd ed. (Lyon: Nicholas Gay, 1637), 467.

[129] Jean Astruc, *Traité des maladies des femmes* [1737], 6 vols (Paris: P. Guillaume Cavelier, 1761), vol. 1, 63.

[130] Jean Astruc, *Traité des maladies des femmes* [1737] (Paris: P. Guillaume Cavelier, 1761), vol. 2, 299–301.

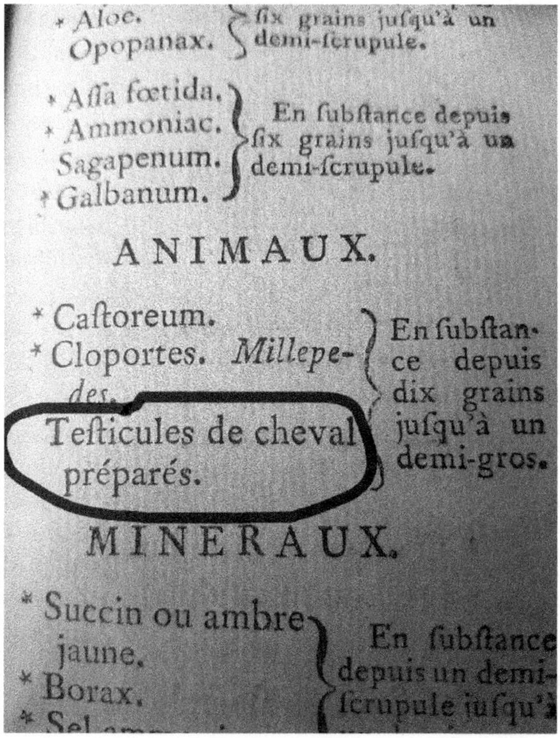

* Aloe.
Opopanax.
ſix grains juſqu'à un demi-ſcrupule.

* Aſſa fœtida.
* Ammoniac.
Sagapenum.
* Galbanum.
En ſubſtance depuis ſix grains juſqu'à un demi-ſcrupule.

ANIMAUX.

* Caſtoreum.
* Cloportes. *Millepedes.*
Teſticules de cheval préparés.
En ſubſtance depuis dix grains juſqu'à un demi-gros.

MINERAUX.

* Succin ou ambre jaune.
* Borax.
En ſubſtance depuis un demi-ſcrupule juſqu'à

Image 1.1 Text description of the dried horse testicles which Astruc prescribed as a pharmacological remedy for infertility in women in Jean Astruc, *Traité des maladies des femmes*, vol. 5 (Paris: P. Guillaume Cavelier, 1761–1765), 143.

and bilious women's menses tended to end abruptly, causing the body to become 'overwhelmed with an uncomfortable plethora' ('le corps se trouve surcharge d'une pléthore incommode'), characterised by headaches and suffocations.[131] Astruc here and in other parts of his six-volume work also warned (nearly sixty years before the much-cited 1774 pamphlet on this topic by the English physician John Fothergill) against the iatrogenic symptoms of the natural cessation of menses in ageing which sometimes occurred with the misuse of purgative and emmenagogic remedies that were appropriate only for the treatment of menstrual suppression during the reproductive years.[132] He noted that some women refused to accept the end of their menses and sought pharmacological intervention (purgatives and emmagogues) to resume them, resulting in uterine haemorrhages, white discharge, or even dangerous cancers and ulcers of the uterus.[133]

[131] Ibid., 305–307. [132] Ibid., 316.

[133] Astruc, *Traité des maladies des femmes*, vol. 1, 156. Discussed by both Annick Tillier, 'Un âge critique: La Ménopause sous le regard des médecins des XVIIIe et XIXe siècles', *CLIO: Femmes, genre,*

Astruc's limited interest in making the final cessation of menses into a specific topic of medical attention was consistent with his views about the expectation of regular menstruation during the reproductive years, based on intercultural comparison and on his ideas about the effects of civilisation on women's reproductive physiology. He took the claims of Jean de Léry about menstruation among South American women to imply that missing menstruation with resultant temporary sterility, contrary to medical convention, should not necessarily be seen as a sign of disease. He went as far as to suggest that the regular monthly cycles of menstruation experienced by women of the urban elites was a product of excess 'civilisation', which he placed in inverted commas to indicate his scepticism of the notion of superiority often ascribed to this this term:

> It is generally known that frugal living country women have fewer periods than those who live in abundance: Most travellers report that among savages, women barely menstruate, or do so very little.[134]

Astruc claimed that the example of the Tupinambá cited by Léry was reflected also in the experience of French peasant women who 'have continued to live in the primary simplicity of nature' ('ont continué de vivre dans la première simplicité de la nature'), whereas 'women of those nations one calls *civilised,* on the contrary, are subjected to abundant and laborious periods'.[135] He also cited here several 'natural' causes for the cessation of menses, which included during pregnancy, but also being older than 45 years of age.[136] Only in women under the age of 45, who were not pregnant, should the physician have any cause for concern about prolonged missing menses which might (but did not necessarily) indicate reduced fertility.[137]

German and Dutch scholars after Titius and Regemann appeared less interested in making the cessation of menses a specialist topic, and instead simply wove it into their general view of the problem—the cessation of menses in women was assimilated as just one (minor) example of the general plethora theory of ageing in both sexes, or as another example of the many ways women generally suffered hysteria during times of uterine change. Another Halle candidate, Alexander Hübner, a student of Michael Alberti, in his 1742 dissertation on second marriages in old men, elaborated in the first of these ways on the notion of the cessation of menses causing plethora.[138] Andreas-Elias Büchner too in his 1750 Halle

histoire, 21 (2005): 268–280 [274]; and more fully Joel Wilbush, 'Menorraghia and Menopause: A Historical Review', *Maturitas*, 10 (1988): 5–26.

134 Astruc, *Traité des maladies des femmes*, vol. 5, 85. 135 Ibid., 85. 136 Ibid., 126.

137 Astruc, *Traité des maladies des femmes*, vol. 2, 300.

138 Alexander Johann August Hübner, *Dissertatio inauguralis medica, de nuptiis senum secundis raro secundis* (Halae Magdeburgicae: Joannis Christiani Hendelii, 1742), 12.

dissertation proposed that women around the 50th year who had ceased menstruating were prone to plethora, with all its attendant problems. However, his work was not specifically about this age group who are only mentioned briefly in a single short section of the dissertation.[139]

While plethora was attributed to ageing in general, it was also associated with stoppages of the menses in women at any age. Christoph Heumann in 1776 appeared to focus on the question again with his Helmstadt dissertation, which referred to diseases of the 'cessation of menses'.[140] The Latin word *cessantibus*, it should be noted, did not necessarily imply permanence and was the same word used to refer to temporary stoppages of menstruation in young women. Heumann's thesis, despite appearances, was not specifically about the final cessation of menses in older women, but like most other medical works on women's reproductive health up until this time, it too was largely about the various reasons for its suppression in women who might be expected to menstruate. However, several pages were here devoted to the question of women around the 50th year, who had ceased menstruating for several months: Heumann claimed that sometimes these women had plethora (as did young women with suppressed menses about whom most of his thesis was focused), as indicated if they reported gout, uterine haemorrhages, haemorrhoids, or being more sensitive of spirit and tense in their bodies ('et quae sensibiliorus animi et tenerioris corporis texturae sunt').[141] Replicating the idea that had by the 1750s also emerged in French medical scholarship, according to which exercise made the final cessation of menses less troublesome, Heumann also distinguished between the ageing of women according to their activity levels social class, and moral virtues—hysteria occurred more often in women who lived lazy and luxurious lives, whereas it rarely happened to rugged and simple women who moved their bodies vigorously ('Foeminae laboriosae simplicique vitae utentes, et corpus congrue moventes, rariori casu illos experiuntur').[142] Also like the French scholars, he claimed that women became more masculine after the cessation of menses, just as men became less so, and likened this convergence of the sexes to the state of androgyny in children ('uterque enim sexus, in senectute decrepita, easdem experitur infirmitates, et eandem similemque, ut ita dicam, hanc secundam infantiam agit, ac primam').[143] Another German thesis from 1796 in Latin from the University of Göttigen, which also might be expected to talk about the final cessation of menses, that of Ludwig Nieymeyer focused entirely on women of menstruating age,

[139] Andreas-Elias Büchner, *De plethora senum ejusque rationali therapeutica tractatione per venaesectionem speciatim suscipienda* (Halae Magdeburgicae: Joannis Christiani Hendelii, 1750), 22.

[140] Christophorus-Augustus-Franciscus Heumann, *Dissertatio medica solemnis de cessante, ob aetatem, mensium fluxu et morbis inde oriundis* (Helmstadii: Schnorrii, 1776).

[141] Ibid., 31. [142] Ibid., 35. [143] Ibid., 37.

using the term *fine* in relation to the 'final purpose' of menstruation, not to its end.[144]

Astruc's renowned 1737 French work on the diseases of women was translated into German in 1768 (and had already been translated into English in 1743), suggesting where Heumann writing in 1776 might have borrowed some of his constitution-specific ideas about managing the final cessation of menses, which extended beyond those of his German (Latin-writing) predecessors.[145] Notably, none of the first specialist French-language works of scholarship on the final cessation of menses, nor even the less specialist French works of this time appear to have engaged with the Halle Latin theses on menstrual stoppage with their new inclusion of older women: aside from Astruc's grudging acknowledgement of some of them in his 1737 bibliography, not a single citation can be found either to Titius, Regemann, Hübner, Büchner, or Heumann, in any of the later French specialist works. There was though a general alignment to broader vitalist and mechanical principles derived from the work of Stahl, Boerhaave, and Hoffmann, among the Montpellier scholars writing at the end of the eighteenth century. So, while the French may not have been the very first ever to identify the final cessation of menses as a topic of medical concern, they were most certainly the first to make it a substantive specialised topic. They possibly did borrow directly from the Latin works of the earlier and contemporary doctoral candidates since these all, to varying degrees, conflated menstrual stoppage with the final cessation of menses, if they talked about the latter at all. The Montpellier vitalist tradition certainly owed much to Stahl's reconfigurations of chemical and mechanical dimensions of the vital force, as well as to the general Halle emphasis on differentiating patients according to age, sex, temperament, activity levels, and other variables.

Midwives and Accoucheurs

By the mid-eighteenth century there was also now a whole other genre of medical writing about women's reproductive health which, as Susan Matterns notes, had frankly nothing to say about the final cessation of menses in older women: midwifery manuals and herbal remedy manuals on women's health written by women.[146] One of the most widely read early modern French works of folk medicine, Marie Fouquet's *Recueil des remèdes faciles et domestiques* of 1685, contained a whole chapter on women's diseases which drew on Fouquet's experience of

[144] Ludwig Heinrich Christian Niemeyer, *De menstruationis fine et usu*. Dissertation (Göttingen: Dieterich, 1796).

[145] Jean Astruc, *Theoretisch-practische Abhandlung von den Frauenzimmer-Krankheiten*, 2 vols (Dresden: Walther, 1768). Jean Astruc, *A treatise on all the diseases incident to women*, trans. J.R. (London: T. Cooper, 1743).

[146] Matterns, *The Slow Moon Climbs*, 270–271.

directing several Paris maternity hospitals in the late seventeenth century.[147] The chapter covered matters relating to childbirth, pregnancy, lactation, breast-care, uterine diseases, as well as suppressed, excessive, or painful menstruation, but had nothing to say about the final cessation of menses in older women.[148] Matterns speculates that menopause may even have become a topic of masculine medical description precisely because it was not already treated by midwives and folk healers.[149] In Chapter 6, we will return to this intriguing question in consideration of how French menopause writers situated their relationship both to folk medical traditions, and to ancient medical custom. Rosalyn Frank describes the seventeenth century as a 'watershed moment for midwives in the city of London', describing the transition from midwifery as a women's space of knowledge to one in which male doctors became increasingly present, and where the transcription of medical knowledge both from specific individuals and from different cultures often occurred without acknowledgement.[150] The historical processes of masculinisation and professionalisation of women's medicine are well described also by both Monica Green and Nathalie Sage-Pranchère.[151] The gender historian Patricia Crawford's study of the sixty-six advertisements of women medical practitioners in London between 1670 and 1710 identified proposed treatments for various menstrual disorders, suppressed menses and infertility, but noted nothing referring to the end of menses in ageing.[152] From the end of the seventeenth century, numerous midwifery works in English had appeared such as Elizabeth Grey's 1653 *Choice Manual*, Jane Sharp's 1671 *Whole Art of Midwifery Discovered*, Sarah Stone's 1737 *Complete Practice of Midwifery*, various anonymous works such as the 1682 *English Midwife Enlarged* and the 1684 *Aristotle's Masterpiece*.[153] There were also numerous works authored by doctors in France, Switzerland, and England who had worked with midwives and recorded their practices, such as the Swiss physician Jacob Rueff's Latin 1554 *De conceptu et generatione hominis*, translated into English as *The Expert Midwife* in 1637, the 1665 *Compleat Midwife's Practice Enlarged* (attributed to Peter Chamberlaine), John Pechey's 1698 *Compleat Midwife's Practice*, and the French doctor Pierre Dionis's 1718

[147] Marie Fouquet, *Recueil des remèdes faciles et domestiques*, 5th ed. (Dijon: Jean Ressayre, 1704); Michel Vernus, *Médecine populaire en Franche-Comté: Petites et grandes histoires des faiseurs de secrets et autres rebouteux* (Pontarlier: Éditions du Belvédère, 2013), 28, 81.

[148] Fouquet, *Recueil des remèdes*, 137–151. [149] Matterns, *The Slow Moon Climbs*, 277.

[150] Rosalyn M. Frank, *The Hidden Face of a Midwifery Treatise from 17th Century England: The Chamberlen Family, Dr. Peter Chamberlen and the Contributions of Huarte de San Juan to The Compleat Midwife's Practice Enlarged* (Creative Common: Roslyn M. Frank, 2016), 3.

[151] Monica H. Green, *Making Women's Medicine Masculine: The Rise of Male Authority in Pre-Modern Gynaecology* (Oxford: Oxford University Press, 2008); Nathalie Sage Pranchère, *L'École des sages-femmes: Naissance d'un corps professionnel 1786–1917* (Tours: Presses universitaires, 2017).

[152] Patricia Crawford, 'Printed Advertisements for Women Medical Practitioners in London, 1670–1710', *Journal for the Social History of Medicine Bulletin*, 35 (1984): 66–70.

[153] Anon., *Aristotle's Masterpiece, or the Secrets of Generations Display'd in all the Parts thereof* [1684] (London: no publisher, 1704).

Traité général des accouchements, translated almost immediately into English as *A General Treatise of Midwifery*.[154] Jean Astruc had authored such a work too, *L'Art d'accoucher*, published in 1766, which was also translated into English the following year.[155] The Paris faculty surgeon-anatomist Pierre Dionis's treatment of the matter of the duration of menses was typical of this entire genre: he simply stated that menstruation began around the age of 14 and ended around the age of 50, from which time women could no longer conceive, with nothing more to be noted about it.[156] But if we were to overlook this clear normalising statement and instead only read the passages in Dionis's work referring to the need for blood-letting to stimulate suppressed menses in women who might be expected to menstruate, it would be easy to assume that Dionis was pathologising menopause. Instead, he was prescribing treatments for what later medicine would call amenorrhea.[157] Dionis did though have other reflections about the diseases of ageing women, as we will consider in Chapter 2. None of the midwifery works surveyed here described the cessation of menses in ageing as a specific era of symptoms, while they all acknowledged that menses ended definitively at a certain time of life. If a view resembling the nineteenth-century concept of symptomatic menopause complex was culturally prevalent from the late sixteenth to mid-eighteenth centuries, one would expect to see at least some mention of it in this substantial corpus of midwife-authored and informed works dealing specifically with women's reproductive health.

Menopause was not innocently 'discovered' by sympathetic doctors finally paying attention to the universal, biologically determined complaints of older women as some scholars have suggested,[158] rather it was a product of the convergence of several new and old medical concepts integrated and propelled by men who were university-trained scholars, engaged in a historically self-conscious pursuit of the newly defined specialisms of hygiene, gynaecology and alienism in the broader context of the emergence of modern biomedical iatromechanical and iatrochemical theories. It was not (*pace* Thomas Laqueur), that doctors were only now discovering women's difference from men at every level of biology: numerous

[154] Jakob Ruf, *De Conceptu et generatione hominis, de matrice et ejus partibus, nec non de conditione infantis in utero et gravidarum cura et officio* (Frankfurt: Tiguri, 1554); Jakob Rüff, *The Expert Midwife, or An excellent and most necessary treatise of the generation and birth of man Wherein is contained many very notable and necessary particulars requisite to be knovvne and practised* (London: S. Burton, 1637); *Dr. Chamberlain's Midwife's Practice: Or, a Guide for Women in that high Concern of Conception, Breeding, and Nursing Children* (London: J. Clowes, 1665); Pechey, *The Compleat Midwife's Practice*; Pierre Dionis, *Traité général des accouchements, qui instruit de tout ce qu'il faut faire pour être habile accoucheur* (Paris: C.-M. d'Houry, 1718); Pierre Dionis, *A General Treatise of Midwifery* (London: A. Bell, 1719).

[155] Jean Astruc, *L'Art d'accoucher réduit à ses principes, où l'on expose les pratiques les plus sûres & les plus usitées dans les différentes espèces d'accouchement* (Paris: P. Guillaume Cavelier, 1766); Jean Astruc, *The Art of Midwifery Reduced to Principles* (London: J. Nourse 1767).

[156] Dionis, *Traité général des accouchements*, 60.

[157] Ibid., 350–351.

[158] Grace E. Kohn, Katherine M. Rodriguez, & Alexander W. Pastuszuk, 'The History of Estrogen Therapy', *Sexual Medicine Review*, 7/3 (2019): 416–421.

historians have established that sexual difference was indeed considered by anatomists and physicians at multiple levels throughout the early modern period.[159] But sex differences in ageing most certainly were radically revised at the close of the eighteenth century, as evidenced by the lack of the sex-specific concept of 'menopause' syndrome, either in name or in distinct conceptual form prior to this time, and by the counter-evidence of a vast corpus of early modern medical works which clearly reflected upon the end of menses in women only to naturalise it as a matter beyond the scope of medical concern.

By the close of the eighteenth century, the works on women's health, both in French and in English, in the genre of midwifery manuals were also clearly known to medical scholars in the major universities. None of these manuals discussed anything like a symptomatic crisis associated with the cessation of menses—an important lacuna which is not addressed at all by those scholars who insist that menopause symptoms were prevalent in early modern medicine. In the nineteenth century too, we will find women-authored works of medicine, which similarly had nothing much to say about women's ageing or the cessation of their menses. Midwifery, admittedly, was a knowledge system concerned primarily with childbirth which might understandably have considered matters of post-reproductive physiology to be beyond its remit. However, reading early modern medical sources through the lens of midwifery holds merit too in reminding us just how much almost all medical specialists writing about women between 1585 and 1750 were distracted by the overwhelming dangers both to women and to their infants which childbearing entailed at this time in history. The menses eventually ending definitively—and most scholars appear to have realised that they must—and the temporary discomforts of this experienced by some elite women (sometimes), must surely have seemed a rather trivial matter in comparison.

It would be easy to produce a short scholarly account of ubiquitous early modern 'menopause' symptomatology by carefully selecting the uncommon sources which briefly described symptoms associated with older women's plethora (common in men as well in younger women), alongside citations from the other far more extensive corpus that merely described suppressed menses in women of reproductive age, with only scant reference to older women. However, there is reason to doubt how much ideas about menstrual suppression were generally extended to the treatment of women approaching the end of their reproductive eras. Numerous important medical works concerning the diseases of women in Latin, French, German, and English published between 1585 and 1750 had frankly nothing to say about secondary effects on women's bodies of the final cessation of menstruation. This was true both in general works of medicine which

[159] Laqueur, *Making Sex*; King, *Midwifery, Obstetrics and the Rise of Gynaecology*; Green, *Making Women's Medicine Masculine*; King, *The One-Sex Body on Trial*; Stolberg, 'Menstruation and Sexual Difference'; Stolberg, 'A Woman Down to her Bones'; McClive, *Menstruation and Procreation*, 5–6.

contained chapters on the reproductive matters, as well as in large and detailed specialist works on the reproductive physiology of women, which from the late sixteenth century became a substantial genre of medical scholarship. Early modern physicians, for the most part, simply did not consider the end of menses a matter of medical concern at all and rather seemed to consider it important that it be understood as an exception to their recommend treatments designed for menstrual suppression in young women. Those who in the late eighteenth century began to apply the notion of a 'critical time' or 'climacteric' to the phenomena of older women's plethora may have provided targets for nineteenth-century postures of decrying traditional myths and championing the modern scientific definition of menopause, as we consider in Chapter 6. Nonetheless, the unique nineteenth-century French fascination with menopause should not be read back onto all earlier medical descriptions of menstrual stoppage.

2

Women's Life Expectancy, Cancer, and the Cessation of Menses

The final cessation of menses as a deadly time for women was one of the most important ideas which French doctors explicitly and repeatedly challenged throughout the nineteenth century. They challenged it in two ways: firstly, by rejecting the supposedly common view that menstrual blood in older women was retained, becoming toxic—an erroneous idea which they attributed variously to the ancients, the Arabs, or to their more recent medical predecessors. From the repetitive nature of these nineteenth-century challenges, it would be reasonable to presume that earlier medicine must itself have widely displayed this toxic view of the final cessation of menses. In fact, this view was very rare in early modern medicine, which more often naturalised this moment in women's lives as not requiring medical attention at all. The other way nineteenth-century doctors evoked an image of themselves as correctors of past medical error in the understanding of menopause was by pointing to new demographic data indicating greater numbers of women surviving into the older age groups. These mortality and morbidity correctives and the purpose they served in the nineteenth-century medicalisation of menopause form the focus of the current chapter. Menopause was not ever widely considered to be a particularly dangerous time for women before the nineteenth century. But as in the notion of toxic blood accumulation, the notion of women's higher mortality around the cessation of menses was most often invoked in order to offer doctors the opportunity to debunk it as a myth that marked their professional identity as moderns, bearing a new bioscientific approach to women's health.

It might be expected that the demographic statistical evidence of women's relative longevity that emerged in seventeenth- and eighteenth-century European science might constrain the rampant medicalisation of women's ageing in modern biomedicine. Daniel Schäfer has suggested a tension did occur in the emergence of biomedical ideas about old age.[1] Certainly, several French demographers we will discuss in this chapter, like Antoine Deparcieux in 1746, Louis-François Benoiston de Châteauneuf in 1818, and Louis Noirot in 1850, explicitly argued

[1] Daniel Schäfer, *Old Age and Disease in Early Modern Medicine*, trans. Patrick Baker (London: Routledge, 2015), 186–187.

The French Invention of Menopause and the Medicalisation of Women's Ageing: A History. Alison M. Downham Moore, Oxford University Press. DOI: 10.1093/oso/9780192842916.003.0003

that the rejection of the medicalisation of the final cessation of menses was a natural conclusion to draw from the mortality data they presented: women in the over 40 or 50 years were not more fragile as evidenced by their greater rates of survival into old age, so there was no need to consider the cessation of menses to be a 'critical time' requiring special medical care.[2] But the view of the cessation of menses as a dangerous time not only provided an important target for doctors' postures of debunking supposedly traditional myths, it also served as a pedagogic case example for the induction of doctoral candidates at the Montpellier, Paris, and Strasbourg faculties into the bioscientific view of women's diseases and of ageing. In these contexts, it helped to justify the inclusion of older women in the emerging specialist fields of hygiene, gynaecology and psychiatry after the 1840s—a theme that is considered throughout this book. It thus helped not only to produce the bifurcation of women's diseases from men's, but indeed also the cleaving of ageing morbidity from mortality.

In the vitalist tradition, exemplified by Georg Stahl and his French followers, the essence of life was presumed to preserve the body both from disease and from death, but the emergence of mortality data showing women living longer than men created a modification of this towards the separation of health and longevity. Vitalists were fascinated by ageing and its many diseases for what it indicated about the waning of the life essence throughout the lifespan but they also viewed women's entire physiology as sicker than men's. Elizabeth Williams describes the 'systematic doctrine of sex differences' to which many vitalist thinkers following Roussel subscribed, in which women's sexual and child-rearing roles were seen as the 'only activities consonant with the character of the female vital force'.[3] Because reproduction was seen as an expression of the vital essence, women's loss of capacity to menstruate and conceive was taken to indicate the beginning of their ageing decline. Because women's physiology and social roles were seen as defined by their sexual, reproductive, and child-rearing roles, the fact of ceasing to menstruate necessarily marked a new life stage for women—one of morbidity, lost purpose, and reduced vitality, though not sufficient to shorten their expected lifespan. The discovery of women's greater longevity, though often posited as a contradiction to the view of menopause as a 'critical age', in fact was accommodated within a medical system which richly pathologised women's ageing as a pedagogic example of the non-equivalence of morbidity with mortality. Rather

[2] Antoine Deparcieux, *Essai sur les probabilités de la durée de la vie humaine, d'où l'on déduit la manière de déterminer les rentes viagères, tant simples qu'en Tontines* (Paris: Frères Guerin, 1746), 83; Louis-François Benoiston de Châteauneuf, *Mémoire sur la mortalité des femmes de l'âge de quarante à cinquante ans, lu à l'Académie des Sciences, dans la séance du 13 mai 1818* (Paris: Martinet, 1822), 2–3.

[3] Elizabeth A. Williams, *A Cultural History of Medical Vitalism in Enlightenment Montpellier* (London: Routledge, 2003), 215–229.

than constraining the medicalisation of menopause, the new demographic fact, as it became assimilated into nineteenth-century French medicine, provided a platform for the elaboration of a unique 'hygiene' of menopause, described in Chapter 5.

In the previous chapter we considered numerous single sentences and short passages about the final cessation of menses in early modern medical texts, some claiming it was a time of illness, though most simply stating that it was a natural process that required no medical care. As we saw, the few negative claims about the final cessation were generally embedded within a much larger concern about the negative effects of suppressed menses in younger women, which was understood to compromise fertility, or were part of the description of sanguine plethora which was understood as a disease of women of all ages and of all older people. But there was another, albeit rare, negative view we have not hitherto considered which played a role in the medical debates throughout the eighteenth century about women's mortality and menopause: this was the recognition of women's increased susceptibility to cancers of the breast, uterus, and ovaries with ageing, which was sometimes attributed to both the temporary stoppage of menses in young women as well as its final cessation in older women. We begin this chapter by considering how prevalent medical claims about the cessation of menses causing cancer in fact were between 1650 and 1800, and how frequently such cancers were associated with women's mortality in the ages between 40 and 50 years. While claims of this kind were rare and by no means representative of either seventeenth- or eighteenth-century medical views of women's mortality, their occasional appearance provided a target for the demographic revolution that reshaped French medical views of women's health and of the diseases of ageing at the turn of the nineteenth century.

By the middle of the eighteenth century, the view of the cessation of menses as a particularly dangerous time had been shown to be false by a significant European-wide demographic statistical innovation around this same time: the counting of sex-differentiated deaths in every age band, which indicated much higher numbers of women than men surviving into all the age bands over 35 years. And yet, in precisely the period when this medical fact became assimilated as a matter of broad medical consensus (between 1775 and 1850), there was also a massive spike in the production of doctoral theses focused on the symptoms and hygiene of menopause or the 'critical age', and the production of the first book-length descriptions of this time in women's lives written by mature clinicians. In fact, the recognition of women's greater longevity did not constrain the rampant medicalisation of women's ageing at all, but rather was woven into the very fabric of its discursive elaboration where it helped to cohere doctors' professional identities and the pedagogic appeal of scientific biomedicine, particularly at the University of Paris.

Cancers of the Breast, Ovaries, and Uterus in the Critical Age of Women, 1650–1850

As we saw in the previous chapter, the Paris obstetrician François Mauriceau in his renowned 1668 book had described in great detail numerous diseases resulting from the suppression of menses, without mentioning whether these applied to women after the final cessation. Importantly, Mauriceau's work barely mentioned the age-related cessation of menses specifically and when he did mention it, it was also to naturalise the process in a work that was predominantly focused on the health of childbearing women. But in one sentence, in his 1694 book of aphorisms, he also claimed that more women died around the age of 45–50 years from cancers they developed because they were no longer benefiting from the healthful effects of menstruation.[4] In another aphorism, he showed why he held this assumption: women who had ceased menstruating due to age were more prone to cancerous ulcers than at other times of life.[5] The same belief is held in broad consensus in current oncological research of the twenty-first century which has found increasing cancer risks of many kinds in all kinds of bodies in every age band over 45 years. What Mauriceau lacked, unlike later scholars beginning the mid-eighteenth century, was access to demographic data indicating how little this threat endangered the majority of older women's lives around the time of the cessation of menses. Some scholars have cited Mauriceau as the ur-example of a ubiquitous early modern pathological view of menopause,[6] but it was actually a very rare claim in the scholarship on the diseases of women and one which Mauriceau himself did not elaborate. The simple claim that the cessation of menses was the indirect cause of more women's deaths than anything else was thereafter rarely repeated by scholars writing about the diseases of women, though a handful of other scholars between 1700 and 1800 referred to the increased risk of female-specific cancers with ageing.

The Paris surgeon Pierre Dionis (1643–1718), the royal surgeon to Louis XIV, described the principal internal cause of breast cancer as a 'vice' of the serum part of the blood, which became acidic and coagulated to form an obstruction of the glands, creating a tumour. He claimed that of the twenty women he had treated with breast cancer, fifteen were aged between 40 and 50 years, around the time of their natural cessation of menses, and that it was a common disease among nuns.[7] He said that in his travels with the French monarchs to other Europe cities, he

[4] François Mauriceau, *Aphorismes touchant la grossesse, l'accouchement, les maladies, et autres dispositions des femmes* (Paris: L. d'Houry, 1694), 18.

[5] Ibid., 114.

[6] Cathy McClive, *Menstruation and Procreation in Early-Modern France* (London/New York: Routledge, 2015), 296.

[7] Pierre Dionis, *Cours d'opérations de chirurgie démontrées au Jardin royal* (Paris: Laurent d'Houry, 1714), 385.

had observed that women with this disease were almost always either old enough to have ceased menstruating, or, if younger, suffered irregular menstruation, which he said confirmed the 'relation' between the breast and the uterus.[8] But he did not propose a specific hypothesis of how the fact of not menstruating or bearing children might influence the breasts to become cancerous, and he clearly included younger women who failed to menstruate among those at risk.

Again in 1742, the *Treatise of Surgical Operations* by the Paris royal surgeon and head of the Charité hospital Henri-François Le Dran (1685–1770) said that one particular type of breast cancer—those which grew slowly, were barely visible, and caused no pain—occurred 'more often in very fat women when their periods have stopped by the time marked by nature'.[9] He thought that uterine cancers were more common in women who had heavy periods, and that they usually occurred when the menses diminished or once they had definitely ended.[10] He said that hard cancerous tumours (*squirres*) formed as a result of the suppression of a habitual evacuation, either haemorrhoidal bleeding or menstruation, here including both young women whose periods were missing and those whose menses had definitively ceased. This was a result of the 'slow or rapid deposit of some vicious humour' that was indicated by symptoms such as migraines, haemorrhages, rheumatic pains, and sweats. Such tumours could only be cured by extirpation of the uterus—a procedure that was often fatal in this era before aseptic techniques and anaesthetics.[11] Le Dran did not claim that women in general were more likely to die following the cessation of menses, nor that such cancers were a major cause of death in older women, nor even that all women's cancers were deadly. Nonetheless, one medical historian has attributed to him the view which he claims was common in the eighteenth century, that 'menopause' (a term which did not even exist at this time) was responsible for breast cancer, citing a work by Le Dran which says nothing of the sort and instead merely describes the qualities of different breast tumours and their treatments.[12] It is surely not a deliberate misattribution, but many unsuspecting medical historians have fallen into the trap of reading current medical models back onto the eighteenth century. The medical concept of increased female-specific cancer risk after menopause is so prevalent in our own time (ever since the mid-twentieth century) that many historians are now unable to imagine that this concept was quite unusual in eighteenth-century and nineteenth-century medicine, and so overemphasise the

[8] Ibid., 383–384.

[9] Henri-François Le Dran, *Traité des opérations de chirurgie* (Paris: Charles Osmont, 1742), 384.

[10] Ibid., 386. [11] Ibid., 388.

[12] Daniel De Moulin, *A Short History of Breast Cancer* (Leiden: Martinus Nijhoff, 1983), 44–46; Henri François Le Dran, 'Du cancer des mamelles', in *Encyclopédie ou dictionnaire universel raisonné des connoisances humaines*, ed. Fortunato Bartolomeo De Felice, 57 vols (Yverdon, 1770–1780), vol. 27, 314–316.

magnitude and generalisability of the short remarks rarely to be found in these earlier historical times.

Jean Goulin's 1771 book on women's health evoked the idea of the time after menstruation as both happier for women since they no longer suffered the ill effects of the menses and it was when their character made them the most valuable to society, though it was a more dangerous time for their health, exclaiming, 'No pleasure without pain!' ('Point de plaisir sans peine!').[13] For this reason, he claimed, women needed more medical attention as they aged, counselling 'precautions that can only be known by consulting an enlightened physician.'[14] But this claim in favour of the medicalisation of women's ageing was still vastly different from those forms emerging in the first half of the nineteenth century with reference to the splitting of morbidity and mortality. For Goulin, the propensity towards illness among older women was also the very same source of danger to their lives. The convergence of medical scholarship on the diseases of women with the demographic discovery of women's greater longevity was not yet in place, though French statisticians themselves had already begun to suggest it.

The Demographic Discovery of Women's Longevity

The investigation of how women's greater longevity came to be discovered and assimilated into nineteenth-century French medical thought helps to explain an apparent paradox in ideas about menopause: it was 'not a disease' and yet required elaborate hygienic management. In offering their anti-pathological insistences about menopause, nineteenth-century French doctors placed great emphasis on what they claimed was a newly recognised fact throughout Europe of women far outnumbering men in all the age groups beyond 35 years. Eighteenth-and nineteenth-century demographic surveys had apparently revealed that not only were women not more vulnerable to disease after menopause but they were in fact far less likely than men to die around the age of 50. It was on these grounds that doctors insisted there was no need to consider the end of menses as a disease risk. Nonetheless, they went to considerable effort to assimilate women's ageing (but rarely men's) into the scope of *hygiène—t*hat peculiar nineteenth-century construct that entailed both a wide spectrum of corporeal and behavioural self-management techniques along with regular visits to the physician.

Eighteenth-century European states were converging on the need to centralise birth, death, and marriage records, despite the risks this posed of making known to other states the number of possible military conscripts in the nation.

[13] Jean Goulin & Anselme L. B. Bréchillet Jourdain, *Le Médecin des dames, ou l'art de les conserver en santé* (Paris: Chez Vincent, 1771), 110.

[14] Ibid., 111.

The Swedish decree of 1736 was the earliest of such policies, resulting in the first comprehensive population data gathered by the vicar, astronomer, and mathematician Pehr Wilhelm Wargentin (1717–1783) and published in 1766.[15] However, diverse attempts to calculate population appeared from the late seventeenth century, and the English physician John Graunt is widely considered the first scholar to have published a scientific work on mortality in 1662.[16] But Gaunt lacked sufficient empirical data to account for sex differentiation in each age, relying on generalising assumptions about the percentages of each group relative to others.[17] The English mathematician and astronomer Edmond Halley's attempts to define life expectancy based on birth and death records in the Hapsburg town of Breslau in 1683 were of a similar character. They came about on the urging of the German polymath philosopher Gottfried Leibniz, who recommended him as a collaborator to the Lutheran theologian and scholar Caspar Neumann, who was the author of an unpublished study of births and deaths in the population of Breslau. The result was Halley's 1683 tables using Neumann's data, which differentiated Breslau mortality according to different ages, but not in relation to the sexes separately.[18] Halley's consideration of the sexes as a single group for the purposes of determining mortality risk was not a product of lacking sex-differentiated data, since Neumann had indeed recorded deaths by sex as well as age. But he appears to have assumed that men constituted 'at least half' of the total population at all ages, without checking to see if this was indeed so, most likely on the assumption that women's deaths in childbirth rendered them the smaller proportion of adults.[19]

Next the Dutch demographer Willem Kersseboom (1691–1771) studied mortality in West Friesland in 1738.[20] But crucially, Kersseboom differentiated his subjects by sex.[21] This simple detail made Kersseboom's study one of the most

[15] Pehr Wilhelm Wargentin, 'Mortalitaten i Sverige, i anledning af Tabell-Verket', *Kongl. Vetenskaps-academiens Handlingar*, 27 (1766): 1–25.

[16] John Graunt & William Petty, *Natural and Political Observations Mentioned in a Following Index, and Made Upon the Bills of Mortality* (London: John Martin, James Allestry, and Tho. Dicas, 1662).

[17] Andrea A. Rusnock, *Vital Accounts: Quantifying Health and Population in Eighteenth-Century England and France* (Cambridge: Cambridge University Press, 2002), 33.

[18] Edmond Halley, 'An Estimate of the Degrees of the Mortality of Mankind, Drawn from the Curious Tables of the Births and Funerals of the City of Breslaw, with an Attempt to Ascertain the Price of Annuities Upon Lives', *Philosophical Transactions*, 17 (1693): 596–610; Jean-Marc Rohrbasser & Jacques Véron, *Leibniz et les raisonnements sur la vie humaine* (Paris: Institut National d'Études Démographiques, 2001), 2–3.

[19] Halley, 'An Estimate of the Degrees of the Mortality of Mankind', 601.

[20] Willem Kersseboom, *Proeven van politique rekenkunde, vervat in drie verhandelingen over de meenigte des volks in de provintie van Hollandt en Westvrieslandt; de probable leeftyt der weduwen, de duurzaamheid der huwelyken, de relatie van de meenigte des volks tegen het getal der geborene, en dat der gehuwde paaren &c. als meede over de waardye van lyfrente in proportie van losrente: waarby gevoegt zyn eenige aanmerkingen op de gissingen over den staat van het menschelyk geslacht &c. begrepen in zeekere inleiding tot de algemeene geographie* (Gravenhage: Jan van den Bergh, 1738).

[21] Ida H. Stamhuis, *Cijfers en Aequaties en Kennis der Staatskrachten. Statistiek in Nederland in de negentiende eeuw* (Amsterdam: Rodopi, 1989), 36.

widely cited in French works on mortality from the 1760s onwards.[22] He found that more women than men died in the age band of 16–27 years, confirming suspicions that childbirth impacted women's mortality more than any other variable.[23] But he also noticed that men's survival advantage diminished throughout the older ages, and that in the oldest ages women appeared to live three or four years longer than men.[24] He also referred to an unfinished 1713 work on probability by the Swiss mathematician Jakob Bernouilli (1655–1705), described by the French royal mathematician Pierre Rémond de Montmort in 1708, which included data collected in London for birth and deaths distinguished by sex.[25]

The demographic works of both Kersseboom and Wargentin were partially translated into French and widely discussed in the late eighteenth century.[26] Wargentin's impact on medicine across Europe, and particularly in France, derived from the magnitude of his discoveries and statistical-methodological innovations, but also from the fact that he was an exceptionally well-connected and cosmopolitan scientist whose voluminous correspondence with other major figures of the Enlightenment republic of letters constitutes a veritable archive all its own. This is evidenced in the many letters he exchanged with the likes of the Swedish botanist Carl Linnaeus, the eminent Swiss naturalist Albrecht von Haller (1708–1777), and the French physicist and philosopher Jean Le Rond d'Alembert (1717–1783), whose mammoth French *Encyclopédie* published between 1751 and 1772 was among the most cited works of the European Enlightenment. Consequently, Wargentin was named an honorary foreign member of the Paris Academy of Sciences in 1748.[27]

In 1741 there had also appeared a work by the German Protestant theologian and demographer Johann Peter Süßmilch (1707–1767), *Die göttliche Ordnung in den Veränderungen des menschlichen Geschlechts, aus der Geburt, dem Tode und der Fortpflanzung desselben* (The Divine Order in the Changes in the Human Race through its Sex, Birth, Death, and Generation), which proposed that women out-survived men at every age for reasons commanded by God, though signalling the age around 49–50 years as portentous for women.[28] Nonetheless, Süßmilch,

[22] E.g. Deparcieux, *Essai sur les probabilités*, 82; Anon., *Encyclopédie, ou dictionnaire raisonné des sciences, des arts et des métiers*, vol. 17 (Paris: Samuel Faulche, 1765), 253.

[23] Kersseboom, *Proeven van politique rekenkunde*, 9.

[24] Ibid., 10–11.

[25] Ibid., 9–10; Pierre Rémond Montmort, *Essay d'analyse sur les jeux de hazard* (Paris: Quillau, 1708), 189.

[26] All the French physicians who cited Kersseboom did so from a partial (now lost) French translation, with the author's name spelt slightly differently: W. Kerseboom, *Essai de calcul politique* of 1748. Rohrbasser & Véron, *Leibniz et les raisonnements sur la vie humaine*, vii–x; C. Behar & Y. Ducel, 'L'Arithmétique politique d'Antoine Deparcieux', in Thierry Martin, ed., *Arithmétique politique dans la France du XVIIe siècle* (Paris: Institut National d'Études Démographiques, 2003), 147–194.

[27] Sten Lindroth, 'History of Science in Sweden', *Isis*, 36/1 (1945): 16–19.

[28] Johann Peter Süßmilch, *Die göttliche Ordnung in denen Veränderungen des menschlichen Geschlechts, das ist, Gründlicher Beweis der göttlichen Vorsehung und Vorsorge für das menschliche Geschlecht aus der Vergleichung der gebohrnen und sterbenden, der verheiratheten und gebohrnen, wie*

like both the German physicians Ernst Stahl and Friedrich Hoffmann before him, dismissed the notion that planetary influences were responsible for the climacteric ages ('Stuffen-Jahre') such as that of the seventh septenary, and noted that mortality statistics did not indicate the septenary years to be particularly dangerous.[29]

Both in France and on a European-wide scale, the demographic discovery of women's longevity was slowly and unevenly disseminated, in part because population data were both complex to interpret and far from systematically gathered in all modern states until late in the nineteenth century. The Swiss statistician Johann Heinrich Waser was prosecuted and executed by his state in 1780 for publishing population data on the inhabitants of Zurich.[30] Only in 1817 did a French Interior Ministry initiative permit the publication of sex-differentiated regional birth and death records, fuelling a spate of new demographic studies from this moment onwards. By 1850 British medicine too had begun to insist on the need to acknowledge women's longevity which defied pre-existing expectations of the end of menses as a dangerous time. In this case, the stimulus was a slow recognition of the work of the Scottish actuary John Finlaison, who had demonstrated a massive state underestimation of the cost of naval spousal pensions due to previous poor data on women's lifespans.[31]

One particularly significant figure in the development of such ideas was the French mathematician Antoine Deparcieux (1703–1768), sometimes referred to as de Parcieux or as Déparcieux, who in 1746 made his name with the publication of an *Essay on Probabilities* which revised state predictions of mortality at different ages for the purposes of calculating annuity payments (*rentes viagères*).[32] Many existing life expectancy tables were misleading, Deparcieux showed, because most people born died as infants under 3 years of age, and their inclusion in the tables misrepresented the probability of those who survived early childhood living into old age. For the purposes of calculating annuity payments, this artefact could produce disastrous financial errors. Deparcieux called for modern states to make use of parish priests to gather local records of births and deaths towards a more accurate determination of annuity calculations, as was the practice in Sweden and had been so crucial in enabling Wargentin's calculations.[33]

auch insonderheit aus der beständigen Verhältniß der gebohrnen Knaben und Mägdens (Berlin: Verlag Daniel August Sohls, 1742), 200–201.

[29] Ibid., 361–363.

[30] Patrice Bordelais, *Le Nouvel Âge de la vieillesse* (Paris: Odile Jacob, 1993), 53.

[31] George Long, ed., *The Standard Library Cyclopædia of Political, Constitutional, Statistical, and Forensic Knowledge: Forming a Work of Universal Reference on Subjects of Civil Administration, Political Economy, Finance, Commerce, Laws and Social Relations, in Four Volumes*, vol. 1 (London: Henry G. Bohn, 1848), 144.

[32] Antoine Deparcieux, *Essai sur les probabilités de la durée de la vie humaine, d'où l'on déduit la manière de déterminer les rentes viagères, tant simples qu'en Tontines* (Paris: Frères Guerin, 1746).

[33] Ibid., 69.

Deparcieux's analysis considered the merits of demographic tables constructed by numerous other scholars for specific towns and regions in England, Switzerland, and the German lands, suggesting a significant improvement which could be made to their methods by differentiating men's and women's mortality at each of the different age bands. He considered this advisable on the grounds that women were more exposed to mortality risk during their reproductive years on account of high rates of death during childbirth,[34] so that women's natural life expectancy was skewed in existing data by this variable and could only truly be ascertained by a more detailed differentiation of populations of women who either had no children or who were already beyond their reproductive years.[35] He pointed to the data of the Dutch demographer Kersseboom demonstrating that nuns lived longer than priests, a differential which needed to be tested in the male and female populations more generally.[36] Deparcieux's work was cited in 1766 by Wargentin, who appears to have paid heed to the sex-distinction recommendation in his own survey.[37] And in 1758, Deparcieux was elected a foreign member of the Royal Swedish Academy of Sciences, roughly ten years after Wargentin had received his own honour by the French Academy of Sciences.[38] The statistical innovation of counting male and female mortality separately was clearly a transcultural development in the history of scientific knowledge, but one in which French scholars were pivotal.

Deparcieux's revised life-expectancy data also revealed something he considered novel and noteworthy: women were not more likely than men to die in their forties or fifties as he said many people assumed in referring to this time as a 'critical age'. And he noted that women who lived as nuns appeared to live longer on average than any group, remarking:

> Everyone thinks that the age of forty to fifty is a critical time for women: I do not know if it is any more so than for men, or more for worldly women or for nuns; but as for the latter, we certainly do not see it in their degree of mortality, compared to others.[39]

Later in the essay, he discussed emerging data from other sources which appeared to indicate that more women than men were surviving into extreme old age. Kersseboom had suggested as much in his 1740 report on the entire population of

[34] Ibid., 56. [35] Ibid., 69. [36] Ibid., 97.

[37] Nathalie Le Bouteillec & Jean-Marie Rohrbasser, eds, *Wargentin: Naissance des sciences de la population* (Paris: Institut National d'Études Démographiques, 2017), 122–124.

[38] Jacques Dupâquier, *L'Invention de la table de mortalité, de Graunt à Wargentin* (Paris: Presses Universitaires de France, 1996), 97.

[39] Deparcieux, *Essai sur les probabilités*, 83.

Holland.[40] Wargentin too had found higher female survival in every age, including the older ages, acknowledging that though women were thought the more fragile sex, it could not be denied that they were less vulnerable to death at every age.[41] An author recorded merely as 'the priest of Saint Sulpice of Paris' had released a report on mortality in his parish in 1745, just as Deparcieux's essay was going to press, which also indicated that more women than men survived into old age among priests and nuns.[42]

Deparcieux's tables attracted the interest both of the Encyclopedists, who cited them in their 1765 entry under *Vie*,[43] and of late eighteenth-century physicians interested in ageing and the life cycles, such as Paul-Joseph Barthez.[44] The Encyclopedists praised Deparcieux for beginning his mortality tables after the age of 3, avoiding the artificial underestimation of adult life expectancy produced by previous inclusions of infant deaths.[45] They also took heed of Deparcieux's remarks that mortality data did not confirm women to have a critical age in their forties or fifties as many supposedly assumed—though as we have seen, in the mid-eighteenth century there were still very few medical scholars who held this view.[46] The Encyclopedists also added to Deparcieux's inclusion of mortality data on priests and nuns by citing at length from the report compiled in 1745 by the fastidious clergy of the Parisian Saint Sulpice church, based on records of the births, baptisms, marriages, and deaths in the parish in the preceding thirty years. This was a report that included records of the deaths of priests and nuns and which showed that nuns enjoyed the greatest longevity of all groups. The report also showed that among the general population, women only had higher mortality than men during the childbearing years between ages 20 and 35.[47] Clearly then, they were not the more fragile sex in ageing, and childbirth still by far trumped any diseases attributed to the cessation of menses as the leading cause of women's deaths.

The Swiss Protestant pastor, jurist, and botanist Jean-Louis Muret (1715–1796) was another important figure in the European-wide development of demography of sex-differentiated population statistics, or what was known at the time as

[40] Willem Kersseboom, *Observatien, waar in voornamentlyk getoont word wat is gelyktydigheid, dewelke vereischt word in alle calculatien, die tot voorwerp hebben de probable leevenskracht van persoonen van eenigen voorgestelden ouderdom. Hier is bygeveen proeve van de constante ondervinding, dat die van de vrouwelijke sexe doorgaans maar eenige weinige jaaren doormalkander langer leven, dan die van de mannelyke* (Gravenhage: Jan van den Bergh, 1740).

[41] Le Bouteillec & Rohrbasser, *Wargentin: Naissance des sciences de la population*, 148–152.

[42] Ms. Joly de Fleury-284, fol. 51, Bibliothèque Nationale de Paris (site Richelieu).

[43] Denis Diderot, ed., *Encyclopédie, ou Dictionnaire raisonné des sciences, des arts et des métiers par une société de gens de lettres*, 17 vols (Neuchâtel: Faulche et Cie, 1765), vol. 17, 249–250.

[44] Paul-Joseph Barthez, *Nouveaux Éléments de la science de l'homme* (Montpellier: J. Martel aîné, 1778), 317.

[45] Diderot, ed., *Encyclopédie*, vol. 17, 251.

[46] Ibid., 253–254.

[47] Ms. Joly de Fleury-284.

'political arithmetic'. He was later cited by influential scholars of population such as the English economist and cleric Thomas Robert Malthus (1766–1834), as well as by numerous French doctors writing about menopause and women's ageing throughout the nineteenth century.[48] Muret's 1766 memoir on the Swiss population of the Vaud region, compared this local data to the studies of Wargentin and Kersseboom, showing that men had the lower survival rate in all ages over 30 years, and adding further weight to the view that women were the more resilient sex in ageing.[49] He refuted the explanation for this, which he attributed to Voltaire, that men's higher mortality in adulthood derived from their propensity to get into fights or to die in battle, showing that even in early infancy, male mortality was consistently higher than female. Such views, he said, also ignored the reality that as many women as men were massacred in wars of religion, most likely referring here to the Thirty Years War (1618–1648), ended by the Treaty of Westphalia, in which between 4.5 and 8 million people, mostly civilians, had died.[50] One of Muret's objectives was to determine whether lifetime mortality rates reflected infant mortality, but he found that although these things often went together, they did not always do so, noting that Lausanne had low life expectancy but high infant survival, while in other towns and cantons it was the reverse.[51] Then in 1780 the Swiss physician Louis Odier published his mortality tables of the Geneva population from 1778 to 1779, which noted that 'the probability of life of women is greater than that of men' from as early as birth and persisting through every age of adulthood.[52] But his data also showed some ages where more men than women survived.[53] Clearly how healthy adults were in ageing played some kind of a role, so the question of how the sexes, or other specific populations, aged differently piqued the curiosity of numerous scholars. How might matters of diet, sleep, sex, exercise, alcohol, emotions, clothing, air and water quality, vaccines, and countless other variables, soon to be clustered together under the complex rubric of 'hygiene', impact the ageing of different bodies and determine their longevity? Nineteenth-century menopause became a terrain for the exploration of precisely these sorts of questions.

[48] Thomas Robert Malthus, *An Essay on the Principle of Population* [1823] (New York: Cosimo Classics, 2010), 200–208. See Rusnock, *Vital Accounts*, 15–39; and Cem Behar, 'Le Pasteur Jean-Louis Muret (1715–1796): De la controverse sur la dépopulation à l'analyse démographique', *Population*, 3 (1996): 609–644.

[49] Jean-Louis Muret, *Mémoire sur l'état de la population dans le pays de Vaud* (Yverdon: F.-B. de Félice, 1766), 30.

[50] Ibid., 35; Geoffrey Parker, 'Crisis and Catastrophe: The Global Crisis of the Seventeenth Century Reconsidered', *The American Historical Review*, 113/4 (2008): 1053–1079.

[51] Muret, *Mémoire sur l'état de la population*, 113, 118–119.

[52] Louis Odier, 'Extrait mortuaire de Genève pour les années 1778 & 1779', *Société établie à Genève pour l'encouragement des arts et de l'agriculture: Mémoires*, 1–2 (1780): 144–156 [147].

[53] Ibid., 146.

Life Cycles and Ageing Morbidity in French Encyclopedism

Another important development in bio-scientific ideas about ageing and the lifespan occurred in France from the middle of the eighteenth century, where purportedly ancient accounts of the life cycle inspired attempts to theorise the patterns of ageing across cultures in the work of the naturalist philosopher Georges-Louis Leclerc de Buffon (1707–1788) and his collaborator Louis-Jean-Marie Daubenton (1716–1799). Both were natives of the region around Dijon, who made their names as renowned figures of Paris science. Daubenton appears to have invented the French term which had currency as a synonym for menopause until the early twentieth century: *l'âge de retour* (the age of turning), as Christine Théré has traced.[54] Buffon's and Daubenton's 1750 third volume of the epic, multi-volume *Histoire naturelle générale et particulière* (Natural History, General and Particular) published between 1749 and 1804, contained several important passages relating to questions of ageing that informed later medical views of menopause. Firstly, there were observations about human physiological variability, including descriptions of hunter-gatherer peoples of Europe, Africa, and Asia, where they hinted that contemporary norms of ageing in Europe differed from those of wild-living and historical humans. Most of these descriptions laboured over ethnographic descriptions of customs, dress, skin colour, and facial features in the obsessive cataloguing of human variation, but the scant remarks about ageing across cultures indicate the beginning of the idea that Europeans in particular were ageing badly due to the nefarious effects of civilisation, luxury, and physical inactivity, although no distinctions were drawn here on the basis of sex differences.[55]

This work was also full of derogatory remarks about various 'races', both their physical features and their moral customs, especially their sexual practices. But whatever the authors thought about how other peoples looked and behaved, they had to admit that many tribal-living peoples seemed to age better and live longer, healthy lives than 'civilised' Europeans. The descriptions are heavily filtered through the lenses of colonial power, belief in European moral and intellectual superiority, and an unabashed racist aesthetics of human beauty. But what is clear here is that Buffon and Daubenton themselves, like the seventeenth- and eighteenth-century European ethnographic observers whose accounts they engaged with, were indeed beginning to see questions of ageing in comparative anthropological terms, concluding that elite Europeans were doing it relatively badly. They offered no specific suggestions for how Europeans might reform themselves to age better, but their remarks about other cultures' old age indicates

[54] Théré, 'Âge de retour et retour d'âge', 55.

[55] Georges-Louis Leclerc Comte de Buffon & Louis-Jean-Marie Daubenton, *Histoire naturelle générale et particulière*, 15 vols (La Haye: Pierre de Hondt, 1750), vol. 3, 148–158.

that they primarily blamed the inactivity and laziness of European elites for their own unnecessarily early demise.

This was clearly not a matter of generally exoticising colonial others as more vigorous because they were more animal-like or more natural, since the remarks of Buffon and Daubenton in the *Histoire naturelle* about patterns of ageing flattered some colonised peoples and not others. There was no question here of a universal 'primitive' longevity. The people of Guinea, they claimed, 'though of solid and very good health, rarely however surpass a certain age', since a Guinean man of 50 years 'is in his country an old man'. The cause for this, they suggested, was probably precocious sexual behaviour and childbearing—debauchery, which they assumed to shorten the lifespan.[56] The Swedes too may be an exception to the European norms, they considered, based on the Latin scholarship of the seventeenth-century Swedish polymath physician Olaus Rudbeck (1630–1702).[57] Most Swedes were tremendously fertile, Rudbeck had claimed, and commonly lived beyond the age of 100 years, with many reaching 140 (though Rudbeck himself managed barely half that!). This idea was found too in the descriptions of the Danes in Claude Jordan's 1693 *Voyages historiques de l'Europe*, which attributed Danish longevity to the fresh air of Nordic climes.[58] Buffon and Daubenton deemed Jordan's speculations worthy of simple reportage, adding that the well-known sexual temperance of the Nordic peoples (on account of their cold climate making it difficult to undress) could be the cause of their greater lifespan; but they doubted Rudbeck's more extreme claims on account of the excessive enthusiasm for his own people shown in the work in question.[59]

The theme of sexual activity accelerating ageing is one we will meet again since it appeared repeatedly in nineteenth-century French works on menopause, most often seen as relevant to women rather than to men. These later texts warned women both that previous debauchery in their youth, as well as attempts to engage sexually after menopause, could be the cause of menopausal health problems ranging from nervous and mental derangement to cancer. But it is striking to see the theme of sex causing decline mentioned in Buffon and Daubenton's work 100 years earlier. This was clearly not a widespread idea, since eighteenth-century medical works generally made no such claim, nor indeed did they have much to say at all about older people having sex given their preoccupation with questions of childbearing wherever sexual physiology was concerned. But the idea was seeded here, we might say, providing precedent for the more generalised suspicion of older women's sexuality in late nineteenth-century French alienism, discussed in Chapter 5.

[56] Ibid., 179.

[57] Olaus Rudbeck, *Atlantica (Atland Eller Manheim)* (Uppsala: Henricus Curio, 1679), 392.

[58] Claude Jordan, *Voyages historiques de l'Europe*, 8 vols (Paris: Nicolas Le Gras, 1693), vol. 8, 229.

[59] Buffon and Daubenton, *Histoire naturelle générale et particulière*, 172. See Olaus Rudbeck, *Olaus Rudbeck's Atlantica* [1684], ed. Axel Nelson, 5 vols (Stockholm: Almqvist & Wiksell, 1937–1950).

Most of Daubenton's third volume concerned experimental observations of human corpses, medical observation of skeletal defects and other questions of teratology, clinical observations of physiological functions, and the cataloguing of the entire French royal cabinet of biological specimens, with only a small section of this volume containing remarks about ageing and human cultural variation, and about the supposedly 'ancient' idea of life cycles. This is important because for Buffon and Daubenton, these were but minor questions, in contrast to the overarching concerns that they became for specialist medical writers in the nineteenth century. Daubenton, however, appears to have remained an important reference for several nineteenth-century doctors writing on menopause. The life-cycle reflections of the *Encyclopédie* were clearly one of the layers contained in nineteenth-century concepts which were laid down in the eighteenth century, some of these recalling even older concepts of early modern and ancient lineage. This should not be taken to indicate an undifferentiated continuity in medical thought, since massive differences in magnitude, content, and treatment distinguished sixteenth- to eighteenth-century ideas about life cycles and ageing from the development of sex-specific menopause symptomatology in the nineteenth century. But nor did the emergence of the modern biomedical account of menopause spring forth spontaneously after 1800.

In the 1782 *Methodical Encyclopedia: Natural History of Animals*, Daubenton also aligned the *âge de retour* to another supposedly popular concept of the *verte vieillesse* (green old age—evoking a mature tree at the beginning of autumn which has not yet lost all its green leaves). This French expression in more recent times has referred to vibrant ageing—of remaining vigorous into old age, a meaning which dates from the early eighteenth century.[60] *La verte vieillesse* may have been an eighteenth-century French rendition of the older Latin expression *cruda senectus* (raw old age), though it is unclear how much currency that Latin term had prior to this. Daubenton protested that this part of the life cycle had been overlooked in the history of medical thought and that there was a need to insist more emphatically on the era in between the 'virile age' and old age. Physiologists made too scant mention of this *senium crudum* in between the two other eras, he thought. A man of 45 was not yet an old man after all, and yet clearly some of his faculties had already begun to decline. There must be a turning point from gradual growth into gradual decline and it was this moment of 'turning' which Daubenton sought to locate.

What was at stake here clearly, was not merely how medicine should periodise the life cycles and characterise the different ages of 'Man' (women were evidently still not figuring in such discussions): it was also the process of ageing, and the idea that this process properly begins at a specific moment, referring to the first

[60] 'Vert' in Anon., *Nouveau Dictionnaire de l'Academie Françoise, dedié au roy*. 2 vols, vol. 2: M–Z (Paris: Coignard, 1718), 769.

functional and external signs of decline. Daubenton claimed that the notion of a 'turn of age' evoked in the term *l'âge de retour* was appropriate here because this was the moment when 'nature begins to go backward' ('la nature commence à rétrograder')—when things begin to degenerate, or become subject to *dépérissement* (wasting, withering).[61] The first things to decline were the plumpness of the skin, which Daubenton attributed to a loss of fat filling it out as well as a loss of elasticity of the skin itself; a decline of acute vision, requiring the use of spectacles; and a weakening of digestive power which he highlighted as a very important area of health concern for those over the age of 45 years.[62] The *âge de retour* began at around the age of 45 until 60 or 65 years, from whence old age proper began and endured until death. But there was no mention here of men and women having distinct patterns of ageing, of the end of menstruation as significant, nor of people of different ethnicities, and his mention of greying beards as one of the superficial signs of ageing suggests that his entire discussion was premised on universalising the model of a European white male subject.[63]

Neither Daubenton, nor any of those who cited him subsequently, provided any specific earlier reference to the term *senium crudum*, even though they all asserted that it was an ancient one. The terms *senium crudum* (or *cruda senectus*) cannot be found in the work of Galen or Hippocrates, nor in Ptolemy, nor in the early eighteenth-century Latin Halle school works referring to the cessation of menses in women. A nineteenth-century French–Latin dictionary focused on terminology used in the work of ancient authors had an entry under *senium*, referring to old age in Tacitus, old-age decline in Pliny the Elder, and to *vergentibus annis in senium* (years on the verge of decline) in Lucretius.[64] But Daubenton mentioned none of these as the source of his reference to the *senium crudum*, and nor are they precisely the same expression. Although Daubenton attended to the question of when ageing begins and how this commencement of decline is detected in bodies, by ignoring sex differences and without any reference to the vast and expanding medical corpus of works on the diseases of women, his ideas failed to produce a view of women's 'critical age' of the kind that appeared in the medical faculties of Montpellier and Paris from the end of the eighteenth century. The continuing early modern astrological reference to climacteric moments and the seventh septenary, and the novel elaboration of the *âge de retour* and the *senium crudum* as the moment when ageing began, constituted merely one layer in the complex medical construction of menopause, though a layer it was

[61] Louis-Jean-Marie Daubenton, 'Introduction', in Diderot & D'Alembert, eds, *Encyclopédie méthodique: Histoire naturelle des animaux*, vol. 1 (Paris: Panckoucke, 1782), lxxiv.

[62] Ibid., lxxv. [63] Ibid., Lxxvi.

[64] L. Quicherat & A. Daveluy, *Dictionnaire latin–français: Contenant tous les mots employés par les auteurs latins et les principales inscriptions latines jusqu'au VIe siècle de notre ère avec renvois aux sources des mots rares*, 46th ed. (Paris: Librairie Hachette, 1910), 1254. The first, and much smaller, edition of this dictionary appeared in 1856 without the *senium* entries.

nonetheless. How then did the cessation of menses become enmeshed with these larger concerns about vital ageing and lifespan? The answer to this question lies in the uptake of ideas about ageing in medical vitalism of the eighteenth century, a field which connected the climacteric concept of critical life stages with the growing medical fascination with the diseases of women.

Vitalism and the Cessation of Menstruation

A significant turning point occurred in the emergence of iatromechanical explanation of ageing and of menstrual cessation in the work of the German physician Georg Ernst Stahl (1659–1734), who was well known in France throughout the eighteenth century and remained so well into the nineteenth, with a new complete works of the Halle luminary appearing in French translation in 1859.[65] In his 1707 *Theoria medica vera*, Stahl had discussed the critical days theory of Galen and Hippocrates, according to which the seventh and fourteenth days of an illness were thought to be turning points, which Stahl credited with some validity.[66] He did not appear to engage with the climacteric-ages concept in the manner of Friedrich Hoffmann,[67] but nonetheless gave a temporal frame to women's generative capacity and menstruation of up to the 'seventh septenary' (age 49), after which he said there would be plethora with copious haemorrhages and mental afflictions.[68] But for Stahl, the significance of the forty-ninth year had nothing to do with the planets, which he considered science had not satisfactorily demonstrated had any influence on human health, despite the persistence of astrological beliefs of this kind.[69] Elsewhere in his magnum opus he took pains to reject the notion that the moon governed epileptic fits, describing such beliefs as vulgar, fantastical, and frankly embarrassing.[70] He also expressed contempt for the mystical belief that menstruation corrupted women's bodies, which he related to the emotional perturbations women themselves experience during their periods, producing a tendency to attribute their distress to nefarious forces in their bodies.[71] Nonetheless, he appeared to take as a given that there would be illnesses associated with the cessation of menses, because perturbations of any kind of change within the body produced disease states: any variation of a tranquil state disturbed both the humours and of the mind.[72]

[65] Georg Ernst Stahl, *Œuvres médico-philosophiques et pratiques de G. E. Stahl*, 6 vols, trans. T. Blondin (Paris: J. B. Baillière, 1859–1864).

[66] Georg Ernst Stahl, *Theoria medica vera: Physiologiam & pathologiam* (Halle: Literis Orphanotrophei, 1707), 386.

[67] Friedrich Hoffmann, 'De annorum climactericorum rationali & medica explicatione', in *Opera omnia physico, tomus quintus* (Geneva: Fratres de Tournes, 1704), 89–94.

[68] Stahl, *Theoria medica vera*, 1099–1100. [69] Ibid., 900. [70] Ibid., 1344–1345.

[71] Ibid., 390–391. [72] Ibid., 1100.

A few years later, in a 1711 work on women's fertility, Stahl proposed an iatromechanical explanation for the final cessation of menstruation in women, emphasising the weakened excretory and vital power of the uterus in ageing, resulting in plethora, hysteria, and abdominal (*hypochondriacos*) pains.[73] Here the vital power that made menstruation and conception possible was thought to be the very same power that stabilised the mind and balanced the humours. Women's ageing was thus the loss of both kinds of health. In 1710 as we saw in the previous chapter, Stahl's student David Titius appears to have been the first doctoral candidate in medicine instructed to write his entire dissertation on the cessation of menses in women both young and old, effectively sweeping up a new inclusion of the age-related cessation of menses into the larger and pre-existing medical topic of menstrual suppression in younger women.[74] Thus began a pedagogic tradition that resulted in hundreds of medical theses on such topics published in France throughout the long nineteenth century, as we consider over the remainder of this book—a tradition which only after 1799 became focused on older women's final cessation of menses. Notably, much of the nineteenth-century French fascination with menopause unfolded after the widely discussed demographic evidence of women's greater longevity.

The Montpellier physician Paul-Joseph Barthez was a crucial eighteenth-century thinker responsible for the incorporation of the Halle school ideas about sex differences and ageing into the emergent vitalist currents of French medicine and undoubtedly the most influential thinker in the modernisation of the Montpellier medical faculty in the second half of the eighteenth century.[75] As Charles Wolfe has noted, eighteenth-century medical ideas about vital force, such as those Barthez invoked, are not entirely assimilable to the later metaphysical designation of 'vitalism', but instead appeared within a variety of thought structures alongside materialist, mechanistic, and holistic accounts of nature.[76] Barthez distanced himself from both a purely mechanistic view of the human body and a metaphysical attribution of the life force to the soul. He situated his approach in the Hippocratic tradition which he claimed was reflected in his concern with 'les forces du Principe Vital de l'homme' (the forces of man's vital principle), their communication or 'sympathies' within a system, their expression in different temperaments and ages, and their extinction in death.

In the 1778 work entitled *Nouveaux Éléments de la science de l'homme* (New Elements of the Science of Man), Barthez considered the mortality data of the

[73] Georg Ernst Stahl, *De sterilitate foeminarum: Dissertatio inauguralis medica* (Halle: Henckel, 1711), 13–15.

[74] David Titius, *De fine mensium initiis morborum variorum opportuno: Dissertatio inauguralis medica* (Halle: Henckelii, 1710).

[75] Williams, *A Cultural History of Medical Vitalism*, 255–275.

[76] Charles T. Wolfe, 'Introduction: Vitalism without Metaphysics? Medical Vitalism in the Enlightenment', *Science in Context*, 21/4 (2008): 461–463.

Swedish demographer Pehr Wilhelm Wargentin,[77] as well as that of Deparcieux. He took these data as evidence of a decline of vitality in ageing as indicated by the rising mortality in each decade after the age of 40 years.[78] He elaborated a vitalist and solidist vision of vitality in humans and other animals, seeing the population data as illustrating the extent to which there must be a vital force of finite quantity in every living being which was depleted throughout its lifetime until there was none left. The late forties in both sexes represented the end of the 'consistent age', he noted.[79] Mortality increased in the decades after 50 or 60, Barthez thought, because 'the radical forces of the Vital Principal have an intensity proportional to the tenacity of life'.[80] Women clearly differed from men in ageing on account of their unique relationship to the vital force of youth which enabled their child-bearing capacity, resulting in their ageing occurring less rapidly than men's and their lifespan extending longer.[81] But Barthez did not speculate about the meaning of women's final cessation of menses for their ageing.

The Paris naturalist Julien Joseph Virey mapped the distinct consideration concisely in his 1800 *History of the Human Species*: life was more dangerous to the young, with mortality reducing in those between 30 and 50 years. For women, however, 'the critical time interrupts this consistent age and separates it into two portions, of which the second is happier'.[82] In another part of this same work, Virey distinguished women from men by their lack of beard and body hair, rounder form, and smaller size, adding footnotes referring to exceptions for each of these characteristics. In the exception to the beard, he noted that some medical scholars had observed 'women become bearded after passing the critical age'.[83] He considered the notion of climacteric years on the septenaries being more dangerous than others, attributing this to Pythagorean thought, but following Barthez, he rejected it, despite affirming that puberty, gestation, and women's critical age represented consistent temporal vulnerabilities for women. By avoiding excess and living a sufficiently orderly life ('on vit d'une manière assez réglée'), even these critical junctures could be expected to pass without incident.[84]

Another who helped connect the dots between the accumulating accounts of women's greater longevity in political arithmetic and the new medicine of sex and age differentiation was the Strasbourg hygiene professor Étienne Tourtelle (1756–1801), who had graduated from the Montpellier Faculty in 1782.[85] In 1796

[77] Pehr Wilhelm Wargentin, 'Mortalitaten i Sverige, i anledning af Tabell-Verket', *Kongl. Vetenskaps-academiens Handlingar*, 27 (1766): 1–25.

[78] Paul-Joseph Barthez, *Nouveaux Éléments de la science de l'homme* (Montpellier: J. Martel aîné, 1778).

[79] Ibid., 319. [80] Ibid., 321. [81] Ibid., 325.

[82] Julien-Joseph Virey, *Histoire naturelle du genre humain*, 2 vols (Paris: F. Dufart, 1800), vol. 1, 407.

[83] Ibid., 340. [84] Ibid., 410.

[85] Étienne Tourtelle, *Theses medicae. Ex theoria. De naturâ, diversitate & viribus mineralium aquarum, medicatarum vocitatarum. Ex Praxi* (Montpellier: Jacques François Couché, 1782).

Tourtelle addressed the paradox of reconciling, on the one hand, the demographic statistics that showed more women than men living to the oldest ages with, on the other hand, the notion that women were more delicate, prone to illness throughout the lifespan, and particularly diseased in old age. Ageing was a process of hardening of the tissues, he said, echoing the mechanistic accounts of eighteenth-century scholars. Women's tissues were softer to begin with and, although the cessation of menses redirected force away from the uterus and caused solidification around the epigastric region, their tissues still rigidified at a slower pace than men's throughout the lifespan, which accounted for their greater longevity.[86] But how then to explain women's greater ageing morbidity? Why did the same softness that protected them from death not also protect them from illness? The answer was that women's *âge critique* caused a solidification of their tissues that was still less dangerous than men's but nonetheless morbid for them: 'Their youth is shorter and more brilliant, but their old age is longer and more troublesome (*fâcheuse*).'[87] Thus was born the ongoing medical paradox of women's combination of greater ageing morbidity and greater longevity relative to men.

The medical hygienist Claude Lachaise, in addition to his work on the population of Paris, also authored another grandiose 500-page work in 1825 on the *Physiological Hygiene of Women* which reveals why many others considered him such an authority of the matter of *l'hygiène* for women around the time of cessation of menses.[88] The book was divided into separate chapters for women's various life phases: childhood, puberty, youth, motherhood, the 'so-called critical age', and old age. Because Lachaise recommended gentle exercise as beneficial to girls in puberty, specifying rides in carriages and on horseback as the two best forms, he earned the gentle scorn of a reviewer who remarked that 'it seems our author has in view only the hygiene of the rich and will deal at another time with the inferior classes of society': for now though, his work remained of interest mainly to the members of high society (*gens du monde*) for whom it was clearly written.[89] In this work too Lachaise reminded his readers of the vast statistical evidence that women were not more vulnerable to death than men around the age of 50, and suggested that doctors treating menopausal women should inform them of their longevity advantage as a means of reassuring them that menopause was no 'critical age'.[90]

[86] Étienne Tourtelle, *Élémens d'hygiène, ou De l'influence des choses physiques et morales sur l'homme, et des moyens de conserver la santé*, vol. 1 (Strasbourg: F. G. Levrault, 1796), 40–41.

[87] Ibid., 34.

[88] Charles Lachaise, *Hygiène physiologique de la femme* (Paris: Mequignon-Marvis, 1825).

[89] Anon., 'Hygiène physiologique de la femme', *Revue encyclopédique ou analyse raisonnée des productions les plus remarquables dans les sciences, les arts industriels, la literature et les beaux-arts* (Paris: Bureau central de la revue encyclopédique, 1825), 468–469.

[90] Lachaise, *Hygiène physiologique de la femme*, 425.

The Assimilation of Women's Greater Longevity and Morbidity into the Medicalisation of Menopause

In the German lands, the minority view of the final cessation of menses as a deadly time had an ongoing genealogy well into the nineteenth century: the Prussian royal physician and Berlin professor of pathology Christoph Wilhelm Hufeland (1762–1836), whose 1825 manual of medical therapy was translated into French in 1836 and read by several French doctors of the mid-nineteenth century, observed that women after the cessation of menses were more prone to cancers as well as a range of other dangerous diseases.[91] Consequently, he thought the designation of women's cessation of menses as a 'critical' time aptly represented its danger to them, since it was the period in which the largest number of women died. This was after the French medical ideas about the critical age and menopause had already become a popular thesis topic. Nonetheless, Hufeland's assertion of women's higher mortality around the age of 50 was also, by this time, already widely contradicted by numerous demographic statistical studies in several European cultures, of which he appeared unaware in his casual remarks about the 'critical age' approaching 50 years. Such ignorance of demography was not possible in France, where sex-differentiated mortality statistics were drilled into medical students' consciousness in the faculties of both Paris and Montpellier from the first years of the nineteenth century and throughout the whole century. Still, not all the early scholars of women's critical age found it convenient to discuss this either.

The eminent Montpellier professor of medicine Joseph-Marie-Joachim Vigarous (1759–1826) who taught at Montpellier in the late 1790s and was also widely cited by Paris scholars, referred in his 1801 published lectures on the diseases of women to an earlier lineage of erroneous ideas that had attributed breast cancer to the final cessation of menses. In this view, for which he cited scholars such as Dionis and Le Dran, suppressed menstrual blood accumulated in the body and by sympathy exercised a nefarious effect on the breasts.[92] This explanation provided in a set of university lectures formed part of the pedagogic tradition emerging in this time which consisted in correcting errors of the medical past. Vigarous helped to establish the norm of invoking the pathological view of menopause only to dismiss it as a traditional myth—a pattern of discourse that would thereafter be repeated in hundreds of French doctoral thesis over the following hundred years. While Vigarous did not blame religion for the error,

[91] Christoph Wilhelm Hufeland, *Enchiridion medicum oder Anleitung zur medizinischen Praxis: Vermächtniss einer fünfzigjährigen Erfahrung* (Berlin: Jonas, 1836), 13; Christoph Wilhelm Hufeland, *La Macrobiotique, ou L'Art de prolonger la vie de l'homme, suivi de Conseils sur l'éducation physique des enfants*, trans. A.-J.-L. Jourdan (Paris: J.-B. Baillière, 1836).

[92] Joseph-Marie-Joachim Vigarous, *Cours élémentaire de maladies des femmes, ou Essai sur une nouvelle méthode pour étudier et pour classer les maladies de ce sexe* (Paris: Deterville, 1801), vol.1, 546.

numerous later Paris scholars certainly did, also sometimes misattributing the idea to popular folk healers in their efforts to claim a modern bioscientific identity in the treatment of ageing women's morbidity, as we consider in Chapter 6.

The renowned Paris professor of medicine and anatomy Louis-Jacques Moreau de la Sarthe (1771–1826) also incorporated discussion of the demographic discovery into his writing on the diseases of women in a way that made it available to numerous later scholars engaged in the project of medicalising women's ageing. In his 1803 *Natural History of Woman*, he described how the cessation of menstruation made women more like men in that their faces became more muscular, their hair thinned and whitened, and their skin lost its softness and lustre, but they also no longer suffered the ills of the menstrual and childbearing years. Nonetheless, he noted, they differed from men in that 'their longevity especially is much more extended' ('leur longévité surtout a beaucoup plus d'étendue'). In ageing, women remained distinct: 'they age, decline and die in their own fashion' ('elles vieillissent, déclinent et meurent à leur manières').[93] A woman's reproductive 'apparatus', from the time of puberty until the critical age, had an 'excess of vitality which becomes for her the source of many indispositions'. The end of menstruation did not represent the end of her vitality even though she now lost the capacity to give new life to the species.[94] Even as Moreau called the end of menstruation 'the death of sex' and the 'critical age',[95] he also noted that women of different constitutions faired variously in the cessation of menstruation, and he indicated that there was much for medicine to understand about which 'favourable circumstances' surrounding older women's lives might allow them the greatest wellbeing. Even Roussel, he remarked, preferred the company of older women, after all.[96] This idea, that women might age better or worse according to how they cared for their bodies and minds and might finally, in their older ages, aspire to greater esteem among men, proved immensely generative for the development of French medical fascinations with menopause throughout the nineteenth century, producing the florid hygiene of women's critical age that we will consider in Chapter 5.

The earliest theses on women's critical age or final cessation of menses, such as those of the Montpellier candidates Jérémie-André Pingault and Joseph Gagnebé, were slow to catch on. Even though they had clearly read Vigarous, they made no mention of the mortality data cited by their master, whereas they observed that cancers of the breast, uterus, and ovaries increased after the final cessation of

[93] Louis-Jacques Moreau de la Sarthe, *Histoire naturelle de la femme, suivie d'un traité d'hygiène appliqué à son régime physiques et moral aux différentes époques de la vie*, 3 vols (Paris: Duprat, 1803), vol. 1, 180–181.
[94] Ibid., 208–209. [95] Ibid., vol. 2, 676. [96] Ibid., 412.

menses, following the word of surgeons such as Dionis, Le Dran, and Vacher.[97] The first Paris thesis, that of Jean-Baptiste Chouffe, pondered the relationship between the ability to menstruate and 'an exuberance of the forces of life' in women but offered no conclusions about the meaning of the final cessation of menses for their ageing.[98] In the work of all the early specialists on the topic up to the 1820s, there was not a single mention made of the growing demographic consensus about women's resilience to death in the older ages, even as the renowned professors to whose work they were exposed at Montpellier, Paris, and Strasbourg, Joseph Vigarous, Louis Moreau de la Sarthe, and Étienne Tourtelle, all made a point of it in their discussions of women's final cessation of menses.[99] The Paris candidate Louis Gardanne who coined the term *la menespausie* in his 1812 doctoral thesis (which became *la ménopause* in his later books on the topic), also had nothing to say about older women's mortality risk. He most likely ignored the topic in the view that it would be inconvenient for his claims to a new specialist field of older women's medicine, rather than neglecting it because he was ignorant of the demographic revolution in scientific understandings of sex-differentiated ageing.[100] The demographic fact of women outliving men in later life clearly did not inspire the first pieces of specialist writing on the final cessation of menses. But the encounter of the two themes produced a surprising surge in new ideas about ageing hygienic prescription for women in menopause from 1820 onwards.

In his 1817 *Essay on Women Considered During their Different Periods of Life*, the Montpellier surgeon Gilbert Joseph Magdeleine Guyot, who worked at the Saint-Éloi military hospital, defined the critical age as one of the significant times when women developed tumultuous, convulsive, and emotive disorders.[101] Girls achieved maturity faster than boys, he thought, because beauty (which completes

[97] Jérémie-André Pingault, *De la cessation des règles* (Montpellier: Tournel, 1799), 15–16; Joseph Gagnebé, *Exposition de quelques maladies qui attaquent les femmes à la cessation des règles.* Thèse (Montpellier: Imprimerie de Tournel, 1801), 12–13.

[98] Jean-Baptiste-P. Chouffe, *Des accidents et des maladies qui surviennent à la cessation de la menstruation.* Thèse (Paris: Croullebois & Gabon, 1802), 10.

[99] I. A. Labretoigne-Lavalette, *Réfléxions sur les maladies qui surviennent aux femmes à l'époque de la cessation des règles.* Thèse (Montpellier: Imprimerie Auguste Ricard, 1805); Henri Lamaze, *Essai sur la cessation du flux menstruel et sur les moyens propres à prévenir les accidents et les maladies qui peuvent affecter les femmes à cette époque* (Paris: Didot Jeune, 1805); J.-J. Nicolon, *Observations sur la ménorrhagie qui survient à l'approche de l'âge critique, et sur l'aménorrhée par vice de conformation.* Thèse (Strasbourg: Levrault, 1808); Jean Baptiste Anglade, *Considérations sur les effets que peut produire la cessation des règles.* Thèse (Montpellier: Jean Martel, 1812); C. A. M. Peloux, *Essai sur l'époque critique et sur les moyens propres à prévenir les accidents et les maladies qui en dépendent* (Paris: Didot Jeune, 1812); Jean-Antoine Poussié, *Réflexions sur l'hygiène qui convient aux femmes arrivées à l'âge de retour.* Thèse (Montpellier: Jean Martel aîné, 1813).

[100] Charles-Pierre-Louis de Gardanne, *Dissertation sur les avis à donner aux femmes qui entrent dans l'âge critique.* Thèse (Paris: Didot Jeune, 1812); Charles-Pierre-Louis de Gardanne, *Avis aux femmes qui entrent dans l'âge critique* (Paris: Gabon, 1816); Charles-Pierre-Louis de Gardanne, *De la ménopause ou de l'âge critique des femmes* (Paris: Méquignon-Marvis, 1821).

[101] Gilbert Joseph Magdeleine Guyot, *Quelques propositions sur la femme considérée dans les différentes périodes de la vie.* Thèse (Montpellier: Jean Martel, 1817), 18.

women) is less difficult for nature to accomplish than strength (which completes men).[102] Women's youth both passed more quickly and was more brilliant than men's, but they also suffered 'premature ageing' after the age of 40, particularly if they did not lead an active and laborious life.[103] Guyot, like Moreau de la Sarthe, charmingly referred to menopause as 'the death of sex' ('la mort du sexe'), adding that women served no purpose once their capacity to give new life had ended.[104] And yet even he acknowledged that despite their 'premature ageing', women after menopause could expect to live longer than men (referring to the Dutch statistician Kersseboom's mortality data, among others).[105] His explanation for this apparent paradox was that women had softer tissues and more temperate characters than men, which preserved their lifespan. Nonetheless, he asserted (now ignoring the statistical evidence of monastic orders, such as Kersseboom's) that women only retained their longevity advantage if they bore children, and that while fewer men lived to old age, only they could live to extreme old age.[106] Mortality data, after all, could be selectively read, attending only to those parts of it which supported one's particular gender ideology.

Notably too, while the statistical innovation of counting male and female mortality separately was clearly a transcultural advancement in the history of scientific knowledge, of which French scholars were a part, they were not its only drivers. However, French physicians were by far the dominant force in a nineteenth-century medical movement that engaged consistently and explicitly with this earlier scientific recognition of women's longevity and which referred to concepts of menopause in relation to sex-specific descriptions of ageing and mortality. The first clear entanglement of the two themes appeared in the memoir on mortality presented by the statistician and demographer Louis-François Benoiston de Châteauneuf (1775–1856) to the Académie des Sciences on 13 May 1818, and published four years later in 1822.[107] This report specifically targeted the notion that women suffered a 'critical age' around 45–50 years—a view which Châteauneuf argued was not supported by any of the accumulating mortality statistics of different places in Europe.

Châteauneuf later worked in the Ministry of Finance under the Restoration, leaving public life just prior to the ascension of Emperor Louis Napoleon III.[108] But prior to this, he had served as a military surgeon in the Napoleonic wars, after training in Paris as the Val-Grâce military hospital. There he was influenced by the younger mathematician and physician Siméon-Denis Poisson, after whom the statistical term 'poisson distribution' is named (used to describe probabilistic

[102] Ibid., 6. [103] Ibid., 18. [104] Ibid., 19.
[105] Ibid., 21–22. [106] Ibid., 22–23.
[107] Louis-François Benoiston de Châteauneuf, *Mémoire sur la mortalité des femmes de l'âge de quarante à cinquante ans, lu à l'Académie des sciences, dans la séance du 13 mai 1818* (Paris: Martinet, 1822).
[108] Amédée Dechambre, *Dictionnaire encyclopédique des sciences médicales*, vol. 9 (Paris: Asselin et Houzeau, 1868), 85.

events distributed in space or time). Poisson had studied at the École Polytechnique in Paris, and had been appointed 'professor of mechanical reason' at the new Paris Faculty of Sciences in 1809, so it seems likely that this was where Châteauneuf made his acquaintance.[109] Both men were trained in the military, where their induction into population statistics was very different from that of the graduates of the Paris medical faculty with their emerging orientation towards the hygienic care of the urban elites. As such, Châteauneuf, like Poisson, had little truck with humoral medicine, Hippocratic aphorisms, or questions that did not bear upon the hard facts of mortality. These were scholars who looked to the mechanistic disciplines such as mathematics and physics to yield new understandings of human physiology. With their induction into concerns about military personnel, they were also acutely aware of the state need for more accurate information about population to determine the *effectifs* (men who could be recruited for active military service). Châteauneuf's role in the Napoleonic Ministry of Finance also primed his perspectives towards demographic matters of financial importance to the state.

Around the same time as his paper delivered to the Académie des Sciences in 1817, Châteauneuf had also begun preparing a report on the mortality of the Paris population. Here too he found similar indication that women in the nation's capital suffered no particular spike in mortality around the age of 50, even though life expectancy was generally lower in the metropolis overall than in the provinces.[110] He then extended these studies into a Europe-wide survey of mortality, incorporating the research of Wargentin and others from as early as 1776.[111] Châteauneuf's loud and insistent message of the 1820s and 1830s was that older women were not the most vulnerable group or the ones whose deaths most impacted French population growth, and that they were not to be fussed over just because their reproductive capacity had ended. The demographic facts did not support any need for special care in menopause because, according to mortality data, it represented no risk. While this was prior to the marked slowing of births that became the worried obsession of French statisticians and politicians in the final decades of the nineteenth century, it also reflected the fact that post-reproductive women's mortality had minimal bearing on the depopulation question which focused increasingly on maternal and infant survival as the means to expand the population.[112] Nonetheless, the belief that the French population was failing to grow sufficiently and that without more growth, prosperity would be

[109] François Arago, 'Notices Bibliographies: Poisson', in *Œuvres complètes de François Arago*, 16 vols (Paris: Gide et J. Baudry, 1854), vol. 2, 593–698.

[110] Louis-François Benoiston de Châteauneuf, *Extraits des recherches statistiques sur la ville de Paris et le département de la Seine* (Paris: Bureau du Bulletin, 1824).

[111] Louis-François Benoiston de Châteauneuf, 'Note lue à l'Académie royale des sciences dans sa séance du 30 janvier 1826, sur les changemens qu'ont subies les lois de la mortalité en Europe, depuis un demisiècle (1775–1825)', *Le Moniteur*, 6 February 1826, 1–10.

[112] Bordelais, *Le Nouvel Âge de la vieillesse*, 86–117.

thwarted, was already common from the end of the eighteenth century, inspired by Montesquieu's claims to this effect.[113] And while infant mortality was widely held to be a major obstacle to population growth, both fertility and life expectancy were also in play. As Andrea Rusnock notes, the question of which ages were the most dangerous times for both sexes was a central concern of population scholars in France from the late eighteenth century onwards, and fuelled numerous concerns about modern lifeways, moral habits, consumption patterns, and other factors that might influence ageing.[114]

When the published version of Châteauneuf's report was released in 1822, there were some important differences from the Académie des Sciences version of five years earlier. The book was more detailed, presenting new empirical evidence tabulated by Châteauneuf himself; it also contained an extended series of claims both about the universality of women's greater longevity and about menopause symptomology. Châteauneuf showed himself adept in both forms of discourse that had competed on the question of women's ageing up to this time: both exemplifying the medical hygienic approach to managing menopause as if it were an illness (even as its status as such was denied) while affirming the statistical accounts of women's mortality risk which implied that they were in no need of any special medical surveillance in ageing. Châteauneuf provided an example to medical clinicians of how they could have their cake and eat it too—both embracing (even championing) the statistical challenge to concepts of women's fragility, while supporting clinicians' role in the management of what was now being defined as a troublesome, but not dangerous, time of life. The work of splitting morbidity and mortality in French medical thought of the nineteenth century was importantly elaborated in relation to women's reproductive ageing.

In one sense, Châteauneuf's work here appears as just one of an entire genre of French medical works of the early nineteenth century which insisted on an anti-pathological view of menopause based on the discovery that men were more vulnerable to death after the age of 50 than were women, at the same time as it prescribed special hygiene for women at this time of life. The Paris faculty candidate Antoine Constant Saucerotte (1805–1884) was another who was quick to seize on existing population data, reproducing similar tables of mortality in his 1823 pre-doctoral work aimed at debunking the idea that women's cessation of menses represented a particularly dangerous time. Its title alone speaks to the anti-pathological view of menopause, referring to 'l'âge prétendu critique' (the ostensibly critical age).[115] The population mortality evidence, on the contrary, Saucerotte argued, suggested that it was men who were the more fragile sex in the period considered a 'critical age'. From the mid-nineteenth century, many

[113] Behar, 'Le Pasteur Jean-Louis Muret', 612. [114] Rusnock, *Vital Accounts*, 157–175.

[115] Antoine Constant Saucerotte, *Nouveaux conseils aux femmes sur l'âge prétendu critique, ou conduite à tenir lors de la cessation des règles* (Paris: Madame Auger-Méquinon, 1828).

menopause doctors now followed this pattern of explanation, taking inspiration from the fact of women's greater longevity to insist on the anti-pathological view of menopause and thus rejecting the idea that women even had a 'critical age' at all. But rather than concluding that menopause was therefore not something that required medical treatment—a reasonable conclusion that many people today consider valid—they proposed that the matter demonstrated older women's need for the newly designated discipline of *l'hygiène* which scholars at the Montpellier, Paris, and Strasbourg faculties were now elaborating. Despite his debunking of the idea of menopause as a dangerous time on population statistical grounds, Saucerotte's work nonetheless insisted on the importance of hygiene for women's ageing. In so doing he referred to and honoured the work of the Paris physician Claude Lachaise (1797–1881) and his philosophy of medicine:

> It is high time to persuade the public to appreciate its own true interests and regard hygiene as one of the forms of knowledge required for a good education: It is more important for the art of conserving one's health than the observation of what is happening with Jupiter or Uranus.[116]

Here we might detect a subtle barb directed at those who considered the lifespan cycles to follow the cycle of the planets which underlay the notion of 'climacteric years', but we might also wonder if it was not a criticism of the very mathematical-astronomer statisticians of the previous 150 years, such as Kersseboom, Wargentin, and Deparcieux, who had actually discovered women's greater life expectancy—in Deparcieux's case, this involved not only taking this fact to show that the end of menses was not pathological, but also not admitting any role for physicians in its treatment. Hygiene, on the other hand, in the model of Saucerotte and others, recuperated the role of the physician in the management of women's ageing, despite the absence of data to support a view of them as more fragile than men.

Lachaise, who clearly inspired Châteauneuf, had devoted a section of his 1822 *Medical Topography of Paris* to the apparent inequality of the sexes in their vulnerability to mortality at all ages. He noted the complexities of deducing such matters without vast amounts of data due to random events that could impact the ratio of men to women in any given time-frame in specific local contexts. He cited two examples of such confounding events: harsh and cold winters which he considered likely to impact women and infants more than adult men; and military conflicts which, in his view, clearly dented the adult male population disproportionately.[117] He noted that Paris women aged between 20 and 25 years had

[116] Ibid., 6.

[117] Claude Lachaise, *Topographie médicale de Paris ou Examen général des causes qui peuvent avoir une influence marquée sur la santé des habitans de cette ville, le caractère de leurs maladies, et le choix des précautions hygiéniques qui leur sont applicables* (Paris: J. B. Baillère, 1822), 215–216.

higher mortality than men of the same age, but remarked also that men's mortality was strikingly higher in this age band than in the previous two, from 10 to 15 and from 15 to 20 years. He speculated that in their twenties, young men were filled with 'a new vigour but lacking the break upon it that comes later with the development of reason and of experience' were thus 'driven by nature toward pleasure' but inclined to abuse its forces, thus succumbing 'to their own excesses'.[118] Lachaise himself was precisely 25 years old when he wrote this, perhaps assuring himself of his newly acquired wisdom. But he did not make explicit what he considered the likely mechanism of death among 20–25-year-old men, merely alluding poetically to its underlying universal cause. This left the reader to choose from among a number of health risks widely recognised at this time: Infectious diseases, including syphilis, drunken brawls with other men, or perhaps that other common practice condemned as being bad for one's health according to the Swiss physician Samuel Tissot: masturbation.[119] Lachaise noted the higher male mortality in all the decades beyond 30 years both in his data and in that of Châteauneuf, but appeared to find this unsurprising: 'Women are found in the tranquillity of domestic life' and enjoyed a level of social protection which men lacked.[120] He too made what was fast becoming an obligatory statement about women's mortality and its implications for concepts of a 'critical age' or menopause: he noted that the 'era of cessation of the menstrual flow' was associated with no particular spike in mortality, 'permitting one to judge exaggerated the unfavourable circumstances ordinarily assumed to apply to women of this age'.[121]

Lachaise also leveraged sex differences in mortality towards another battle in which he was engaged with rival physicians both past and present. He rejected the view which he attributed to the eighteenth-century *savant* Raynal, that regular arduous physical activity preserved the lifespan.[122] This was nothing but a convenient fiction, Lachaise thought, through which elites condescended to reassure the fatigued masses who spent their whole lives in backbreaking labour. Here he leaned upon the claims of the physician Charles Londe, whose 1821 introduction to *Medical Gymnastics* had argued that vigorous and repetitive movements exhausted the vital force, causing early death, a stress against which the comforts of civilisation were protective.[123] The proof of this, Lachaise thought, was surely the fact that women everywhere significantly outlived men in the ages above

[118] Lachaise, *Topographie médicale de Paris*, 214.

[119] See Thomas W. Laqueur, *Solitary Sex: A Cultural History of Masturbation* (New York: Zone Books, 2003), 39–95.

[120] Lachaise, *Topographie médicale de Paris*, 223–224. [121] Ibid., 225.

[122] Ibid., 233. This was probably the historian and traveller Guillaume-Thomas Raynal (1713–1796), author of the multi-volume *Histoire philosophique et politique des établissemens et du commerce des Européens dans les deux Indes*, 6 vols (Geneva: Jean-Leonard Pellet, 1780).

[123] Lachaise, *Topographie médicale de Paris*, 233; Charles Londe, *Gymnastique médicale, ou l'exercice appliqué aux organes de l'homme, d'après les lois de la physiologie, de l'hygiène et de la thérapeutique* (Paris: Crouillebois, 1821).

60 years, and since women do no tiresome physical work, clearly its complete avoidance was better for the preservation of the lifespan.[124] The young Lachaise, as his reviewers had observed, was himself so contained within the bubble of Parisian bourgeois society as not to realise that his presumed norm of physical inactivity among older women contradicted the constant demands for labour among the vast majority of people of all ages and sexes in this era, located as they were in subsistence farming lifeways.

The next earliest scholars to refer to refer to women's longevity advantage in discussion of the cessation of menses did so only obliquely, without specific reference to population statistical data. Jacques Devers's Paris thesis of 1822 remarked that menopause made women more like men both in refining their character and in making them susceptible to the same kinds of diseases, in contrast to their youth when they were more distinct in their morbidity patterns and in their looks.[125] Once there was no more menstruation, he claimed, women acquired 'an inexhaustible fund of life' and were 'less subject than men to the infirmities of old age', even becoming more beautiful in some cases on account of the improved vitality they acquired. This was evidence, Devers thought, that the fertile uterus created a huge 'energy deficit' in women's bodies, and with the cessation of its functions, they benefited from a new 'force of vitality'.[126] Other scholars, such as the Strasbourg candidate Poirson in 1827, dismissed eighteenth-century ideas about dangerous cancers being more common in women after menopause, arguing that most of those found in older women had originated many years earlier and only later became painful or detectable.[127]

One of the earliest doctoral students to pick up on the idea of using statistical evidence to defend the need for medical treatment of women's ageing morbidity—counterpoised to their low mortality risk—was the Paris candidate Duplessis in 1828. He seized on Châteauneuf's argument that the dangers of menopause had been exaggerated by previous and popular medicine and were not supported by mortality statistics, while focusing his entire thesis on the 'hygienic care that women demand at this time'.[128] The Lyon candidate Pétrequin, on the other hand, only referred to mortality in his 1836 thesis on menstruation in the form of a quip in which he proposed that the lifespan of 'woman' was actually a mere twenty-five years from puberty to menopause (assuming the reproductive age as between 15 and 40 years) after which 'she ceases to be one'.[129] The Montpellier candidate

124 Lachaise, *Topographie médicale de Paris*, 233–234.

125 Jacques Devers, *Essai sur la cessation des règles*. Thèse (Paris: Didot le Jeune, 1822), 9.

126 Ibid., 10.

127 Hubert Quirin Franklin Poirson, *Dissertation sur la ménespausie*. Thèse (Strasbourg: F. G. Levrault, 1827), 7.

128 E. Duplessis, *De l'âge critique et des soins hygiéniques que réclament les femmes à cette époque* (Paris: Didot Jeune, 1828), 8.

129 Joseph-Pierre-Éléonor Pétrequin, *Recherches sur la menstruation*. Thèse (Paris: Didot le Jeune, 1836), 13.

Joseph-Hortense Houlès took the matter more seriously again in 1843, describing a different relationship to ageing between the sexes throughout the lifespan: women matured more rapidly, and while both sexes experienced an 'âge de retour' around 50 years, women lost their charms and energy before men, but men's vitality fell 'rapidly into ruins' after this, making their march towards death faster.[130] Nonetheless, his entire thesis was about the hygiene women needed in the time of menopause.

One reason for the revival of the mortality question in doctoral theses after 1840 was that it had been well integrated into Paris medical pedagogy by this time and cited by several eminent pedagogic figures: the Paris professor of medicine Marc Colombat de l'Isère (1797–1851) raised the matter in his *Treatise on the Diseases of Women* in 1838, referring to the statistical evidence of both Murat and Châteauneuf as an indication that the 'critical age' was not a dangerous time for women.[131] He also confirmed Châteauneuf's view that women's longevity advantage did not mean that one could afford to ignore the critical age which required specific hygienic regimes. And he cited the now widely claimed 'fact' that peasant women aged better than their elite urban counterparts as the sign that only correct hygiene could confer the natural longevity advantage for city women.[132] The major figures of hygiene at the Paris faculty, Michel Lévy (1809–1872) and Louis Alfred Becquerel (1814–1862), also made a point of women's greater longevity in their works of public and private hygiene published in the 1840s and 1850s.[133]

Another key figure in Paris medical pedagogy to discuss the mortality statistics of Muret, Châteauneuf, Lachaise, Saucerotte, and Finlaison was the clinical head at the Paris faculty, Adam Raciborski (1809–1871). In his 1844 book on women's physiology *From Puberty to the Critical Age*, he remarked that it was uncontroversial that women held the longevity advantage over men, although he repeated the claim that breast cancer was most common in women around the time of menopause.[134] The mature Paris clinician and author of several books about women's health, ageing, and longevity Sébastien Guyétant (1777–1865) also discussed sex-differentiated mortality statistics in all of his various works published between 1836 and 1870.[135] 'The time of the cessation of the menstrual flux is not

[130] Joseph-Hortense Houlès, *De la ménopause considérée au point de vue de l'hygiène*. Thèse (Montpellier: Isadore Tournel, 1843), 6–7.

[131] Marc Colombat de l'Isère, *Traité des maladies des femmes et de l'hygiène spéciale de leur sexe*, 2 vols (Paris: Labé, 1838), vol. 1, 58.

[132] Ibid., 59.

[133] Michel Lévy, *Traité d'hygiène publique et privée*, 2 vols (Paris: J.-B. Baillière et fils, 1844–1845), vol. 2, 491; Louis Alfred Becquerel, *Traité élémentaire d'hygiène privée et publique* (Paris: Labé, 1851), 575, 634–635.

[134] Adam Raciborski, *De la puberté et de l'âge critique chez la femme, au point de vue physiologique, hygiénique et médical* (Paris: J. B. Baillière 1844), 347–348, 343.

[135] Sébastien Guyétant, *Le Médecin de l'âge de retour et la vieillesse: Conseils aux gens du monde, qui ont passé l'âge de quarante-cinq ans* (Paris: Dufey, 1836), 73–75; Sébastien Guyétant, *Nouvelles considérations sur la longévité humaine* (Paris: Chez l'auteur, 1863), 83.

as lethal as is commonly believed and does not deserve to inspire so much fear,' he proclaimed in his posthumously published 1870 book on the 'âge de retour' and old age addressed to 'upper-class people' ('les gens du monde'). 'All the same,' he said, 'we approve of women voluntarily taking precautions at this time to preserve their health and augment their chances of longevity.'[136] Guyétant differed from many doctors of women's health writing about their ageing in that he also prescribed an elaborate regime of hygienic practices to men over the age of 50 years.[137] Nonetheless, he still reduced women's ageing to the cessation of menses while insisting that it was the moment when their hygienic focus should begin: 'Man and woman... walk unevenly [*à pas inégaux*] toward old age, and one [*l'une*] arrives there much earlier than the other.'[138]

French demographers of the mid-nineteenth century continued to gather further data supporting claims about women's higher life expectancy which was again leveraged to propose that older women were more resilient than men, but only if they lived according to the rules of *hygiène*. Louis Noirot's 1850 study of the lifespan of the population of greater Dijon, some '24,500 souls,' was widely cited in French medical works about sex-differentiated ageing after this time.[139] His corrective to supposedly prevailing assumptions about the vulnerability of older women was poignantly argued on the basis of his data on the Dijonnais, who he said were renowned for their longevity and healthy lifeways. Noirot saw the hygienic model of menopause care that had already established itself in French medical practice as excessively prescriptive and in need of modification in response to the scientific data, remarking that: 'Statistics provide useful support for hygiene, giving mathematical sanction to its precepts, formulating its results, and indicating the direction in which its efforts should be especially exerted.'[140] Whatever doctors might believe about women's ageing on the basis of casual observations and popular hearsay, the numbers did not lie.

Noirot repeated the argument made by Deparcieux in the 1740s that the high level of infant mortality prior to the nineteenth century massively skewed overall life expectancy, provoking the belief that few people lived beyond the age of 35 before recent times.[141] Populations with low life expectancy due to high infant mortality could nonetheless have many elderly individuals.[142] In his statistical tables, he was able to show clearly that life expectancy had improved among the Dijonnais during the nineteenth century. He proposed that this was due variously to the increased prosperity of the lower classes, improved infant survival due to advances in medical knowledge, the spread of hygienic understanding among the

[136] Sébastien Guyétant, *L'âge de retour et la vieillesse: Conseils au gens du monde* (Paris: L. Brunet, 1870), 56.
[137] Ibid., 28–50. [138] Ibid., 79.
[139] Louis Noirot, *Études statistiques sur la mortalité et la durée de la vie dans la ville et l'arrondissement de Dijon depuis le 19e siècle jusqu'à nos jours* (Paris: J. Baillière, 1850), 12.
[140] Ibid., 2. [141] Ibid., 7. [142] Ibid., 22.

population, and more salubrious and better ventilated housing. And he predicted that the recent improvements in urban sanitation—in particular the provision of fresh, public fountains fed by spring water from 1840, and the channelling of clean water in the mid-1840s from the river Suzon, replacing an open sewer running through the city into a tiled and covered aqueduct—would further increase local lifespans.[143]

In the introduction to his study, Noirot alluded to the revelation in his data that sex distinction was one of the circumstances that 'leads to a large difference in longevity'.[144] But it was in the fourth chapter of this work that he elaborated his statistical corrective to the view of women as the more fragile sex. Noirot, like other demographers throughout Europe, had found both higher male birth-rates and death-rates across all ages in the period of his study, including even the reproductive years when women's mortality peaked relatively due to deaths in childbirth. Consequently, there were fewer men than women in the overall adult population, and far higher numbers of women than men among the Dijonnais octogenarians and nonagenarians (744 vs 428), with only a single man among the eight recorded centenarians. 'Vainly,' he noted, 'have we searched to explain this phenomenon in depicting the life of men as "stormier, more subject to the influence of destructive agents, charged with tiring labours, stimulated by political passions, the victims of the vicissitudes of war, of all kinds of dangers".' Noirot considered that there was proof of something inherent to physiological sex differences at stake in the evidence from monasteries. Here, priests leading peaceful, protected, and entirely non-combatant lives identical to those of nuns nonetheless all died younger than their female counterparts.[145] In fact, with the risk of childbirth removed in the study of nuns, who constituted an ideal childless female population for the purposes of calculating natural female life expectancy without this single greatest risk to their survival, their longevity advantage appeared even starker.

By 1850, the mention of women's advantage in mortality statistics had become obligatory for specialist scholars writing about menopause where it performed the role of confirming their scientifically informed biomedical professional identity through the correction of supposedly ancient and popular ideas about menopause as a dangerous time. At the same time, it posed no obstacle to the elaboration of hygienic prescriptions on which women's health in ageing was said to depend. The Paris candidate Louis Chandelux heavily stressed this in his 1850 thesis, titling a chapter with the rhetorical question: 'Is the age of menopause a perilous time in the lives of women?' He claimed that this was a 'popular' (*vulgaire*) opinion which scientific medicine had debunked (citing Moreau de la Sarthe, Saucerotte, Lachaise, Finlaison, Brierre de Boismont, and Raciborski) but

[143] Ibid., 24–32. [144] Ibid., 4. [145] Ibid., 39–40.

which nonetheless haunted and frightened women who continued to imagine menopause as a 'fatal moment'.[146] In 1859, the Paris candidate Gustave Plihon referred to menopause health as a topic of continuing medical controversy, while acknowledging that mortality data had consistently revealed the age from 45 to 55 years as less dangerous for women than for men.[147] Menopause was thus 'not a disease, but a state that renders one apt to contract numerous diseases'.[148] Another Paris student, Bernard Puyo, in 1865 discussed the mortality data of Muret, Benoiston de Châteauneuf, and Lachaise, noting that menopause did not increase women's risk of death. Nonetheless, it was a 'physiological fact' that exposed women 'to a thousand dangers' if they did not place their trust in doctors and observe hygienic prescriptions.[149]

The mature Montpellier professor of medicine Émile Bertin reinvigorated the question of how the end of fertility and menstruation impacted the vital force of women's economy in his 1866 book on the hygiene of menopause, asking 'Does menopause change... the vital mode of women and thus create new physiological conditions and new morbid aptitudes', or could it 'on the contrary, heal afflictions that have been resistant...?'[150] He cited the work of earlier demographers from France, Switzerland, England, and the German lands, nonetheless warning against too much optimism about women's ageing from this population data.[151] He even included his own mortality table comparing sex differences without saying from whence this data derived or to which populations it referred. This was similar to other population tables of the time and showed men's mortality to be higher than women's at all ages. But Bertin interpreted as significant the fact that more women died after 50 years than between 40 and 50 years, which he said indicated that menopause was still a somewhat dangerous time requiring observation of the array of hygienic prescriptions on which his book focused.[152] The utility of citing the demographic fact of women's longevity persisted into the 1870s: the Paris candidate Victor Force noted in his 1877 thesis that menopause was 'popularly known as a critical time, an *âge de retour*, a turn of age', but medicine knew better from the mortality data. Nonetheless, menopause was 'an important fact in the economy of woman' and often resulted in numerous infirmities.[153]

[146] Louis Chandelux, *L'Âge critique de la femme (ménopause)*. Thèse (Paris: Irgnoux, 1850), 20–21.
[147] Gustave-Adolphe Plihon, *De la ménopause (âge critique)*. Thèse (Paris: Rignoux, 1859), 5.
[148] Ibid., 6.
[149] Bernard-Grégoire-Émile Puyo, *La Ménopause*. Thèse (Paris: A Parent, 1865), 5.
[150] Émile Bertin, *De la ménopause considérée principalement au point de vue de l'hygiène* (Montpellier: C. Coulet/Paris: Adrien Delahaye, 1866), 87.
[151] Ibid., 62, 119–120. [152] Ibid., 125–126.
[153] Victor Force, *Du Rhumatisme à la ménopause*. Thèse (Paris: A. Parent, 1877), 6.

French Medicine in a Global Context

The news of women's higher life expectancy certainly spread throughout European cultures, but the notion that women nonetheless needed medical care for the menopause transition was slow to gain traction outside France. An American work published around the same time as Lachaise's *Hygiène physiologique* was that of the renowned Philadelphia obstetrician William Potts Dewees *On the Diseases of Females* of 1826.[154] Dewees was an adjunct professor of midwifery at the University of Pennsylvania when he wrote this work (which appeared in multiple editions throughout the nineteenth century) and he held the chair in obstetrics there from 1834 to 1841. This work lacked several of the key features of Lachaise's approach—both the division of a woman's life into highly distinct phases, and recommendations for the hygienic management of normal female ageing. It was a work devoted almost entirely to pathologies of the female reproductive system in relation to menstruation and childbirth. What Potts-Dewes had to say about the cessation of menses was brief and of a similar character to what the English physician John Fothergill had written in the previous century—that is, to remark that the cessation of menstrual flow around the age of 50 was non-pathological and should therefore not be medicated; that some women, particularly those living a life of 'idleness', were prone to dreadful symptoms during the transition towards the complete cessation of menstruation; and that women approaching menopause were inclined to worry if their period became lighter or less regular but should be dissuaded from the erroneous belief that the blood was noxious and would cause disease if not expelled.[155] This work referred to none of the considerable French scholarship on the subject of women's 'critical age' that had appeared over the previous twenty-seven years, except for a brief mention of Gardanne (mistaking him for the obstetrician Gardien), suggesting that Dewees even here was referring to the French scholarship via a second-hand source.[156] But he did include a footnote referring to the population tables cited so frequently in French medical writing on menopause, and Dewees considered this important evidence against an approach to older women that assumed their routine need for medical treatment.[157] His hygienic recommendations focused largely on physical activity, and appeared to apply only to women who complained of symptoms around the time of their menses ending. French hygiene for older women was clearly not spreading to the USA in this period, even as news of women's greater life expectancy certainly did.

One the other hand, the English physician Edward Tilt, referring to the actuary work of John Finlaison, mentioned the fact of 'longevity being attained more

[154] William Potts Dewees, *Treatise on the Disease of Females* (Philadelphia: H. C. Carey & I. Lea, 1826).
[155] Ibid., 92–94. [156] Ibid., 92. [157] Ibid., 94 footnote.

frequently by women than by men' in the 1870 third edition of the *Change of Life* treatise, first published in 1856.[158] But he objected to the uses made of this fact by the French-speaking demographers Châteauneuf and Odier when they concluded that it meant there was therefore no need for doctors to fuss over women around the time of their end of menstruation, or to characterise the end of menses as a dangerous time of life.[159] Tilt viewed this as an 'erroneous interpretation of statistics', since these authors equated the 'critical period' with fatality. While menopause was not a more fatal moment, Tilt argued, it was nonetheless a moment of health crisis, requiring medical care. This was the clearest statement yet in English sources of the split between morbidity and mortality in relation to treatment of older women.

The first German specialist work on menopause by the Austrian gynaecologist Enoch Kisch in 1874 also cited the work of Muret, Deparcieux, Châteauneuf, Lachaise, and Saucerotte as scholars who had all debunked the notion of women's critical age as a dangerous time, and showed through demographic statistics, that it was instead men who were more likely to die around the age of 50.[160] Kisch too produced his own table showing the mortality of men and women between the ages of 30 and 60 in both five- and ten-year age bands, comparing Sweden, England, Belgium, the Netherlands, Bavaria, and giving the average of them all. In all of these places, women mostly survived in slightly greater numbers than men in every age band.[161] Nonetheless, Kisch, like Tilt and like the many French doctors before them all whom we consider in Chapter 5, advised women to practice 'hygiene' in the climacteric age: he recommended gentle purgative treatments to relieve plethora and avoid constipation, observation of a strict diet and exercise programme, and avoidance of all mental strain and emotional disturbance.[162] The split between morbidity and mortality that had been produced through the French assimilation of women's greater longevity within the hygienic medicalisation of women's ageing and cessation of menses was indeed now becoming disseminated on a transnational scale.

[158] Edward John Tilt, *The Change of Life in Health and Disease: A Practical Treatise on the Nervous and Other Affections Incidental to Women at the Decline of Life* [1857], 3rd ed. (London: J. Churchill, 1870), 9.

[159] Ibid., 2–3.

[160] Enoch Heinrich Kisch, *Das klimakterische Alter der Frauen in physiologischer und pathologischer Beziehung* (Erlangen: Ferdinand Enke, 1874), 72, 76–77.

[161] Ibid., 73. [162] Ibid., 171–173.

3
Crises, Critical Ages, and the 'Invention' of *la Ménopause*, c.1770–1812

Throughout the nineteenth-century efflorescence of the complete concept of menopause, references to it as a 'critical time' were ubiquitous, sometimes in rejecting this term as over-pathologising, though more often reclaiming it as justifying an appropriate insistence on the prescription of hygienic advice and on women's medical surveillance in ageing. Menopause retained a strong continuity with the earlier, non-sex-specific concepts of critical periods, which referred to ancient Ptolemaic hebdomal climacteric cycles of health vulnerability that recurred every seven years, the worst junctures being the seventh septenary (age 49) and the great climacteric (age 63).[1] And certainly, hebdomal divisions of the lifespan persisted in later medical works that elaborated on menopause, with the age of 49, as the seventh septenary, most frequently invoked. In a highly generative article published in 2015, Christine Théré locates late eighteenth-century naturalist contributions as important in this development, showing that scholars such as Louis-Jean-Marie Daubenton, Denis Diderot, Jean-Noël Hallé, and Jean-Claude de La Métherie reanimated the notion of lifespan crises while largely maintaining existing non-sex-specific concepts of ageing based on either the Ptolemaic septenary climacterics or on the four ages of Isadore de Seville: it was not here that the concepts of menstrual cessation and of lifespan climacterics were fused.[2] As we saw in Chapter 1, the fusion had already to some degree been suggested by German and Dutch scholars writing in Latin between 1700 and 1780, who assimilated the final cessation of menses to the larger medical concern with suppressed menses in young women, referring to both as a critical time of hysteria, vapours, or hypochondria, and redefining all matters relating to absent menstruation as signs of climacteric crisis.

As Théré remarks, several important French figures contributed in only brief and fragmentary ways to this emerging association. Notable among them is the Aquitaine-born and Montpellier-trained, Parisian medical writer and journalist Pierre Roussel (1742–1802), author of a tremendously successful 1775 *Système*

[1] Max Engammare, *Soixante-trois: La Peur de la grande année climactérique à la Renaissance* (Geneva: Droz, 2013); Daniel Schäfer, *Old Age and Disease in Early Modern Medicine*, trans. Patrick Baker (London: Routledge, 2015).

[2] Christine Théré, 'Âge de retour et retour d'âge: L'Asymétrie entre les sexes dans les discours médicaux en France (1770–1836)', *CLIO: Femmes, genre, histoire*, 42 (2015): 54–75 [56–60].

The French Invention of Menopause and the Medicalisation of Women's Ageing: A History. Alison M. Downham Moore, Oxford University Press. © Alison M. Downham Moore 2022. DOI: 10.1093/oso/9780192842916.003.0004

physique et moral de la femme (Moral and Physical System of Woman), which sharply differentiated the biology and psychology of the sexes, with significant effects on subsequent French medical accounts of sex-differentiated ageing.[3] This was a work published in eight French editions between 1795 and 1869, and by 1786 it had already had been translated into German, with an Italian translation following in 1829 (in turn released in several editions throughout the nineteenth century), and a Spanish translation in 1851.[4] Medical historian Anne Vila describes it as a 'watershed publication', which synthesised the development of medical ideas about sensibility in the work of Pierre-Jean-George Cabanis, Claude-Adrien Helvétius, and others, making nervous function the basis for a new anthropology of the sexes.[5] Also, as Elizabeth Williams notes, this important work linked the vitalist and mechanist approaches of both Stahl and Boerhaave to the attempts by the Montpellier doctors to revolutionise medicine by making it more sex-, age-, temperament-, and climate-specific.[6] Roussel certainly adapted the prevalent eighteenth-century concept of *sensibilité* to the new iatromechanist and materialist thrust of biomedicine, relocating it as inscribed in women's biology—not alterable by education.[7] Unlike Astruc, Roussel adamantly insisted on the universal regularity of the menstrual cycle from the age of 14 to the age of 45 or 50, and viewed it as an undeniable indicator of a woman's health; and though he too noted the ethnographic reports of Léry and others indicating wide variability across cultures, he insisted that neither cultural differences nor the cycles of the moon were factors in menstruation—instead it was a fundamental matter of the 'animal economy'.[8] Roussel also suggested that Astruc and others had overlooked the importance of the organs themselves in regulating women's bodies, and that plethora alone could not explain all the complexities of menstruation.[9] Nonetheless, he too conceded that country women had less abundant menstruation compared to women who engaged in the 'vices of high society' ('les vices de

[3] Pierre Roussel, *Système physique et moral de la femme* (Paris: Chez Vincent, 1775).

[4] Pierre Roussel, *Physiologie des weiblichen Geschlechtes*, trans. C. F. Michaelis (Berlin: Weissenfels, 1786); Pierre Roussel, *Sistema fisico e morale della donna*, 2 vols (Naples: Raffaelle Manzi, 1829); Pierre Roussel, *Sistema fisico y moral de la mujer* (Barcelona: D. A. Gaspar, 1851).

[5] Anne C. Vila, 'Sex and Sensibility: Pierre Rousseau's *Système physique et moral de la femme*', *Representations*, 52 (1995): 76–93. See also Kathleen Anne Wellman, 'Physicians and Philosophes: Physiology and Sexual Morality in the French Enlightenment', *Eighteenth-Century Studies*, 35/2 (2002): 267–277; and Anne C. Vila, 'Visceralism and the Superior Mind in French Medicine and Literature, 1750–1850', in Manon Mathias & Alison M. Moore, eds, *Gut Feeling and Digestive Health in Nineteenth-Century Literature, History and Culture* (New York: Palgrave, 2018), 133–154.

[6] Roussel, *Système physique et moral*, 182, Elizabeth A. Williams, *The Physical and the Moral: Anthropology, Physiology, and Philosophical Medicine in France, 1750–1850* (Cambridge: Cambridge University Press, 1994), 55–58.

[7] Sean M. Quinlan, *The Great Nation in Decline: Sex, Modernity and Health Crises in Revolutionary France, c.1750–1850* (Aldershot: Ashgate, 2007), 47–49.

[8] Roussel, *Système physique et moral*, 178–180, 196. On the concept of 'animal economy', see Charles T. Wolfe & Motoichi Terada, 'The Animal Economy as Object and Program in Montpellier Vitalism', *Science in Context*, 21/4 (2008): 537–579.

[9] Roussel, *Système physique et moral*, 206.

grandes sociétés'), and that both a lack of exercise and an overabundance of poor-quality food explained most of the bodily ills from which elite women suffered at all ages.[10] He also suggested something like a proto-evolutionary account of menstruation, suggesting that humans had not always required it but had adapted to it over history, though for what reason he did not wager a guess.[11]

Indeed, the long-range impact of Roussel's influence on the development of ideas about women's reproductive physiology can be seen rippling through some of the key debates in the rapid coherence of the complete concept of menopause that occurred between the 1790s and 1812 through the contest played out between Montpellier and Paris doctoral students. The plethora model of menstruation found in the first Latin theses under Stahl during the first half of the eighteenth century had allowed limited potential for the elaboration of the final cessation of menses as a distinct pathological state, since all older people were thought to suffer plethora anyway, and the associated symptoms, such as gout, were not even more common in women. But the purely iatrochemical model proposed by Daniel Duncan had also allowed limited scope for the medicalisation of women's final cessation of menses. On the other hand, the increasing emphasis on women's nervous physiology proved tremendously generative for two strands of thought in nineteenth-century menopause medicine: first, the view that the uterus, by virtue of its 'sympathy' with nerves in other parts of the body, could generate symptoms of a spectacular variety of different kinds, effectively encompassing any complaint of older women, either physical or psychological; second, the view that, as the more nervous sex, women in ageing were necessarily affected by nervous disorders such as hysteria, vapours or hypochondria, or—after the 1840s—degenerate madness and erotomania. Roussel in fact said nothing about women's cessation of menses, and specified that women's *vieillesse* did not even begin immediately from the moment they could no longer conceive. But he considered women to begin ageing earlier than men, since they reached puberty earlier, and considered their dread of losing their beauty in old age (*not* their end of menses, *pace* Stolberg) to be 'l'enfer des femmes' ('women's hell').[12] In elaborating a view of menstruation as definitive of femininity, Roussel implied its cessation to be also a loss of women's particularity and sensibility, as well as a form of degeneration to an earlier stage of the historical development of humanity before the sexes had differentiated. He was undoubtedly read this way by subsequent medical writers on the topic of menopause. Roussel's work thus proved tremendously generative for the development of medical and psychiatric ideas about sex differences and ageing in general throughout the nineteenth century.[13]

[10] Ibid., 189–196, 204. [11] Ibid., 202. [12] Ibid., 84–85.

[13] Nicoletta Diasio, 'Maillage des temps et gouvernement des corps dans la construction des rapports d'âge et de genre', *SociologieS: Dossiers, genre et vieillissement* (2012): <http://journals.openedition.org/sociologies/4118>; Cécile Charlap, *La Fabrique de la ménopause* (Paris: Publications CNRS, 2019), 51.

Another figure whose ideas clearly had a tremendous influence on the emergence of hygienic concepts of sex differences in ageing in both Paris and Montpellier, without himself having much to say about menopause, was the renowned medical scholar Pierre-Jean-Georges Cabanis (1757–1808), raised in the Limousin but trained in Paris.[14] Indeed, philosophy scholar Rose Goetz proposes that Cabanis opened an entirely new horizon of the 'sciences of ageing', while the feminist scholar Nicole Mosconi attributes the origin of modern sexist ideas about women's cognitive capacities to Cabanis's account of feminine weakness.[15] On the one hand, in his 1802 *Rapports du physique et du moral de l'homme* (Relation of the Physical to the Moral in Man), Cabanis conveyed the early modern Ptolemaic concept of climacteric ages in septenary junctures, claiming that both men and women suffered a 'critical age' around 49 or 50, which coincided for women with the cessation of menses, but was nonetheless a dangerous time for men too.[16] On the other hand, here he defined the cessation of reproductive capacities as a fundamental shift in the function of the organism akin to that which occurred in puberty: 'The individual enters a new order of things when he loses the capacity to reproduce, just as when he acquired it.' But these phases were particularly 'marked' in women, while gradual and even in men, hence the post-reproductive passage of women brought 'painful turns' ('retours pénibles').[17]

And yet none of these influential scholars can entirely help us explain the emergence of the increased attention given to the final cessation of menses after the 1770s, when numerous French medical scholars in both the Paris and Montpellier medical faculties began converging on the insistence of the need for greater differentiation in the treatment of different types of people, specifically with reference to the sexes in ageing. Indeed, by the time Cabanis was writing about older women's *retours pénibles*, there were already several specialist works on women's 'critical age' produced by doctoral students at the University of Montpellier; and even before them, a number of influential works on the diseases of women began differentiating women's ageing from men's, producing an emphasis on the need for medical surveillance of older women. The 1771 popular medical guide *Le Médecin des dames* by the Paris medical professor and Encyclopedist Jean Goulin (1728–1799) already showed signs of moving in this

[14] Noted also by Annick Tillier, 'Un âge critique: La Ménopause sous le regard des médecins des XVIIIe et XIXe siècles', *CLIO: Femmes, genre, histoire*, 21 (2005): 268–280.

[15] Rose Goetz, 'Les Âges de la vie dans les rapports du physique et du moral de l'homme de Pierre-Jean-Georges Cabanis', *Le portiQue: Revue de philosophie et de sciences humaines*, 21 (2008). Doi: 10.4000/leportique.1713; Nicole Mosconi, 'Aux sources du sexisme contemporain: Cabanis et la faiblesse des femmes', *Le Télémaque*, 39 (2011): 115–130.

[16] Pierre-Jean-Georges Cabanis, *Rapports du physique et du moral de l'homme: Cinquième mémoire: De l'influence des sexes sur le caractère des idées et des affections morales* [1802], *Œuvres complètes de Cabanis* (Paris: Bossanges Frères/Firmin Didot), vol. 4, 477–482.

[17] Ibid., 481.

direction.[18] Goulin celebrated the increasing popularisation of medical knowledge to which he himself contributed, noting its particular benefits for educated women who could now understand their own bodies without risk of offence to their *pudeur*.[19] He claimed that ageing brought changes to the temperament, as well as in employment and ways of living, making adjustments necessary in each of the five stages of life: childhood, adolescence, puberty, virility, and caducity (also calling this last stage the 'advanced age' and the 'decrepit age').[20] He referred only vaguely to 'the cessation of the faculties' in women, presumably implying menstruation and fertility, and emphasised that one's health in this age depended upon 'the life one has led and the abuse one has committed upon one's temperament' up until that time, particularly with reference to the damaging effects of 'uncontrolled passions' ('passions déréglées').[21] He considered women who did not menstruate to be most prone to rheumatism due to an abundance of blood (plethora), particularly if they were 'too sedentary'.[22] However, most of his discussion of women's ageing related to gout, which he acknowledged was more common in men, but from which he considered women could suffer too in old age (if they did not regulate their passions). Referring to what was now quite an old-fashioned humoral concept, he proposed that the main change in ageing was 'the loss of natural heat' requiring greater 'conservation of health'.[23] He described a particular type of catarrh to which women were prone in old age, caused by 'the suppression of some evacuations'—but these seem likely to be bowel-related, since the solution he recommended was coffee sweetened with sugar, or tobacco, which were common remedies for intestinal constipation.[24] While Goulin specifically affirmed the need to differentiate the sexes in ageing here, both the suggested theoretical grounds and the practicalities of doing so in therapeutic terms remained quite underdeveloped.

One particular English work also had an important impact in stimulating French medical ideas about women's specific ageing in the final decades of the eighteenth century: John Fothergill's short essay, and the first English work devoted to the question of the cessation of menses in older women, published as a pamphlet in 1774, and which was translated into French in 1778.[25] As Christine Théré notes, while Fothergill himself had no specific word for the final cessation of menses, his French translators assimilated his remarks about it to the terms *temps critique* and *période critique*.[26] Fothergill himself naturalised the cessation of menses as a normal life process that required no specific medical attention, so

[18] Jean Goulin, *Le Médecin des dames, ou l'art de les conserver en santé* (Paris: Chez Vincent, 1771).
[19] Ibid., v–vi. [20] Ibid., vii, 265. [21] Ibid., 265–272.
[22] Ibid., 271. [23] Ibid., 272–273. [24] Ibid., 274.
[25] John Fothergill, 'Of the Management Proper at the Cessation of the Menses', [1774] in *The Works of John Fothergill*, ed. J. Coakely Lettsom (London: Charles Dilly, 1783), 201–222.
[26] Théré, 'Âge de retour et retour d'âge', 60; John Fothergill, *Conseils pour les femmes de quarante-cinq à cinquante ans, ou conduite à tenir lors de la cessation des règles* [1778], 2nd ed. (Paris: Gabon, 1778), 19, 34.

it is ironic that his pamphlet provided fuel for the French medicalisation of menopause for over 120 years after its publication. But anti-pathological arguments in this period, as we shall see, were not always a sceptical tool for resisting medical treatment and were instead sometimes leveraged precisely to insist on a wide-ranging program of hygienic precautions and abstentions. Like the earlier French scholar Daniel Duncan, Jean Astruc in 1737, and Jean Goulin who was writing around the same time as Fothergill, the English physician emphasised that purgative medicaments should not be used to attempt to resume menstruation in women over 45–50 years, adding that such medicaments could themselves cause the very complaints of haemorrhagic bleeding of which some women complained in the 'decline of life'.[27]

The tone of Fothergill's tract, like Astruc's remarks, certainly seems to suggest that by this time at least some doctors, charlatans, folk healers, or women themselves were attempting to medicate away the final cessation of menses, through the misapplication of medical practices intended for younger women with 'untimely stoppage' which was associated both with hysteria/vapours and with infertility. From the early modern sources discussed in Chapter 1, however, it is clear that no physician advocated such a practice for older women, and indeed others before Fothergill (Freind, Duncan, and Astruc) had specifically excluded it, insisting that the age-related cessation of menses was part of the natural life course (or God's will) that should not be interfered with. Nonetheless, French doctors writing about menopause throughout the nineteenth century, particularly those trained in Paris, ubiquitously cited Fothergill in support of the implied view that the iatrogenic medication of menopause was part of ancient and folk chemical traditions that modern scientific, mechanistic biomedicine had only recently debunked. In doing so they drew not only on his perspective in their own anti-pathological insistences, but even made the anti-chemical stance a central theme of both pedagogic induction and professional identity.

Fothergill's contribution to medical thought about the cessation of menses is widely cited as one of the most important publications by most scholars who have worked on the comparative history of menopause.[28] However, the impact of his work was certainly not immediate, and it is clear from the earlier writings of Duncan and Astruc, and the contemporaneous work of Goubelly and Chambon de Montaux, that the French did not require Fothergill to give them the idea of focusing on women at this life stage. The critique of the widespread use of purgatives for all sorts of medical conditions in general was also common in French

[27] Fothergill, *Conseils pour les femmes de quarante-cinq à cinquante ans*, 204.

[28] Théré, 'Âge de retour et retour d'âge', 54–75; Louise Foxcroft, *Hot Flushes, Cold Science: A History of the Modern Menopause* (London: Granta Books, 2011), 92–120; Tillier, 'Un âge critique'; Michael Stolberg, 'Von den "Stufenjahren" zur "Menopause": Das Klimakterium im Wandel der Zeit', *Wurzburger Medizinhistorische Mitteilungen*, 24 (2005): 41–50; Joel Wilbush, 'Menorraghia and Menopause: A Historical Review', *Maturitas*, 10 (1988): 5–26.

medicine by this time, having been subject to an oft-cited, scathing Latin book about the question as early as 1714 by the Reims physician Philippe Hecquet, Dean of the Paris Faculty of Medicine in the early eighteenth century.[29] But by focusing on Fothergill's version of the purgative objection, the new Parisian scholars writing about women's critical age after 1802 could sustain the rejection of earlier figures such as Astruc and Duncan, who represented styles of medicine now considered old-fashioned: Duncan because he gave Catholic religious grounds for his analysis of women's physiology, and Astruc because he was vitalist and humoralist in ways the new mechanistic and materialistic focus increasingly eschewed.[30]

By 1779, the Swiss physician Samuel-Auguste Tissot was already complaining that the term *l'âge critique* applied to women's cessation of menses was inappropriate because it implied that this change was dangerous, causing women to worry unnecessarily about its approach.[31] Citing only Fothergill and none of the many earlier French authors who had explicitly naturalised the final cessation of menses, Tissot himself insisted that it generally occurred 'without any incident' ('sans aucun accident'), such that most women passed through it without even noticing it.[32] The ones to blame for the catastrophising view of women's critical age, Tissot thought, were those wedded to the 'chemical opinion' which viewed menstrual blood as venomous, poisoning the woman's body once it could not exit the body through menstrual flow. This view was not found among the ancients, he noted, before instead bizarrely blaming it on 'the Arabs'.[33] Although some women experienced symptoms after menses ended, he acknowledged, these were not caused by self-poisoning but by plethora, or by irritation of the nerves similar to that seen in women before their periods.[34] Tissot might have been expected to better understand the Montpellier concept of critical periods, which (as we will soon show) referred not to dangerous times but to transitory healing crises: He had studied at Montpellier himself in his youth. But, as Elizabeth Williams notes, he held negative views of his teachers there, and often denigrated the faculty afterwards.[35]

Adding to growing scepticism of the 'vulgar' practice of designating women's final cessation of menses a 'critical time', a short thesis in Latin was produced in 1786 by the Paris doctoral candidate Joseph-Pierre Deslandes, which focused

[29] Philippe Hecquet, *De purgandâ medicinâ a curarum sordibus* (Paris: Chavelier, 1714); Anthelme Balhasar Baron Richerand, *Nouveaux Éléments de physiologie* (Paris: Richard, Caille et Ravier, 1812), vol. 1, 325.

[30] Elizabeth A. Williams, *A Cultural History of Medical Vitalism in Enlightenment Montpellier* (London: Routledge, 2003), 120.

[31] Noted also by Théré, 'Âge de retour et retour d'âge', 60.

[32] Samuel-Auguste Tissot, *Traité des nerfs et de leurs maladies* (Paris: Théophile Barrois le jeune, 1779), vol. 2, Partie 1, 103.

[33] Ibid., 104. [34] Ibid., 106–108.

[35] Williams, *A Cultural History of Medical Vitalism*, 60.

entirely 'On Diseases of the Cessation of the Monthly Flux'.[36] Like Fothergill (but also like Astruc), he warned against the overuse of purgative medications for menstrual stoppage, which he said not only could not cure plethora, but instead would draw copious blood back into the uterus.[37] Deslandes listed a wide variety of symptoms from which women could suffer at this time of life, including epigastric swelling, painful haemorrhoids, intestinal grumbling, constipation, fevers, vapours, hysteria, and melancholy, as well as uterine haemorrhages, polyps, and other growths.[38] He cited no other works, so it is unclear what he had read, but his thesis was remarkably similar to other Latin theses produced by German and Dutch scholars throughout the eighteenth century, beginning with Stahl's students at the Halle faculty. These works all assimilated the final age-related cessation of menses to their temporary stoppage in women of reproductive age, viewing both through the lens of the Stahlian hydraulic account of plethora. Clearly, though, Deslandes was also aware of the growing French medical discourse of the final cessation as variously troublesome according to temperament, with the worst ills of this time mainly affecting idle women of the large cities, especially 'our Paris', which, he said, was where plethora was particularly common.[39]

But not all the significant contributions to the emerging medicalisation of women's final cessation of menses came out of the University. In the 1780s and 1790s, Nicolas Chambon de Montaux (1748–1793), who was head of the Salpêtrière hospital in 1786 and briefly mayor of Paris in the winter of 1792–1793, became one of the most prolific scholars of women's health, also referring to the cessation of menses in ageing. In none of his numerous books about women's health did he mention Fothergill's pamphlet. He may well have been unaware of it, since its primary vogue was among the professors and students of the Paris faculty from the late 1790s onwards, whereas Chambon's own *licence* was earned in 1780. Chambon was highly influential in French medicine and spanned two different worlds of concepts about women's health. Like Goubelly, he shared in the widespread approach to women's health wherein both pregnancy and childbirth (with their many attendant dangers) mattered far more than all other medical questions about women (such as their end of menstruation). But he was part also of a new generation that arose in the final decades of the eighteenth century, which began to view ageing women as targets for increased medical concern. Chambon de Montaux published a work on the diseases of women in 1784, a major two-volume work on the diseases of girls in 1785, and a final work on the diseases of pregnancy to complete his trilogy on women's health also in 1785.[40] Like John Freind's work, Chambon's 1785 book on girls devoted several chapters

[36] Joseph-Pierre Deslandes, *An morborum, cessante mensium fluxu, therapeia, quae difficillema, rationali medicina duce, felicior?* (Paris: Quillau, 1786), 2.

[37] Ibid., 6. [38] Ibid., 2, 4. [39] Ibid., 2.

[40] Nicolas Chambon de Montaux, *Des maladies des femmes*, 2 vols (Paris: Rue et Hôtel Serpente, 1784); Nicolas Chambon de Montaux, *Des maladies des filles*, 2 vols (Paris: Rue et Hôtel Serpente,

to the problems related to suppressed menses. He considered this to result in putrefaction in the uterus through the accumulation of blood, leaning heavily on Hippocrates for support, while also doubting Galen's explanation of the capacity of the uterus to suffocate the visceral organs as the cause of hysterical vapours.[41] But nowhere in any of this discussion, as might be expected, were older women mentioned.

His 1784 work on women, on the other hand, had contained a section devoted to the age-related final cessation of menses. Nonetheless, most of this book too focused on matters of pregnancy and childbirth, rather than on older women.[42] Several chapters discussed the suppression of menses, again focusing entirely on women of reproductive age.[43] Even the separate large section devoted to 'the cessation of periods' was still nonetheless devoted primarily to matters of temporary menstrual suppression, not the final cessation. This section is virtually identical to the entire separate book on *Chronic Diseases upon the Cessation of Menses*, published posthumously under Chambon's name in 1798.[44] Even here, in a book which appears, on the surface, to be about what later became known as menopause, we find the cessation of menses being still discussed mostly in relation to the problem of temporary menstrual suppression during the reproductive years. Notably though, the 1798 posthumous work did now begin with a new short introductory chapter—not clearly Chambon's own words—which referred to this cessation as a particular 'critical' era in a woman's life. This period was characterised, according to the chapter, by 'hypochondriac' complaints such as diarrhoea and uterine disorders, as well as palpitations, and 'chez quelques-unes, des sueurs fréquents' ('among a few women, frequent sweats').[45] This 1798 text referred to a variety of either non-specific symptoms of ageing in general, to non-specific gynaecological disorders, or to general illnesses, such as epilepsy, haemorrhoids, abdominal pains, fatigue, inflammatory fevers, skin conditions, tumours, cancers, loss of sensation in the extremities, loss of eyesight, hysteria, nightmares, sleep disturbance, and *la gêne universelle* (general discomfort).[46]

Overall, in Chambon's work on women's health, concerns with ageing women appear relatively minimal. Like so many other medical writers of the seventeenth and eighteenth centuries, he attended primarily to the many grave dangers that awaited French women in pregnancy and childbirth before the modern era. He treated disruptions of menstruation in young women as a central problem, because they may indicate either reduced fertility or gynaecological diseases. And

1785); Nicholas Chambon de Montaux, *Les Maladies de la grossesse* (Paris: Rue et Hôtel Serpente, 1785).

41 Chambon de Montaux, *Des maladies des filles*, vol. 2, 106–199.

42 Ibid., vol. 1, xxvii.

43 Ibid., 171–202.

44 Nicholas Chambon de Montaux, *Maladies chroniques à la cessation des règles* (Paris: Dugour et Durand, 1798).

45 Ibid., 1–3.

46 Chambon de Montaux, *Des maladies des femmes*, vol. 2, 184–485.

like the Halle scholars of the early eighteenth century, he included the final cessation of menses as a subtopic of the larger theme of menstrual disorders of the reproductive years. Like the work of the English physician John Fothergill (but without citing him), the 1798 text warned against the 'abuse of purgative medicaments' to treat uterine obstructions (such as tumours), which he claimed were dangerous and unlikely to succeed.[47] The treatments he recommended varied widely depending on the complaint. Tumorous obstructions might be treated with blood-letting, but these were of limited value in general and Chambon recommended against using them simply because a woman had ceased to menstruate, reserving them only for the treatment of uterine haemorrhages.[48]

Some years earlier, another (now emeritus) Paris medical professor, Jean-Baptiste-Claude Jeannet des Longrois, saw the tremendous potential in engaging with both Fothergill's iatrogenesis challenge and Chambon de Montaux's hygienic suggestions for the medicalisation of older women. In 1787, he published the first in what thereafter became a massive nineteenth-century genre of French works of a similar prophylactic kind, *Conseils aux femmes de 40 ans* (Advice to 40-Year-Old Women).[49] Jeannet referred to a woman's forties as her *verte vieillesse*, claiming to have borrowed this term from an unnamed early modern author, most probably André du Laurens in 1594.[50] Notably, though, du Laurens had used the term to refer to the ages between 50 and 60 in men and women, without any reference to menstruation or its ending.[51] This was typical of the way in which eighteenth-century French medical scholars repurposed and assimilated past unisex medical concepts quite different from their own dimorphic view of the sexes, without recognising these crucial differences, in order to suggest a continuous inheritance—a tendency Sabine Arnaud notes too in her 2015 monograph on the history of hysteria.[52] Jeannet also elaborated floridly on the theme of 'peasant women do it better': he explained that the fatigue, sadness, hypochondria, hiccups, asthma, vapours, hysteria, fainting, vomiting blood, cancer, flatulence, heart palpitations, jaundice, and nymphomania of urban women over the age of 40 were products of a nervous system derangement of the 'animal economy', and were caused by a lack of exercise, fresh air, and simple living.[53] Here though too, Jeannet struggled to find symptoms specific to women over 40 which were not also, he said, a feature of young women's nervous disorders. Menstruation was a product of plethora and became particularly acute when the menses was suppressed or in the days leading

[47] Ibid., 66–68. [48] Ibid., 198–200.

[49] Jean-Baptiste-Claude Jeannet des Longrois, *Conseils aux femmes de 40 ans* (Paris: Méquignon, 1787).

[50] Ibid., 2.

[51] André du Laurens, *Discours de la conservation de la veuë: Des maladies mélancoliques des catarrhes, & de la vieillesse*, 3rd ed. [1594] (Rouen: Claude le Villain, 1600), 246.

[52] Sabine Arnaud, *On Hysteria: The Invention of a Medical Category Between 1670 and 1820* (Chicago: University of Chicago Press, 2015), 1–5.

[53] Jeannet des Longrois, *Conseils aux femmes de 40 ans*, 56, 24–194.

up to a woman's period, but it did not appear any more so for women after the menses had definitively ended.[54] He referred briefly to the end of menstruation as the moment when women entered their 'critical age',[55] but nonetheless referred in the title of his work to women of 40 years. This transition was thus defined neither by the fact of the cessation of menses nor as a physiological crisis, but simply by reaching a certain numerical age, no longer even determined by the seven-year cycles of the astrological climacteric. Indeed, by most eighteenth-century accounts, 40 would be unusually early for the final cessation of menses, with most authors agreeing on the most common age falling between the ages of either 45 and 50 or 50 and 55. Without naming Fothergill, Astruc, or any of the other many early modern writers who naturalised women's cessation of menses, Jeannet des Longrois nonetheless explicitly rejected the view that 'at the critical age' one should simply 'let nature do its work' ('laisser agir la nature'), which he considered an erroneous approach. Nature could only act on simple ills, he objected, and women's diseases were anything but simple.[56]

Claude André Goubelly was another Paris professor of medicine whose two-volume 1785 work on women's health included ideas about the final age-related cessation of menses as a minor topic in its second volume: *Connoissances nécessaires sur la grossesse, sur les maladies laiteuses et sur la cessation des règles* (Necessary Knowledge of Pregnancy, of the Diseases of Lactation and of the Cessation of Periods).[57] As a *docteur régent* of the Paris medical faculty, Goubelly's patient body included poor women treated as part of the charitable mission of his role.[58] He thus had a broader experience of different kinds of women from all the social classes of late eighteenth-century France, which is reflected in his account of what he called the *temps critique* and its dependence on temperament, activity, past health conditions and pregnancies, corpulence, as well as city or country living.[59] He associated an even wider age range with the *temps critique* than Jeannet des Longrois, from 32 to 42 years. The earlier incidences were in bilious and melancholic women, those who lived 'sumptuously', in the town, or lived a sedentary life, bathed in cold water, were separated from their husbands, or suffered domestic sorrows; but he considered that whenever the critical time occurred, it would last 4–5 years.[60] He listed symptoms in many women during this phase which were similar to those ascribed in the rest of the work to menstruating, lactating, and pregnant women, as well as those who had just given birth. Goubelly generally considered menstruating, pregnant, and lactating women to be prone to

[54] Ibid., 56–58. [55] Ibid., 2. [56] Ibid., 9.

[57] Claude André Goubelly, *Connoissances nécessaires sur la grossesse, sur les maladies laiteuses et sur la cessation des règles; ouvrage utile au sexe, et aux gens de l'art*, 2 vols (Paris: Chez l'auteur, 1785).

[58] On the *docteurs régents* see Isabelle Coquillard, 'Les Docteurs régents de la Faculté de Médecine de Paris et la fourniture de soins aux "bons pauvres malades" dans les paroisses parisiennes (1644–1791)'. *Revue historique*, 4/668 (2013): 875–904.

[59] Goubelly, *Connoissances nécessaires*, vol. 2. [60] Ibid., 372.

hysteria, inflammation, and spasms, while in the *temps critique* there would be epigastric pains, greater nervous sensitivity, sorrow, a tendency to cry more, corpulence (*embonpoint*), a yellowing of the skin, and sometimes cancers. Strikingly, though, in this chapter, Goubelly fiercely insisted on the necessity of medical surveillance for women in the beginning of their critical time which might be considered a crying call for the creation of a new medical discipline of gynaecology:

> A woman must take the precaution of letting herself be touched by her *Accoucheur*, so that he may ensure that the uterus or the neighbouring parts are not affected by engorgement. Such a woman who, in this time, believes herself to be in perfect health and does not wish to take precautions and refuses the assistance of Medicine often carries inside her, without realising it, a cancer or the germ of a disease that will cost her life. Alas, how many respectable mothers has death taken away because this precaution was not taken![61]

Goubelly also provided a long list of hygienic interventions and treatments for women to follow, including purgative medications, enemas, easy to digest foods, fasting in the morning, frugal living, exercise (more important at this age than ever), dry and temperate air, sleep from 10 p.m. and rising early at the same time each morning, blood-letting from the feet or arms (depending on constitutional type), and the use of leeches (though not on the labia, which he considered inappropriate in the critical time).[62]

The Meaning of Crisis in Montpellier Vitalism

As we have seen, Tissot considered the 'critical age' to be an excessively negative designation for women's final cessation of menses, as did numerous later Paris scholars of the early nineteenth century. But another meaning of 'crisis' and 'critical times' had been emerging in the Montpellier vitalist tradition since the mid-eighteenth century of which both the Swiss and Parisian physicians were either unaware, or which they deliberately snubbed as part of their broader rivalry with the Montpellier faculty. The influential Montpellier professor Théophile Bordeu (1722–1776) described a wide range of conditions considered 'crises' in his widely cited 1756 work on pulses indicative of different temperaments and critical physiological states—a highly influential work that was republished in eight subsequent editions up to 1786.[63] Each major organ had its own impact on the pulse, including the uterus, provoking Bordeu to remark that 'women furnish in their

[61] Ibid., 375. [62] Ibid., 376–381.
[63] Théophile Bordeu, *Recherches sur le pouls, par rapport aux crises* (Paris: De Bure l'aîné, 1756).

different periods a striking example of this influence of a particular organ on the pulse'.[64] Women's reproductive changes were repeatedly described throughout this work as examples of 'crises', defined by their very own unique pulse patterns. Such crises occurred in puberty,[65] prior to menstruation,[66] during suppression of the menses in the reproductive years,[67] during pregnancy and childbirth,[68] and around the time of the final cessation of menses.[69] While Bordeu had the most to say about the pulses found in pregnant and birthing women, he also signalled the first menstruation and the final cessation of menses as particularly influenced by the uterus with its singular effect on the pulse.[70] Sensitive women underwent haemorrhagic bleeding, coughing up blood, or nosebleeds after the final cessation of their menses, he said, indicating not plethora, but a distinct and singular critical state.[71] Bordeu here, like Stahl, Hoffmann, and their students, had begun adding the final cessation of menses to the existing list of all the other menstruation-related changes in women defined as critical states and described in an established literature. But unlike the others, he emphasised that the crisis of the final menstruation was not assimilable to all the others and constituted its own unique critical transition from one state to another.

Importantly though, Bordeu did not define critical states as pathological, nor all women's pathological states as critical. In his case examples, he described three women aged between 40 and 50 who were 'about to lose their periods', and who all had irregular pulses indicative of crisis, which resolved into calmer pulses as soon as their menses had definitively ended.[72] Another woman, aged 46, had suffered shivering and headaches with agitation, exhibiting an irregular pulse. This too resolved after the suppuration of her ear.[73] But he remarked of the 'nervous and convulsive illnesses of women' that although these too had particular pulse patterns (irregular, weak) which might suggest they represented a crisis, in fact these patients were generally not considered to be in a 'critical' state in the true sense, since this required an excretory element which nervous illnesses did not generally exhibit. Moreover, remedies such as blood-letting, repeated purgatives, and enemas masked the true pulse of a critical state and worked against the natural progression of the crisis.[74] Thus, neither mechanical nor chemical treatments were appropriate in many critical uterine states. There were clearly some illnesses to which this did not apply, though, and Bordeu also described the use of abundant suppuration of a swollen leg in an 'old woman' afflicted with asthma whose respiratory crises appeared to have been resolved by this treatment.[75] This view related to the ancient Hippocratic work *The Crises*,[76] and to Dutch physician

[64] Ibid., 459. [65] Ibid., 467. [66] Ibid., 186, 356. [67] Ibid., 59, 99.
[68] Ibid., 90, 185, 192, 196. [69] Ibid., 94, 261. [70] Ibid., 467. [71] Ibid., 416.
[72] Ibid., 261. [73] Ibid., 261–262. [74] Ibid., 378, 469. [75] Ibid., 343.
[76] Hippocrates, *The Crises*, in *The Prognostics and Crises of Hippocrates*, trans. Henry William Ducachet (New York : James Eastbury & Co., 1819), 81–119.

Herman Boerhaave's Hippocratic aphorisms on which Gerhard van Swieten (1700–1772) had written a lengthy commentary. This commentary appeared in French translation in 1775, and the 1779 fifth edition of Bordeu's highly influential *Recherches sur le pouls* is riddled with references to it. Here Bordeu drew out the important implication of Van Swieten's corrective of Galen's critical days theory relative to acute diseases (which was by this time widely viewed as false), and refocused instead on the Hippocratic concept of crises in relation to chronic conditions, in which 'critical evacuations' signified turning points in the disease progression which should not be disrupted by medical intervention.[77]

The notion of crisis as a positive change linked to secretions was also central to an important work of Montpellier medicine published in 1775, Dominique Raymond's *Treatise of Diseases that are Dangerous to Treat*, which reappeared in two more editions in 1808 and in 1816.[78] Raymond recounted a standard plethora-hydraulic view of menstruation which he timed from the start of the second to the end of the seventh septenary of women's lifespan—referring to the Ptolemaic astrological divisions of the lifespan into seven-year periods, each marked by a climacteric or crisis year.[79] Although Raymond said nothing explicit about the final cessation of menses, among the diseases that he said did not require treatment and which should best be left to run their course, he included several of the conditions later listed as symptoms of the critical age in nineteenth-century works on menopause: uterine haemorrhages without any accompanying symptoms, and white vaginal discharge. He said he had seen women swimming in blood who recovered just fine, while all the negative outcomes of such conditions he had seen in fact resulted from attempts to suppress the haemorrhage. Even symptomatic haemorrhages were not to be treated in the case of acute illness, he said, since they were 'often critical and very healthy' ('souvent critiques & très-salutaire').[80]

By way of illustration, he recounted a case example of a 50-year-old woman who was thin and pale and who had ceased menstruating several years before, who developed uterine haemorrhages which did not respond to the standard treatment of blood-letting from the arm, a rich diet of large meals, and soothing astringent remedies. She became worried when urination became painful and 'there was something on the vulva'. Raymond reassured her that nature would take its course and that whatever was stuck inside her 'would be delivered'. The next day indeed she expelled a 'foreign body' which he analysed as a fibrous,

[77] Gerard van Swieten, *Commentaires sur les aphorismes d'H. Boerhaave, de la connaissance et de la cure des maladies*, trans. M Moublet, 6 vols (Lyon: Frères Perisse, 1775), vol. 2, 392–397; Théophile de Bordeu, *Recherches sur le pouls par rapport aux crises* [1756], new ed., 3 vols (Paris: Didot Jeune, 1779), vol. 3, 2e Partie, 364, 389–396, 411, 416, 433–436, 473, 515.

[78] Dominique Raymond, *Traité des maladies qu'il est dangereux de guérir*, 2 vols (Avignon: F. B. Merande, 1757).

[79] Ibid., vol. 1, 274–275. [80] Ibid., 281.

sticky mass of flesh weighing about ten ounces which 'stank intolerably'.[81] Sweating too could be divided between 'critical' or 'symptomatic'—the first kind followed from internal causes and was generally 'benevolent' and 'healthy', just as other secretions of leukorrhea, vomiting, or haemorrhoidal bleeding were often 'healthy' and even 'necessary' and should not be treated.[82] In Raymond's 1816 posthumously published *Selected Consultations of Several Renowned Doctors of the University of Montpellier*, there were also cases of older women with haemorrhoidal bleeding, or coughing up blood, which he considered as compensation for their loss of menses, and this too was taken to be a positive critical symptom.[83]

The notion of crisis as something categorically positive (and for which medicating was contraindicated—particularly in relation to women's diseases), was clearly circulating in French scholarship of the mid- and late eighteenth century, as indicated by a curious text authored by the idiosyncratic Italian-French abbot, lawyer, magnetist, and playwright Claude Paumerelle (b. 1746). It was a work on the philosophy of vapours published in 1774, appearing in a second edition ten years later, and which Sabine Arnauld has contextualised in her 2009 re-edition of this work.[84] The 1784 version of Paumerelle's book published in Cyprus, included a 'Treatise on Crises', which had not been part of the original edition, and which appeared alongside the main text in which the author evoked a positive vision of the vapours as a kind of performative suffering to be encouraged, since it made pretty aristocratic women more charming and their own lives more enjoyable. The treatise offered a clear representation of the emerging mechanistic explanation of the vapours as a pathological physical imbalance akin to hysteria which caused symptoms such as epigastric pain, migraines, haemorrhagic bleeding, diarrhoea, and countless other unexplained ailments. It also summarised well the focus of the Montpellier school's account of critical states or crises of health. 'Whoever says crisis says secretion!...No perfect crisis without secretion', exclaimed Paumerelle.[85] Secretions included everything encumbering, and consequently rejected by the body, including vomit, menstruation, haemorrhoids, sweat, and blood-noses.[86] This account of crisis emphasised its mechanical nature as a product of 'irritability'.[87]

On the other hand, the one figure who most fleshed out Bordeu's vitalist account of the relation between healing crises and menstrual matters in ways that probably encouraged further pursuit of the idea of the 'critical age' was Philippe

[81] Ibid., 287–288.
[82] Dominique Raymond, *Traité des maladies qu'il est dangereux de guérir*, new ed. (Paris: Brunot-Labbe, 1816), 45, 73, 84, 297, 335.
[83] Anon., *Consultation de plusieurs médecins célébrés de l'Université de Montpellier sur des maladies aigues et chroniques*, 9 vols (Paris: Durand & Pissot fils, 1748–1750), vol. 8, 322, 419.
[84] Claude Paumerelle, *La Philosophie des vapeurs* (Lausanne: J. Fr. Bastien, 1774); Claude Paumerelle, *La Philosophie des vapeurs*, ed. Sabine Arnaud (Paris: Mercure de France, 2009).
[85] Claude Paumerelle, *La Philosophie des vapeurs*, 2nd ed. (Paphos: Royez, 1784), 14–15.
[86] Ibid., 15. [87] Ibid., 18.

Pinel (1745–1826), a Montpellier graduate who became a renowned professor of medicine at the Paris faculty and who is considered a founding figure in the emergence of modern psychiatry.[88] Pinel gave lectures in internal pathology at the Paris faculty during the entire period in which the first specialised theses on the final cessation of menses at the faculty were produced (1802–1816). Almost all cited him. His most successful work, the 1797 *Nosographie philosophique*, considered Stahl's fascination with sanguine hydraulics and the 'vital tonic movement' that animated it.[89] Sharing Bordeu's scepticism of plethora as an explanation of menstruation, he followed Barthez's account of 'sympathies' between the blood vessels toward the view of 'critical haemorrhages' as a form of healing crisis, taking menstruation as an example, the characteristics of which were instructive in relation to all other kinds of haemorrhages.[90] So long as they were moderate, he noted, haemorrhages produced no 'state of debility', and even relieved the common 'sentiment of stupor and heaviness' that generally preceded them. Artificial haemorrhages created via blood-letting, on the other hand, could lead to uncontrolled bleeding, while measures taken to stop a naturally occurring 'critical haemorrhage' could put the patient in a state of languor, or in a 'hectic fever'.[91] Menstruation was sometimes observed outside the time frame in which it was expected, both in childhood and 'at an advanced age', he noted; and those who suffered haemorrhoidal bleeding in their youth were prone to other chronic diseases between the ages of 40 and 50. But stimulant treatments that sought to provoke menstruation were a 'fertile source of the worst evils' ('une source féconde de maux les plus graves').[92] Pains and anxieties ceased following an 'eruption of blood', indicating that the 'excretion of blood' was 'healthful' ('salutaire'), and should not be perturbed by the 'inappropriate use of astringents',[93] which could lead to oedema, hypochondria, hysteria, or hectic fever.[94]

Consistent with his vitalist perspective on the dynamics of the blood and his view of menstruation and other haemorrhages as 'critical', Pinel considered suppression of menstruation generally far more dangerous than excess bleeding.[95] But where did this leave women, who, due to age, no longer menstruated at all? Here Pinel coined a phrase that would be quoted, or rather plagiarised, countless times by medical scholars of menopause for the next century. He began by characterising the final cessation of menses as the most natural thing in the world, before sharply distinguishing between two different kinds of experience of the change:

[88] Dora B. Weiner, '"Le Geste de Pinel": The History of a Psychiatric Myth', in Mark S. Micale & Roy Porter, eds, *Discovering the History of Psychiatry* (New York: Oxford University Press, 1994), 232–242.

[89] Philippe Pinel, *Nosographie philosophique, ou la méthode de l'analyse appliquée à la médecine*, vol. 1 (Paris: Maradon, 1797), 247.

[90] Ibid., 241–248. [91] Ibid., 245. [92] Ibid., 246. [93] Ibid., 252.

[94] Ibid., 264. [95] Ibid., 281.

> Women who have lived following the wish of nature, who have been mothers and have led an active and laborious life, generally go through the critical age without danger, and without experiencing notable woes; but those who have lived in idleness and eaten to excess, those who have abused aromatic substances and spirits...experience afflictions of a singularly varied nature in the time of their cessation.[96]

They might have blood in their urine,[97] vomit blood,[98] suffer rheumatic pains, eye, or ear, or visceral symptoms,[99] or suffer 'very vivid emotional afflictions, especially around the usual time of the evacuation of the blood'.[100] Indeed, Pinel's remarks about the effect of the cessation of menses on women's nerves, both here and in other works, were highly generative for scholars elaborating ideas about the vapours, hysteria, and hypochondria in the critical age, as we consider in Chapter 5. The work of building a highly gender-dimorphic view of ageing, focused on women's final cessation of menses, was here, in Pinel's work, already begun. But it was through the many specialist doctoral theses published on the topic that menopause came to be made into recognised topic of clinical care and medical importance, and to be named as a specific symptomatic phenomenon that was increasingly divorced from its various eighteenth-century origins in climacteric theories of the life cycle, in vitalist accounts of critical times, and in the earlier medical description of young women's vapours, plethora, and uterine disorders.

Specialist medical theses that focused on the topic of crises and critical periods were also produced in a significant number at the Montpellier faculty throughout the first half of the nineteenth century, reiterating their positive, vitalist, self-healing, and secretory definition. J. B. F. Létu's Montpellier thesis of 1816 expressed it thus:

> ...one must consider crisis to be a salutary, necessary, indispensable movement, solicited by nature for the reestablishment of the order which characterises health. It is a sort of reaction of the vital forces which changes the order of functions established by the illness, in order to bring them back to the natural state.[101]

Crisis was thus part of the body's efforts to heal itself, and the use of medications could easily derail its progress. Létu warned against the habitual purging and blood-letting that some people liked to practise 'at certain times of the year', which he said weakened the organism.[102] Crises followed patterns of the number

[96] Ibid., 285. [97] Ibid., 258. [98] Ibid., 263.
[99] Ibid., 286. [100] Ibid., 263.
[101] J. B. D. Létu, *Essai sur la doctrine des crises et des jours critiques dans les maladies aiguës*. Thèse (Montpellier: Jean Martel aîné, 1816), 7.
[102] Ibid., 15.

seven, he insisted, while noting that numbers had become an unreasonable obsession to some of the ancient medical scholars. Hence, crisis occurred at the age of seven months when the infant's teeth broke through, at the age of 7 years when these teeth fell out and were replaced by adult ones, at 14 with the advent of puberty, at 21 with the cessation of growth, and at 49 'or at the end of the seventh septennial' which was when, 'the system of forces begins to experience a striking debility'. Here he did not differentiate the sexes here at all.[103]

A similar thesis was produced the following year by the Paris doctoral candidate P. F. T. Jacob, which provided even more explicitly vitalist/animist grounds for the view of crisis as healthful.[104] Crises were nature healing itself via a 'principle of movement, harmony, the action of the functions, the coursing of the forces toward conserving life... the existence of which is incontestable'.[105] Strong, robust bodies in the throes of acute crisis thus required few medications because 'they traverse with haste their diverse periods', nature needing few external supports. Medication was for chronic illness, when nature had become fatigued and had given up its quest to return to health and so needed to be rescued.[106] Jacob doubted that crisis always had to entail bodily fluids. Nonetheless, uterine haemorrhages were a clear example of a crisis, Jacob said. He recounted a case in which a woman with chronic pulmonary complaints who had never menstruated was given a purgative medication which caused her to develop an itchy anus, haemorrhoids, and then heavy uterine haemorrhagic bleeding, after which she was cured of her chronic illness. Age, sex, temperament, climate, and the seasons all had a marked influenced on crises.[107] But old people were less prone to them, as were those who lived in cold places.[108]

Crises and critical states also featured significantly in French medical pedagogy, as suggested by the numerous doctoral theses written on these themes throughout the early and mid-nineteenth century, with the topic seemingly batted back and forth between the schools of Montpellier and Paris throughout this time.[109] It remained an important topic in late eighteenth- and in nineteenth-century medicine in both the iatromechanist and iatrochemical currents, since what defined a critical state was both a movement of matter toward the return to equilibrium, and a secretory shedding that could be pharmacologically influenced. The 1792 *Encyclopédie méthodique* acknowledged the difficulty of defining the term 'critical' given the variety of concepts to which it was now attached in medicine, citing both the 'critical days' within a fever (Galen's idea), and the *temps*

[103] Ibid. 18.
[104] P. F. T., Jacob, *Essai sur la doctrine des crises*. Thèse (Paris: Didot Jeune, 1817).
[105] Ibid., 7. [106] Ibid., 8. [107] Ibid., 12. [108] Ibid., 10.
[109] Dussault, *Essai sur les hémorrhagies actives du système muqueux considérées comme crises dans les maladies aiguës*. Thèse (Paris: Didot Jeune, 1818); Nicolas-Marie Grévin, *Essai sur les crises*. Thèse (Montpellier: Jean Martel, 1825); François Simon, *Essai sur les crises*. Thèse (Paris: Didot le Jeune, 1831); Julien Poussié, *Essai sur les crises et leur existence dans les maladies*. Thèse (Montpellier: Ricard, 1840); Jean-Louis Solier, *Essai sur les crises*. Thèse (Montpellier: Boehm, 1857).

critique of women, here referring to puberty, menstruation, and pre-menstrual states, but making no mention whatsoever of the final cessation of menses in older women. As Christine Théré notes, while late eighteenth-century uses of the term *temps critique*, such as that found in the 1792 Encyclopedia (Théré cites the 1798 edition), referred not to menopause but to puberty, menstruation, or the pre-menstrual state, by the early nineteenth century such works listed both meanings of the term, including its new use as a synonym for the final cessation of menses.[110] What defined all critical states was that they were moving the patient from one state to another—they were always uncomfortable moments of transition—and they generally entailed secretions or excretions.[111]

A similar account of crises is found too in the 1801 published lectures of the renowned Montpellier professor of medicine Joseph-Marie-Joachim Vigarous (1759–1826), who lectured on the diseases of women at Montpellier in the late 1790s.[112] He used the term 'critical', not to refer to either menstruation or the cessation of menses, but to distinguish different kinds of evacuations and how doctors should respond to them. Critical states were those which medicine should not treat since they would resolve themselves naturally if left unhindered. It was important to distinguish 'critical sweats' from 'symptomatic ones', he said: only the latter required treatment.[113] The critical kind could be recognised by the lax and soft skin, red face, shivering, tightened belly, suppression of urination, and soft, undulating pulse.[114] Flows of blood were always critical too—both the habitual menstrual flux, as well as the bleeding of haemorrhoids in men or women—and their suppression was thus often a cause of inflammatory fevers.[115] By definition though, the final cessation of menses did not fit this criteria, since it heralded the beginning of a new permanent state, rather than being an interruption of a resuming one, which probably explains why Vigarous took no interest in defining this time of life as particularly problematic for women. It was certainly not from Vigarous that the idea emerged of treating women's final cessation of menses as a troublesome 'critical age'.

This idea of positive crises persisted in Montpellier medicine throughout the early nineteenth century and continued to be subject to a specialist doctoral scholarship. In 1825 the surgeon Nicolas-Marie Grévin defended his Montpellier thesis, *Essai sur les crises*,[116] exemplifying the fluid movement between the Montpellier disciplines of surgery and medicine that had existed since the eighteenth century, unlike the professional divisions found still (though not for much

[110] Thére, 'Âge de retour et retour d'âge', 59.

[111] *Encyclopédie méthodique*, vol. 5 (Paris: Pancoucke, 1792), 219–232.

[112] Joseph-Marie-Joachim Vigarous, *Cours élémentaire de maladies des femmes, ou Essai sur une nouvelle méthode pour étudier et pour classer les maladies de ce sexe*, 2 vols (Paris: Deterville, 1801).

[113] Vigarous, *Cours élémentaire de maladies des femmes*, vol. 2, 236.

[114] Ibid., 239. [115] Ibid., 232.

[116] Grévin, *Essai sur les crises.*

longer) in Paris at that time, as Elizabeth Williams has described.[117] Grévin had previously served as a military surgical assistant (*chirurgien aide-major*) in an Italian hospital, as well as for the French army stationed in the northern Alps, and had been a surgical extern of the Paris Hôtel-Dieu. He indicated that his father had taught at the Paris faculty, while his brother worked as a doctor at Aubenas in the Rhône-Alpes region.[118] Grévin's thesis reflected the Montpellier emphasis on resisting the tendency to over-medicate or aggressively intervene in the self-regulating wonder of the vital force. He referred to distinct ages or 'degrees, times or periods', not only in human lives but in those of all plants and animals, describing this as an ancient doctrine that should 'lead us to determine the circumstances when the doctor must act or remain a tranquil spectator of the efforts of nature'.[119] Grévin leaned on Hippocrates in support of the view that doctors must 'respect the medicating efforts of nature' itself, while also recognising when it was necessary to intervene to divert a disease from a 'viscous direction'. Crisis was 'the effect of nature chasing its defeated enemy' and was therefore broadly to be considered 'a change for the better'.[120] Medicine suffered two most common forms of error, he said. The first stemmed from hubris or 'blind confidence', which was very dangerous (perhaps referring both to the non-medically trained surgeons and the iatromechanist obsession with blood-letting, leeches, and enemas), and the second was random, wishful polypharmacy (likely referring both the iatrochemical overuse of purgative and emetic herbs in official medicine and to the still vastly prevalent use of herbal formulas among popular folk healers).[121]

The Paris faculty in 1830 even ran a prize competition on the theme of crises and critical periods, in which contestants had to 'prove, by facts exclusively observed in one of the clinical medical rooms, to what extent the doctrine of crises and of critical days is well founded'. But the competition was thwarted—perhaps ironically—by the political crisis of the July revolution that year and the prize was never awarded.[122] The competition did, however, stimulate the production of theses on the question at both the Montpellier and Paris faculties, including that of François Simon, whose 1831 Paris thesis was again entitled *Essai sur les crises*,[123] and that of a Boulenger whose 1831 Paris thesis had exactly the same title as Jacob's 1817 Paris thesis but focused mainly on the Galenic idea of 'critical days' in acute illness.[124] Boulenger did not appear to engage with the Montpellier vitalist concept of crises as a period of positive adaptation at all, but he cited 'the menstrual flow' as one of twenty-seven common critical times observed in medicine.[125] Another Paris thesis on haemorrhages, submitted in 1818 by Dussault

117 Williams, *A Cultural History of Medical Vitalism*, 61.
118 Grévin, *Essai sur les crises*, 2. 119 Ibid., 3.
120 Ibid., 11. 121 Ibid., 6.
122 Simon, *Essai sur les crises*, v. 123 Ibid.
124 P. F. T. Jacob, *Essai sur la doctrine des crises*. Thèse (Paris: Didot Jeune, 1817).
125 J.-B.-M.-N.-D. Boulenger, *Essai sur la doctrine des crises*. Thèse (Paris: Didot le Jeune, 1831), 25.

(citing Hoffmann), had also proposed that women's regular menstrual haemorrhages demonstrated the principle that such critical times often resolved favourably.[126] Simon's work, though produced at the Paris faculty, nonetheless also clearly took up the Montpellier idea of crises as 'happy solutions to illness with the aid of some organic secretion'.[127]

Another Montpellier thesis by surgeon-physician Julien Poussié defended in 1840 elaborated on the crisis model of disease that medical hygiene was designed to address. He did so not according to an idea of critical days, which, he said, had been rejected long before, even by Galen himself. He referred instead to the new model that focused on internal changes in the organism throughout both the day and the life course, including 'revolutions of ageing, puberty, fever, sleep, blindness and deafness' which all played a part in 'critical' phenomena impacting human health.[128] Intriguingly, Poussié offered a mapping of the question of crises in the history of medicine among the preceding generation of European scholars, among the ancient scholars, and according to contemporary solidist and humoralist commitments. The concept of crises had suffered some embarrassing episodes in the history of medicine, Poussié acknowledged, citing both the Ptolemaic septenary idea that attributed great power to the number seven, and the Dutch chemist Van Helmont's adherence to the influence of the moon, which Bordeu had soundly dismissed.[129] But the idea of crises also attracted major partisans such as the Armenian-Italian chemist Giorgio Baglivi (1668–1707), the Paris professor of medicine Jacques Houllier (*c.*1504–1562), and the Dutch physician Gerard van Swieten (1700–1772). Poussié defined the humoralist approach to crisis as characterised by four conjectures: first, that health improvements were often preceded by a critical phase; second, that if a crisis was not complete, the disease could return; third, that the state of the organism in crisis was pathological and not its normal state; and finally, that crisis was something more than merely a morbid state. The classic example of the humoral crisis, Poussié said, was that occurring before the first menstruation or before the appearance of lactation, which was resolved by the flow of blood and of milk respectively. The solidist view of crises, exemplified by the Paris medical professor Auguste-François Chomel's 1824 *Elements of General Pathology*, was far less encouraging, confining these merely to the progression of acute illnesses, referring to the 'critical days' in fevers, an idea derived from Galen.[130] Only humoralists based their recognition on the 'interior curative work of nature', making their perspective a fitter vehicle for the explication of crisis.[131] Poussié, like the other Montpellier scholars, defined

[126] Dussault, *Essai sur les hémorrhagies*, 12, 17. [127] Simon, *Essai sur les crises*, 8.
[128] Poussié, *Essai sur les crises*, 30–31. [129] Ibid., 11.
[130] Ibid., 14–15; Auguste-François Chomel, *Éléments de pathologie générale* (Paris: Crochard, 1824), 395.
[131] Poussié, *Essai sur les crises*, 17.

crisis as a 'favourable change', but which could be divided into 'good or bad, safe or dangerous', as well as 'perfect or imperfect'.[132] All excretions and secretions, including menstrual blood, belonged to the material crises, while the revolutions of ageing, fevers, and sleep belonged to the immaterial crises.[133]

The First Specialist Medical Works on Women's Critical Age

While crisis scholarship increasingly intersected with the cohesion of specialist medical works on women's final cessation of menses, the specialist view of age-related menstrual cessation as itself constituting a 'critical time' did not depend on these other developments. Even before this substantial corpus of vitalist works on crises appeared, the concept of women's final cessation of menses as a 'critical time' had already begun to cohere among doctoral candidates at the Montpellier faculty. The first specialist medical thesis in French focused entirely on the final cessation of menses, by the Montpellier candidate Jérémie André Pingault, appeared in 1799. This phenomenon was now firmly labelled as a 'critical age', some thirteen years before the Paris thesis of Charles-Pierre-Louis de Gardanne took credit for the modern medical neologism *la ménopause*.[134] This student from the Aquitaine *département* of Vienne who later taught at the University of Poitiers,[135] provided one of the most detailed mechanistic explanations of the known physiology of menstrual cessation. Providing an expansive account of its possible symptoms and of its treatment, he drew on the lessons of the professor Joseph-Marie-Joachim Vigarous who lectured on the diseases of women at Montpellier in the late 1790s and authored a book on this topic;[136] on the ideas of Petiot, who lectured in internal medicine (without holding a professorial position); on the writings of Georg Stahl, John Cullen, John Fothergill, and, like all good *montpelliérains* students—on the Hippocratic corpus.

In 1801, just as the two volumes of the lectures of Vigarous became available to scholars throughout France, another Montpellier thesis, by Joseph Gagnebé from the Lot *département* in the south of France, and supervised by the physiology professor Charles-Louis Dumas (1765–1813), also addressed 'the illnesses which attack women upon the cessation of the period'.[137] Gagnebé, referring mostly to the work of Chambon de Montaux, gave a temperament-based account of the *accidens* of which women might suffer at this time—but only if they had

[132] Ibid., 26–27. [133] Ibid., 30.

[134] Jérémie-André Pingault, *De la cessation des règles* (Montpellier: Tournel, 1799).

[135] *Annuaire statistique du département de la Vienne pour 1833* (Poitiers: Saurin Frères, 1833), vol. 1, 198.

[136] Joseph-Marie-Joachim Vigarous, *Cours élémentaire de maladies des femmes, ou Essai sur une nouvelle méthode pour étudier et pour classer les maladies de ce sexe*, 2 vols (Paris: Deterville, 1801).

[137] Joseph Gagnebé, *Exposition de quelques maladies qui attaquent les femmes à la cessation des règles*. Thèse (Montpellier: Imprimerie de Tournel, 1801).

previously been prone to menstrual suppression, difficult pregnancies, or other psychological (*morales*) or physical diseases. Sanguine women in this case would suffer haemorrhoids, uterine haemorrhages, and skin infections (*érysipèles*); lymphatic women would suffer oedema, cysts, and cancers of breasts and uterus; while nervous women would suffer vapours, spasms, and convulsions. Healthy women would simply observe a gradual diminution of the menstrual flow until it ceased altogether, along with a little fat gain if they were temperamentally disposed to this.[138] While most women in general were 'pituitary', sanguine or melancholic women could also manifest signs of bilious temperament once they ceased menstruating, similar to that of men, because the vital forces that had once been directed to the uterus now dispersed throughout the body.[139]

Gagnebé, although using the term *époque critique* to describe the final cessation of menses, nonetheless appears to have misunderstood the strict Montpellier definition of critical periods, which referred to positive transitory states of healing or adaptation, instead describing the 'critical age' as commencing around 45–50 but extending for the remainder of women's lives, hence also providing case examples that referred to women as old as 60.[140] This rather expansive definition of the critical age as simply all of life following the cessation of menses allowed the term to capture a much wider range of diseases than could otherwise be ascribed to the transitory 'crisis' of the body adapting to its state of no longer menstruating. By referring to the now widely recognised correlations between age in general and the prevalence of cancers, Gagnebé also associated 'the critical age' with dangerous cancers of the breasts and uterus observed more commonly in older women in general. He appears to have adopted the fallacy of attributing this to the end of menstruation from the 1740 dissertation of the Besançon surgeon Gilles Vacher on breast cancers, in which the latter had claimed that the final cessation of menses was a 'frequent cause' of such cancers since they were more common in older women, but without providing any explanation of a mechanism by which these cancers might relate to the loss of menstruation.[141]

By 1802, the topic of women's critical age had become a central concern now of the Paris faculty, which was not about to let this theme become dominated by the southerners. Jean-Baptiste Chouffe, who had studied under both Hallé and Pinel, began his thesis on the cessation of menses by considering the importance of the genital organs in the pubertal development of the differences between men and women, as a prelude to proposing that it was fertility which defined the sexes, and without which they were practically indistinguishable.[142] Quoting Hallé, he proposed that 'woman is the nervous part of the human race, and man is the

[138] Ibid., 4–5. [139] Ibid., 5. [140] Ibid., 3, 14.

[141] Gilles Vacher, *Dissertation sur le cancer des mammelles, ou Sans recourir à aucune hipotése, on donne une véritable idée de la nature* (Besançon: Jean-Baptiste Charmet, 1740), 38.

[142] Jean-Baptiste-P. Chouffe, *Des accidents et des maladies qui surviennent à la cessation de la menstruation*. Thèse (Paris: Croullebois & Gabon, 1802), 2–5.

muscular part'.[143] Chouffe joined the growing chorus of enthusiasm for women fulfilling 'their duties as mothers' on threat of a miserable critical age later if they did otherwise. The period from 45 to 50 was when 'woman sees the season of pleasures disappear', to be replaced by numerous ills, unless she acted preventively by living according to the 'laws of hygiene'.[144] Aggravating factors for '*accidens*' around the cessation of menses included: 'nervous susceptibility that makes the influence of the passions more intense', lymphatico-sanguine temperament, laziness, opulence, late nights spent gambling, large gatherings, the abuse of alcohol, immoderate use of coffee, bad food, celibacy, excesses of sexual pleasure, menstrual abnormalities in one's youth, bleeding during pregnancy, a tendency toward white discharge, frequent abortions, or previous illnesses relating to menstruation.[145] Chouffe also described four case observations of patients, all aged between 49 and 55, who suffered various headaches, hot flushes, and sleep disturbances as their menstrual cycles came to an end, including one who was treated unsuccessfully by Pinel with blood-letting and an emetic drink.[146] He also described one of Hoffmann's reported cases of a Dutch woman in her fifties with plethora who was prescribed purgative medication and blood-letting, also unsuccessfully.[147]

The prescription of purgatives to women during the cessation of menses was also the subject of a new round of protest in this same year at Paris, with the 1803 thesis of J. N. Gilbert, which took aim at those who 'only know to use pharmaceutical means', and mostly only purgatives.[148] Gilbert drew on an old reference to Giorgio Baglivi's criticism of purgative overuse,[149] revivifying a late seventeenth-century warning by bringing Fothergill's late eighteenth-century tract to bear on the question of purgatives as a problem specific to women around the cessation of menses.[150] Then, in 1805, a new edition of Fothergill's text was published in French by the Paris press Crochard, whose offices were located in the rue de l'École de Médecine.[151] It might seem odd that so much fuss was still being made of this short essay by an English doctor written in 1774, given that the criticism of purgative use with women's cessation of menses was already to be found in the work of Astruc and that criticisms of purgative abuse in general had been a common topic of medical discussion since the late seventeenth century. But unlike any of these previous iterations, Fothergill's essay had hinted at something

[143] Ibid., 6. [144] Ibid., 9. [145] Ibid., 30–31.

[146] Ibid., 19–28 [20–21]. [147] Ibid., 22.

[148] J. N. Guilbert, *Des purgatifs à la cessation des menstrues*. Thèse (Paris: Imprimerie de la Bibliothèque Médicale, 1803), 3.

[149] Giorgio Baglivi, *De praxi medica ad priscam observandi rationem revocanda. Libri duo. Accedunt dissertationes novae* (Leiden: Fredericum Haringium, 1700).

[150] Guilbert, *Des purgatifs à la cessation des menstrues*, 5.

[151] Charles-François-Simon Giraudy, *Conseils aux femmes sur les moyens de prévenir ou d'arrêter les suites fâcheuses de leur temps critique par le Docteur Fothergill de Londres, traduit de l'anglais* (Paris: Crochard, 1805).

which the Paris scholars clearly found very exciting: the idea that modern physicians whose training was balanced between the different medical disciplines (not only pharmacy) might begin to constitute a new kind of speciality in older women's health, which was needed to combat the popular beliefs driving prevalent and inappropriate forms of pharmacy that might be used to treat menopause. In Chapter 6 we revisit Fothergill's impact in France in the context of medical denigrations of popular practitioners known as empirics, charlatans, and women folk healers (*commères*), who were all accused of irresponsible and poor-quality polypharmacy, as well as of midwives who were accused of botching births, with later consequences for women's menopause.

A third Paris thesis this same year on the cessation of menses was that of Pierre Béclard, which proposed that since women's biological function was so absolutely determined by their childbearing capacities, it was inevitable that the end of these capacities would be 'one of the most critical' periods of their lives. Here he used the word 'critical' not in the *montpelliérain* sense, but as a synonym simply for 'terrible' or 'morbid'.[152] Béclard recounted what was to become very much a standard narrative of naturalising statements about the final cessation of menses and warnings against purgative use to combat it, both borrowed from Fothergill. He also included assertions about older women effectively becoming men since menstruation defined them as a sex,[153] as well as references to Pinel's remarks about lazy women who had enjoyed too much sexual pleasure, alcohol, aromatic substances, and revelry, therefore suffering menstruation disorders in their youth and an early and miserable critical age.[154] This was then followed by a detailed inventory of all the diseases from which older women had been observed to suffer, supplied as symptoms of the cessation of menses. By way of example, Béclard repeated a case observation from Pinel's lectures describing a woman of 48 who had suffered menstrual suppression in her youth, contracted gonorrhoea in her thirties, and began vomiting blood and experiencing fever which worsened after she turned 45, becoming permanently hysteric when her menses ended.[155]

Béclard's and Pinel's remarks about women becoming men once they ceased menstruating also received a significant boost from another important medical professor at the Paris faculty, Jacques-Louis Moreau (de la Sarthe) (1771–1826). His 1803 *Histoire naturelle de la femme* (Natural History of Woman), like the works of both Roussel and Cabanis, attracted numerous citations throughout the nineteenth century in scholarship on menopause.[156] Moreau acknowledged women's greater longevity,[157] while also insisting on the 'excess of vitality' of

[152] Pierre A. Béclard, *Essai sur les maladies auxquelles les femmes sont le plus fréquemment exposées à l'époque de la cessation des menstrues*. Thèse (Paris: Pancoucke, 1802), 3.

[153] Ibid., 5–7. [154] Ibid., 17. [155] Ibid., 30.

[156] Jacques-Louis Moreau de la Sarthe, *Histoire naturelle de la femme, suivie d'un traité d'hygiène appliquée à son régime physique et moral aux différentes époques de la vie*, 3 vols (Paris: Duprat, 1803).

[157] Ibid., vol. 1, 181.

women's genital organs, which 'reacted more strongly to the different ages' of 'menstrual revolution'—both puberty and the *temps critique*.[158] The loss of reproductive capacities not only made women more similar to the 'opposite sex', but also freed them to pursue their own ends (*la vie individuelle*), rather than serving others,[159] which in turn made them more interesting company for men.[160] Moreau too cited Fothergill—not in order to agree with his warnings against purgatives, but rather to agree with his long list of symptoms from which women could be expected to suffer in the critical time, particularly loss of energy, abdominal pains, and hot flushes.[161] He referred to the change rather alarmingly as 'the death of sex' ('la mort du sexe'), connoting at once the loss of sexed difference, the loss of sexual desire, and the loss of desirability.[162]

Influential though Moreau de la Sarthe was, his remarks appeared scattered over just a handful of pages in just one volume of this hefty work. The pursuit of women's critical age as a specialist topic, for now, remained the task of doctoral students. The Paris faculty assigned the thesis topic to another two candidates in 1805, within two years of those of Béclard, Chouffe, and Gilbert.[163] One was by L. J. S. Jallon, who had taught anatomy and obstetrics at the Orléans College attached to the Hôtel-Dieu Hospice during his doctoral studies. His *Essai sur l'âge critique* used the notion of crisis too in its more negative sense, as 'that stormy period in the lives of women' ('cette période orageuse de la vie des femmes').[164] Jallon blamed sedentary habits, 'prolonged passions', uterine diseases, venereal infections, difficult pregnancies, and both abuses or privations of sexual relations for the later ailments of the critical age. He defined different problems according to humoral temperament, just like Montpellier scholars.[165] The solution here too was to mimic the peasant ways of physical labour.[166] But he also listed a range of medical treatments and prescriptions, including specific diets for each constitutional type, and the use of blood-letting, purgative medications, cauterisation, and other cures for uterine pathologies (medicines, herbal teas, injections into the uterus, and compresses).[167] In contrast to the Montpellier theses to date, Jallon's work was far less theoretically developed, but went much further in elaborating the therapeutic dimensions of menopause medicine, seemingly blissfully unaware of how controversial some of these treatments had already become—especially purgatives, but also to some extent phlebotomy. This was far from the vitalist approach of letting nature do its work, but it also revealed much about how older women were in fact being treated by Paris doctors now that the 'critical age' had become part of their university curricula.

158 Ibid., 208–209. 159 Ibid., 209.
160 Ibid., 412. 161 Ibid:, 410–411. 162 Ibid., 676.
163 L. J. S. Jallon, *Essai sur l'âge critique des femmes*. Thèse (Paris: Didot Jeune, 1805); Henri Lamaze, *Essai sur la cessation du flux menstruel et sur les moyens propres à prévenir les accidents et les maladies qui peuvent affecter les femmes à cette époque* (Paris: Didot Jeune, 1805).
164 Jallon, *Essai sur l'âge critique des femmes*, 6.
165 Ibid., 34. 166 Ibid., 36. 167 Ibid., 69–91.

The other Paris thesis of 1805, by Henri Lamaze, from the *département* of Corrèze in the Limousin, emphasised the particularity of the diseases affecting women's generative organs, from which they suffered in addition to all the illnesses common to both sexes. Women were simply the sicker sex.[168] All the uterine changes produced 'accidens': puberty, pregnancy, childbirth, lactation, and the critical age—an idea that became most generative during the mid-nineteenth century in Parisian claims about women's mental pathologies, as we consider in Chapter 7.[169] Most women ceased menstruating around the age of 45–50, Lamaze said, though he noted that both Haller and Stahl had cited cases of women continuing to menstruate into old age. Nonetheless, as Astruc (and Pinel) had indicated, if a woman still bled from the uterus after 50, cancer should be suspected.[170] Fothergill was enlisted in support of a naturalising view of the cessation of menses, which was ordinarily without danger among women who had 'fulfilled the wishes of nature' ('rempli le vœu de la nature') and who did some exercise, as was the case of the ideal peasant woman.[171] The greater a woman's indulgence of voluptuousness in youth, the worse would be her critical age.[172]

Also in 1805, I. A. Labretoigne-Lavalette the younger, son of the Montpellier medical professor Ignace Labretoigne-Lavalette (who had completed his doctorate on stroke treatment at Montpellier in 1758),[173] offered his own 'reflections on the diseases that occur in women at the time of the cessation of menses'.[174] He defended the idea of the final menses as a 'critical time', only surpassed by those other critical times that were menstruation itself and pregnancy. Only women from the cities, especially those who had never married, experienced a 'violent disturbance' ('une violente secousse') causing numerous diseases around this time of life. The end of the menses 'changed the order of things in the animal economy' causing a certain 'commotion', but it also coincided with the beginning of old age, which itself brought an increased number of illnesses.[175] The problem, he noted astutely, was how to distinguish those illnesses which were directly caused by the cessation of the menses from those which had nothing to do with it. It was important not to overlook any diseases that were related, he thought, but there was also the danger of 'grouping together a host of diseases of which the cessation of menses may not be the only determining cause, and which could equally have resulted from an erroneous regime' (dietary or other).[176] He made a point of

[168] Lamaze, *Essai sur la cessation du flux menstruel*, 5. [169] Ibid., 6.
[170] Ibid., 6. [171] Ibid., 8–9. [172] Ibid., 9.
[173] Ignace Labretoigne-Lavalette, *Quaestio medica eaque therapeutica sub hac verborum serie: an in apoplexia emetica semper convenient?* (Montpellier: Jean Martel, 1758).
[174] J. A. Labretoigne-Lavalette, *Réfléxions sur les maladies qui surviennent aux femmes à l'époque de la cessation des règles*. Thèse (Montpellier: Imprimerie Auguste Ricard, 1805).
[175] Ibid., 5–6. [176] Ibid., 7.

rejecting the plethora hydraulic view of menstruation, which he said had been discredited by Bordeu. Illnesses caused by the loss of menses were not, then, due to plethora, but to the sympathetic influence of the uterus on other organs.[177]

The Montpellier thesis of Antoine Leyral in 1806 focused instead on 'prophylactic' care for women around the time of their final menstruation.[178] Leyral, also from a family of doctors, had a combined background in surgery and medicine in the military hospital system in the Corrèze, undertaking his Montpellier studies under Louis Dumas, J.-B. Timothée Baumes, Nicolas Berthe, and J.-M.-J. Vigarous. He described both the first and the last menstruation as 'critical periods' which required the patient to exercise caution.[179] The final menses brought 'no troubles at all, because this event would not disrupt the harmony reigning between the diverse orders of life'. So long as women worked their bodies, bore children, and avoided 'allowing themselves to be consumed by the passions that society produces', they would be 'almost protected from all dangers once they ceased to be fertile'. The dangers arose only from 'luxury, limpness (*mollessse*) and city ways (*mœurs des villes*)'.[180] Leyral described an account which he associated with 'the Stahlians' (including Bordeu) of illnesses associated with the cessation of menses, which came in four kinds: diseases of the uterus itself; hypochondriac afflictions; rheumatic (*fluxionnaires*) diseases; and rheumatic-spastic (convulsive) disorders.[181] But he warned against the error produced when all the diseases of older women were taken to define the list of illnesses caused by the 'critical age', noting that Philippe Pinel had criticised a certain author (Fothergill) who 'in enumerating these diseases, had almost made a complete nosology of them'.[182] Leyral too claimed that 'no one believes anymore today that the periods are the necessary effect of plethora', but he also considered that without recourse to the 'periodic haemorrhages' of menstruation, blood could force its way out of the body in other ways, manifesting as ulcers, mucous secretions, other kinds of haemorrhages (nose-bleeds, haemorrhoids), skin complaints, as well as rheumatic pains, colic, and nervous pains.[183]

Thomas Guillit de Chatellus's Montpellier thesis of 1807 addressed 'the modifications brought upon the economy of woman by the first appearance and the final cessation of the periods'.[184] This thesis developed the idea that it was the moments of uterine change that most impacted the vital organisation of women's bodies, referring explicitly to Cabanis's statements about this, and defining the cessation

[177] Ibid., 8–9.

[178] Antoine Leyral, *Essai sur la prophylactique des femmes parvenues à l'époque de la cessation des règles*. Thèse (Montpellier: Imprimerie Auguste Ricard, 1806).

[179] Ibid., 3. [180] Ibid., 4. [181] Ibid., 7.

[182] Ibid., 5. Pinel, *Nosographie philosophique*, vol. 1, 290.

[183] Leyral, *Essai sur la prophylactique*, 10–11.

[184] Thomas Guillit de Chatellus, *Recherches physiologique et médicales sur l'influence et les modifications qu'apportent dans l'économie de la femme et la première apparition et la cessation absolue des règles*. Thèse (Montpellier: Auguste Ricard, 1807).

of menses as a kind of second puberty.[185] He also referred to Roussel's remarks in confirming that women did not become 'old' as soon as they ceased to be fertile.[186] Guillit de Chatellus distinguished two roles of the uterus as both an 'external organ' (meaning, local) and a 'vital organ' with systemic effects through its many sympathies with the other organs.[187] Like others, he referred to differences of temperament impacting women's experience of this time of life, which he situated not around the seventh septenary as others had done, but about the eighth septenary of 56 years, which he said corresponded to Stahl's *senectus prima* or *âge de retour*.[188] Though much of his thesis focused on the vapours and hysterical symptoms which affected some women at this time of life, he considered the inertia into which the uterus fell to provide relief from existing nervous symptoms.[189] Nonetheless, only women who had lived simple and virtuous lives could expect to experience a trouble-free cessation of menses.[190] He suggested that 'degenerate fluids' could accumulate in the body once the avenue of menstrual release ended, prescribing blood-letting as a remedy, but not purgative medications, which he said almost everyone agreed now were a bad idea.[191]

François-Pierre-Prosper Vernière's Montpellier thesis on the 'dangers of the critical age' of 1811 also cited Roussel's brief remarks in pointing to the importance of menstruation in defining the feminine vital force. Without menstruation, women 'acquired the constitution of men'.[192] But he took the equation of menstruation with femininity toward its most negative conclusion, condemning women after the end of menses to a state of uselessness, wrinkles, sagging breasts, loss of nobility of purpose and of harmony in health.[193] He claimed a stark difference too between rural and urban women, claiming that the latter reached their critical age as early as 38, while those in the countryside ceased menstruating between the ages of 45 and 50. He cited Fothergill's text in support of a naturalising view which promised a peaceful transition to old age for those had followed 'the wishes of nature' (meaning, they had children), had not been lazy, sedentary, either gluttonous or undernourished, drunk too much alcohol, taken too many hot baths or consumed too many hot beverages, engaged in tumultuous passions or excesses of venereal pleasure, had abortions, or long, difficult childbirths.[194]

There were several Paris theses on women's critical age too in the years 1808 and 1809.[195] But by 1808, the topic had also already spread to other regional medical faculties, as indicated by the example of the mature clinician J. J. Nicolon,

185 Ibid., 28. 186 Ibid., 49–50. 187 Ibid., 31.
188 Ibid., 50. 189 Ibid., 54. 190 Ibid., 55. 191 Ibid., 57.
192 François-Pierre-Prosper Vernière, *Aperçu des dangers de l'âge critique* (Montpellier: Jean Martel aîné, 1811), 3, 7.
193 Ibid., 4. 194 Ibid., 4, 7–8.
195 E. D. Ménissier, *Considérations générales sur quelques maladies qui affectent les femmes à l'âge critique*. Thèse (Paris: Didot Jeune, 1808); Honoré-Jean Verne, *Essai sur la cessation des menstrues et sur quelques maladies qui attaquent les femmes à cette époque critique*. Thèse (Paris: Didot Jeune, 1809).

who defended his doctoral thesis on the topic of menorrhagia during the 'critical age' at the University of Strasbourg.[196] He had formed his thesis from copious clinical notes of twenty years' practising medicine as either an *officier de santé* or a surgeon.[197] On the basis of his observation of the heavy bleeding that he considered to constitute menorrhagia, he placed the 'critical age' rather approximatively between the ages of 38 and 48.[198] Consequently, his case examples referred to young, even pregnant women, as well as those approaching the final cessation of menses.[199] This thesis was followed by another at Strasbourg in 1811 by Louis-Joseph Windrif,[200] which referred to no other works on the topic except for general principles derived from Haller and the naturalising stance borrowed from Fothergill. Windrif, like others, evoked the notion that since menstruation defined women's nature, its loss meant they became 'assimilated to men' from whom they now differed 'only in form'.[201] It contained no treatment advice aside from the recommendation that doctors dissuade women from their common view that menstruation was needed to cleanse their bodies.[202]

In 1812, J. B. Anglade approached the topic again in his Montpellier thesis, leaning heavily instead on the teachings of Montpellier scholar Vigarous.[203] He remarked that there was already a significant divergence of medical opinion about the matter of ailments relating to the final cessation of menses, with some physicians being attached to the idea that the diagnosis of every form of illness emerging around this time of a woman's life should be connected to the effects of the cessation of menses. The opposing view, on the other hand, suggested that since the cessation of menses was 'a phenomenon as natural as its apparition, it was better to count on the wise foresight of nature', and to regard most illnesses coinciding with the cessation of menses as unrelated to the functions of the uterus.[204] He implicitly cautioned against generalising to all women from clinical observations of the most symptomatic patients, observing astutely that if the cessation of menses mostly occurred 'according to the general order of nature, and consequently without the least trouble', doctors would be none the wiser for it, since these women would hardly warrant medical attention.[205] The two major effects of the cessation of menses, he said, were firstly that the blood flow to which a woman had been accustomed for some thirty years was now suppressed; and secondly,

[196] J.-J. Nicolon, *Observations sur la ménorrhagie qui survient à l'approche de l'âge critique, et sur l'aménorrhée par vice de conformation*. Thèse (Strasbourg: Levrault, 1808).
[197] Ibid., 1. [198] Ibid., 3. [199] Ibid., 4, 14,
[200] Louis-Joseph Windrif, *Essai sur les phénomènes de l'âge critique chez la femme; sur les principaux accidens que l'on remarque à cette époque, et sur les moyens de les prévenir*. Dissertation (Strasbourg: Levrault, 1811).
[201] Ibid., 2. [202] Ibid., 32.
[203] Jean Baptiste Anglade, *Considérations sur les effets que peut produire la cessation des règles*. Thèse (Montpellier: Jean Martel, 1812).
[204] Ibid., 5–6. [205] Ibid., 6.

that a woman was thereafter free of 'all the more or less dangerous impressions to which she was exposed' as a result of regular menstruation.[206]

Anglade noted that women who were too young to be experiencing the final cessation nonetheless often nonetheless had times of suppressed menses, with the two forms of suppression barely distinguishable from one another. In both cases, those women prone to plethora reported symptoms of 'constant suffocations, troubled breathing' and other lung complaints, heat palpitations, digestive complaints, and disturbed sleep. But, he said, while repeated blood-letting was a common prescription for suppressed menses in young plethoric women, such a treatment would be disastrous to women after the final cessation of menses, and was not advisable.[207] Anglade, like Leyral, remarked that because chronic illnesses occurred more often in older people, they could appear to coincide with the cessation of menses.[208] He noted the emergence of works by medical scholars (without naming anyone, but suggesting Fothergill) who were vociferously opposed to the use of purgatives in treating symptoms of the final cessation of menses, but who defended these for specific indications of plethora in some older women, as well as the use of leeches applied to the anus, cervix, vulva, or inner thighs whenever one suspected localised plethora of the genital organs.[209] Anglade accepted the now common view that illnesses in other parts of the body associated with cessation of menses could be caused by the sympathetic influence of the uterus through the nerves. But he also proposed that other organs in turn could negatively influence the uterus, and that it was they, and not the cessation of menses, that caused many of the uterine symptoms of older women.[210]

In the same year as the publication of Anglade's comparatively subtle and original considerations, there were another three specialist Paris theses on the final cessation of menses, as well as a fourth which treated it as part of an overview of all the questions of women's health relating to the uterus, from puberty until the critical age.[211] The thesis of C. A. M. Peloux, from a family of surgeons, was highly moral in tone, developing the theme of the Montpellier theses which had prescribed the childbearing and otherwise unstimulating peasant way of life as the ideal for corrupt city women to mimic, warning them against a wide range of self-indulgent behaviours throughout their lives that would supposedly determine their miserable 'critical age'. Peloux suggested that historically barbarian peoples had chased women away once they reached this time of life, or even

[206] Ibid., 15. [207] Ibid., 17. [208] Ibid., 16.
[209] Ibid., 20. [210] Ibid., 24.
[211] C. A. M. Peloux, *Essai sur l'époque critique et sur les moyens propres à prévenir les accidents et les maladies qui en dépendent* (Paris: Didot Jeune, 1812); Charles-Pierre-Louis de Gardanne, *Dissertation sur les avis à donner aux femmes qui entrent dans l'âge critique.* Thèse (Paris: Didot Jeune, 1812); J. A. Transtour, *Considérations générales sur quelques maladies qui affectent les femmes à l'âge critique.* Thèse (Paris: Didot Jeune, 1812); Joseph Capuron, *Traité des maladies des femmes, depuis la puberté jusqu'à l'âge critique inclusivement.* Thèse (Paris: Croullebois, 1812).

massacred them, virtue-signalling his own horror and outrage at such a treatment of the part of humanity who had given birth to its very leaders.[212] His reassurances of a peaceful critical age, which he acknowledged was possible, applied only to those women who had 'followed the wishes of nature', and lived frugal lives in the countryside and fresh air.[213] Woe be to those worldly women (*femmes du monde*) who were 'accustomed to a soft and idle life amidst a sickly atmosphere, whose health was damaged by the fire and turmoil of passions, by the profusions of delicacies, by the abuse of perfumes, of fermented liqueurs and by revelling in a thousand pleasures'.[214]

Capuron intoned in a similar fashion against women of dissolute morals whose critical age would punish them for having 'violated the laws of hygiene' and eschewed 'the precepts of clean morals'.[215] He seemed particularly concerned about women who were 'naturally passionate and voluptuous', who instead of moderating their tendencies, sought out 'tender liaisons, amorous intrigues, lascivious paintings, obscene books', and 'licentious conversations', which were all ill advised behaviours for those approaching the cessation of menses.[216] He too cited Fothergill's warning against the use of purgative medications, but made no mention of the many Montpellier scholars who been writing about the critical age or cessation of menses over the previous fourteen years, nor of Astruc's remarks about purgatives in the critical age dating from 1737.[217] Capuron captured perfectly the novel paradox of the emerging Parisian discourse about menopause. He explicitly naturalised it ('nothing is more natural than the cessation of the menses')[218] and rejected a variety of medical treatments which he claimed were conventional,[219] while also prescribing a wide range of hygienic interventions informed by strident moral assertions about different kinds of women according to social class, urban or rural lifeways, and moral virtues.[220] This was no simple matter of excessive 'medicalisation', nor indeed of depathologisation (as it pretended), but of which specific kind of medicine suited the treatment of this 'natural' life stage and which kind of woman was deemed to have merited a healthy experience of ageing.

Charles-Pierre-Louis de Gardanne's thesis was the one of the four of 1812 which would thereafter massively dominate the attention both of medical reviewers in its own time and of medical historians of menopause thereafter. It too was hardly original; its claim to fame was that its author proposed a single-word neologism to replace the cumbersome formulation 'the final cessation of menses': *la menespausie*, later modified to the more elegant *la ménopause* in his 1821 book based on the thesis, *De la ménopause, ou de l'âge critique des femmes* (On Menopause, or

[212] Peloux, *Essai sur l'époque critique*, v. [213] Ibid., 12. [214] Ibid., 11.
[215] Capuron, *Traité des maladies des femmes*, 126. [216] Ibid., 231. [217] Ibid., 240–241.
[218] Ibid., 126. [219] Ibid., 126, 230. [220] Ibid., 210, 231, 235–241.

the Critical Age of Women).[221] Gardanne claimed that his neologism was the only truly non-pathological designation, based on a strict definition of the object to which it referred as the cessation of menses.[222] Both the *temps critique* and the other less common *âge de retour*, he complained, echoing Tissot though without citing him, were terms which evoked danger, and so served only to worry women unnecessarily about this natural period of their lives, as they were prone to do anyway.[223] Given that much of the existing scholarship on the critical age came out of the University of Montpellier, it seems possible that Gardanne was here implicitly attacking the rival faculty, which had long been the object of much resentment at the Paris faculty since the end of the seventeenth century, on account of the royal favour in which the Montpelliérains had been held since the time of Louis XIII.[224] However, his attempted displacement of the 'critical age' was based on a misconception of the Montpellier concept of crises. He appears to have been entirely unaware both of the Montpellier theses published before his own on the topic, and of the vitalist concept of crises and critical times elaborated both in Montpellier and in Paris, which viewed these as positive, transitory adaptations in the movement from one mode of vital organisation toward another. Gardanne also suggested that the neologism was needed to eliminate what he claimed was a proliferation of terms all referring to the same thing: 'critical era, cessation of menses, disappearance of menstruation, the turn of age, the age of decline, the elderly spring (*verte vieillesse*), woman's hell, woman's winter, the death of sex, the critical time', remarking, 'one becomes lost in this maze of terms'.[225] In fact, though, Gardanne was conflating a number of different designations here, and several seem to have been entirely confected in order to show the need for his neologistic reduction. The 'woman's hell' derived from Roussel, who used it to refer not to the cessation of menses at all, but to women's fear of losing their beauty in ageing.[226] Similarly Jeannet des Longrois had used the term *verte vieillesse* in 1787 to refer to women in their forties, himself borrowing from a sixteenth-century scholar who had not used it to discuss either women or the cessation of menses.[227] Throughout the nineteenth century, the term was most commonly used to refer to healthy ageing in men and women, not to its sex-specific crisis, as for instance when at the funeral of 58-year-old Jean-Baptiste Maugras in 1830, the historian Charles du Rozoir said of him that 'everything led us to hope that he would prolong his *verte vieillesse*' when a brief illness suddenly

[221] Charles-Pierre-Louis de Gardanne, *De la ménopause ou de l'âge critique des femmes* (Paris: Méquignon-Marvis, 1821).
[222] Théré, 'Âge de retour et retour d'âge', 54–55.
[223] Gardanne, *Dissertation sur les avis à donner aux femmes*, v.
[224] Williams, *A Cultural History of Medical Vitalism*, 60.
[225] Gardanne, *Dissertation sur les avis à donner aux femmes*, ix.
[226] Roussel, *Système physique et moral*, 84–85.
[227] Jeannet des Longrois, *Conseils aux femmes de 40 ans*, 2; Laurens, *Discours de la conservation de la vene*, 246.

removed him on 17 February;[228] or as when the Abbé Bonnot in 1889 celebrated the fifty-year wedding anniversary of Mr and Mrs Charié-Marsaines by remarking that God had rewarded their piety with a *verte vieillesse* free of the many pains of existence that typically accompanied such a long life and marriage.[229]

In the next chapter we will return to Gardanne's themes, which differed little from those found in countless other theses throughout the nineteenth century claiming a new scientific modernity and providing broad hygienic advice for the management of older women's lives. Menopause, as it was now sometimes called, or the critical age, as it more often continued to be called, remained a popular topic of medical description and pedagogy: Between 1812 and 1930, more than 200 additional specialist works by doctoral students, established clinicians, medical professors, and medical popularisers were authored on it, with substantial subsections on the theme also appearing in general medical reference works and in general works on women's health or on medical hygiene. We end this chapter with Gardanne because after 1812 the sheer volume of works produced on the topic of menopause became so great as to prohibit exhaustive discussion, although their exhaustive reading has informed the analysis provided here. There would be little to be gained from citing all these works in any case—few of the many French theses and books to follow contained substantial innovation, mostly repetitively echoing the themes of earlier scholarship from both Montpellier and Paris, at times even blatantly plagiarising from it. No precedent or contemporaneous tradition in any other language yet came even close to the tremendous nineteenth-century French outpouring of medical writing on the topic of women's final cessation of menses, although a handful of specialist English, American, and German works appeared in the second half of the nineteenth century.[230] But as we saw in the previous chapters, several conceptual layers derived from diverse early modern traditions appear to have sedimented into something that might be considered a viable substrate for the medicalisation of women's final cessation of menses by the late eighteenth century. Thus began a long French tradition of insisting that the end of menses was not, per se, a risk to women's health, while at the same time offering heavily prescriptive and proscriptive hygienic advice that included management of sleep, movement, diet and digestion, sexuality, dress,

[228] Charles du Rozier, *Notice historique sur Maugras* (Paris: Brunueax, 1843), 4.

[229] *Cinquantième anniversaire du mariage de M. et Mme Charié-Marsaines: souvenir du 29 avril 1889* (Paris: E. Plon Nourrit et Cie, 1889), 3.

[230] Edward John Tilt, *The Change of Life in Health and Disease: A Practical Treatise on the Nervous and Other Affections Incidental to Women at the Decline of Life* (London: J. Churchill, 1857); Enoch Heinrich Kisch, *Das klimakterische Alter der Frauen: Physiologischer und pathologischer Beziehung* (Erlangen: Ferdinand Enke, 1874); Cohnstein, 'Zur Physiologie der Menopause', *Archiv für Pathologische Anatomie und Physiologie und für Klinische Medizin*, 61/1 (1874): 100–109; Siegfried Kracauer, *Die Melancholie der Frauen nach dem Climacterium.* Dissertation (Breslau: F. Jungfer, 1882); Ernst Börner, *Die Wechseljahre der Frau* (Stuttgart: Ferdinand Enke, 1886); Julius Brühl, *Über die psychischen Störungen des Klimakteriums.* Dissertation (Würzburg: A. Memminger, 1887); Andrew Fay Currier, *The Menopause* (New York: D. Appleton & Co.: 1897).

alcohol and coffee consumption, conditions of habitation, cosmetic usage, and warnings about the use of medications and services of folk healers, along with the assertion that this time of a woman's life 'requires the doctor's full attention.'[231]

In Chapter 1 we considered a range of early modern sources in which the final cessation of menses was acknowledged and naturalised, with the first scant smatterings of something resembling a negative view of it in the work of the late seventeenth-century Scottish-French Montpellier-trained physician Daniel Duncan. Duncan explicitly denied the value of medicating the final cessation or menses in any form. But by the time of Gardanne's neologisms in 1812 and 1821, the idea that a woman approaching menopause required medical supervision and treatment was already established, in different forms, in both Paris and Montpellier medicine. How, then, was this leap made? In part it was made through the assimilation of the final cessation of menses to all the other uterine changes thought to cause vapours, hysteria, and hypochondria, which was a feature of medical writing on these themes throughout the eighteenth and early nineteenth centuries at Halle, Paris, and Montpellier, as we consider in Chapter 5. In part too, though, it was fuelled by a mistranslation of different concepts of crisis and critical times between two kinds of medical tradition, and by the rivalry between the two largest medical faculties in France. The Montpellier view of menstrual changes as critical times leading to positive adaptation of the organism to a new mode of vital organisation was entirely lost on Parisian scholars of menopause, who instead fixated on these terms for the performance of a new kind of anti-pathological insistence that marked them as scientifically modern. That the Montpellier faculty took this response as a challenge to be answered is indicated by the wave of new Montpellier theses on women's critical age over the four decades following Gardanne's and the other 1812 Paris dissertations, but waning after the 1860s.[232] Strasbourg scholars, too, had entered the fray from as

[231] Gardanne, *Dissertation sur les avis à donner aux femmes*, 20–36.

[232] Jean-Antoine Poussié, *Réflexions sur l'hygiène qui convient aux femmes arrivées à l'âge de retour*. Thèse (Montpellier: Jean Martel aîné, 1813); Nicolas Broye, *Considérations sur la cessation des règles*. Thèse (Montpellier: Jean Martel Aîné, 1813); Jean-André Selvy, *Dissertation sur la métrorrhagie, ou hémorragie utérine qui a lieu dans l'âge critique*. Thèse (Montpellier: Jean Martel aîné, 1814); Louis Gubian, *Considérations générales sur l'état physiologique de la femme parvenue à l'âge critique, et sur les moyens hygiéniques qui lui conviennent*. Thèse (Paris: Didot Jeune, 1816); Jean-Antoine-Placide Jaumes, *Aperçu sur diverses maladies qui peuvent affecter les femmes à l'âge du retour* (Montpellier: Jean Martel aîné, 1816); Jean-Charles-Auguste Laville, *Considérations générales sur les causes et les moyens préservatifs des maladies des femmes à l'époque de la cessation des menstrues*. Thèse (Paris: Didot Jeune, 1816); Gilbert-Joseph-Magdeleine Guyot, *Quelques propositions sur la femme considérée dans les différentes périodes de la vie*. Thèse (Montpellier: Jean Martel, 1817); Sucrion Ramondene, *Considérations sur l'état de la femme à l'époque de la cessation des règles*. Thèse (Montpellier: Jean Martel, 1820); Jean-Claude Giraud, *Essai sur la ménespausie ou cessation des menstrues*. Thèse (Montpellier: Jean Martel, 1824); Jacques-Philippe Labarraque, *Aperçu physiologico-pathologique sur la menstruation en général, et quelques conseils d'hygiène pour l'âge critique en particulier*. Thèse (Montpellier: Jean Martel aîné, 1827); Joseph-Hortense Houlès, *De la ménopause considérée au point de vue de l'hygiène*. Thèse (Montpellier: Isadore Tournel, 1843); Edouard de Massia, *Âge critique chez la femme*. Thèse. (Montpellier: Boehm, 1851); Jacques Laugier, *De la ménopause (âge critique)*. Thèse (Montpellier: Jean Martel aine, 1861); Émile Bertin, *De la ménopause considérée principalement au point de vue de l'hygiène* (Montpellier: C. Coulet/Paris: Adrien Delahaye, 1866). Also discussing menopause as part of

early as 1808, as we saw, and continued to address the critical age question throughout the 1820s and 1830s, often ignoring all of the existing scholarship produced by the other two French faculties to engage instead with the emerging interest in women's diseases of ageing in English and German medicine.[233] The Paris scholars responded in turn with a veritable flood of at least forty new books and theses focused entirely or substantially on menopause throughout the period between 1813 and 1865, slightly less than one every year.[234] This might not seem

studies of both men's and women's critical ages were: Jean-Antoine Boude, *Quelques propositions sur l'hygiène des vieillards et des gens faibles*. Thèse (Montpellier: Jean Martel aîné, 1813), and François-Hyacinthe Teysset, *Quelques généralités sur l'hygiène des vieillards*. Thèse (Montpellier: Jean Martel, 1825).

[233] Prosper-Louis Sauvé, *Réflexions sur l'âge critique, et particulièrement sur le régime le plus convenable pour préserver les femmes des accidens qui ont coutume de survenir cette époque de leur vie*. Thèse (Strasbourg: F. G. Levrault, 1826); Hubert Quirin Franklin Poirson, *Dissertation sur la ménespausie*. Thèse (Strasbourg: F. G. Levrault, 1827); Louis-Marie-André Jeannin, *Considérations physiologiques, pathologiques et hygiéniques sur l'âge de retour des femmes*. Thèse (Strasbourg: F. G. Levrault, 1830).

[234] J.-P. Gravis, *Dissertation sur la cessation des menstrues, et sur les conseils à donner aux femmes pour les préserver des accidents ou maladies dont elles sont menacées à cette époque*. Thèse (Paris: Didot Jeune, 1813); Claude-Martial Bardout, *Considérations générales sur la cessation du flux menstruel, et sur les précautions à prendre pour en prévenir les accidens ou les maladies*. Thèse (Paris: Didot Jeune, 1816); Charles-Pierre-Louis de Gardanne, *Avis aux femmes qui entrent dans l'âge critique* (Paris: Gabon, 1816); Jean-Charles Auguste Laville, *Considérations générales sur les causes et les moyens préservatifs des maladies des femmes à l'époque de la cessation des menstrues*. Thèse (Paris: Didot Jeune, 1816); Etienne-Léandre Hébert, *Dissertation sur la cessation des règles, les accidens auxquels la femme est alors exposée, et les précautions qu'elle doit prendre pour les éviter* (Paris: Didot Jeune, 1817); P. N. Glinel, *Sur l'âge critique des femmes; Dissertation médico-physiologique* (Paris: Didot Jeune, 1818); Antoine-Alexandre Olive, *Dissertation inaugurale sur la première menstruation, l'âge critique et les soins hygiéniques que réclament les femmes à ces deux époques*. Thèse (Paris: Didot Jeune, 1819); Joseph-François Garnier, *Considérations sur l'âge critique, et sur l'hygiène des femmes à cette époque*. Thèse (Paris: Didot Jeune, 1820); P. Armand, *Considérations sur l'âge critique des femmes, et sur les moyens de prévenir les maladies qui peuvent survenir à cette période de la vie*. Thèse (Paris: Didot Jeune, 1820); Albert Assegond, *De la femme considérée à l'âge critique; changements physiologiques qui s'opèrent dans on état physiques et moral, et de l'application des règles de l'hygiène à cette principale époque de la vie*. Thèse (Paris: Didot Jeune, 1821); Alexis-François Aulagnier, *Nouveau recueil d'observations et de consultations sur les maladies des femmes, et spécialement sur celles qui se déclarent vers l'âge critique* (Paris: l'auteur, 1821); Gardanne, *De la ménopause ou de l'âge critique des femmes*; Jacques Devers, *Essai sur la cessation des règles*. Thèse (Paris: Didot le Jeune, 1822); C. L. Junod, *De l'époque critique chez les femmes et des précautions à prendre pour en prévenir et combattre quelques accidens ou maladies*. Thèse (Paris: Didot Jeune, 1822); N. N. Firmin Lemoyne, *Considérations générales sur les phénomènes qui se manifestent à la cessation du flux menstruel et sur le régime que doivent adopter les femmes pour franchir heureusement cette époque*. Thèse (Paris: Didot Jeune, 1824); Pierre-Jean-Baptiste Bertrand, *Dissertation sur l'aménorrhée définitive ou âge critique des femmes sur les accidents auxquels elles sont exposées à cette époque, et sur les moyens thérapeutiques, hygiéniques et prophylactiques les plus appropriés à leur situation* (Paris: Didot le Jeune, 1824); S. G. Chazal, *De l'hygiène des femmes à l'époque de la cessation des menstrues*. Thèse (Paris: Didot Jeune, 1826); Joseph-Paul Lefèvre, *Considérations générales sur la ménopausie, ou cessation naturelle des menstrues*. Thèse (Paris: Didot Jeune, 1826); E. Duplessis, *De l'âge critique et des soins hygiéniques que réclament les femmes à cette époque*. Thèse (Paris: Didot Le Jeune, 1828); Antoine Constant Saucerotte, *Nouveaux conseils aux femmes sur l'âge prétendu critique, ou conduite à tenir lors de la cessation des règles* (Paris: Madame Auger-Méquinon, 1828); Guy-François Marvaud, *Considérations générales sur la cessation des règles et sur l'âge faussement appelé critique*. Thèse (Paris: Didot Jeune, 1829); Stanislas-Victor-Amédée Navet, *Propositions sur le tempérament de la femme, sur sa menstruation et sur son âge critique*. Thèse (Paris: Didot Jeune, 1830); Lucien-Hector Docé, *Dissertation sur la cessation des menstrues vulgairement appelée âge critique, et sur les moyens hygiéniques que réclame la santé de la femme à cette époque*. Thèse (Paris: Didot Jeune, 1831); P. Maurice, *De la ménespausie*. Thèse (Paris: Didot Jeune, 1832); Charles-Victor Harreaux, *Essai sur une variété d'hypcondrie particulière aux femmes de l'âge*

huge compared other major topics in the history of nineteenth-century medicine. But it is striking considering that it referred to what most agreed was only a period of three to five years in women's lives, to what was by everyone's insistence 'not a disease', to what many agreed was often entirely asymptomatic, and correlated with no increased mortality, a fact that was also well understood by most scholars writing about it throughout this time, as we saw in the previous chapter. After the 1840s, Parisian scholars also responded—as did a few in Strasbourg—to the surge of new Montpellier publications by turning menopause into a new topic of degeneration psychopathology, as we consider in Chapter 7. Paris medicine of the mid and late nineteenth century emphatically medicalised the final cessation of menses, catastrophising the loss of menstrual function and listing a wide variety of serious medical and psychiatric problems attributable to it. It misconstrued the vitalist view of critical times as positive transitions, blaming both these and the folk practices of charlatans, empirics, and *commères* for pathologising menopause. Menopause had become a battleground in the struggle for scholarly preeminence between two rival faculties (neither of which allowed women to train as doctors), spurring the generation of a vast ocean of words, representing an entire new class of medical specialism, all dedicated to the meaning of women's reproductive ageing, but largely penned by young men as part of their pedagogic induction into the newly competitive world of clinical practice.

critique. Thèse (Paris: Imprimerie et fonderie de Rignoux et Cie, 1837); Auguste Nicaise, *Essai sur l'âge de retour chez la femme.* Thèse (Paris: Imprimerie et fonderie de Rignoux et Cie, Imprimeurs de la Faculté de Médecine, 1838); Louis-Marie Lafontaine-Margariteau, *Conseils hygiéniques aux femmes depuis leur naissance jusqu'à l'âge critique, ayant pour but principal de les préserver de la leucorrhée (fleurs blanches), ou de la diminuer si elle existe.* Thèse (Paris: Didot le Jeune, 1835); Joseph-Pierre-Éléonor Pétrequin, *Recherches sur la menstruation.* Thèse (Paris: Didot le Jeune, 1836); Sebastien Guyétant, *Le Médecin de l'âge de retour et la vieillesse: Conseils aux gens du monde, qui ont passé l'âge de quarante-cinq ans* (Paris: Dufey, 1836); Charles Menville, *Conseils aux femmes à l'époque de l'âge de retour, ou de l'âge critique, et de moyens de combattre et prévenir les maladies qui peuvent survenir à cette époque de la vie* (Paris: Germer Baillière, 1839); Adam Raciborski, *De la puberté et de l'âge critique chez la femme, au point de vue physiologique, hygiénique et médical* (Paris: J. B. Baillière 1844); Jean-Baptiste-Louis Poquillon, *De la ménopause, ou de l'âge dit critique chez la femme,* Dissertation (Paris: Rignoux, 1846); Ch.-Aug.-Dés. Ripeault, *De la ménopause.* Thèse (Paris: Rignoux, 1848); Jean-Baptiste Nosely, *Dissertation sur l'âge critique.* Thèse (Paris: Rignoux, 1848); Bernard-Eugène Gérard, *De l'âge critique chez la femme, et des maladies qui l'accompagnent.* Dissertation (Paris: Rignoux, 1849); Louis Chandelux, *L'Âge critique de la femme (ménopause).* Thèse (Paris: Irgnoux, 1850); Joseph Stéphane Baron, *De la ménopause (âge critique).* Thèse (Paris: Rignoux, 1851); Henri-Eugène Rocque, *Essai sur la physiologie et la pathologie de la ménopause.* Thèse (Paris: Rignoux, 1858); Marie-Gustave Léopold Chéneaux, *De la menstruation et de la ménopause, au point de vue de la physiologie et de l'hygiène.* Thèse (Paris: Rignoux, 1859); Virginie Messager, *Guide pratique de l'âge critique, ou Conseils aux femmes sur les maladies qui peuvent les attaquer à cette époque de leur vie, et sur les moyens de combattre ces maladies, mais surtout de les prévenir; suivis de Réflexions et d'observations sur les maladies laiteuses* (Paris: chez l'auteur, 1859); Gustave-Adolphe Plihon, *De la ménopause (âge critique).* Thèse (Paris: Rignoux, 1859); Jacques Laborde, *Quelques considérations sur la puberté chez la femme et sur la ménopause.* Thèse (Paris: Rignoux, 1860); Théophile-Charles-Emmanuel-Édouard Auber, *Hygiène des femmes nerveuses, ou Conseils aux femmes pour les époques critiques de leur vie* (Paris: Germer Baillière, 1864); Desmarres, 'Clinique opthalmologique: Amaurose cérébrale double, due à la suppression de l'époque menstruelle.—Guérison. Par M. le Docteur Xavier Galezowski', *Gazette des hôpitaux civils et militaires* (1864): 138; Bernard-Grégoire Emile Puyo, *De la ménopause.* Thèse (Paris: A. Parent, 1865).

4

Menstruation, Vapours, Hypochondria, and Hysteria

'Vous ne pouvez pas vous figurer combien le mot vapeur est riche en signification.'

('You cannot imagine how rich the word vapours is in signification.')
Claude Paumerelle, *La Philosophie des vapeurs*, 1774.[1]

One of the pathways through which the final cessation of menses became pathologised in modern biomedicine derived from its marginal association with three categories of nervous diseases which flourished in medical writing from the end of the seventeenth century, enduring into the nineteenth century: the vapours, hysteria, and hypochondria. Often all three of these terms were used interchangeably, although some scholars insisted on their differentiation both in cause and in treatment. The associations were marginal in the sense that none of these three nervous pathologies was particularly thought to affect older women or women who had ceased to menstruate, who, as noted in our first chapter, attracted barely any attention generally in the burgeoning scholarship on the diseases of women prior to the 1780s. Nonetheless, because nervous pathologies from this time onwards were increasingly discussed in relation to young women's menstruation, plethora, pre-menstrual times, pregnancy, and suppressed menses, post-menstruating women were sometimes now also included in the grouping of states of uterine change which made women more susceptible to these pathologies. Nervous diseases, many eighteenth-century doctors thought, were a product of luxury and civilisation—urban life, stale air, sedentary lifeways, overeating, exotic foods and beverages, licentiousness, and corporeal laziness. Many of the nineteenth-century ideas of nervous pathologies in menopause as resulting from the confluence of uterine change with the effects of modern affluent lifeways were directly imported from eighteenth-century works describing hysteria, hypochondria, and the vapours without any reference to older women. By the mid-eighteenth century, a medical view emerged of urban elite women in modern civilisation as generally more prone to nervous diseases, most of all during times

[1] Claude Paumerelle, *La Philosophie des vapeurs* [1774], 2nd ed. (Paphos: Royez, 1784), 5.

The French Invention of Menopause and the Medicalisation of Women's Ageing: A History. Alison M. Downham Moore, Oxford University Press. © Alison M. Downham Moore 2022. DOI: 10.1093/oso/9780192842916.003.0005

of uterine change—puberty, menstruation, pregnancy, childbirth, lactation, and the final cessation of menses, via the 'sympathies' of the uterus with other organs and particularly with the nervous system and the brain.

As several recent French scholars have noted, the late eighteenth century represented a marked shift in medical ideas about women's diseases, away from early modern accounts of pregnancy as a 'nine-month long illness', towards a view of puberty and the 'critical age' as peak moments of crisis and pathology in the female lifespan, with the childbearing years increasingly idealised as the pinnacle of women's health.[2] At the same time, numerous doctors, cognisant of emerging statistical data on mortality, insisted upon the continued danger that childbearing represented to women, naturalising the end of menses and the demise of fertility as the passing of the most dangerous time, as we saw in Chapter 2. From around the mid-nineteenth century, a new version of the idea that women's reproductive organs deranged their minds or nervous systems became most concentrated at the Paris faculty, where it intersected with the rise of alienism and developed into an elaborate theory of menopausal nervous and mental pathologies, with an emphasis on 'erotic mania' (discussed in Chapter 7). From the 1770s to the 1850s, Montpellier scholars, while making important contributions both to medical writing on the vapours and to the emergence of medical description of the cessation of menses, in fact often kept these two fields largely apart from one another. In this period, Montpellier scholars sometimes included the final cessation in descriptions of times when uterine sympathy disturbed women's nerves, but just as often insisted that the vapours and hysteria were less common in women once their menstruation ended. In the second half of the nineteenth century, the Montpellier scholars' influence waned due both to the centralisation of state support for medical pedagogy, and the development of competing faculties in other regional centres.[3] After 1840, the Montpellier faculty barely participated at all in the new ideas about menopause as a specific time of mental or nervous illness, only occasionally protesting against this view which had gathered so much force in the rise of Paris alienism. The critical age remained a pedagogical topic at Montpellier, but much less than it had been between 1799 and the 1830s. The fewer works after this time from Montpellier focused on anti-pathological hygienic advice, before joining the growing tide of research on ovarian physiology and opotherapy in the early twentieth century.[4]

[2] Elsa Dorlin, *La Matrice de la race: Généalogie sexuelle et coloniale de la nation française* [2006] (Paris: La Découverte/Poche, 2009), 131; Nicoletta Diasio, '"Habillée de temps": La Femme à l'âge critique dans le discours médical au tournant du XIXe siècle', in Virginie Vinel, ed., *Féminin/masculin: Approches anthropologiques des catégories et des pratiques médicales* (Strasbourg: Cahiers du portiQue, 2007), 101–129.

[3] Williams, *A Cultural History of Medical Vitalism*, 322–332; Matthew Ramsey, *Professional and Popular Medicine in France, 1779–1830* (Cambridge: Cambridge University Press, 1988), 71–97.

[4] Émile Bertin, *De la ménopause considérée principalement au point de vue de l'hygiène* (Montpellier: C. Coulet/Paris: Adrien Delahaye, 1866); Pierre Alaize, *Le Rôle de la fonction interne de l'ovaire et les*

Uterine and Ovarian Reductionism

Paradoxically, although the term used for the notion of a unique female mental illness derived from the Latin *hystericus*, referring to the uterus, nineteenth-century medical specialist writing on menopause hysteria actually emerged contemporaneously with an international revision of the role of the uterus in gynaecological thought, towards a new account of the ovaries as the main driver both of women's sexual desire and pathology.[5] The small size of uteruses observed in anatomical studies of elderly women's corpses since the sixteenth century had been taken to support a view of the cessation of menses as primarily a process of uterine atrophy. This view endured until the 1830s, after which the focus slowly began shifting throughout the nineteenth century towards a new emphasis on the ovary as the more important organ which declined in ageing. By the 1840s, many doctors of women's health were now converging on the view that it was generally the ovaries, not the uterus, which governed women's reproductive functions. Nonetheless, this corrective was far from universally accepted, and by the mid-nineteenth century, menopause as a time of nervous pathology had become its own specialist topic in the formation of Parisian degenerationist psychiatry, often with reference to the idea of uterine sympathy, as we consider in Chapter 7. The larger shift in physiological understanding away from the uterus and towards the ovaries certainly impacted ideas about women's reproductive organs perturbing their nerves, for some scholars, by casting doubt on the very concept of the genital origins of nervous disease. That concept nonetheless grew in influence, represented by a strident dogma in French psychiatry of the late nineteenth century, which associated menopause with hysteria, mania, hypochondria, and sexual perversion.

The ovarian revision was incomplete throughout the nineteenth century. It remained contentious well until the early twentieth century, with continuing references to the uterus in much French, German, and British medical writing on women's reproductive physiology, hysteria, women's sexuality, and menopause. In some works, it was specifically the ovaries that were said to shrink, atrophy, or ossify in menopause, thus disturbing the nervous system in the way that the uterus had been thought to do.[6] As early as 1758, the Strasbourg-native,

essais d'opothérapie ovarienne en pathologie nerveuse et mentale (Montpellier: Imprimerie générale du Midi, 1906); Adolphe Charreire, *Myomes et ménopause, atrophie, dégénérescences malignes, indications*. Thèse (Montpellier: G. Firmin, Montane & Sicardi, 1907); Pierre Nicolau, *Contribution à l'étude des métrorragies de la ménopause (métrorragies d'origine ovarienne)*. Thèse (Montpellier: Firmin & Montane, 1912).

[5] Ornella Moscucci, *The Science of Woman: Gynaecology and Gender in England, 1800–1929* (Cambridge: Cambridge University Press, 1993), 33–35.

[6] Adame Raciborski, *Traité de la menstruation; ses rapports avec la fécondation, l'hygiène de la puberté et de l'âge critique, son role dans les différentes maladies, ses troubles et leur traitement* (Paris: J. B. Baillière et Fils, 1868), 6–7.

Göttingen-based scholar Johann Georg Roederer (1726–1763) had described the anatomical changes in ovarian physiology associated with post-reproductive ageing in women.[7] The knowledge for the shift from a uterine to ovarian focus in relation to menopause was thus available from that time onwards, but the shift only definitely occurred after the 1890s. Prior to this time, and throughout the nineteenth century, almost all French medical works on menopause cited the supposedly Hippocratic aphorism: 'Propter uterum mulier tota morbus est' ('the uterus is the source of all women's diseases'), as we examine in Chapter 6.[8] In 1844, the Paris physician and medical historian Achille Chéreau (1817–1885) proposed that the Hippocratic aphorism needed revising in recognition of the emerging understanding of ovarian influences on the entirety of female physiology, suggesting the alternative: 'Propter solum ovariuni, mulier est id quod est.'[9] This was later edited into more correct Latin by the German physician and sceptic of Darwinism Rudolf Virchow, in the 1880s, as 'Propter ovarium solum mulier est quod est' ('woman is what she is solely because of the ovary').[10] In 1880, Dr Raoul Bossi asserted that 'It is the ovary, the female analogy of the male testicle, which performs the highest functions of the genital apparatus; the uterus is but a receptacle.'[11] Here the language of genital 'analogy' between the sexes, historian Thomas Laqueur's 'one-sex' conceptual layer, appears to have played an ongoing role. But in other works, the uterus continued to be emphasised in menopause symptomatology.[12] Uterine determinism was too prevalent and too central to gynaecologists' pedagogical and professional identity to be displaced so easily. Some collated the two organs into a single network, avoiding the question of which governed the other, or which more directly impacted women's overall health and disease.[13] Even after this shift had occurred, as Anne Fausto-Sterling remarks, debates about women's sexual anatomy in the history of modern medicine continued to refer to the Hippocratic uterine expression, proposing revisions of its Latin construction according to the mechanism now being posited as primary. The British obstetrician William Blair-Bell proposed in 1916 a further revision along the lines of the endocrinological shift in gynaecology/obstetrics:

[7] Johann Georg Roederer, *Icones uteri humani observationibus illustratae* (Göttingen: Vandenhoeck, 1758), 40.

[8] Or with the alternative sentence structure 'Mulier propter uterum tota morbus est': e.g. C. Leblanc, *Essai sur la métrite aiguë de la matrice ou inflammation* (Paris: Didot le Jeune, 1823), title page.

[9] Achilles Chéreau, *Mémoires pour servir à l'étude des maladies des ovaires* (Paris: Fortin, Masson, 1844), 91.

[10] Cited in Victor C. Medvei, *A History of Endocrinology* (Lancaster: MTP Press, 1982), 215.

[11] Raoul Boussi, *Étude sur les troubles nerveux réflexes observés dans les maladies utérines* (Paris: V. Adrien Delahaye, 1880), 36.

[12] Louis de Seré, *La Virilité à l'âge critique chez l'homme et chez la femme* (Paris: A. Delahaye et Lecrosnier, 1885), 17; Guyétant, *L'Âge de retour et la vieillesse*, 139.

[13] Pierre Berthier, *Des névroses menstruelles, ou la menstruation dans ses rapports avec les maladies nerveuses et mentales* (Paris: Delahaye, 1874), 5.

'Propter secretiones internas totas mulier est quod est' ('a woman is only as she is because of her internal secretions').[14] In all cases, the claim persisted that women were only women because of one or another component of their reproductive function, with the implication that in menopause, some essential defining condition of femininity was lost altogether. By this stage the early twentieth century there were growing international conversations about reproductive physiology and menopause, and the French were joined by new German, British, and American discourses about it.[15] But whichever organ was thought to be the locus of control over women's behaviour, it was always some part of the reproductive system that was cited: woman was still always nothing more than her youthful, functioning genital organs

As medical historian Victor Medvei noted, these perspectives all assumed a mechanism of control in which the nervous system mediated both physiology and behaviour via the ovaries, uterus, or both organs, implying an electrical impulse, rather than the type of sanguine mechanism that had dominated early modern views of menstruation as plethora. Only at the turn of the twentieth century did emerging developments in endocrinology suggest to some gynaecologists that the ovaries, as glandular organs, might be responsible for the production of hormonal products circulating in the bloodstream that mediated (but did not alone control) both reproductive physiology and sexual behaviour.[16] In the context of the nineteenth-century insistences that women's character was determined by their reproductive organs (or their secretions), it is perhaps unsurprising that French texts were undermined in their attempts to normalise a healthful vision of menopause, creating powerful tensions in their work that made their hygienic assurances to women appear empty.

Vapours, Hysteria, and the Assemblage of Menopause

We turn now to consider how the nineteenth-century assemblage of ideas connecting the end of menstruation with nervous pathology was brought about by the convergence of diverse strands of medical ideation about women which were elaborated throughout the long eighteenth century—with enduring legacies

[14] A. Fausto-Sterling, *Sexing the Body: Gender Politics and the Construction of Sexuality* (New York: Basic Books, 2000), loc7343 note 52. B. W. Bell, *The Sex-Complex: A Study of the Relationship of the Internal Secretions to the Female Characteristics and Functions in Health and Disease* (New York: William Wood & Co., 1916), 129.

[15] Birgit Panke-Kochinke, *Die Wechseljahre der Frau: Aktualität und Geschichte (1772–1996)* (Opladen: Leske & Budrich, 1998); Moscucci, *The Science of Woman;* Fausto-Sterling, *Sexing the Body*; Foxcroft, *Hot Flushes, Cold Science*; Houck, *Hot and Bothered*; Margeret M. Lock, *Encounters with Aging: Mythologies of Menopause in Japan and North America* (Berkeley: University of California Press, 1993).

[16] Medvei, *A History of Endocrinology*, 215.

throughout the nineteenth century as well. The presence of the final cessation of menses in medical writing on the vapours, hysteria, and hypochondria during the long eighteenth century was scant but distinguishable. This allowed the first generation of scholars writing on women's critical age or menopause in the final decades of the century, and especially in the first half of the nineteenth century, to lean on eighteenth-century scholars in ascribing nervous diseases to this time of life. This was so even though none of these scholars themselves considered the cessation of menses to be a particularly important time for nervous diseases (although Pinel, on the cusp of the nineteenth century, came closer than any of the others, as we will discuss in this chapter). The claim that the 'critical age' was the cause of nervous diseases was also contested by numerous other scholars who argued that, on the contrary, the cessation of menses alleviated nervous pathologies that impacted women only during the time of peak uterine activity, in their reproductive years.

As Sabine Arnaud has shown in relation to hysteria during this time, a new account of hysteria as a uniquely feminine and nervous disease was reconstructed during the eighteenth century. Hysteria was described with reference to diverse concepts presented as derived from the ancients, and thus as having deep foundations in the history of medicine.[17] By the early nineteenth century, a similar process would occur with menopause, as we consider in Chapter 6, with physicians repeatedly claiming that medical tradition had always catastrophised the negative symptoms of the final cessation of menses. While hysteria was a central topic in French medicine after the 1750s, and then in French psychiatry throughout the nineteenth century and beyond, the vapours, by Arnaud's authoritative account, flourished from roughly 1689 to 1789,[18] although some use of the term as a synonym for hysteria endured into the nineteenth century.[19] Hypochondria was clearly part of the discourses of hysteria and the vapours, but was also a more general term that could refer to any diseases of the abdomen (below the ribs, as the Latin word describes) in men or women. Alternatively, it was sometimes used in a more specific sense to refer to nervous disorders of presumed digestive origin, though nineteenth-century texts on menopause it was sometimes given a special place as the nervous disease of women approaching the final cessation of menses.[20] Throughout most of the eighteenth century until the 1770s, however, it was rarely used in relation to older women, and never, it seems, in relation to the end of menstruation specifically.

[17] Sabine Arnaud, *On Hysteria: The Invention of a Medical Category Between 1670 and 1820* (Chicago: University of Chicago Press, 2015), 1, 9–13.

[18] Ibid., 4.

[19] Clair Antoine, *Essai sur les vapeurs en général, et sur l'hystérie en particulier* (Montpellier: Jean Martel aîné, 1814); Louis-Charles-Edouard Lapasse, *Hygiène de longévité, guérison des migraines, maux d'estomac, maux de nerfs et vapeurs* (Paris: Victor Masson/Garnier Frères, 1861).

[20] Charles-Victor Harreaux, *Essai sur une variété d'hypocondrie particulière aux femmes de l'âge critique*. Thèse (Paris: Rignoux et cie., 1837).

vapours and the nineteenth-century elaboration of menopause. Even in the second half of the eighteenth century, the vapours were still never considered to impact older women specifically, and in fact were more often discussed as a problem of young women and even of men. But strikingly, the themes listed as causes of the vapours in eighteenth-century medical works were very similar to the proposed causes of menopausal symptoms described by nineteenth-century doctors, who sometimes even still referred to such symptoms as vaporous.[36] The vapours—like plethora—although clearly not menopause, represented one of the numerous conceptual layers in the substrate of ideas from which the French notion of menopause germinated. The 1758 *Treatise on the Vaporous Afflictions of the* [Female] *Sex* by the royal physician Joseph Raulin (here using *le sexe* as a synonym for women), elaborated how European bodies, especially female ones, now ubiquitously suffered from the effects of modern civilisation in the form of vapours, which he more or less equated with both hysteria and hypochondria. The primary culprit, Raulin thought, was sedentary life and the lack of exercise in urban and elite women:

> I have given but a simple idea of the necessity of exercise and of the inconvenience of laziness; however, if one casts one's eye upon the way of life of Ladies of our time, one will not be surprised if the majority are overheated, covered in pimples, bothered by heat in the viscera, exhausted by white discharge, by extraordinary bleeding even at an advanced age—since bleeding at such an age is never in the natural order of things. Often there is suppression, and always obstruction in the viscera and a great irritability of the nervous type. Hence vapours, from hence hypochondriac afflictions.[37]

Raulin clearly saw disorders of discharge and bleeding as proximate causes of the vapours in women, including older women, which were distantly explained by the lazy and dissolute lifeways of the elites of modern Europe. While this might have led him to consider all women who had permanently ceased menstruating even more susceptible to vapours, like Hunauld, he was altogether uninterested in the idea that specific life phases were causes of this disease, instead focusing primarily on what he called 'external' causes, especially the matter of life habits.

[36] Examples include Joseph Gagnebé, *Exposition de quelques maladies qui attaquent les femmes à la cessation des règles*. Thèse (Montpellier: Imprimerie de Tournel, 1801), 5; Charles Menville, *De l'âge critique chez les femmes, des maladies qui peuvent survenir à cette époque de la vie et des moyens de les combattre et de les prévenir* (Paris: Imprimerie de Bourgogne et Martinet, 1840), 44; Théophile-Charles-Emmanuel-Édouard Auber, *Hygiène des femmes nerveuses, ou Conseils aux femmes pour les époques critiques de leur vie* (Paris: Germer Baillière, 1864), 220; and especially Louis-Charles-Edouard Lapasse, *Hygiène de longévité, guérison des migraines, maux d'estomac, maux de nerfs et vapeurs* (Paris: Victor Masson/Garnier Frères, 1861).

[37] Joseph Raulin, *Traité des affections vaporeuses du sexe, avec l'exposition de leurs symptômes, de leurs différentes causes, et la méthode de les guérir* (Paris: Jean-Thomas Hérissant, 1758), 97.

Raulin's ideas about the vapours being caused by various external forces extended into some extraordinary claims about foreign influences on women's bodies in modern civilisation. Alongside sedentary mores, he considered the consumption of colonial products such as tobacco, coffee, tea, and chocolate as among the principal causes of the vapours and general ill health. Such products, while long favoured by peoples of the Orient and South America, were damaging to Europeans, he claimed.[38] Tea was all very well for Asians whose blood was thick, but it caused Europeans to urinate and sweat excessively and was especially bad for old people.[39] *Café au lait*, much in vogue among ladies of the day, nonetheless gave them white vaginal discharge (*fleurs blanches*), he asserted. Chocolate was a healthy drink in its original form, but was corrupted by French adaptations of it, such as the practice of serving it sweetened with sugar, and flavoured with cinnamon, clove, vanilla, ambergris, and musk.[40] In a remarkable reverse-victim discourse, Raulin claimed that tobacco, along with syphilis, was the vengeance of those conquered by colonial powers, whom he blamed for the 'gift of venereal disease' and characterised as installing their habits in Europeans and bequeathing pernicious plants to them.[41]

Raulin also helped to develop one of the central themes of medical discourses about women's health that became most common after his time, remaining so throughout the nineteenth century: the comparison of peasant women who engaged in constant physical activity with urban elite women who lived lazy and inactive lives. In Raulin's account, it was the latter lifestyle which made one susceptible to the vapours.[42] 'Women in whom education was gained at the cost of a too delicate life, who have been nourished far from exercise, in the bosom of pleasures, have nerves so tender that the slightest thing perturbs them and puts them into convulsion.'[43] In the nineteenth century, numerous doctors drew upon the exact same distinction to account for the symptoms of menopause, of which women of the countryside were said never to suffer, but which tormented the spoilt elites of the city with their soft beds, luxurious habits, and lazy lifeways. It is quite clear that, although the eighteenth-century vapours were not specifically related to women's ageing or the cessation of menses, many of the same ideas about their causation were transferred directly to the new menopause aetiology half a century later.

Notably, too, Raulin did consider that among the symptoms of vapours were disorders of vaginal secretion or blood flow, including unnatural bleeding in older women—implying those who would be expected no longer to menstruate. Here a similar hydraulic model to that which had underpinned the Halle school's description of plethora was brought into play. Liquids were separated from solids

[38] Ibid., 76–80. [39] Ibid., 76–77. [40] Ibid., 81.
[41] Ibid., 84. [42] Ibid., 96. [43] Ibid., 112.

in the process of digestion, 'the juices that nature does not adopt become foreign from the moment they are separated', at which moment they must be excreted, otherwise they became corrupted, 'becoming obstacles to nature and the cause of illness'.[44] Sweat, urine, and faeces could all become obstructed, causing disease in both sexes, but nothing affected those of nervous temperament more than perturbations of menstruation. Heavy menstruation was particularly a cause of the vapours, but so too were delayed or suppressed menses.[45] Women were thus more prone to vapours on account of menstruating (or of failing to), but they were also 'naturally disposed to convulsive perturbations' due to their greater sensitivity and the impressionability of their nervous fibres. 'Famous authors have observed that the disposition of the vessels of women's lower belly is often one of the causes of their vaporous afflictions', he remarked, here equating the vapours with hysteria.[46] He said that the corpses of women who had long been afflicted with the vapours, when opened, were found to have tumours of the uterus. But one woman he had examined after her death was also found to have a large polyp in the left ventricle of the heart.[47] Notably, Raulin's detailed description of the many forms of menstrual pathology included no mention of women who had ceased menstruating due to age.[48] While he certainly considered the uterus to be the most important culprit in the causation of the vapours, all the other visceral organs were also salient, with the intestines, the ventricles, the mesentery, the pancreas, the liver, and the spleen also all attracting their own separate chapters in his book.[49] Vapours could disseminate to any part of the body through a kind of 'metastasis', 'where the reverse mechanism which had brought them to the lower belly from the chest, from the head' could also redistribute them into other organs.[50]

Another important influence which helped to cement the associations of menstrual stoppage with nervous pathologies was the work of the Irish-French scholar Gérard Fitzgerald (1686–1748) who migrated to Montpellier, where he became an influential professor of the diseases of women there during the 1720s and 1730s. He wrote very little himself but taught a great deal, and his Latin lectures were transcribed by his students and published after his death, both in Latin and in French translation.[51] Importantly, Fitzgerald, although he discussed nervous and other diseases associated with the suppression of menstruation, carefully distinguished between suppression in women of reproductive age and the natural cessation of menses with ageing. His copious remarks about the dangers of suppressed menses, he said, were only relevant to those women 'who were of an

44 Ibid., 98–99. 45 Ibid., 104. 46 Ibid., 111. 47 Ibid., 134–136.
48 Ibid., 395–406. 49 Ibid., 140–175. 50 Ibid., xii.
51 Gérard Fitzgerald, *Tractatus pathologicus de affectibus feminarum praeternaturalibus* (Paris: J. Neaulme, 1754); Gérard Fitzgerald, *Traité des maladies des femmes* (Paris: Duchesne, 1758). See Louis Dulieu, *La Médecine à Montpellier*, vol. 3: *L'Époque classique*, 1er partie, 288–289 and 2ème partie, 760–761; Williams, *A Cultural History of Medical Vitalism*, 68.

age to have periods'.[52] He considered the suppression of menstruation during pregnancy problematic since, while most of the blood served to nourish the infant, there was often an excess which infused the vessels and mixed with humours of the neighbouring regions, causing disorder.[53] But it does not appear to have occurred to him to extend this theory to women after their menstruation had definitively ceased. Much of his interest in women's health was focused on the problem of chlorosis (later defined as iron deficiency) which could render women sterile, and he noted that this condition was more severe in older than in young women, but also considered that this was because the disease had been present for many years—it was not in itself a disease of ageing.[54]

Other scholars, both in France and in England of the 1760s and 1770s, began connecting the vapours partially to matters of unusual uterine bleeding, vaginal secretions, pregnancy, childbirth, and menstrual suppression. Jean Maria's Lyon dissertation of 1759 focused precisely on this theme, using the terms *les vapeurs*, *l'hypochondrie*, and *l'hystérie* interchangeably, though nuancing a wide variety of diverse pathologies for them all according to the different temperaments.[55] Six years later, an English work by the Edinburgh physician Robert Whytt, *Observations on the Nature, Causes and Cure of those Disorders called Nervous, Hypochondriac or Hysteric*, had a significant impact in French medicine, where it helped to discredit the vague concept of vapours in favour of the supposedly more specific hysteria and hypochondria.[56] The gradual loss of medical esteem for the term 'vapours' after this time was not only a product of Whytt's scorn for the overuse of the word—the satirical *La Philosophie des vapeurs* by the playwright Claude Paumerelle published in 1774 (cited at the start of this chapter) exposed the absurd popular meanings attributed to this term, making it a dubious basis for biomedical aetiology or terminology.[57] Whytt's book appeared in French translation in 1767, only two years after the original. It was greeted enthusiastically in France no doubt in part because it implicitly scoffed at the humoralist approach found in works on the vapours over the past 100 years, which had since given way to more solidist emphases focused on the nerves. It also expanded on the highly fashionable topic of nervous 'sympathy' and 'irritability'. Whytt reiterated the view already found in French scholarship that women were the more nervous and mobile sex, and therefore more prone to nervous diseases; but he also importantly listed menstrual suppression or diminution among the occasional causes of hysteria, clearly and explicitly including the natural cessation of

[52] Fitzgerald, *Traité des maladies des femmes*, 20. [53] Ibid., 320. [54] Ibid., 21–22.

[55] Jean Maria, *Dissertation sur les vapeurs, pertes de sang, pertes blanches, grossesses et couches* (Lyon, 1759).

[56] Robert Whytt, *Observations on the Nature, Causes and Cure of those Disorders, which have been commonly called Nervous, Hypochondriac or Hysteric; To which are prefixed some Remarks on the Sympathy of the Nerves* (Edinburgh: T. Becket & P. A. De Hondt, 1765).

[57] Paumerelle, *La Philosophie des vapeurs*.

menses in ageing. Any 'change of the circulation in the womb' could irritate the nerves, Whytt claimed, making pregnancy as well as the final cessation of menses both peak moments for hysterical vapours.[58] This was via a mechanism of 'sympathy' between the womb and the nervous system, since when the vessels of the womb were engorged with blood, they would stimulate the surrounding nerves, which in turn would transmit their irritation to other parts of the body. Menstruation was not caused by a general state of plethora, he acknowledged, but when a body that was accustomed to rid itself of an accumulation of blood suddenly lost its capacity to do so, the whole organism would suffer nervous complaints.[59] This was why both women in whom menstruation had ceased for whatever reason, as well as men or women whose haemorrhoidal flow had stopped, were likely to suffer nervous diseases.[60] Menstrual blood was particularly nefarious to retain, though, Whytt thought, and became acrid when it could not exit, causing especially negative effects on the nerves.[61]

Not deterred by Whytt's criticism of the all-encompassing definition of every disease as 'vaporous', the Lyon professor of medicine and surgery Jean-Baptiste Pressavin, who had trained in Paris, authored a much-cited treatise on the vapours in 1770 which, like Whytt's book, described the moments of uterine change in puberty, menstruation, and childbirth as among the many possible causes of epilepsy, 'false epilepsy' (a single-episode form of epilepsy), or vapours.[62] Pressavin certainly did not consider all nervous pathologies to be more common in women. He included an entire chapter on priapism in men (uncontrollable, often painful, constant erection), classing it as a physiological spasm of the nerves of the penis, in contrast to satyriasis, which he viewed as simple debauchery.[63] Nonetheless, like earlier scholars, Pressavin considered women more prone to nervous disorders in general on account of their more delicate constitutions and more elastic nerve fibres;[64] and throughout his treatise, he presented perturbations of the womb (during puberty, childbirth, and with suppressed menses) as the most important cause of women's nervous pathologies.[65] The remedy differed according to the kind of disturbance—blood-letting if the cause was plethora; purgatives if the cause was a disturbance of the humours; tonic medicines if the cause was excessive laxity of the nervous fibres; and diluent remedies (*délayants*) and baths if the fibres were too rigid.[66] If epilepsy was caused by menstrual suppression, the clinical focus should be on restoring the function of the womb with different emmenagogues.[67] Hysterical vapours too were cured by emmenagogues

[58] Robert Whytt, *Les Vapeurs et maladies nerveuses, hypocondriaques ou hystériques reconnues & traitées dans les deux sexes*, 2 vols (Paris: Vincent, 1767), vol. 1, 494–496.
[59] Ibid., 497–499. [60] Ibid., 494. [61] Ibid., 504.
[62] Jean-Baptiste Pressavin, *Nouveau Traité des vapeurs, ou traité des maladies des nerfs, dans lequel on développe les vrais principes des vapeurs* (Paris: La Veuve Reguilliat, 1770), 89–96.
[63] Ibid., 63–72. [64] Ibid., 203–205, 233.
[65] Ibid., 89–90, 101, 110, 122, 128. [66] Ibid., 117–118. [67] Ibid., 122.

administered along with iron-rich remedies (*martiaux*).[68] Pressavin considered heavy menstruation a cause of convulsive asthma via 'irritation of the womb's nerves', which was communicated to the nerves of the chest. The remedy for this was simply blood-letting.[69] Women were also prone to hysterical colic and to the vapours if their menses were overdue and suppressed, which was caused by retained blood distending the nerves of the womb—or by plethora.[70] Women could also suffer this problem after childbirth, but in both cases, Pressavin considered that no remedy was needed, since these conditions would cure themselves with the eventual expulsion of the blood.[71] He recommended a topical omelette (made of eggs, milk, breadcrumbs, onion, and saffron) applied to the belly for premenstrual cramps, along with an elixir of cinnamon quills, lemon-balm, castoreum, laudanum, and opium syrup.[72]

Notably, Pressavin's treatise contains no mention whatsoever of women's final cessation of menses. Nonetheless, it is not hard to see how later scholars viewed his work as supporting their case for the classification of menopause as a time of nervous pathology, seamlessly extending Pressavin's notion of uterine perturbation as a cause of hysteria, epilepsy, the vapours, or hypochondria to the final cessation of menses—as both Hecquet and Whytt, and indeed the earlier Halle scholars, had all done. Pressavin claimed that it was rare for a woman suffering any form of gynaecological problem, including ulcers, tumours, or cancer, not also to have hysterical vapours.[73] He also referred to the—by now standard—hygienic differentiation of healthy, active peasant women versus lazy, affluent, and voluptuous urban women with poor diet, which thereafter became a central theme of nineteenth-century claims about menopause symptomatology.[74]

The ample mechanistic rationale for nervous pathologies provided by Pressavin can help us to appreciate how women in every stage of uterine change, and in relation to their modern lifeways, were increasingly targets of French medical ideas from this time onwards. He followed both the Swiss naturalist Albrecht von Haller (1708–1777) and the English physician Francis Glisson (1597–1677) in reiterating the concept of 'irritability' as an elastic property of the nerves which made them potentially capable of a reaction greater than their own underlying force—hence their capacity for pathology.[75] He also followed Haller in the view that while elasticity was inherent to animal fibres, sensitivity was foreign to them and was elicited by outside stimulation from the environment.[76] This explained

[68] Ibid., 168. [69] Ibid., 175–176. [70] Ibid., 181, 253, 274.
[71] Ibid., 181–182. [72] Ibid., 183. [73] Ibid., 255. [74] Ibid., 256.
[75] Ibid., ix–x; Albrecht von Haller, *Elementa physiologiae corporis humani*, vol. 8, Part II (Berne: Sumptibus Sumptibus Societatis Typographicae, 1766); Francis Glisson, *Tractatus de natura substantiae energetica, seu de vita naturae* (London: Flesher, 1672).
[76] Pressavin, *Nouveau Traité des vapeurs*, xi.

why women, whose fibres were now thought more elastic than men's, were both more prone to nervous pathology in general and more susceptible to the nefarious effects of the lifeways of industrial modernity and affluence, which were thought to over-sensitise their delicate nervous systems. Likewise, other major figures of French thought in the period between 1777 and 1802, such as Pierre Roussel, Claude-Adrien Helvétius, and Pierre-Jean-George Cabanis, reiterated the view of women's specific nervous perturbation by the stimulus of civilisation.[77] Helvétius too recalled the naturalistic characterisation of women's religious ecstasy as vapours, which had been a feature of late seventeenth-century debates about the *convulsionnaires*, remarking that 'hysterical women and those subject to the vapours are the most prone to ecstasies and visions'.[78] Later in the nineteenth century, the theme of women's nervous diseases in menopause expressed as religious fervour would re-emerge as 'symptom' of ageing decline.[79]

Another Montpellier scholar, Edme-Pierre Chauvot de Beauchêne (1749–1824), with his 1781 book on women's nervous diseases (published in four different editions up to 1798), further helped to develop the association of the final cessation of menses with all the other uterine changes which many already agreed caused vapours, hysteria, or hypochondria in women.[80] Beauchêne provided the most nuanced account of various nervous diseases of women yet published in French or any other language, detailing highly specific symptomatologies and treatment regimes for them all. While Pressavin had suggested that the vapours were particularly a problem of civilisation and luxury, Beauchêne went much further in suggesting that nervous diseases were entirely historically novel, appearing only in recent times in large towns, especially Paris. He provided the most florid exegesis yet on the theme of how modernity, luxury, and urban life disturbed the nerves of women, and how simple, hard-working peasant women were free from all such disturbances. Most women in large towns now had the vapours, he declared, whereas they were rarely ever seen in the countryside.[81] Life in the city was problematic for women, both because the sensitivity of their organs often exceeded their organs' own internal force[82] and because city women

[77] Pierre Roussel, *Système physique et moral de la femme* (Paris: Chez Vincent, 1775); Claude-Adrien Helvétius, *Œuvres complètes*, vol. 4 (London: No publisher named, 1777); Pierre-Jean-Georges Cabanis, 'Rapports du physique et du moral de l'homme: Cinquième mémoire: De l'influence des sexes sur le caractère des idées et des affections morales' [1802], *Œuvres complètes de Cabanis*, vol. 3 (Paris: Bossanges Frères/Firmin Didot, 1824), 293–365.

[78] Helvétius, *Œuvres complètes*, vol. 4, 304. 'Les femmes hystériques & sujettes aux vapeurs sont les plus sujettes aux extases & aux visions'.

[79] Esquirol, *Des maladies mentales*, vol. 1, 503; Michel-Victor Barbier, *De l'influence de la menstruation sur les maladies mentales*. Thèse (Paris: Rignoux, 1848), 14; Henri Guimbail, *De la folie à la ménopause*. Thèse (Paris: A. Delahaye, 1884), 27, 29, 49–50, 69–70.

[80] Edme-Pierre Chauvot de Beauchêne, *De l'influence des affections de l'âme dans les maladies nerveuses des femmes, avec le traitement qui convient à ces maladies* [1781], 2nd ed. (Montpellier & Paris: Méquignon, 1783).

[81] Ibid., 1–2, 7–9. [82] Ibid., 17.

woke too late in the day to enjoy the fresh morning air, exercised insufficiently, and ate almost constantly, including copious desserts and liqueurs which made 'a great impression on their nerves'.[83] Beauchêne alluded to the theory of sympathy between the uterus and brain, but said nothing about different ages of women in his mechanistic account.[84] He reiterated Astruc's view that regular menstruation was not necessary for good health and that weak, delicate women almost always had heavy periods.[85] Nonetheless, he listed many nervous diseases that could result from suppressed menses, for which the treatment should not be bloodletting but acrid enemas, half-baths, ligatures, friction of the limbs with tincture of cantharides, cupping with a scarificator, vesicatory (a blistering agent), with a view to drawing movement away from the uterus.[86] Most curiously though, his case observations included three women around the age of 45–50 years, whom he specified to be 'in the era of their critical time'.[87]

A close look at Beauchêne's cases helps us to see how a wide variety of different conditions in women in their forties and fifties were by now both being categorised as nervous pathologies and being associated with the 'critical time' of the final cessation of menses. One case-observation concerned a woman 'around 45 years of age', who since 'arriving at the era of her critical time' had been suffering spasms, convulsions, fainting, poor appetite, and disturbed sleep for several years. She had received little treatment, Beauchêne said, because her symptoms were assumed to be the result of her menses ending.[88] This intriguing remark suggests a curious juncture in the history of Montpellier medicine. The cessation of menses was now taken to be the cause of a wide variety of health problems in women around 45–50 years of age, but was also often still naturalised as a 'crisis' in the Montpellier sense of something that would resolve itself favourably if left alone, hence requiring no treatment. But the new categorisation of so many different conditions as 'nervous', of which Beauchêne was a proponent, created a tension with the naturalising approach. Beauchêne diagnosed this woman with 'an extreme mobility in the entire nervous system', and hypothesised that a 'mass of humours' most likely around the womb was the cause of a vicious sensitivity of the viscera, which was transmitted via sympathy to the nerves of the brain. He treated her with a mostly vegetable diet, lots of fruit, light white beer, dandelion juice, and various mineral waters, which 'purged' her of a copious black bile, after which she was cured.[89] Another of his cases described a 48-year-old woman who had passed 'the critical time' in her thirties and had had blood and burning sensations with her urination ever since, along with pain throughout the kidneys, lumbar, buttocks, and thighs. Beauchêne

83 Ibid., 31–35. 84 Ibid., 44–54. 85 Ibid., 118.
86 Ibid., 123–126. 87 Ibid., 126–128, 157–158, 167–171.
88 Ibid., 126–127. 89 Ibid., 127–128.

diagnosed her with mucosal degeneration of the blood, with possible kidney stones, and prescribed her a vegetable diet, iron, mineral waters, and strong purgatives, including hemlock and cinchona at high doses.[90] Another woman he treated, aged 45, who had always had irregular periods only recently developed abdominal pain, white discharge interspersed with heavy and painful bleeding, as well as colic, poor digestion, spasms, and convulsions.[91] Before coming to Beauchêne, she had been treated with much blood-letting, baths, and gentle, calming remedies, to no avail. She was diagnosed with a uterine polyp and recommended for surgical ligature, and Beauchêne was called upon to treat the nervous aspects of her illness.[92] He treated her firstly with aromatic and purifying herbs such as thyme (*serpolet*) and marjoram, beef bile and cinchona, followed by repeated vaginal flushing with corrosive mineral waters, abdominal compresses, and enemas of coffee with a few drops of Hoffmann's elixir, or of opium. He prescribed a mustard of grated horseradish to be taken with every meal, and a diet of dark meats, egg yolks, game meats, ripe fruits, white wine, and watery coffee; soups, floury products, white meats, fish, and legumes were strictly forbidden. After two months of this regime, her nervous symptoms were cured, and her uterine mass had 'melted'.[93]

These fascinating case examples show how the new mechanistic concept of women's nervous pathologies related to uterine sympathy with the brain merged with humoral and chemical models of constitution-specific ageing among the Montpellier-trained physicians of the late eighteenth century. Unsurprisingly, it was at this medical faculty that the tangled complex of old and new medical ideas first cohered into a view of women's final cessation of menses as a unique form of critical transition—not at the Paris school so often emphasised in existing scholarship on French menopause and where Gardanne coined the modern neologism in 1812. But it was far from obvious how doctors should respond to the 'crisis' of the end of menstruation, and works both on the end of menses and on women's nervous pathologies still contained no clear recommendations for the treatment of women at this life stage, nor even any clear statement of a need for such treatment. By the 1780s there were also now the first discussions of general physical symptoms associated with the final cessation of menses: the French translation of Fothergill's complaint about older women using purgatives had appeared (1778), there was Chambon de Montaux's inclusion of the 'critical age' in the times of women's uterine perturbation (1784), and Jeannet des Longrois's *Conseils aux femmes de 40 ans* (1787).

[90] Ibid., 157. [91] Ibid., 167–168. [92] Ibid., 169. [93] Ibid., 171–172.

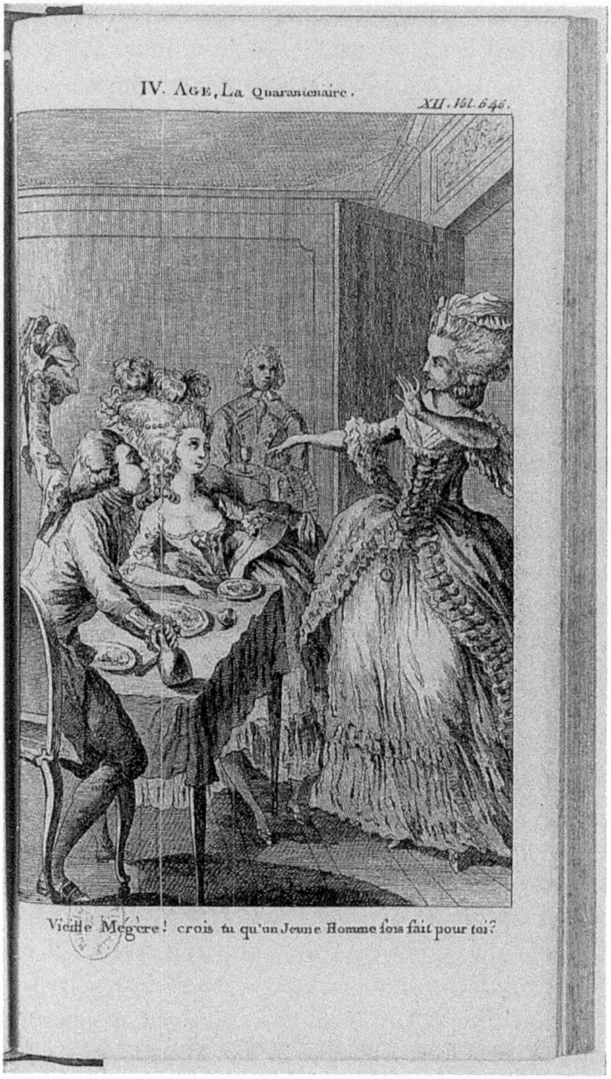
IV. Age, La Quarantenaire.
XII. Vol. 646.
Vieille Megère! crois tu qu'un Jeune Homme sois fait pour toi?

Image 4.1 Louis Binet, 'Les Six Ages de la fille: 4ème âge, la quarantenaire', in Louis Binet, Louis Berthet, Louis Papin, Nicolas-Edmé Restif de la Bretonne, *Illustrations de Les Contemporaines ou Aventures des plus jolies femmes de l'âge présent* (Paris: No publisher identified, 1780–1782). Courtesy of the Bibliothèque Nationale de France.

The Nineteenth-Century Assimilation of Vapours and Hysteria to Emerging Discourses of Menopause

It was a small step from this emerging medical convergence about hysterical vapours to the notion that the 'critical time' of uterine change around 45–50 might also make women prone to nervous diseases. The first Montpellier theses to focus on the end of menses and the critical age therefore listed hysteria, hypochondria, and the vapours in the long list of symptoms thought to befall certain elite city women when their menses ended.[94] The first generation of Paris scholars followed suit. It was possible to claim the cessation of menses as time of uterine activity while also accommodating the physiological theory of it as a process of uterine atrophy, by stretching the time frame that counted towards the critical transition. In 1802, the thesis of Jean-Baptiste Chouffe claimed that since the end of menses usually occurred gradually, there was often a long period during which the regular cycle had begun to degenerate but occasional bleeding still persisted, in which the nervous system was commonly disturbed.[95] The causes were nervous temperament, obesity entailing constipation, excess sexual pleasure, and soft beds.[96] Chouffe alone, of all the specialist scholars writing in French on the topic of women's final cessation of menses, cited the early eighteenth-century work of Stahl's student David Titius.[97] After this generation, it was scarcely possible any more to refer to women's nervous pathologies as vapours, which was increasingly viewed as a popularised and imprecise designation. But that vapours were now also increasingly understood in French culture to refer to nervous pathologies of older women is suggested by the Paris theatrical comedy, *La Femme de quarante ans, ou Les Femmes à vapeurs* (The Woman of 40 Years, or The Women with Vapours), performed at the Palais-Royal in 1805.[98]

Although eighteenth-century elaborations of hysteria, the vapours, and hypochondria had only a little to say about older women or the final cessation of menses as part of a larger general theory of women's nervous sensitivity, many nineteenth-century specialist scholars of menopause drew upon these precedents in developing the sex-specific concepts of women's ageing, often writing as if the more general thesis of uterine sympathy was itself the same elaborate symptomatology of menopause which they themselves now described. This historical conflation (still made by many current historians of medicine), in which different past concepts are collapsed into contemporary terms, was itself a form of instrumentalisation of the past in the invention of menopause medicine to instantiate novel nineteenth-century medical concepts through the insistence on continuity with tradition. At the same time, however, and in tension with these claims to continuity, many doctors also insisted that menopause medicine was a rupture with the traditional medical error of seeing women's 'critical age' as itself a pathology—often via misreading of, and underhanded attack on, the Montpellier

[94] Jérémie-André Pingault, *De la cessation des règles* (Montpellier: Tournel, 1799), 16–17; Joseph Gagnebé, *Exposition de quelques maladies qui attaquent les femmes à la cessation des règles*. Thèse (Montpellier: Imprimerie de Tournel, 1801), 4–5, 15–16.

[95] Jean-Baptiste-P. Chouffe, *Des accidents et des maladies qui surviennent à la cessation de la menstruation*. Thèse (Paris: Croullebois & Gabon, 1802), 19.

[96] Ibid., 44. [97] Ibid., 36.

[98] C. A. Faciolle, *La Femme de quarante ans, ou Les Femmes à vapeurs: Comédie en un acte et en prose, représentée pour la première fois, à Paris, sur le théâtre des Variétés, au Palais-Royal* (Paris: Delauney, 1805).

medical school's emphasis on crises, as we considered in the previous chapter. In general, it was those doctors and alienists proposing that menopause made women especially prone to nervous diseases who were more inclined to claim continuity with the medical past. Several steps contributed to the assimilation of hysteria, vapours, and hypochondria to the emerging concept of menopause, resulting eventually in the menopausal erotic madness thesis that flourished in the second half of the nineteenth century (the focus of Chapter 7). Prior to this, though, scholars in the Paris, Montpellier, Lyon, and Edinburgh faculties were all instrumental in the early development of connections made between hysteria, the vapours, hypochondria, and women's final cessation of menses.

In 1807 there was the widely read posthumous publication of the medical consultation notes of the eminent Montpellier scholar Paul-Joseph Barthez (1734–1806), with a second edition appearing only three years later, which represented a record of Barthez's Paris clinic in the mid-1770s.[99] Barthez was not a scholar of gynaecology, and his theoretical writing had little to say about women's physiology at all. But his case notes tell a different story, and were certainly read by nineteenth-century menopause scholars as prefiguring their medicalisation of women's final cessation of menses. Among Barthez's forty cases collected in this two-volume edition, there was just one woman (Consultation VII in volume 1) whom he described as 'close to the age when her menses might be expected to end' ('elle approche du temps où l'on a lieu de croire que ses règles finiront'—her exact age is not given).[100] This eminent figure of eighteenth-century medicine thus became available for nineteenth-century scholars to lean upon in legitimising the medicalisation of the final cessation of menses. But a close reading of this case, and of Barthez's other consultation subjects, suggests that the concept of women suffering a critical age relating to the final cessation of menses was entirely absent from Barthez's own treatment practices and rationales, even though he certainly emphasised differentiating patients on the basis of sex, age, temperament, and other variables. In the case in question, Barthez in fact made no remarks about the woman's stage of life as contributing to her condition. She is described under the heading 'Nervous disease caused by excessive menstrual flux' and is diagnosed with vapours related to her excessive menses, a causal relation which Barthez took to be indicated by the fact that for sixteen years in her youth she had very few periods and suffered none of her current symptoms.[101] In other cases of much younger women with suppressed menses, he noted that such suppression was not necessarily problematic, and that far worse problems could be caused by trying to medicate the menses to return.[102] He appears only to have treated suppressed menses in the event of specific symptoms associated with

[99] Paul-Joseph Barthez, *Consultations de Médecine*, ouvrage posthume, 2 vols, ed. J. Lordat (Paris: Michaud et Frères, 1810).

[100] Ibid., vol. 1, 120–130.

[101] Ibid., 122.

[102] Ibid., 131–135. Also, vol. 2, 270.

them, rather than as something which itself needed to be treated. He considered the woman in Consultation VII to be suffering not from anything recognisable as equivalent to menopause, but instead from general exhaustion due to her heavy menses, which he said was a known cause of hysteria. But he also evoked the 'orgasm of the blood' ('l'orgasme du sang') responsible for the plethora of the vessels of the womb that resulted in menstruation, which in this woman's case was clearly excessive. Her treatment required a three-part approach: firstly, moderating 'the movements of the orgasm of the blood toward the womb' using tempering and revulsive remedies, including enemas and laxatives to draw force away from the uterus;[103] secondly, an analeptic (restorative) diet, entailing easily digestible foods, was needed to combat exhaustion; thirdly, the vapours must be alleviated using specific remedies aimed at each individual vaporous symptom.[104] For flatulence, she was prescribed a vitriolic elixir in cold water; for heat in the head, a tea of aniseed and ginger; for palpitations, Hoffmann's mineral liqueur; and for her shoulder-blade pain, an ointment of camphorated oil with liquid laudanum and the topical application of oily liniment of ammonia.[105]

Barthez's consultation notes make for fascinating reading indeed, not least for the detailed treatment information he provided. It is also clear that Barthez did not prescribe the same treatments for similar conditions in different individuals, let alone providing universal advice to people classified by numeric age-brackets or specific stages of development. His treatments were instead highly individualised based on specific symptoms, as well as sex, age, humoral temperament, behavioural habits, and histories of past diseases, including previous responses to past medical treatment. Nothing could be more foreign to Barthez's way of operating than to tell all women whose menses were ending how to behave. Nor did he appear to see either vapours or hysteria as more common among this group relative to men or to younger women. Indeed, women between the ages of 45 and 55, or who are described as ceasing to menstruate due to age, are barely represented at all in the two volumes of his consultation notes. The single case observation discussed above is an outlying—and in any case ambiguous—exception. The remedies Barthez prescribed to women for both the vapours and hysteria appeared anything but onerous: in one example of vapours, the main remedy is a small glass of Spanish wine with a few grains of saffron or a little tincture of ambergris, and an anti-hysteric elixir consisted of rose-water, lemon balm, and musk with sugar and a carnation syrup.[106]

Notably though too, Barthez described numerous men aged in their forties and fifties whom he also considered to be suffering from the vapours,[107] including several aged precisely 49 years. Consultation XXXI presents the case of a man about to turn 50 who had 'abused venereal pleasures' since he was 13 years old

[103] Ibid., vol. 1, 125. [104] Ibid., 124. [105] Ibid., 129.
[106] Ibid., 135, 193. [107] Ibid., Consultation I, 33–45; additional observations I and II, 46.

and had had an 'immoderate' consumption of wine for some years. Barthez diagnosed him with vapours based on his vertigo, fainting spells, sleep disturbance, oedema of the leg, cold sweats, and hot flushes, as well as a pain in his penis after sexual relations.[108] He was prescribed moderate blood-letting, cauterisation on the leg, daily enemas, tobacco scented with white sage and rosemary (to be chewed), a vitriolic elixir, warm vinegar footbaths before bed, specific foods (whey with mustard, chicken or veal broth), and was told to moderate his sexual relations—and never to have such relations after dinner.[109] Another man who, having turned 49, suffered violent fevers and hypochondriac pains for three or four years, is described as undergoing a 'crisis' from which he recovered following copious bilious vomiting. Barthez considered the man to be weakened by a venereal virus he had contracted in his twenties and never truly shaken, with the 49th-year crisis representing *la Nature* surmounting and weakening this virus by exciting critical evacuations.[110] Men's haemorrhoidal blood flow was also considered to be a sort of critical evacuation, whose stoppage was related to symptoms of both plethora and the vapours.[111] A man of sanguine temperament aged 42 who had always been 'subject to haemorrhoidal flow' and enjoyed good health suddenly began suffering a sore throat and coughing up blood, coinciding with the cessation of his haemorrhoidal bleeding.[112] This man was diagnosed with plethora and prescribed blood-letting from the arm. Barthez considered him to require some form of bleeding, seeing the coughing-up of blood as a direct attempt by the body to compensate for the loss of haemorrhoidal flow—*crachements de sang* were a sort of 'haemorrhoids of the mouth'.[113]

The Montpellier scholars at the turn of the nineteenth century were still not always inclined to pathologise the final cessation of menses, though they did take an increased interest in questions of sex-specific ageing, often relating them to the growing concern with nervous diseases. In Years 8 and 9 of the Revolutionary Calendar (1799–1801)—when the Montpellier students Jérémie-André Pingault and Joseph Gagnebé produced the first medical theses in French focused entirely on women's final cessation of menses—another Montpellier student, Joseph-Damien Liaubet, wrote a thesis on the by now quite unfashionable topic of the vapours.[114] All three were students of the physiology professor Charles-Louis Dumas (1765–1813) and of Joseph-Marie-Joachim Vigarous (1759–1826), who

[108] Ibid, vol. 2, 144–155: Consultation XXXI; 213–225: Consultation XXXVI.

[109] Ibid., 144–155.

[110] Ibid., 224–225.

[111] Ibid, vol. 1, 53–54. On this theme see Michael Stohlberg, 'Menstruation and Sexual Difference in Early Modern Medicine', in Andrew Shail & Gillian Howed, eds, *Menstruation: A Cultural History* (New York: Palgrave, 2005), 90–101.

[112] Barthez, *Consultations de médecine*, vol. 1, 138–140.

[113] Ibid., 139–140.

[114] Jérémie-André Pingault, *De la cessation des règles* (Montpellier: Tournel, 1799); Joseph Gagnebé, *Exposition de quelques maladies qui attaquent les femmes à la cessation des règles*. Thèse (Montpellier: Imprimerie de Tournel, 1801); Joseph-Damien Liaubet, *Dissertation sur la névropathie ou vapeurs*. Thèse (Montpellier: Imprimerie de Coucourdan, 1801).

lectured on the diseases of women at Montpellier.[115] Unlike most eighteenth-century writers on the theme, Liaubet appeared to refer to the vapours not as a specific pathology, but rather as a broad term to describe various forms of nervous pathology (*névropathie*), of which the most important were hysteria, defined as a perturbation of the nervous system deriving from the uterus, and hypochondria, a similar perturbation caused by the digestive organs.[116] Age, sex, and temperament influenced susceptibility to the vapours, and while women were, as usual, said to be the most prone, the only age that mattered was childhood, when all the fibres of the body were most sensitive to outside impressions. The only temperament that made a person more likely to have the vapours was that of lax, pituitary, dry, bilious, and melancholic (*picrocole*) men.[117] Other causes included bad diet, viral illnesses, fevers, venereal diseases, heavy menstruation, excesses of sexual pleasure but also sexual abstinence ('because they produce the same effects'), intemperance, overeating, and the consumption of foods that caused bloating and gas.[118] Sedentary life was also a major cause of both nervous and all other diseases, while women who did not exercise, and who read novels that inflamed their imagination, were also very susceptible to the vapours.[119] Strong emotions of all kinds were a trigger, but also luxurious odours, such as rose, musk and ambergris.[120] Among the treatments were refreshing herbal teas, whey, boiled meats, and Hoffmann's bitter elixir, which remained in vogue.[121]

Bernard Lamothe's thesis on the same topic produced at Montpellier the following year likewise had nothing to say about women's end of menstruation as a stimulus for the vapours.[122] The 1807 Montpellier thesis of Thomas Guillit de Chatellus was one of the first works to assert explicitly that the final cessation of menses actually reduced women's likelihood of developing hysteria by relieving them of the 'nervous and spasmodic afflictions' from which they tended to suffer due to menstruation.[123] This was because 'the uterine organ being less subordinate to external causes, thus deprived of its excessive irritability, no longer reacts upon the sensitive organs to the same degree'.[124] Different women experienced the change differently, Guillit de Chatellus noted, on account of their diverse temperaments and degrees of physical activity; but some women 'acquired a new vigour at this time' because the inertia of the uterus caused their entire economy

[115] Joseph-Marie-Joachim Vigarous, *Cours élémentaire de maladies des femmes, ou Essai sur une nouvelle méthode pour étudier et pour classer les maladies de ce sexe*, 2 vols (Paris: Deterville, 1801).

[116] Liaubet, *Dissertation sur la névropathie ou vapeurs*, 7. [117] Ibid., 12–13.

[118] Ibid., 14. [119] Ibid., 17. [120] Ibid., 19–22. [121] Ibid., 24–26.

[122] Bernard Lamothe, *Dissertation sur l'hystéricie ou vapeurs hystériques en général*. Thèse (Montpellier: Jean Martel aîné, 1802).

[123] Thomas Guillit de Chatellus, *Recherches physiologique et médicales sur l'influence et les modifications qu'apportent dans l'économie de la femme et la première apparition et la cessation absolue des règles*. Thèse (Montpellier: Auguste Ricard, 1807), 51.

[124] Ibid., 54. 'L'organe utérin moins subordonnée alors aux cause externes, privé lui-même de cette excessive irritabilité, ne réagit plus sur les organes sensitifs avec le même degré d'énergie.'

to function more like that of a man.[125] Over the next twelve years, another two Montpellier doctoral students also writing about the vapours or hysteria similarly departed from the tendency in eighteenth-century works to include the cessation of menses in the list of times when women might be expected to suffer nervous diseases.[126] The 1808 Paris thesis of L. J. F. Monnet, who was from the Drôme department of the Auvergne-Rhône-Alpes region, referred to hysteria as that disease which was 'popularly known as vapours', inspiring an almost identical Montpellier thesis in 1809.[127]

In the first decade of the nineteenth century, then, it seems a Paris–Montpellier consensus had been reached, at least on the matter of proper medical terminology. Thereafter, few major works of French alienism or general medicine used the now defunct 'vapours' to describe nervous pathologies, instead primarily referring increasingly to hysteria or hypochondria.[128] There was a relative consensus that the cessation of menses signalled the end of the danger to women from uterine disturbance of their nerves. Monnet in 1808 remarked that 'hysteria normally manifests in women from the age of puberty up until that of 45 to 50 years, the period of the menstrual cessation, and one observes it very rarely before the first and after the last of these two times'.[129] Melancholy, nervous, or lascivious women all were more prone to it, but the greatest susceptibility was among women who from childhood had led a sedentary existence.[130] Monnet and Guillit de Chatellus represented a view briefly common in the period from the final years of the eighteenth century until around 1819, during which specialist writing on hysteria as a disturbance of the nerves caused by the sympathetic influence of the uterus interacted with the physiological concept of the cessation of menses as uterine atrophy. This combination produced the view of the cessation of menses not as a time of susceptibility for nervous diseases, but on the contrary as curing or reducing the likelihood of hysteria. Although this view persisted in later scholarship, it was not to remain dominant throughout the nineteenth century.

The Emergence of Menopausal Nervous Pathology

One of the most esteemed figures of the Montpellier medical faculty, who then went on to become a leading figure in Paris, was the well-known early pioneer of

[125] Ibid., 51.

[126] Antoine Clair, *Essai sur les vapeurs en général, et sur l'hystérie en particulier* (Montpellier: Jean Martel aîné, 1814); Daniel Dagassan, *Dissertation sur l'hystérie, vulgairement connue sous le nom de vapeurs* (Montpellier: Jean Martel aîné, 1819).

[127] L. J. F. Monnet, *Dissertation sur l'hystérie, appelée vulgairement vapeurs* (Paris: Didot Jeune, 1808); Dagassan, *Dissertation sur l'hystérie.*

[128] One exception was Louis-Charles-Edouard Lapasse, *Hygiène de longévité, guérison des migraines, maux d'estomac, maux de nerfs et vapeurs* (Paris: Victor Masson/Garnier Frères, 1861).

[129] Monnet, *Dissertation sur l'hystérie*, 11–12.

[130] Ibid., 12.

the medical description of mental pathologies Philippe Pinel (1745–1826). Pinel was the author of the widely cited *Nosographie philosophique* of 1797, as well as the 1800 *Traité medico-philosophique sur l'aliénation mentale*—both works printed in multiple editions and cited by numerous French menopause doctors throughout the nineteenth century.[131] Pinel was also an early proponent of clinical pedagogy, which hospitals in Paris (but not those in other regional centres) were required to provide to medical students in the second half of the nineteenth century.[132] He did not write about women's health in particular, but he did spend the early part of his career working at the Salpêtrière women's hospital in Paris, and he considered women roughly twice as likely to suffer nervous disorders as men, most commonly in the form of hysteria or hypochondria.[133] He said that it was menstruation and pregnancies that made women more susceptible to mental alienation—an idea that, as we will see in the next chapter, had tremendous tenacity throughout the nineteenth and twentieth centuries.[134]

Nonetheless, Pinel dismissed the idea that the uterus controlled all of women's physiology. He insisted that neither this organ nor any other could be blamed for the spasmodic symptoms found in nervous disorders such as hysteria, which, he thought, might emanate simply from the force of the muscles themselves or from the nerves.[135] Hypochondria could be trigged by the abuse of opium, 'an intemperate life', the sudden adoption of sedentary habits, suppression of the menses, difficult births, or by 'the excessive sampling of the cabinet of the pleasures of love'.[136] Hysteria was most often found in 'young ardent girls' but also in those of all ages 'devoted to either a voluntary or forced continence', such as married women whose husbands were absent, or young widows who ate indulgently ('se livrent à la bonne chère') and read lascivious books. Heavy or irregular menstruation could also cause it, as could difficult pregnancies and childbirths.[137] Hysteria or hypochondria were not particular features of women in the critical age, but nor did Pinel dismiss the possibility that they might occur throughout the lifespan: he

[131] Philippe Pinel, *Nosographie philosophique, ou la méthode de l'analyse appliquée à la médecine*, 3 vols (Paris: Maradon, 1797); Philippe Pinel, *Traité medico-philosophique sur l'aliénation mentale* (Paris: Richard, 1800).

[132] Philippe Pinel, *La Médecine clinique rendue plus précise et plus exacte par l'application de l'analyse, ou Recueil et résultat d'observations sur les maladies aiguës, faites à la Salpêtrière* (Paris: Brosson, Gabon et Cie, 1802); Joy Harvey, '"Faithful to its Old Traditions?" Paris Clinical Medicine from the Second Empire to the Third Republic', in Caroline Hannaway & Ann La Berge, eds, *Constructing Paris Medicine* (Amsterdam: Rodopi, 1998), 313–336 [326].

[133] Pinel, *Nosographie philosophique*, vol. 2, 10.

[134] Philippe Pinel, *Traité medico-philosophique sur l'aliénation mentale* [1800], 2nd ed. [entièrement refondue et très-augmentée] (Paris, J. A. Brosson, 1809), 30, note 1.

[135] Pinel, *Nosographie philosophique*, vol. 2, 51. [136] Ibid., 24–25.

[137] Ibid., 48–49. 'L'hystérie en général est plus ordinaire aux jeunes filles d'une constitution ardente aux personnes du sexe de tout âge vouées à une continence volontaire ou forcée, aux jeunes veuves qui se livrent à la bonne chère et à des lectures lascives, aux femmes mariées pendant une longue absence de leurs époux. Une menstruation laborieuse ou irrégulière, des accidens pendant la grossesse, les couches, peuvent aussi produire l'hystérie.'

also considered *vesanies*—non-febrile departures from reason ('égaremens d'esprit non fébriles')—to afflict specific kinds of people according to natural disposition, age, and sex. Like most Montpellier-trained scholars in this period, he complained that others too often confused this condition with hypochondria, hysteria, or melancholy.[138]

Pinel's scant remarks about the effects of the final cessation of menses in his earliest work referred to no specific mental or nervous pathologies but only to skin eruptions, which he said indicated that it was important for women to follow a dietary regime through this 'stormy period' ('époque orageuse').[139] However, in the 1809 second edition of his 1800 treatise, he added that complicated nervous afflictions in general could occur in some women following childbirth, from alcohol abuse or head injuries, or due either to menstrual suppression or to its natural cessation with age.[140] Elsewhere in the same text, he discussed how sensitivity made people more susceptible to mental illness, becoming 'extreme at certain times in the life of women, such as in puberty, during pregnancy and childbirth, and during that which is called the '"critical age"'.[141] Calling this time also *l'âge de retour*, he described it as 'the saddest and most melancholy' time, during which 'frivolous pleasures and attractions dissipate', describing one of his patients in the 'critical epoch' who had become melancholy but was relieved of her 'spasmodic contractions, frightening worries and state of stupor' by the prescription of 'a simple diet, varied bodily exercises, and diverse forms of distraction'.[142] The final cessation of menses was thus assimilated here into the spectrum of possible causes of women's nervous illness, but was also, importantly, described as amenable to hygienic intervention.

Pinel also helped to develop the concepts of nervous disorders both as hereditary and as inherently connected to sexual morals—ideas that would be widely discussed in psychiatric writing of the late nineteenth century, where sexual variations were often thought to constitute mental or nervous illnesses that were the product of inheritance or 'genetic taint'.[143] In Pinel's use of the idea, inheritance and sexual immorality were both cited among several possible causes of nervousness (rather than as a complete explanation), along with drunkenness, 'certain vivid moral affections', cutaneous eruptions, head lesions, as an after-effect of other illnesses, profound chagrin, confounded love, extreme religious principles—and the sudden suppression of a haemorrhage, implying here both amenorrhea or the final cessation of menses.[144] There were too many examples of madness

[138] Ibid., 395. [139] Ibid., 193.

[140] Pinel, *Traité medico-philosophique sur l'aliénation mentale*, v, xxi, 418.

[141] Ibid., 11–12. [142] Ibid., 51–52.

[143] For instance: Charles Féré, *La Famille névropathique: Théorie tératologique de l'hérédité et de la prédisposition morbides et de la dégénérescence*, 2nd ed. (Paris: F. Alcan, 1898).

[144] Pinel, *Traité medico-philosophique sur l'aliénation mentale*, 4. For an interesting discussion of the puzzle of translating *affections morales* in this context (as moral/ethical, or otherwise affective) see Louis C. Charland, 'Benevolent Theory: Moral Treatment at the York Retreat', *History of Psychiatry*, 18/1 (2007): 61–80 [76].

running in families over several generations for doctors not to consider that it might be hereditarily transmitted, Pinel remarked.[145] The origin of mania could also develop 'at an advanced age', its 'late explosion' determined by 'other life circumstances'.[146] He described two anatomical specimens of deceased maniac women he had examined, one of a woman aged 49 when she died, the other aged 54, remarking that they confirmed his suppositions about mania as caused by 'profound moral affections', and about 'the periods of age when there is the greatest chance of contracting it'.[147]

The age of 50 appeared in another live case example—this time of a man who worked in the public service, retiring when his brother was reduced to a state of dementia; the man himself developed 'an immoderate ardour for venereal pleasures', visited 'places of debauchery', abandoned himself 'to every excess', and eventually developed a delirium in which he imagined himself a god.[148] Nonetheless, Pinel said, in his time at the Salpêtrière patients presenting with indications of hereditary conditions were deemed incurable, and thus were not generally admitted for treatment.[149] He took a jab too at the empirics, women folk healers (*bonnes femmes*), and even skilled doctors (*médecins habiles*) who claimed to heal symptoms of hypochondria, invariably failing, but attempting multiple 'futile treatment plans'.[150] Such accusations became common in later denigrations of folk healers treating older women, as we consider in Chapter 6.

Philippe Pinel's ideas about nervous hysteria and menstruation (discussed in the previous chapter) were clearly tremendously generative for the development of ideas about menopause mental pathology among the generation of doctors he directly helped to train. The much cited 1838 psychiatric work by his student Jean-Étienne Dominique Esquirol, *Traité des maladies mentales*, assimilated women at the 'critical time' into the larger definition of the conditions of life in both sexes that inclined people towards nervous and mental illnesses such as *lypémanie* (melancholy) and demonomania (the delusion of being possessed by evil spirits). The miseries of ageing constituted precisely such a trigger for their activation in women, the more nervous sex in general:

> Arriving at the critical time, abandoned by the world, passing from boredom to sadness, the woman falls into melancholy [*lypémanie*], often of a religious kind.... weakness of spirit, ignorance and prejudices, have, in a manner of speaking, fashioned her in advance for such an illness.[151]

145 Pinel, *Traité medico-philosophique sur l'aliénation mentale*, 13. 146 Ibid., 15.
147 Ibid., 466. 148 Ibid., 15–16. 149 Ibid., 445. 150 Ibid., 24.
151 Jean-Etienne D. Esquirol, *Des maladies mentales considérées sous les rapports médical, hygiénique et médico-légal*, vol. 1 (Paris: J. B. Baillière, 1838), 503.

Like Pinel, Esquirol had received his doctorate from Montpellier (in 1805), but shortly after this worked at the Salpêtrière hospital in Paris, there becoming a protégé of Pinel. Esquirol's primary focus in relation to women's madness was on puberty and menstruation, with menopausal transition merely added on to the larger spectrum of disorders thought to befall women during all moments of uterine change: 'Among women of all classes, menstruation, whether struggling to become established, suppressed, or finally ceasing in the critical time, is one of the most common causes of mania.'[152] He claimed to have observed both how young women who were mad due to suppressed menses, became cured once their menses resumed, and how the final cessation of menses in older women could definitively cure them of mental disorders of which they had suffered their whole lives up to that time.[153] Esquirol's treatise contained several case studies of women between the ages of 40 and 50 who suffered from melancholy and delusions. These women, as in the male cases he cited, appeared to consume large amounts of alcohol daily, though Esquirol did not appear to count this among the triggers of their conditions, instead viewing it as a 'need' that persists in the mentally ill.[154] His mentor, Pinel, considered the propensity towards alcohol abuse to be often 'hereditary'.[155] One of Esquirol's patients, Madame P., 'arriving at the critical time', began consuming liqueurs for a stomach-ache, later moving on to distilled spirits (*eaux-de-vie*); she spent several years in a state of drunkenness before being found dead one day without any sign of 'derangement of her organs'. Similarly, the 50-year-old wife of a wine merchant began drinking wine, then liqueurs, then distilled spirits, spending every night in a state of complete drunkenness; Madame B., aged 42, began consuming large amounts of wine, became sad, fatigued, and had stomach-aches, then became paranoid that enemies wished her ill. She was treated with blood-letting and became convulsive, anorexic, and hallucinatory, beginning to drink even more heavily, but then was finally cured once her menses resumed.[156]

Another student of Pinel was the Paris alienist Étienne-Jean Georget (1795–1828), who in his short life wrote prolifically about both nervous and mental pathologies. His 1821 two-volume work on the physiology of the nervous system focused much on hysteria, hypochondria, epilepsy, and nervous asthma, referring repeatedly to women's 'critical age' as one of the times when all of these diseases became more common.[157] His work focused much on genital-nerve physiology, examining how venereal desires and sensations were driven by the

[152] Ibid., vol. 2, 140. [153] Ibid., vol. 1, 95. [154] Ibid., vol. 2, 81.

[155] Pinel, *Traité medico-philosophique sur l'aliénation mentale*, xxi.

[156] Esquirol, *Des maladies mentales considérées sous les rapports médical*, vol. 2, 77–78.

[157] Étienne-Jean Georget, *De la physiologie du système nerveux et spécialement du cerveau, recherches sur les maladies nerveuses en général et en particulier sur le siège, la nature et le traitement de l'hystérie, de l'hypochondrie, de l'épilepsie et de l'asthme convulsif*, vol. 1 (Paris: J.-B. Baillière, 1821), 184–185.

brain via the nervous system.[158] He was a major critic of the genital theory of hysteria, mocking eighteenth-century works on the vapours for subscribing to the idea that the uterus could derange the nervous system, which he called 'absurd'. In Georget's view, the functions of the uterus were merely menstruation and gestation—to expel the menstrual flow and to contain and then eject the foetus.[159] Nonetheless, he affirmed that the 'critical age' was a time 'productive of vapours, madness, hysteria, hypochondria and other disorders of this genre', but expressed frustration with the lack of a satisfactory mechanism provided for the correlation of nervous pathologies with the cessation of menstruation—a moment when women became more like men and so might be expected to display less of the feminine predilection for nervous diseases.[160] Whereas men, advancing in age, acquired more power, money. and dignity, the opposite was true for women, he noted, for whom the loss of youth and beauty represented a demotion in the social order.[161]

One indication that ideas about women's nervous and mental disorders in times of uterine change (puberty, menstruation, pregnancy, and menopause) were becoming more widely discussed throughout the nineteenth century is that they increasingly appeared in new forms of medical writing. One such example is the naturalist and anthropologist Julien-Joseph Virey's 1828 two-volume *Philosophical Hygiene*, which addressed the challenges posed to human health by modern civilisation, providing medically informed hygienic advice on how to live a healthy life.[162] 'Generally, there is more hereditary madness in women than in men, but their alienation is less murderous and less tenacious,' he remarked.[163] Virey transmitted here to a general educated readership the emerging medical view that women's insanity was more often hereditary, and that it was often caused by changes in the reproductive organs:

> Among insane women, it is not rare to find various organic diseases in their ovaries or their uterus, principally when their madness is erotic, or due to jealousy, or caused by sequelae of childbirth, or by derangements of menstruation.[164]

Nonetheless, Virey's message was a call to resist the temptations of modern civilisation, which reduced vitality through an excess of 'softness and luxury' that made women delicate, convulsive, or spasmodic.[165] This was a clear inheritance of the claims from the eighteenth-century vapours literature, about the impact of modernity and luxury on women's delicate nervous systems, requiring hygienic management. Others were distinctly more deterministic about women's inherited reproductive physiology, extending this into concepts of their nervous doom in ageing.

[158] Ibid., vol. 2, 159–181. [159] Ibid., 239–240.
[160] Ibid., vol. 1, 196. [161] Ibid., 196–197.
[162] Julien-Joseph Virey, *Hygiène philosophique, ou De la santé dans le régime physique, moral et politique de la civilisation moderne*, 2 vols (Paris: Crochard, 1828).
[163] Ibid., vol. 2, 265. [164] Ibid., 265–267. [165] Ibid., 12.

Menopausal Hypochondria and Hysteria

From the very beginning of the invention of *la ménopause*, several doctors proposed that one of the most common causes of its diverse symptoms must in fact be hypochondria.[166] In the eighteenth century, hypochondria, as we saw, was often listed as identical to hysteria and the vapours, or else was distinguished as its own unique form of nervous pathology with similar external symptoms. Generally, however, it was rarely thought to be particular to women, since its point of origin was thought to be not the uterus but the digestive organs. By the early nineteenth century, this word now carried the connotation of weak character, just as it does today, but it was also classed as a distinct mental or nervous pathology (rather than purely as a form of worrying). In the latter sense it was often also related to diverse abdominal diseases—anything below the ribs, as the Latin word indicated—including problems of digestion, uterine and ovarian tumours, other menstrual problems, as well as genital and urinary disorders. Hypochondria occurred in menopause, then, both because it entailed uterine change and because it was a time of nervous perturbation that women supposedly dreaded. The menopause neologist Gardanne had remarked in his 1812 Paris thesis that 'the approach of menopause makes such an impression on women that their imagination is quick to create vain chimeras which bring great disturbance to their entire animal physiology; they become morose, worried, taciturn'.[167] Joseph-François Garnier's Paris thesis of 1820 was even more emphatic, proposing that worrying about the diseases purported to occur in the critical age might actually be the very cause of the disorders of which women complained.[168]

The much cited 1817 *Elements of General Pathology* by the Charité doctor and Paris faculty professor Auguste Chomel, which was published in five French editions and translated into both English (1856) and Spanish (1868), remarked on the increasingly popular use of the term *l'âge critique* or *temps critique* to refer to women's final cessation of menses as a time of tumultuous nervousness, noting that 'there is no one who does not agree about the influence of these climacteric

[166] Charles-Pierre-Louis de Gardanne, *Dissertation sur les avis à donner aux femmes qui entrent dans l'âge critique*. Thèse (Paris: Didot Jeune, 1812), 18; Joseph-François Garnier, *Considérations sur l'âge critique, et sur l'hygiène des femmes à cette époque*. Thèse (Paris: Didot Jeune, 1820), 8; Auguste François Chomel, *Éléments de pathologie générale* [1817], 2nd ed. (Paris Crochard, 1824), Gustave-Adolphe Plihon, *De la ménopause (âge critique)*. Thèse (Paris: Rignoux, 1859), 22–30; Prosper-Louis Sauvé, *Réflexions sur l'âge critique, et particulièrement sur le régime le plus convenable pour préserver les femmes des accidens qui ont coutume de survenir à cette époque de leur vie*. Thèse (Strasbourg: F. G. Levrault, 1826), 3; André Castan, *Hygiène de l'âge de retour* (Paris: J. B. Baillière et Fils, 1901), 196–241; Jean-Baptiste Nosely, *Dissertation sur l'âge critique*. Thèse (Paris: Rignoux, 1848), 5; Émile-Joseph-Amédée Valleteau de Moulliac, *Contribution à l'étude de l'âge critique chez l'homme* (Bordeaux: A. Destout aîné, 1907), 20–21.

[167] Charles-Pierre-Louis de Gardanne, *Dissertation sur les avis à donner aux femmes qui entrent dans l'âge critique*. Thèse (Paris: Didot Jeune, 1812), 18.

[168] Joseph-François Garnier, *Considérations sur l'âge critique, et sur l'hygiène des femmes à cette époque*. Thèse (Paris: Didot Jeune, 1820), 8.

periods on the constitution and on health'.[169] Another Paris doctoral thesis by Charles-Victor Harreaux, defended in 1837, proposed as its main argument that hypochondria was the nervous disorder *par excellence* of the menopausal woman, claiming that after several years of clinical study in hospitals, he was struck by a unique form of it that was particular to women of the *âge de retour*.[170] The Paris physician Sébastien-Didier L'Héritier, who later became a medical consultant to Napoléon III, wrote in his 1836 *Complete Treatise on the Diseases of Women* that it was the very fear of menopause which caused the physiological symptoms seen in women at the 'critical age'. He navigated perfectly between simultaneously pathologising and anti-pathological stances with the sentence, 'While it is true that the cessation of women's periods exposes them to a quite large number of incidents, it is not less true that these incidences have been exaggerated.'[171] Similarly, Jean-Baptiste Nosely complained in his 1848 Paris thesis of 'the imaginary dangers surrounding the critical age, the fears which are born and which grow increasingly as the time approaches, only ceasing once it has definitively passed.'[172] If there was one feature of menopause that all doctors agreed was a problem, it was women's worrying about it, which could itself cause abdominal symptoms such as pain, haemorrhagic bleeding, constipation, or even cancer. From these ideas about menopausal hypochondria, only a small step was needed to situate menopausal symptoms within the other large medical rubric of female-specific health that flourished in this same period: hysteria.

Hysteria was more controversial, however, because it evoked the genital origin of nervous disease, which was increasingly doubted. Throughout the nineteenth century, many alienists and gynaecologists suggested that hysteria was common in menopause, while others claimed that menopause could actually cure it. In 1802 the Paris professor of anatomy Jean-Baptise Louyer-Villermay (who later became royal surgeon to both Louis Philippe and Napoleon III) added his aristocratic weight to the positive claim, citing Hoffmann's consultation records which accounted for eleven cases of hysteria of which five were in puberty, five were in the 'critical age', and only one was in her twenties.[173] But Joseph-Marie-Joachim Vigarous, the renowned Montpellier professor, had asserted the opposite opinion only one year earlier. He was among a growing cohort of scholars who did their medical degrees at Montpellier and initially taught there, but were later taken on as professors at the Paris faculty. Their attractiveness to the Parisian scene was in part on account of their nuanced work in disambiguating hysteria from other

[169] Auguste François Chomel, *Éléments de pathologie générale* [1817], 2nd ed. (Paris Crochard, 1824), 75, note 1.

[170] Harreaux, *Essai sur une variété d'hypocondrie particulière aux femmes de l'âge critique*, 5.

[171] L'Héritier, *Traité complet des maladies de la femmes*, 141.

[172] Nosely, *Dissertation sur l'âge critique*, 5.

[173] Jean-Baptiste Louyer Villermay, *Recherches historiques et médicales sur l'hyponcondrie isolée, par l'observation et l'analyse, de l'hystérie et de la mélancolie* (Paris: Mequignon, 1902), 49.

women's pathologies that merely resembled it—in particular hypochondria (which, by focusing on the epigastric region, potentially encompassed many of the uterine pathologies more common in older women) and the 'vapours that that rise up from retained menstrual blood or semen toward all parts of the body'.[174] Vigarous's influential elementary lectures, published in two volumes by a Parisian press in 1801, specified that true hysteria, deriving from the nefarious influence of the uterus over the body, afflicted women and girls only from the 'epoch of puberty until that of forty to forty-five years'. He emphasised:

> It is in this interval only that the uterus is subject to acquiring a degree of force that can become abnormal, and which communicating to other parts of the body via its numerous means of sympathy, necessarily produces symptoms as varied as are its means of communication...[175]

Vigarous began a trend among doctors who, though they were inclined to ascribe many aspects of young women's physiological and psychic experience to hysteria, explicitly excluded women beyond the age of about 45 years from this category of diagnosis. Vigarous said this was because 'toward the age of forty to fifty years, the mass of the forces of the other organs increases relative to those of the uterus, which no longer has any particular life, nor any activity and therefore remains without influence'. Women in this era 'seem to acquire a foundation of inexhaustible life; the time of peril is past; they are no longer subject to the particular ills of their sex; and they acquire the constitution of Man just as he in turn begins to lose it'.[176] Women only became more solid late in life, while men were solidified from the beginning and had more years to develop blockages of their arterial system: this, he said, was why women enjoyed greater longevity.[177] Vigarous was fascinated by the process of ageing, and commented repeatedly throughout his lectures on the differences between the physiology of children and that of older people. Children's blood was more acidic, circulated more freely, and rarely stagnated, whereas 'in the mature age, and especially in old age, this liquid becomes susceptible to contracting every degree of putridity and a true alkaline degeneration'.[178] Such comparisons formed the basis of his speculations about the physiology of the ageing process.

Vigarous also clearly distinguished between menstrual suppression in young women and the cessation of menses in ageing, in contrast to the earlier work of the Halle scholars, who tended to conflate them, as we saw in Chapter 1:

[174] Joseph-Marie-Joachim Vigarous, *Cours élémentaires de maladies des femmes, ou Essai sur une nouvelle méthode pour étudier et pour classer les maladies de ce sexe*, vol. 1 (Paris: Deterville, 1801), 457–458.

[175] Ibid., 459. [176] Ibid., 47. [177] Ibid., 48. [178] Ibid., 334.

> One cannot call the menses suppressed when they have not yet appeared at the tender age, when the uterus does not yet enjoy its action, nor is yet awakened; nor at the advanced age when, as we have seen, this evacuation stops entirely never to resume, and the uterus loses its activity, its influence.[179]

On the other hand, hypochondria could afflict older women too, Vigarous suggested, communicating its 'stasis of the humours' from the epigastric region to other parts of the body via the portal vein. Here he cited the eminent German vitalist Georg Stahl, whose work remained an important influence on the Montpellier scholars in this period.[180] The distinction between hypochondria and hysteria was salient for Vigarous because the treatments for each were diametrically opposed: while the hypochondriac would benefit from 'much exercise, calming remedies, spirits, volatiles, stomach remedies, aromatics, neutral salts, mineral waters, bitters and especially the martials (iron)', these very remedies would be damaging to the hysteric, who instead required blood-letting, narcotics, nitrites, antiepileptics, refreshing/cold water, and whey.[181] Notably here (again contradicting the accounts of some recent historians), it was not older women who were thought to need blood-letting on the view that their menstruation was now stuck inside them, but rather young menstruating 'hysteric' women who were prescribed phlebotomy. 'Hypochondriac' older women were prescribed iron, while young menstruating women were not, which seems counter-intuitive to twenty-first-century reasoning which relates blood-loss to iron deficiency. Eighteenth-century reasoning about matters of women's health simply cannot be understood through present-day premises.

The matter of women's hysteria or hypochondria in menopause had also commonly been evoked in the new genre of specialist works on menopause that began emerging from the first decade of the nineteenth century and which endured well into the twentieth. Here menopausal nervous disorders appeared as just a part of a long list of possible symptoms from which women might suffer during the transition, when the menses were disrupted and irregular, but had not yet definitively ceased, and for some time afterwards. More often, doctors writing about menopause in the first half of the nineteenth century focused on physiological symptoms such as abdominal pain, back pain, joint pain, headaches, fatigue, hot flushes, constipation, gout, weight gain, or insomnia, but also added nervousness, melancholy, jealousy, hysteria, vapours, hypochondria, epilepsy, and mania to the already long list of symptoms of this thing they insisted was 'not a disease'. As early as 1805, L. J. S. Jallon, in his Paris thesis, had considered hysteria to be just one of the possible mental effects of the critical age in women, along with 'hypochondria, melancholy, mania and epilepsy'.[182] Gardanne, who coined the term

[179] Ibid., 91. [180] Ibid., 451. [181] Ibid., 450–451.

[182] L. J. S. Jallon, *Essai sur l'âge critique des femmes*. Thèse (Paris: Didot Jeune, 1805), 63.

la ménopause, had included a whole section on hysteria among its symptoms in his 1816 book expanding on his doctoral thesis, describing it as a 'nervous affliction of the womb'.[183] Sébastien-Didier L'Héritier claimed in his 1836 *Treatise on the Diseases of Women* that hysteria was common among women of the 'critical age', while also acknowledging that many other doctors regarded it as pertaining only to young women.[184] The 1837 Paris thesis of Harreaux, as we saw, made a more aggressive statement of the link between hysteria and menopause, proposing that it was the same diversion of nervous energy towards the uterus in hysterics that caused most of the symptoms of menopause of which women complained. But because the menopausal woman had an atrophied uterus, he argued, this diversion of nervous energy produced melancholic symptoms and hypochondria rather than the convulsive symptoms of the hysteric.[185]

The mechanistic model of the uterus governing women's reproductive physiology as a phenomenon of uterine atrophy remained common in the first half of the nineteenth century. Through the mechanistic theory of sympathies between the uterus and the nervous system, it was drawn upon to account for the mental pathologies of pubescent, pregnant, menstruating, and menopausal women, even though there were those like Georget who had dismissed this idea in the 1820s. In 1842, Brierre de Boismont could still insist that 'the uterus maintains numerous sympathies with the economy; there is no region, organ or function that cannot manifest its ties to this important viscus'.[186] After the Paris professor Achille Chéreau published his major 1844 work on ovarian physiology, the view of menopause as producing an atrophy of the uterus began to be substantially displaced by the model of ovarian depletion, as reflected in Chéreau's assertion of the ovaries as the primary organ of generation in women, analogous to the testicles in men. In Chéreau's view, the uterus was a mere 'appendage' ('annexe') of the ovaries, which functioned as the primary secretory and governing organs of the female reproductive system from puberty until the end of the 'âge de retour', after which they 'weaken' ('s'affaiblisssent') and 'wither' ('se flétrissent').[187] Nonetheless, the uterus would not be so readily dismissed by many of the medical scholars theorising about menopause and nervous diseases.

Of those still committed to the uterine atrophy model, some imagined that with the power of the uterus diminished hysteria would be lessened; others, such as Harreaux, argued that the loss of uterine governance over women's physiology

[183] Charles-Pierre-Louis de Gardanne, *Avis aux femmes qui entrent dans l'âge critique* (Paris: Gabon, 1816), 403–405.

[184] L'Héritier, *Traité complet des maladies de la femme*, 146.

[185] Harreaux, *Essai sur une variété d'hypocondrie particulière aux femmes de l'âge critique*, 5–16.

[186] Brierre de Boismont, *De la menstruation*, 239.

[187] Achille Chéreau, *Mémoires pour servir à l'étude des maladies des ovaires; Première mémoire* (Paris: Fortin & Masson, 1844), 1–2; 27. Although Chéreau appears to have envisaged a series of memoirs of which this publication would be merely the first, in fact he did not write any further volumes.

combined with the maintenance of the organ within their bodies produced an aberrant influence of a weak and dysfunctional organ that nonetheless persisted in trying to exercise control.[188] Harreaux was an outlier in this period, however: most doctors and doctoral students throughout the 1830s and 1870s continued to see both hypochondria and hysteria as among an array of equally vaguely defined pathologies that could befall women in menopause, rather than as the underlying cause of all menopausal symptoms or a condition to which menopausal women were especially susceptible. Gustave-Adolphe Plihon's Paris doctoral thesis of 1859, for instance, similarly to the earliest theses by Gagnebé, Pingault, Chouffe, and Jallon, listed hysteria as one of several nervous symptoms from which women suffered in the critical age, along with epilepsy and hypochondria ('vapours' was no longer a credible term).[189] The mature Parisian clinician Ernest Barié, in his book of 1877, cited the English physician Edward John Tilt in support of the view that the majority of menopausal women suffered mild nervous disorders, with some of particularly nervous temperament suffering 'serious neuroses', including hysteria, epilepsy, or chorea (involuntary movements and tics).[190] He nonetheless took a step further towards the view of all the nervous symptoms of menopause as hysterical, remarking that 'we will not insist upon menopause as producing unique neuroses; these are for the most part just different manifestations of the same illness: hysteria'.[191] Menopause, then, did not produce its own unique forms of mental pathology, but it certainly could bring on mental pathologies of the kind observed in young hysterical women. Nonetheless, Barié also recognised a large body of scholarship claiming that hysterical symptoms most commonly eased after menopause, citing the work of Vigarous (1801), Dubois d'Amiens (1837), Brierre de Boismont (1842), Landouzy (1846), Hardy and Béhier (1850–1858), and others.[192]

Certainly, there were many who now flatly disagreed that hysteria or any mental pathologies were due to sexual behaviour, or more likely to occur during menstruation or the 'critical age', or after menopause, seeing such claims made by others as frankly erroneous. Hector Landouzy, a graduate of the Paris faculty who was an adjunct professor at the Reims medical school when he authored his 1846 *Traité complet de l'hystérie*, had much to say about the predisposing factors for women to succumb to mental or nervous illness.[193] He differed from many in

[188] Harreaux, *Essai sur une variété d'hypcondrie particulière*, 17–18.

[189] Plihon, *De la ménopause*, 22–30.

[190] Ernest Barié, *Étude sur la ménopause* (Paris: V. Adrien Delahaye, 1877), 49–50; Edward J. Tilt, *The Change of Life in Health and Disease* (Philadelphia: Lindsay & Blakiston, 1871).

[191] Barié, *Étude sur la ménopause*, 121.

[192] Ibid., 122. Joseph-Marie-Joachim Vigarous, *Cours élémentaire*, vol. 1; F. Dubois d'Amiens, *Histoire philosophique de l'hypochondrie et de l'hystérie* (Paris: Deville Cavellin, 1833); Brierre de Boismont, *De la menstruation*; Hector Landouzy, *Traité complet de l'hystérie* (Paris: J. B & G. Baillière, 1846); A. Hardy & J. Béhier, *Traité élémentaire de pathologie interne* (Paris: Labé, 1850–1858).

[193] Hector Landouzy, *Traité complet de l'hystérie* (Paris: J. B. Baillière, 1846).

seeing a greater danger of the development of hysteria with sexual abstinence, rather than sexual excess; he claimed to have witnessed cases cured by sexual union, noting that it was almost never found in prostitutes.[194] He did not agree that amenorrhea could cause hysteria, dismissing outright the notion that the uterus had any action on the nervous system, or the power to provoke mental pathologies.[195] Nor did he agree that menopause was a cause of hysteria, remarking that 'Gardanne must have been blinded by the speciality of his subject' to believe such a thing. On the contrary, he said, it was more common to see already existing cases of hysteria cured by the final cessation of menses. He reluctantly allowed that the 'extinction of the periodic haemorrhage', in combination with other illnesses and emotional troubles experienced by women at this time of life, might sometimes manifest in hysterical symptoms. But menopause alone, he thought, was not sufficient for this.[196]

Many of the medical specialists in gynaecological diseases also remained unconvinced of claims of menopause-induced nervous pathologies, seeing these as just another form of catastrophising of a harmless natural process. To some extent this division related to the long competition between the Paris and Montpellier faculties, with the Paris faculty becoming increasingly influenced by the growth of alienism and its theories of women's nervous and mental pathologies, and the Montpellier faculty remaining aligned with the anti-pathological and preventive-health concepts of medical hygiene and adaptive 'critical times'. Sometimes such debates focused on the growing critique of uterine reductionism. The Montpellier-trained alienist Pierre Berthier (1830–1877) expressed humble but grave doubts in 1874 about the idea that mental pathologies derived from women's reproductive organs, noting that 'the uterus itself seems only to be a place of deposit destined to receive the foetus', and that it is the ovaries that 'seem to radiate all influences that the genital organs exert on the organism of women'.[197] Nor did he appear to consider the decline of the ovaries as making women more inclined towards nervous or mental pathologies as they aged. The Montpellier gynaecology professor Amédée Courty, in his 1866 *Practical Treaty of Diseases of the Uterus*, acknowledged that menopause could produce mild 'nervous' symptoms such as hot flushes, vertigo, palpitations, bad moods, and hysteria; but he also insisted that it was nothing to be too concerned about and that 'in general, the cessation of the menstrual flux occurs without danger', sometimes merely taking a while 'for the economy of the body to return to equilibrium'.[198]

In 1868, the renowned Paris gynaecologist Adam Raciborski (1809–1871) confirmed the ovarian-demise model of menopause, leaning on eighteenth-century

[194] Ibid., 184–186. [195] Ibid., 183. [196] Ibid., 196.

[197] Pierre Berthier, *Des névroses menstruelles, ou La Menstruation dans ses rapports avec les maladies nerveuses et mentales* (Paris: Delahaye, 1874), 5.

[198] Amédée Courty, *Traité pratique des maladies de l'utérus, des ovaires et des trompes* [1866] (Paris: P. Asselin, 1872), 355.

Göttingen Latin anatomical observations of the desiccation and withering of the follicles of de Graaf in older female cadavers, as in the work of the Strasbourg obstetrics scholar Johann Georg Roederer and of the eminent Swiss physiologist Albrecht von Haller.[199] Raciborski insisted that menopause was unjustifiably feared, misquoting Roussel's designation of 'l'enfer des femmes' (which referred to women's fear of becoming less beautiful as they aged). Nonetheless, women during the critical age could not simply 'dispense with a wise hygienic direction.'[200] Raciborski, one of the most cited Paris scholars of women's reproductive health in the second half of the nineteenth century, authored several works, including an 1844 book on women's health 'from puberty to the critical age', an 1856 book about the role of menstruation in gynaecological pathologies and their therapeutics, and the 1868 treatise on menstruation for which he was most known, all published by the eminent press Baillière.[201]

Raciborski's most important contribution to ideas about menopause was to criticise what he presented as his predecessors' overemphasis on sanguine plethora, which he proposed should be replaced by a new definition of menopausal plethora as a pathology of the nervous system. This 'nervous plethora' was what became more common once the menses definitely ceased, because the 'nervous ganglionic system' no longer had ovulation to occupy it. This was not the case with temporary stoppages of menses during the reproductive years, Raciborski specified, which conformed to the classic sanguine model. The distinction was important because the treatments for the two were not the same.[202] But the nervous plethora thesis also liberated alienists and gynaecologists from the need to explain older women's hysteria by accommodating the shift from a uterine atrophy model to a mechanism of ovarian decline which was becoming increasingly widely recognised.

Indeed, the idea that women's nervous pathologies were the result of changes in their genital organs at all was increasingly doubted by many medical scholars. Some at the University of Paris flatly disagreed with the claims about menopause hysteria and madness. The Charité hospital doctor Pierre Briquet included a chapter on 'the influence of age' in his 1859 book on hysteria where, similarly to the Montpellier scholars from early in the century, he remarked that 'it rarely

199 Adam Raciborski, *Traité de la menstruation, ses rapports avec l'ovulation, la fécondation, l'hygiène de la puberté et de l'âge critique* (Paris: J. B. Baillière, 1868), 261; Johann Georg Roederer, *Icones uteri humani observationibus illustratae* (Göttingen: Vandenhoeck, 1759), 40; Albrecht von Haller, *Elementa physiologiae corporis humani*, vol. 8, Part II (Berne: Sumptibus Sumptibus Societatis Typographicae, 1766), 34.

200 Raciborski, *Traité de la menstruation*, xvii.

201 Adam Raciborski, *De la puberté et de l'âge critique chez la femme, au point de vue physiologique, hygiénique et médical* (Paris: J. B. Baillière, 1844); Adam Raciborski, *Du rôle de la menstruation dans la pathologie et la thérapeutique* (Paris: J. B. Baillière, 1856); Raciborski, *Traité de la menstruation.*

202 Raciborski, *Traité de la menstruation*, xv.

affects young girls prior to puberty or women after menopause'.[203] The 1880 Paris thesis of Raoul Boussi said that among women in good health, both menstruation and menopause 'evolve silently', identifying the problem as one of 'the present era' in which 'poor health among women is becoming the rule and good health the exception'. He claimed never to have seen even a single case of any uterine affliction causing 'an attack of nerves',[204] adding that 'the physiological and pathological influence of the genital organs on the nervous system has been exaggerated'.[205]

Moreover, even though many now claimed the cessation of menses as a likely moment for hysterical symptoms, curiously this did not reinforce notions of either hysteria or the critical age as uniquely female-specific. 'Virile hysteria' emerged as an important addition to scholarship on hysteria around this time, as indicated by Charcot's 1890s work on the topic, just as ideas about men's critical age retained their place in medical scholarship on reproductive ageing.[206] Pierre Marie, who had headed Charcot's clinic during the early 1880s, claimed that men's hysteria in Paris was epidemic, counting 525 cases versus 172 in women during the month of May 1889.[207] Men's hysteria between the ages of 40 and 50 was noted by several authors, who attributed it to degeneration: such tendencies were inherited and latent until some later trigger activated them. This could be trauma, intoxication, or the 'critical age'.[208] One no longer needed a uterus to be hysterical: the shift towards the definition of hysteria as a disease of the nervous system, not the reproductive organs of women, meant that men, along with menopausal women whose genital organs were deemed atrophied, could now be diagnosed with the disorder. Degeneration provided an alternative rationale both for hysteria and for the mental pathologies newly defined as common among menopausal women in Parisian psychiatry after the 1850s, as we discuss in Chapter 7.

The Longevity of Menopausal Nervous Pathologies

Following decades of medical disagreement about women's mental and nervous health around the time of menopause, the Paris neurologist Paul Sollier's 1893

[203] Paul Briquet, *Traité clinique et thérapeutique de l'hystérie* (Paris: J. B. Baillère et Fils, 1859), 52–53.

[204] Raoul Boussi, *Étude sur les troubles nerveux réflexes observés dans les maladies utérines* (Paris: V. Adrien Delahaye, 1880), 89.

[205] Ibid., 124.

[206] Jean-Marie Charcot, *Leçons sur l'hystérie virile, introd. par M. Ouerd* (Paris: Le Sycamore, 1984); Mark Micale, *Hysterical Men: The Hidden History of Male Nervous Illness* (Cambridge, Mass.: Harvard University Press, 2008), 117–227.

[207] Pierre Marie, 'L'Hystérie à la consultation du Bureau Central des Hôpitaux de Paris—Étude statistique', *Progrès médical*, 10 (27 July 1889), 68–69, cited in Jean-Marie Charcot, *Leçons du mardi à la Salpêtrière: Policlinique 1888–1889*. Notes de cours de M. M. Blin (Paris: Bureaux du Progrès médicale/E. Lecrosnier & Babé, 1889), 285, and in Micale, *Hysterical Men*, 183.

[208] Meurisse, *Syndrome utérin et manifestations hystériques*, 67. On male hysteria, in addition to Micale, *Hysterical Men*, see Olivier Douville, 'Folie hystérique et hystérie virile', *Figures de la psychanalyse*, 1/27 (2014), 25–33. doi:10.3917/fp.027.0025; and Nicole Edelman, *Les Métamorphoses de l'hystérique: Du début du XIXe siècle à la Grande Guerre* (Paris: La Découverte, 2013), 147–178.

Practical Guide to Mental Illnesses pronounced on the remaining non-consensus with a corrective to what he described as 'what is generally believed' (that menopause is not a disease and could be managed simply with healthy living): menopause, on the contrary, he claimed, was indeed 'one of the times when melancholy most frequently appears'.[209] In his 1901 work on hysteria, he noted that 'menstrual troubles are almost the rule in hysteria', but in fact focused far more on male hysteria than on that of older women.[210] The types of mental pathologies had by now been fairly neatly sorted: young women (and now men) were the true hysterics, while menopause was characterised sometimes by hysteria but more often by melancholy. Sollier (1861–1933) was secretary of the Société Medico-psychologique and *chef de clinique* at the Paris medical faculty, having previously been an intern of both the Bicêtre hospice and the Salpêtrière hospital under Charcot. Although he was rejected by the Académie de Médecine due to his rivalry with the eminent psychologist Pierre Janet, he was much cited by other neurologists and psychiatrists throughout the early twentieth century. His confirmation of the menopause mental pathology thesis can thus probably be taken as an indication of its broad acceptance in this milieux at the *fin de siècle*, at least among Paris psychiatrists.[211]

Despite the increasing emphasis on hysteria as a purely nervous disorder, genital theories of its origins did not disappear entirely, permitting the continued ascription of a wide variety of diseases in women to menstrual cessation. Case notes reported in works published by clinicians in this period provide a window into how women continued to be diagnosed with menopausal hysteria according to the genital model. The Belgian doctor Émile Berger (1855–1926), whose work on *Ocular Disorders of Genital Origin* appeared in 1905 (with the assistance of the Paris professor of gynaecology, Robert Loewy), described his treatment of an unmarried woman of 48 who was anaemic, the daughter of a very nervous father and a mother with gout.[212] Her periods had ceased precociously at the age of 32 after a miscarriage, and she had been very nervous ever since. Berger identified 'hysteric stigmata' on examining her, which explained her visual colour distortions, pain, and excessive tearing from her left eye, 'which make her life intolerable'. Injections of cocaine into her eye, or of sodium cacodylate (to correct anaemia) intravenously, only aggravated her symptoms, and while corrective convex lenses improved the patient's vision, she rejected them.[213] Other patients apparently reported conjunctivitis during menopause, though again Berger noted only one case of it in what he described as 'premature menopause' at age 41. This

[209] Paul Sollier, *Guide pratique des maladies mentales: Séméiologie, pronostic, indications* (Paris: G. Masson, 1893), 27, 136.

[210] Paul Sollier, *L'Hystérie et son traitement* (Paris: Félix Alcan, 1901), 280.

[211] Martha Evans, *Fits and Starts: A Genealogy of Hysteria in Modern France* (Ithaca, NY/London: Cornell University Press, 1991), 64–65; Edelman, *Les Métamorphoses de l'hystérique*, 263–283.

[212] Émile Berger, *Les Troubles oculaires d'origine génitale chez la femme* (Paris: Félix Alcan, 1905).

[213] Ibid., 64–65.

woman too appears to have suffered vision problems throughout her life which became worse in midlife, coinciding with her abrupt cessation of menses.[214]

At the very end of the nineteenth century, medical disagreement about hysteria during menopause continued, becoming itself an object of scholarly observation. In 1895, graduating from the Paris faculty just one year before his death at the age of 89, the Lille obstetrician Bernard Meurisse (1808–1896) remarked politely that 'the influence of menopause as an aetiological cause of hysteria is variously evaluated by [different] authors'.[215] He attributed the confusion to the peculiar episodic pattern of hysteria, leaning on Grasset for support: women did not appear to develop new mental pathologies at this time of life, but could experience a resurgence of earlier episodes that had previously been 'dormant or disappeared'.[216] Meurisse was still content to attribute the genesis of women's mental pathologies to the influence of the uterus; he just did not agree that menopause constituted one of the times when this was especially likely to happen.

Nonetheless, while a clear divergence of medical opinion about menopausal hysteria had by this time become apparent to all, the view of menopause as a vulnerable phase for mental pathologies also remained consistently ensconced in specialist scholarship on hysteria, along with puberty, pregnancy, and during menstruation. These were all considered times when susceptible women might succumb to the illness, and collections of case histories now typically included at least one example of a menopausal patient. D. Scialom's 1902 Montpellier medical dissertation on hysteria, for instance, detailed the case example of a woman aged 51 who was a dressmaker living a sedentary life, and whose 'neural disorders' and kidney stones emerged during menopause, having 'appeared right at the time of the disappearance of her period'.[217]

Conclusion

The nexus of ideas which connected the final cessation of menses to nervous pathologies and aberrant sexual desires had already acquired an ill-defined protoform in eighteenth-century medical thought. This began with the Latin theses of the Halle scholars trained under Stahl and Hoffmann who first listed hysteria and nymphomania among the signs of plethora in women both young and old, citing the final cessation of menses as one of the times when nervous pathologies of

[214] Ibid., 65.

[215] Bernard(-Clovis) Meurisse, *Syndrome utérin et manifestations hystériques* (Lille: L. Quarré, 1895), 66.

[216] Ibid.

[217] D. Scialom, *Associations névroso-organiques (hystérie et neurasthénie)* (Montpellier: G. Firmin, Montane et Sicardi, 1902), 35; Ernest Monin, *Les Troubles nerveux de cause sexuelle* (Paris: O. Doin, 1890), 43–47.

genital origin could occur. These were rather scant references, as we saw in Chapter 1, to something that was barely distinguishable as either unique to women or unique to ageing; and very few of the first French doctors to elaborate substantially on women's critical age were even aware of these Halle precedents.[218] Nineteenth-century theories of menopausal nervous illness drew parallels with pubescent girls, menstruating and pregnant women, and ageing men. But the image of the manic or hysterical menopausal woman nonetheless gained distinct traction in medical ideas, both in the emergent discipline of alienism/psychiatry and in specialist scholarship on menopause and women's reproductive health, including in the emergent discipline of gynaecology; in the wider field of medical hygiene; and in the popular medical advice-literature that became more common in the last two decades of the nineteenth century.

Importantly, during the mid-nineteenth century, as ideas about menopausal nervous pathologies were being challenged and redefined, so too was the medical understanding of women's reproductive physiology. This was expressed in the slow drift away from the view (based on seventeenth-century readings of Hippocrates) of the uterus determining all of women's physiology. Instead, there was a turn towards a focus on the ovaries as the primary secretory organ of women's conceptive capacity and sexual desire. In this context, hysteria, insofar as it was still understood as a nervous disorder caused by the uterus, no longer appeared consistent with what was increasingly understood to be the mechanism of the cessation of menses: not the atrophy of the uterus, but the uneven decline of the ovarian secretions which were now thought to influence women's entire physiology instead.[219] Increasing numbers of medical accounts of hysteria in the second half of the nineteenth century viewed it as a purely nervous disorder, similar to epilepsy, rather than as a mental pathology of genital origin. In practice, this permitted the ongoing (if controversial) attribution of hysteria and other nervous pathologies to the symptomatology of menopause. With both the decline of the uterine model of hysteria and the development of concepts of the end of menses as a 'critical age', it thus remained possible to refer to menopausal hysteria, hypochondria, melancholy, or mania (less so the vapours). All were thought to be stimulated by periods of stress or change in the organism and women's physiology throughout the lifespan was defined as constantly subject to such disturbances.

[218] The sole exception in 1805 being Chouffe, *Des accidents et des maladies qui surviennent à la cessation*, 36.

[219] Micale, *Approaching Hysteria*, 25.

5
Women's Ageing and Medical Hygiene
Between Montpellier and Paris

> 'J'ai jugé à propos d'instruire les femmes elles-mêmes; de leur apprendre à s'étudier, à se connoître & même à se pouvoir gouverner par leurs propres conseils, comme elles auroient pû faire sans la conduite des Médecins.'
>
> ('I have judged it appropriate to instruct women themselves; to teach them to study themselves, to get to know themselves, and even to be able to govern themselves by their own advice, such as they would be able to do without the guidance of doctors.')[1]
>
> Pierre Hunauld, 1756.
>
> 'On ne saurait trop recommander les précautions hygiéniques aux femmes qui approchent de l'âge critique.'
>
> ('One cannot recommend hygienic precautions enough to women approaching the critical age.')[2]
>
> Sébastien-Didier l'Héritier, 1838.

From as early as the middle of the eighteenth century, doctors of women's diseases began considering that women were more often ill, and aged faster and more poorly, and were therefore in need of a higher level of both medical surveillance and self-care, captured in the concept of *l'hygiène*. Initially, statements about hygiene proposed that women themselves could mostly be educated to nourish and nurture their bodies in a preventive health sense, such that they would have little need for doctors to treat them at all, as the Paris vapours scholar Pierre Hunauld suggested in the quotation above. The Montpellier faculty inducted all medical doctoral candidates throughout the eighteenth and early nineteenth century into the vitalist idea that human bodies could heal themselves through the power of the vital force within, so long as the 'laws of nature' were obeyed in the sense of eating enough but not too much food—mostly of the fresh kind found in

[1] Pierre Hunauld, *Dissertation sur les vapeurs et les pertes de sang* (Paris: Jean-Noel Leloup, 1756), xv.

[2] Sébastien-Didier l'Héritier, *Traité complet des maladies de la femme, étudiées sous les rapports physiologique, nosographique et thérapeutique* (Paris: Bulletin du Bureau Clinique, 1838), 148.

The French Invention of Menopause and the Medicalisation of Women's Ageing: A History. Alison M. Downham Moore, Oxford University Press. DOI: 10.1093/oso/9780192842916.003.0006

peasant diets—breathing fresh air, drinking clean water, having the correct amount of sleep, exercise, and sexual relations; and for women, bearing children, and avoiding nervous perturbations to which it was thought they were more sensitive. Later, the Paris faculty went even further, developing a highly gender-dimorphic account of the need for hygiene based on a vision of the uniquely dreadful properties of women's ageing, in particular. Unlike Montpellier, Paris had its own dedicated Chair of Hygiene from 1794 and devoted substantial expertise to questions of preventive health, both public and private, throughout the first half of the nineteenth century.[3] Nonetheless, the general hygiene scholars there were largely uninterested in the critical age of women until the 1820s, though specialist theses defended on the topic there, like those in Montpellier, often included hygienic advice for women approaching the critical age: here the role of doctoral candidates was clearly one of helping to flesh-out emergent concepts of hygiene for women approaching the final cessation of menses. The very first specialist theses on the final cessation of menses or critical age produced in Montpellier during the revolutionary period were rich in hygienic content, and the first wave of Paris candidates increasingly approached the topic in a similar manner, adding the familiar theme of the need for urban women to live like peasants to avoid the ravages of menopause. The peasant model of women's health, as we saw in the previous chapter, had first emerged as the solution to the 'vapours' in eighteenth-century medicine.

The new specialist doctoral works (in both faculties) identified older women as particular targets of hygienic care for several reasons. Firstly, women in general were thought more sensitive than men and so needed more hygienic care, and older people in general were thought more vulnerable to disease and so needed hygienic care more than the young. But the time around the cessation of menses itself now also constituted a life 'crisis' that perturbed the organism and made one more susceptible to disease. As we saw in Chapter 3, the concept of crises and critical evacuations had been developed by Montpellier-trained scholars such as Théophile de Bordeu and Philippe Pinel who conveyed them to Paris medicine; but the Paris doctoral candidates appeared to have misunderstood the vitalist underpinnings of crises in the Montpellier tradition, seeing them instead as purely negative and dangerous episodes. By the 1820s, the idea of medical hygiene in relation to older women's health was becoming significantly more catastrophising, with the 'critical age' around 45–50 years being proposed as a particularly delicate time in which 'one cannot recommend hygienic precautions enough', as the Parisian doctor Sébastien-Didier l'Héritier insisted in 1838.[4]

[3] Erwin H. Ackernecht, 'Hygiene in France, 1815–1848', *Bulletin of the History of Medicine*, 22/2 (1948), 117–155 [119].

[4] L'Héritier, *Traité complet des maladies de la femme*, 148.

One reason that hygienic approaches to health were part of the Montpellier school approaches, even though it had no dedicated chair of hygiene until 1864, was on account of the ongoing influence of vitalism in the tradition of the German physician Georg Ernst Stahl (1659–1734) whose work had been a major influence on the mid- and late eighteenth-century Montpellier scholars Théophile de Bordeu (1722–1776), and Paul-Joseph Barthez (1734–1806), and particularly, via the interpretation of Stahl by François Boissier de Sauvages (1706–1767).[5] The core idea of vitalism, that there was a life force which animated bodies, suggested to doctors that the resources lay within patients to heal themselves, so long as severe disharmony had not already taken root. As we saw in Chapter 3, the Montpellier vision of crisis proposed that such periods of health vulnerability occurring in the bodies of urban patients could resolve favourably of their own accord given the appropriate lifestyle modifications. As Laurence Brockliss and Colin Jones showed, the unique French approach to hygiene as a matter of preventive health became an important topic of medicine throughout the eighteenth century.[6] But it was only around the turn of the century that it became the central idea of managing women's final cessation of menses, particularly in works produced at the Montpellier medical faculty, but also soon too in Paris where many Montpellier scholars migrated or were published.

When French doctors, both in Montpellier and in Paris, talked about hygiene, they were effectively describing an approach to medicine that was largely preventive, emphasising the different ages, sexes, humoral constitutions, as well as the character of the individual, climate, and other contextual variables that must be managed in determining the best method of caring for oneself.[7] The role of the doctor in such a vision was essentially pedagogic and advisory, helping the patient to treat herself by avoiding those disharmonious conditions, or by managing the natural life-course crises—such as the 'critical age' of the final cessation of menses was understood to be. The doctor must also know how to treat the sick, but the concept of hygiene invested tremendous hope in the capacity of individuals to understand their own health needs and manage these themselves. Even women, who were commonly thought weaker and less rational than men, were seen as able to treat their own health hygienically. In fact, as the quotation of Pierre Hunauld cited at the start of this chapter indicates, many doctors were interested in helping women, in particular, to manage their own health in the view that, as the more sensitive sex, they both needed hygienic interventions more than men,

[5] Silvia Waisse, Maria Amaral, & Thereza Cer Galvão, 'Roots of French Vitalism: Bordeu and Barthez, between Paris and Montepellier', in Ana M. Alfonso-Goldfarb, ed., *História, Ciências, Saúde—Manguinhos*, 18/3 (2011). <http://scielo.br>; Louis Dulieu, *La Médecine à Montpellier*, vol. 3: *L'Époque classique* (Avignon: Presses Universelles, 1983), 602–605.

[6] Laurence Brockliss and Colin Jones, *The Medical World of Early Modern France* (Oxford: Clarendon, 1997), 441–473.

[7] Gérard Seignan, 'L'Hygiène sociale au XIXe siècle: Une physiologie morale', *Revue d'histoire du XIXe siècle*, 40 (2010), 113–130.

and would also be more physiologically responsive to them. Older bodies too were generally thought to need greater hygienic care, which made older women a likely intersectional target for such recommendations.

The Emergence of Ideas about Women's Ageing and Hygiene: Between Montpellier and Paris

The concept of hygiene and the need for it in relation to ageing and life crises became an important pedagogic topic of its own at the Montpellier faculty in the first two decades of the nineteenth century, where it encountered the other interest in women's diseases blossoming since the final decades of the seventeenth century, and particularly following the influence of Jean Astruc (1684–1766). Both areas were increasingly integrated into the vitalist commitment to differentiating bodies on the bases of age, sex, constitution, and other variables, with a view towards personalised practices of clinical care. Numerous doctoral theses in the first decades of the nineteenth century now advanced the cause of the hygienic management of patients, including of women in the critical age.[8] But the matter of medical hygiene was not left to the doctoral students alone. The great Montpellier-trained Paris professor of physiology Pierre-Jean-Georges Cabanis (1757–1808) included hygiene among the ten crucial medical disciplines in his 1804 work on 'revolutions' in the history of medicine.[9] His widely read 1805 *Rapports du physique et du moral de l'homme* (Man's Relations of the Physical and the Moral) described the importance of regimes in hygienic self-care, remarking that a good system of living (*plan de vie*) could 'considerably improve a person's physical constitution', while a bad one could alter, or even destroy it irredeemably.[10] As we considered in Chapter 3, Cabanis made only scant remarks about women's critical age, and it was instead the 1775 *Système physique et moral de la femme* of Pierre Roussel that had the most profound impact on Paris medical ideas about women's ageing following the cessation of menses.[11] But Roussel was neither a practising doctor nor a hygiene specialist, and his account of women's ageing morbidity held little suggestion of how an individual might manage their cessation of menses as a 'critical time' through specific interventions of diet, intoxicants, physical activity, sleep, sex, emotional stimulus, and other

[8] André Mathieu, *Quelques propositions sur l'hygiène en général*. Thèse (Montpellier: Publisher not identified, 1807); Jean-Louis-Victor Combres, *Dissertation sur la médecine conservatrice, ou l'hygiène* (Montpellier: Jean Martel, 1813); F.-Hyacinthe Teysset, *Quelques généralités sur l'hygiène des vieillards*. Thèse (Montpellier: Jean Martel, 1825).

[9] Pierre-Jean-Georges Cabanis, *Coup d'œil sur les révolutions et sur la réforme de la médecine* (Paris: Crapart, Caille & Ravier, 1804), 362–371.

[10] Pierre-Jean-Georges Cabanis, *Rapports du physique et du moral de l'homme*, vol. 2 (Paris: Crapelet, 1805), 12.

[11] Pierre Roussel, *Système physique et moral de la femme* (Paris: Chez Vincent, 1775).

variables—that theme which became so dominant in almost every medical thesis or book written on menopause throughout the nineteenth century. So, if we want to understand how the hygienic view of managing menopause came into being and came to hold so much cultural currency in nineteenth-century French medicine, we need to look at those works about hygiene which first integrated women's ageing into their field of concerns. Perhaps unsurprisingly, the influence of the Montpellier medical school was crucial in drawing together several of the separate, generative strands of thought about women's ageing which had appeared in the final decades of the eighteenth century. But while rivalries between the two largest medical faculties in France helped to drive the proliferation of hygienic ideas about women's ageing, the movement of scholars from the provinces to Paris, the publication of books by regional scholars with Paris presses, and the national success of Montpellier figures such as Barthez, Bordeu, Pinel, and Roussel all facilitated an important cross-flow of ideas that made vitalist ideas about gender, ageing, and hygiene very much a national set of themes.[12]

Dr Gabriel Jouard's 1804 *Nouvel Essai sur la femme considérée comparativement à l'homme*, which was an essay on the biology of women compared to that of men, was a new, expanded edition of his Paris medical thesis of 1803.[13] A central theme in it was the development of Roussel's attempt to describe the distinctness of women at every physiological and behavioural plane. Jouard proposed that the marked differences between men and women, particularly at the level of anatomy and reproductive physiology but also in every tissue right down to the cellular level, constituted a defining feature of humanity, declaring: 'Of all the animals that have two separate sexes, the human species is that in which the two individuals present the most differences between them.'[14] Much of Jouard's book was about all these many differences both in physiology and in spirit. Nonetheless, old age stood out as a shocking exception to the general rule:

> I have said that in every era of life, woman differs from man. Up to the present, I have examined her in her happy age of development and the brilliant age of her physical perfection. There is another age, an age of pain and bitterness for her...[15]

Old age erased the differences between men and women which distinguished human beings from other animals, he said. But it was especially in women that

[12] Elizabeth A. Williams, *The Physical and the Moral: Anthropology, Physiology, and Philosophical Medicine in France, 1750–1850* (Cambridge: Cambridge University Press, 1994), 67.

[13] Gabriel Jouard, *Nouvel Essai sur la femme considérée comparativement à l'homme principalement sous les rapports moral, physique, philosophique* (Paris: Chez Crochard, 1804); Gabriel Jouard, *Essai sur quelques points de l'histoire naturelle médicale de la femme, considérés sous les rapports physique, anatomique, physiologique, avec des applications à la pathologie*. Thèse (Paris: S. A. Huguelet, 1803).

[14] Jouard, *Nouvel Essai sur la femme*, 66.

[15] Ibid., 22–23.

the loss of characteristics of the 'empire of sex' were seen.[16] The most 'deplorable' of the many changes to take place in ageing women was seen in their 'moral comparison' ('rapport moral') with men, he said. What women had in their youth and which was lost to them in old age, appeared to transfer over to men who became even more beautiful and interesting as they aged.[17] Like others, he implied the cessation of menses to begin a permanent state analogous to the 'anaphrodisia' that existed prior to the age of menstruation, and during which a woman's genital organs held no influence over her.[18] Men, on the other hand, once maturing sexually, remained always influenced by their sex—indeed, the difference in how women lost their 'empire of sex' with age while men did not prompted Jouard to wonder if men and women were not in fact two entirely different species.[19] Clearly, in losing their differentiation from men, ageing women were already less human than before by virtue of no longer conforming to the feature that distinguished humans from other animals. On the other hand, Jouard said that he had less often seen calcification of the arteries in the corpses of old women compared to men the same age.[20] Clearly women did not age more poorly in every respect, even for Jouard who held their prospects of vitality in old age in such low regard. He, like Roussel, also did not appear to consider that there was anything a woman could or should do to manage her dehumanising ageing, which he presented as beginning with the cessation of menses, but without proposing this change to constitute a specific period of life crisis, implying that once begun, the bad times would simply endure for the rest of her life.

One of the most important figures to integrate ideas about women's ageing into the newly emerging hygienic prescriptions recommended for managing the final cessation of menses was the Strasbourg hygiene professor Étienne Tourtelle (1756-1801), who had graduated from the Montpellier Faculty in 1782.[21] His *Eléments d'hygiène* of 1797 was republished in numerous versions and editions up to 1868, including an 1809 English translation published in the USA.[22] This identical French work was also published as the *Traité d'hygiène*, with the Paris hygiene professor Jean-Noël Hallé (1754–1822) included as a co-author, and was incorporated thus as one of the volumes of various 1830s multi-volume medical encyclopedias, such as that published in 1837 and edited by the Paris professor

[16] Ibid., 23. [17] Ibid., 24. [18] Ibid., 68.
[19] Ibid., 69. [20] Ibid., 102.

[21] Étienne Tourtelle, *Theses medicae. Ex theoria. De naturâ, diversitate & viribus mineralium aquarum, medicatarum vocitatarum. Ex Praxi* (Montpellier: Jacques François Couché, 1782). See Rudolf Gerhard, 'Santé publique et éducation: Notions d'hygiène sociale au XVIIIe et au XIXe siècle: Étienne Tourtelle (1756–1800), Jules Levy (1805–1872), Jules Rochard (1819–1896)', *Histoire des sciences médicales*, 17/A1 (1982), 146–150.

[22] Étienne Tourtelle, *Elémens d'hygiène, ou De l'influence des choses physiques et morales sur l'homme, et des moyens de conserver la santé*, 2 vols (Strasbourg: Chez F. G. Levrault, 1797); Étienne Tourtelle and George Williamson, *Elements of hygiene (Principles of health) or, A treatise on the influence of physical and moral causes on man, and on the means of preserving health* (Baltimore: J. Robinson, 1809).

Isidore Bricheteau (1789-1861).[23] One notable difference between Tourtelle's 1797 treatise and all the posthumously published versions of this work, beginning with the 1815 third edition of it, was the inclusion of a long slab of direct quotation from Roussel's 1775 *Système physique et moral de la femme*—indeed the entire section dealing with women's ageing which Roussel called 'l'enfer des femmes' ('women's hell') both because it resulted in the loss of their beauty and desirability to men, and because women suffered more illness and debility in their ageing than men.[24]

In his original 1796 hygiene treatise, Tourtelle already had much to say about the hygiene of women, and particularly in relation to their ageing after the final cessation of menstruation.[25] Therefore, it seems likely that many of the doctoral students specialising in menopause or the critical age at both Montpellier and Paris between the late 1790s and 1860s were influenced by his ideas more than any of the Paris hygiene specialists of the late eighteenth and early nineteenth century, who in dismissing all of women's ageing as a miserable time about which nothing could be done, left little inspiration for the development of detailed hygienic regime for the management of the cessation of menses. Tourtelle subscribed to that view found already in multiple eighteenth-century works on the vapours and hysteria, that all the times of uterine change, including menstruation, pregnancy, childbirth, lactation, during the suppression of menses, and around the final cessation of menses—all of which he referred to as *temps critiques*—made women prone to nervous diseases, including gastric (hypochondriac) complaints; hence at these times, all chagrins and excitement should be avoided.[26] He declared: 'The time of life when the periods cease is critical for women, like when they began.' At this time, the uterus 'projects itself onto other parts and produces more or less serious incidents, according to the general disposition of the body'. Thus it was the time of life when 'one sees the largest number of women affected by chronic diseases and die'.[27] But such concerns were not applicable to peasant women, he declared, since they were free of the many problems resulting from the 'dysregulated habits' ('mœurs... déréglées') of city women ('citadines').[28] The idea that only lazy, decadent city women suffered symptoms with the cessation of menses had already been transferred from the vapours works to women around the around the age of 40 by Jeannet de Longrois in the

[23] Étienne Tourtelle & Jean Noël Hallé, *Encyclopédie des sciences médicales*, VII: *Hygiène*, ed. M. Bricheteau (Paris: Bureau de l'Encyclopédie, 1837).

[24] Étienne Tourtelle, *Élémens d'hygiène, ou De l'influence des choses physiques et morales sur l'homme, et des moyens de conserver la santé* [1796], 3rd ed., Tome 2 (Paris: Rémont et fils, 1815), 333–336.

[25] Étienne Tourtelle, *Élémens d'hygiène, ou De l'influence des choses physiques et morales sur l'homme, et des moyens de conserver la santé*, vol. 1 (Strasbourg: F. G. Levrault, 1796).

[26] Étienne Tourtelle, *éléments d'hygiène, ou De l'influence des choses physiques et morales sur l'homme, et des moyens de conserver la santé*, vol. 2 (Str asbourg: F. G. Levrault, 1796), 194–196, 266.

[27] Ibid., 267–268. [28] Ibid., 268.

1787 *Conseils aux femmes de quarante ans*, and had been reiterated by Philippe Pinel in 1797.[29] It remained a staple theme thereafter in the entire corpus of books and theses about menopause published throughout the nineteenth century, as we shall see.

It is doubtful how much Hallé had to do with any version of Tourtelle's hygienic treatise since, apart from the addition of the Roussel quotation in the 1815 version which included Hallé as an author, neither this version, nor any of the later re-editions, differed markedly from Tourtelle's 1797 original. Hallé lectured on hygiene at the Paris faculty at the very end of the eighteenth century and throughout the first decade of the nineteenth century, resulting in numerous hygiene doctoral theses on the topic being written in the period just after Gardanne's work on menopause in 1812, including the 1818 theses of Charles Moulinet on the hygienic care of the elderly, and that of T. M. Tillionbois de Valleuil on the hygiene of women during pregnancy.[30] In contrast with the specialist theses around this same time, none of the Paris general hygiene students appeared to have engaged with the emerging concern about women's 'critical age', 'âge de retour', or menopause as it was now called, though Moulinet notably cited Roussel's account of women's more rapid and morbid ageing compared to men.[31] But if menopause was not yet incorporated into general Paris hygiene in the way it was already becoming in Montpellier by the end of the eighteenth century, nonetheless, the first and most subsequent specialist works on women's critical age or menopause at both faculties were filled with hygienic prescriptions, as we consider in the second part of the chapter.

In addition to Tourtelle, there were several other hygiene scholars in Paris during the 1820s and 1830s who also engaged with Roussel's generative but non-clinical remarks about women's ageing morbidity and contributed to the emergent specialist scholarship on the final cessation of menses. One was the Paris medical professor Claude Lachaise (1797–1881), who had been a student of Montpellier-trained Jean-Étienne Dominique Esquirol (himself a disciple of Philippe Pinel). Lachaise wrote several works about ways to improve the health of women, about how to correct spinal scoliosis in children and about the topography of Paris and urban hygiene in which he had shown his own statistical evidence of women's

[29] M. Jeannet des Longrois, *Conseils aux femmes de quarante ans; dans l'ordre social, les femmes ont à souffir de mille dépendances; comme dans l'univers physique, de mille infirmités* (Paris: Méquignon, 1787), 5–6; Philippe Pinel, *Nosographie philosophique, ou la méthode de l'analyse appliquée à la médecine*, vol. 2 (Paris: Maradon, 1797), 332.

[30] T. M. Tillionbois de Valleuil, *Essai sur l'hygiène des femmes considérées pendant la grossesse, l'accouchement et les couches* (Paris: Didot Jeune, 1818); Charles Moulinet, *Essai sur l'hygiène des vieillards* (Paris: Didot Jeune, 1818).

[31] Moulinet, *Essai sur l'hygiène des vieillards*, 8, 12.

greater survival in the older age groups.[32] He also wrote, under the rather thinly disguised pseudonym Claude Sachaile, about Paris doctors whom he 'judged by their works.'[33] Lachaise's 1825 *Hygiène physiologique de la femme* shows just how pointedly he was inclined to judge his colleagues and predecessors. It was effectively a strident corrective to Roussel's attempt to define women's physiological specificity and ageing.

Men and women were indeed fundamentally differentiated by their experience of ageing, he said, just not in the way that Roussel thought. Men changed so gradually and constantly that they did not even notice themselves ageing, while women were completely different: 'Each of the principle periods of her existence is marked by disturbances (*secousses*) that render her life positively stormy (*orageuse*).'[34] While puberty was full of discomforts, and childbearing threatened her life at every turn, the end of a woman's fertility marked a new era of danger—a time either of death, or 'the manifestation of chronic illnesses' that medicine was not likely to be able to cure.[35] Women's 'entire lives were but a fabric of revolutions that placed them, at every moment, on the edge of a precipice that constantly threatens to collapse.'[36] He said that Roussel had 'sacrificed precision for the charms of style' and had been misguided when he asserted that women's greater longevity was due to their vital qualities being 'more exquisite than robust, more mobile than capable of moving', but refrained from offering his own opinion about why more women than men appeared to be living to old age.[37] He complained that Roussel, like most others who contemplated the differences between men and women, failed to consider the single most important difference which was actually in the social opportunities available to each sex, pointing to the 'innumerable inconveniences to which the feminine sex is subject in terms of what our social institutions assign to her.'[38]

Lachaise, as we saw in Chapter 3, was indeed one of those attending closely to the demographic scholarship of the past hundred years that had suggested women everywhere to be less likely than men to die in their fifties (citing Wargentin, Murat, Odier, Krafft, Déparcieux, and Benoiston de Châteauneuf, whose comparative mortality tables he even reproduced in his own book). He berated his current medical colleagues for failing to do proper research on the question of what influenced different women's disease propensities in the critical age.[39]

[32] Claude Lachaise, *Hygiène physiologique de la femme ou de la femme considérée dans son système physique et moral* (Paris: Mequignon Marvis, 1825); Claude Lachaise, *Topographie médicale de Paris ou Examen général des causes qui peuvent avoir une influence marquée sur la santé des habitans de cette ville, le caractère de leurs maladies, et le choix des précautions hygiéniques qui leur sont applicables* (Paris: J.-B. Baillère, 1822).

[33] Claude Sachaile, *Les Médecins de Paris jugés par leurs œuvres, ou Statistique scientifique et morale des médecins de Paris* (Paris: Chez l'auteur, 1845).

[34] Lachaise, *Hygiène physiologique de la femme*, ii–iii. [35] Ibid., iii. [36] Ibid., iv.

[37] Ibid., vii, xiii. [38] Ibid., vi. [39] Ibid., 411–412.

Medicine still understood almost nothing about the ovaries, he remarked,[40] and he complained fiercely about the uterine reductionist model of women's physiology (attributed to Van Helmont and to Hippocrates), which remained so often cited by medical scholars.[41] He criticised Moreau de la Sarthe for producing a book about women's health that was useful neither to doctors nor to women themselves.[42] Gardanne's book on menopause was barely any better, he suggested, since in 'looking to exploit popular opinion', the author had failed to provide a proper medical account of the physiological changes produced by the cessation of menses.[43] The main error of all existing works on menopause, he said, was the tendency to exaggerate the number and danger of illnesses that might occur, including all the possible diseases of ageing that could appear after the final cessation of menses but which were unrelated specifically to it.[44] Moreover, he said that most of the diseases attributed to the cessation of menses were actually pre-existing conditions that had simply recurred. A disease could only be counted as essentially caused by the critical age if it resolved itself and disappeared once the time had passed and equilibrium was restored.[45] Only a few conditions met that criterion, he thought, namely 'sanguine plethora' producing uterine haemorrhages, white vaginal flow (leukorrhea), and 'several cerebral and nervous afflictions'.[46]

Overall, he suggested that medicine had quite failed women and that what passed for hygienic advice was often reducible merely to 'a few vague exclamations about the use of corsets, the taking of baths, and the advantages of exercise'. For all that had been written about the sexual perturbations women suffered in puberty, maturity, and in the critical age, there was no agreed hygienic approach, and instead only 'controversies' and 'exaggerated opinions'.[47] Lachaise nonetheless himself also considered menopause to be a sort of whole-body physiological crisis, similar to the Montpellier view of critical times, one of the 'diverse epochs when the animal economy adopts different nuances, and seems even, in certain individuals, to reform itself down to its foundations'.[48] Women should thus 'submit themselves to a new series of precautions' at this moment, to protect their lives.[49]

He admitted that his own approach to the hygiene of women's cessation of menses was hardly original, and indeed reproduced the standard discourse of how menopause symptoms did not happen to women of the countryside because they lived closer to nature; therefore, the solution for urban women was to try to emulate peasant lifeways as much as possible. For him, this meant primarily following 'the wishes of nature' (bearing children in one's youth), and not giving

[40] Ibid., 402. [41] Ibid., xxii. [42] Ibid., xiv.
[43] Ibid., 394. [44] Ibid., 394–395; 419. [45] Ibid., 420. [46] Ibid., 421.
[47] Ibid., xx–xxi. [48] Ibid., viii. [49] Ibid., 417.

over to excess in both 'the pleasures of love and of the table'.[50] Illnesses at this time of life were most impacted by either 'excess or privation of the pleasures of love', as well as certain intellectual dispositions and past histories of illness.[51] The most important change of menopause, he said was that food became more energetic to the body, producing the tendency to thicken around the waist. This was because the shrinkage of the uterus (he rejected the term 'withering', since the change was a simple reduction in size, not in quality), permitted more energy to become available to the other organs.[52] It was mainly only women of sanguine temperament who needed to take precautions, though women of extreme cerebral or nervous susceptibility would also be prone to headaches, palpitations, and intestinal irritations.[53] Warm baths, whey, and light infusions of linden and orange blossom were prophylactic measure he recommended to everyone. In the event of plethoric conditions, he recommended gentle purgatives at low dose, such as neutral salts dissolved in prune juice, along with blood-letting. Nervous women should use light antispasmodics, baths, and enemas to prevent hypochondria, hysteria, spasmodic pains, palpitations, fainting and flatulence, hot flushes, intestinal pains, and painful spasms of the uterus.[54]

Although Lachaise was unusual in his scepticism of multiple forms of biological reductionism in medical ideas about women's nature prevalent at this time, he was not alone among hygienists of the early nineteenth century in wondering how many of the differences between women and men might actually be products of culture and education, rather than biology. François Ribes (1800–1864), who was a professor of the Montpellier medical faculty during the 1830s, like Lachaise, was dissatisfied with the existing understanding of women's physiological 'nature'. In 1836, he encouraged other medical scholars to pursue questions of women's health as a model for the development of medical hygiene in general, according to a vitalist principle that viewed sexual functions as the expression of the very same force of life itself.[55] Women were the sensitive half of humanity, without which there would be disharmony, he claimed, and men too often made the mistake of seeking their own qualities in women and finding them defective as a result. But sex differences did not imply, Ribes thought, that women were unequal to men or should be treated with less sovereignty, and he recommended doctors to focus their efforts on nourishing women's faculties, their education, and the hygienic conservation of their health throughout their lifespan.[56] To assume that women's inferior position was a product of their physiology, he remarked, was akin to the aristocracy claiming a natural right to rule over others, aligning his proto-feminist position to the politics of revolutionary repub-

[50] Ibid., 410. [51] Ibid., 420. [52] Ibid., 403.
[53] Ibid., 422. [54] Ibid., 426–427.
[55] François Ribes, *Discours sur la vie de la femme, prononcé à l'ouverture du cours d'hygiène de la Faculté de médecine de Montpellier* (Montpellier: Sevalle-Castel, 1836), 3–6.
[56] Ibid., 6–8.

licanism.[57] But Ribes wrote nothing about menopause or women's ageing. Lachaise too, who held a similarly sceptical view of the common arguments made about women's fragility and morbidity, only managed to reproduce a short list of general hygienic measures already being recommended to older bodies, while discouraging doctors from attributing all the diseases of ageing to the cessation of menses. The sceptical view was simply not generative towards the florid medicalisation of women's critical age in the face of the demographic recognition of their ageing resilience. Unsurprisingly then, it was not the dominant perspective brought to bear on the matter, and had it been so, the rampant fascination of French medicine with menopause would most likely never have flourished.

By the 1820s–1830s there were certainly plenty of other scholars though who attributed all the diseases of ageing ever found in women to the cessation of menses occurring around the age of 45–50 years. The Montpellier-trained doctor Alexis-François Aulagnier (1767–1839) who practised in Marseille and wrote on colic, nutrition, and other topics, also wrote two books on the diseases of women's cessation of menses or 'critical age'—the first self-published in 1821, and the second published in 1824 by the reputable Parisian press Gabon (located in the rue de la Médecine).[58] Aulagnier provides perhaps an example of the phenomenon described by medical historian Elizabeth Williams of Montpellier doctors needing multiple strategies for generating income given the competitiveness of medical practice in the south.[59] His 1821 work was begun as a serialised set of twelve pamphlets, available by mail order from the author himself to be released over several years, costing 1 Franc 40 cents each—quite a high price even for a substantial medical book at this time. By comparison, cheeses, which were widely regarded as having an 'indispensable' nutritional value, sold in Paris for 1 Franc 25 cents per kilo (enough protein for four or five adult meals) in the first decades of the nineteenth century up until 1843.[60] But only the first two pamphlets appear to have been released before Gabon took over publication of the entire manuscript as a single book costing just 75 cents—a more usual price for a short work of medical advice; and this book included a short chapter on the symptoms of the cessation of menses with ageing, which Aulagnier called 'nature's final crisis'.[61] But despite its pretence to offering detailed recommendations for women in the critical age, much of Aulagnier's work (both the serial pamphlet and the book

[57] Ibid., 8.

[58] Alexis-François Aulagnier, *Nouveau recueil d'observations et de consultations sur les maladies des femmes, et spécialement sur celles qui se déclarent vers l'âge critique* (Paris: l'auteur, 1821); Alexis-François Aulagnier, *Considérations sur l'âge critique qui amène la suppression absolue du flux périodique* (Paris: Gabon, 1821–1824).

[59] Elizabeth A. Williams, *A Cultural History of Medical Vitalism in Enlightenment Montpellier* (London: Routledge, 2003), 35.

[60] Gustave Bienaymé, 'Le Coût de la vie à Paris à diverses époques', *Journal de la société statistique de Paris*, 37 (1896): 375–390 [379].

[61] Aulagnier, *Considérations sur l'âge critique*, 12–22 [15].

versions) actually described diseases of women of all ages, including during puberty and pregnancy, with a major focus on vaginal discharges (leukorrhea and blennorrhoea).[62] Like other Montpellier scholars, he provided a detailed pharmacological differentiation of treatments for diverse disease presentations, and like others he reiterated the uterine reductionist view of women's physiology.[63] But a specialist work on menopause it was not, and if any women had subscribed to his serialised version looking for hygienic prescriptions for the critical age, they would probably have been sorely disappointed. That he abandoned the series after the second pamphlet is probably a sign that it was generating far too little commercial success for it to be worth the expense of printing it.

Medical hygiene focused on preventive health and the differentiation of people based on age, sex, class, and temperament remained an important topic in the Montpellier faculty throughout the early and middle of the nineteenth century, influencing Paris medicine too through the many Montpellier graduates who found positions in the capital. The Montpellier professor Michel Lévy (1809-1872), who later became director of surgical medicine at the Val de Grâce military hospital in the fifth arrondissement of Paris, was clearly one such important influence on other scholars in the development of medical concepts of hygiene. Like others, he defined hygiene as a kind of preventive healthcare in which the role of doctors was to guide patients towards the avoidance of illness with a view to annulling the need for direct medical treatment—a position that was particularly appealing to those, like Lévy, who had left Montpellier for more abundant patient markets in the capital. His 1844-1845 two-volume *Traité d'hygiène publique et privée* ran into six editions up to 1879 and was widely cited by all the other scholars focused on medical hygiene throughout the second half of the nineteenth century, both in Montpellier and in Paris.[64] Lévy, as we saw in Chapter 2, was one of those doctors who took the evidence of women's greater longevity to be reason to doubt the concept of menopause as a 'critical time', and like Lachaise, he considered that most of the diseases other doctors associated with this time in women's lives were actually existing conditions or disease of ageing in general rather than products of the cessation of menses specifically. The only true menopausal diseases, he said, were uterine haemorrhages, leukorrhea, haemorrhoids, plethora, congestion of the lower belly, and irritation of the uterus, as well as nervous vapours, hysteria, and melancholy, and sometimes eczema and other skin conditions.[65]

He said that 'only hygiene' could effectively protect women from the 'morbid imminence' of this 'revolution of age' that would otherwise endure indefinitely.[66]

62 Ibid., 1–12; Aulagnier, *Nouveau recueil d'observations*, 9–46.
63 Ibid., 6–8.
64 Michel Lévy, *Traité d'hygiène publique et privée*, 2 vols (Paris: J.-B. Baillière et fils, 1844–1845).
65 Lévy, *Traité d'hygiène publique et privée*, vol. 1, 270–271; ibid., vol. 2, 491.
66 Ibid., vol. 1, 271.

The 'formula' here was eating a humectant diet with little sustenance—mostly made up of vegetables and dairy—avoiding all alcoholic and aromatic beverages, taking light exercise in the fresh air, and dressing in warm clothes 'that lightly provoke the skin and decentralise the forces that converge toward the uterus'.[67] Women in Paris were far more likely to have leukorrhea than those in Marseille, he claimed. It was caused by uterine disturbances of all kinds, but also by masturbation, venereal excess, previous miscarriages, uterine polyps, use of excessive toiletry products ('l'usage vicieux de toilette'), or by either smallpox or measles.[68] Levy's book certainly did not provide a detailed inventory of hygienic prescriptions such as one finds in other works on the cessation of menses by this time, but his was also a work of general hygienic medicine about both public questions (contagious diseases, sanitation, industrialisation) and private health matters of all sexes and ages.

Even the influential Montpellier professor of medicine and criminologist Alexandre Lacassagne (1843-1924) in his early career was part of his faculty's insistence on hygienic care tailored to the sexes and ages. In his 1874 *Précis d'hygiène*, written when he was 30 years old and before making his name throughout Europe as the French counterpart to the Italian alienist Cesare Lombroro, Lacassagne defined 'the laws of hygiene' appropriate for the different categories of bodies following the model of Lévy. Citing a version of the Van Helmont Hippocratic aphorism that reduced women to the uterus (but attributing this saying, to the other famous Dutch physician Gerard van Swieten), he affirmed that hygienic remedies for women must also follow from the principle of women's greater sensitivity and plasticity. (as Lachaise, following Tourtelle, had remarked): women entered puberty and began ageing faster than men because their 'growth and diminution have a greater speed'.[69] Throughout the manual, nonetheless, he recommended similar hygienic interventions to young and old, men and women, referring to appropriate nutrition, avoiding extremes of cold or heat, engaging in muscular exercise, ensuring a clean, well-ventilated habitation with pure air and avoiding contagious diseases. His only mention of menopause referred to uterine pathologies, as one of the challenges unique to women, along with anaemia that could be suffered with menstruation, and due to the birth and lactation elements of pregnancy.[70] Women were not singled out as requiring greater hygienic management in ageing than men, but rather were distinguished by their greater responsiveness to such interventions, and by the particular pattern of their needs according to the influence of the uterus. Much later in life, Lacassagne returned

[67] Ibid., 272. [68] Ibid., 191–192.
[69] Alexandre Lacassagne, *Précis d'hygiène privé et sociale* (Paris: G. Masson, 1874), 510.
[70] Ibid., 510.

again to questions of ageing in both men and women, but here too took little interest in women's specificity or cessation of menses.[71]

Parisian versions of the growing chorus of ideas about older women's need for hygienic management between the 1830s and 1870s became considerably more catastrophising and less empathic. The Paris doctor and hygienist Marc Colombat de l'Isère (1797–1851) was an important contributor to the idea that women required a whole specialist field of hygienic care, publishing a three-volume treatise on this between 1838 and 1843 with the reputable Paris medical press Labé.[72] The argument Colombat made about why women needed three whole volumes of hygiene advice specific to them was by now a familiar one for anyone exposed to the substantial late eighteenth-century French intellectual tradition of radically distinguishing the sexes, who had read either Roussel or any of the many eighteenth-century medical works on the vapours: women were born 'weak and sensitive' and their entire lives were nothing but a 'series of physical and moral changes.... a long suite of modifications and revolutions', all of which required medical attention.[73] The 'general rule' about the sexes and ageing, he said, was that men were slower to develop at puberty and slower to degrade throughout the lifespan, while the old age of woman was 'as hasty as her puberty is precocious'. This, he thought, was indicated by the pattern of fertility's emergence and decline which represented the character of the very 'vital force that regulates the organic system and the organs that constitute it'.[74]

Women's periods of change were all more 'stressful' ('pénibles') than those of men on account of their 'very delicate and nervous' constitution.[75] He discussed the scholarly debates about the meaning of menstruation that formed such a major topic in eighteenth-century medicine, noting the variability of ages at which women began and finished menstruating across cultures and in different climates, acknowledging that some women who never menstruated were healthy and even still fertile nonetheless.[76] But he also represented menstruation as necessary for women's 'health, vitality and beauty', describing its cessation with ageing as 'the death of sex' ('la mort du sexe').[77] Menstrual stoppage caused 'a mass of symptoms', including languor, difficulty breathing, poor circulation, 'perverted, depraved' tastes and appetites, swollen limbs and face, jaundice, 'painful palpitations', fainting, anxiety, weakened senses, laziness, and heaviness. If menstruation became irregular it was accompanied by sympathy of the womb with other organs, resulting in hysteria, catalepsy, convulsions, spasmodic diseases, leukorrhea, pulmonary diseases, and haemorrhages.[78] The final cessation of menses represented a slowing down of the circulation of blood and humours. It was

[71] Alexandre Lacassagne, *La Verte Vieillesse* (Paris: A. Rey, 1920).

[72] Marc Colombat de l'Isère, *Traité des maladies des femmes et de l'hygiène spéciale de leur sexe*, 3 vols (Paris: Librairie médicale de Labé, 1838), vol. 1.

[73] Ibid., 17–18. [74] Ibid., 18–19. [75] Ibid., 25.

[76] Ibid., 29–31, 39–41. [77] Ibid., 33. [78] Ibid., 54–55.

thus 'the most cruel' time for women and so was rightly called 'l'âge de retour, temps critique, enfer des femmes'—here citing Roussel's expression about women's ageing in general but, like others, assigning it more specifically to their cessation of menses.[79] Blood no longer travelled to the organs of gestation and instead filled the upper parts of the body which resulted in vertigo, headaches, hot flushes, red and swollen eyes, troubled sleep, agitation, irritable limbs, pain in the lumbar region and lower belly, gnawing and itching of the vulva and anus, and the sagging and loss of colour of skin and breasts. If the pulse was 'rebounding', this indicated plethora.[80] Some women breezed through this time, he acknowledged, but others 'as in puberty, their sensitivity augments, they are tormented by vapours and hysteric attacks', and became taciturn, sad and worried.[81] For other women, there were cancers of the uterus, vagina, rectum, breasts or ovaries, chronic metritis, uterine haemorrhages, fibroid tumours and polyps of the vagina or uterus, ulcerations, and other growths of these organs.[82] While the critical age was not the most dangerous time for women, he acknowledged, referring to the recent consensus among demographers about women's greater longevity, Parisian elite women nonetheless particularly needed to observe a suite of hygienic measures to survive this time of life.[83] Older urban women were thus the group most in need of hygiene even if they were more resilient than men in terms of mortality.

Colombat evoked the now familiar idea of the final cessation of menses as representing a massive 'revolution' of woman's entire economy, akin to that of puberty, only 'less fun and no less stormy'. It was the moment when women were 'obliged to cede to time's empire', and how women experienced this devastating moment was influenced by climate, constitution, way of life ('la manière de vivre'), social status, and general state of health, all of which indicated that 'hygienic precautions' could ameliorate the ravages of the critical age.[84] This meant not only avoiding the remedies of charlatans (discussed in our next chapter), but also eating a diet with 'little nourishment', focused on white meats, vegetables (chicory and spinach), cooked sour fruits or raw ripe ones, and avoiding spices, stews, dark or salted meats, coffee, tea, alcoholic spirits, and any other 'exciting' or hard-to-digest foods. Sleep, exercise, dress, entertainment, air quality, bodily excretions, bedding, as well as 'passions of the soul' and coitus, must all be strictly managed.[85] Frequent enemas were recommended, blood-letting from the arm and purgatives should be used in the case of sanguinary plethora—though not the drastic aloetic kind of remedies.[86] He said both that women worried too much about the critical age, needing reassurance from their doctors that it was a natural process, but also that 'one cannot advise women too much' about

79 Ibid., 48–49. 80 Ibid., 52. 81 Ibid., 53.
82 Ibid., 57. 83 Ibid., 59.
84 Marc Colombat de l'Isère, *Traité des maladies des femmes et de l'hygiène spéciale de leur sexe* (Paris: Librairie médicale de Labé, 1843), vol. 3, 1096.
85 Ibid., 1097–1099. 86 Ibid., 1100–1101.

'infractions of the laws of hygiene' which could bring death to women at the very moment they began to enter 'a more tranquil life and an existence less exposed' to the largest danger (implying childbirth).[87]

Colombat was an eclectic medical scholar, publishing on numerous topics as well as authoring works of theatre and poetry. While he denigrated practitioners of traditional medical remedies, he was a promoter of new pharmacological substances entering the European market through global colonial trade, publishing an entire book in 1832 about the benefits of Amazonian Copaiba balm (derived from the oily resin of leguminous trees in the Copaifera genus of South America), which he had formed into flavourless pastilles in collaboration with a pharmacist named Corriol in the rue de Sèvres. He recommended these particularly for women's gynaecological and venereal diseases—blennorrhagia and leukorrhea, which referred respectively to the yellow and white forms of vaginal discharge; the white form was widely considered to be a symptom of menstrual disorders and of the critical age.[88] He was thus perhaps one of the first doctors to wed a commercial pharmaceutical interest to ideas about older women's need for medical treatment. His treatise on women also provided an extensive account of all the emerging gynaecological surgeries being practised experimentally still rarely but with increasing frequency in Paris hospitals, including the (almost always lethal) hysterectomy for the treatment of uterine cancer and for fibroid polyps which were recognised to be non-cancerous.[89] He also said that nymphomaniac hysteric conditions should sometimes be treated with clitoridectomy, and that hypertrophic growth of the labia was treated with surgery too.[90] It is unclear if Colombat himself ever practised any such surgeries as he may simply have been collating all the existing scholarship on gynaecological procedures known to medicine by this time. But his work curiously evokes an early proto-version of the psycho-pharmaco-technological nexus of practices that later emerged in the treatment of menopausal women—both in the psychiatric definition of sexually active older women as maniacs and perverts (discussed in Chapter 7), and in the dual prescription of hysterectomy with chronic pharmacological treatment which emerged in the 1890s and which remains common still in gynaecological practice of our own time relative to women in midlife (discussed in Chapter 10).

Around 1850, numerous works of Paris hygiene focused on women's health, including passages about the cessation of menses, which was still most often referred to as the 'critical age', despite Gardanne's neologism holding greater respectability. For doctors wishing to appeal to a wider readership, the neologism

[87] Ibid., 1102.

[88] Marc Colombat de l'Isère, *Le Baume de copahu sans odeur ni saveur désagréables, administré sous la forme de dragées dans la blennorragie et la leucorrhée* (Paris: chez les principaux libraires, 1832), 18; Colombat de l'Isère, *Traité des maladies des femmes*, vol. 3, 1098.

[89] Colombat de l'Isère, *Traité des maladies des femmes*, vol. 2, 667–715, 774–799.

[90] Ibid., 1018–1030.

was perhaps seen either as too technical or insufficiently generative. The Paris doctor Hippolyte Pierre Crosilhes, like Colombat and others, likened the cessation of menses in ageing to the commencement of menstruation in puberty as the two great moments of physiological revolution in women's lives. In his 1850 treatise on the hygiene and diseases of women, he declared: 'There are two great periods in the life of woman one has understood to be so important as to attribute to them the term "critical times".' This was because, as an 'ancient author' had affirmed, the uterus was the direct or indirect cause of most of women's diseases.[91] He too asserted that women, arriving at the 'critical age', must adhere 'scrupulously' to the 'rules of hygiene', avoiding all concerts, balls, and other events, alcohol, stimulating foods or beverages, exercising regularly and following a similar restrictive dietary regime to that outlined by Colombat.[92] Unusually though, Crosilhes seemed to think that once the menstrual periods had definitively ceased, a woman had overcome the time of danger and no longer needed to observe any particular hygienic prescriptions. For post-menopausal women, he seemed mainly concerned that they abstain from wearing too much make-up in the effort to disguise their age, which he said did not fool anyone and was suitable only for stage actresses.[93]

The insistence on women having a specific need for hygienic care around the cessation of menses was certainly integrated then into general Paris hygiene texts and works on the diseases of women by the mid-century, remaining an important layer of medical ideas about women's ageing thereafter. Nonetheless, most influential hygienists from this time on focused on new forms of scientific evidence, such as demographic statistics, and on the large-scale health problems of urban life, and were considerably less interested in the idea of the 'critical age'. Notably, the 1851 *Treatise of Private and Public Hygiene* by the renowned Paris hygienist Louis Alfred Becquerel (1814–1866), which ran into eight editions up to 1883, had frankly nothing to say about women's cessation of menses whatsoever, focusing instead on general hygienic advice for all ages, sexes, and social classes.[94] He referred to Daubenton's six ages, which included that of the 'age de retour' from age 45 to 60 years, but revised this to his own list of seven ages, differentiating infancy from early childhood and early from late childhood—Daubenton had collapsed them all; but also, crucially, he deleted the 'age de retour' altogether, proposing instead a single large 'adult age' from 20 to 60 years.[95] This was not because Becquerel took men's lifespan to be the human norm, ignoring women, as many eighteenth-century works about ageing had tended to do; on the contrary, he referred in numerous places to the differing mortality ages of men and

[91] Hippolyte Pierre Crosilhes, *Hygiène et maladies des femmes* (Paris: Moquet, 1850), 2.
[92] Ibid., 14–15. [93] Ibid., 16.
[94] Louis Alfred Becquerel, *Traité élémentaire d'hygiène privée et publique* (Paris: Labé, 1851).
[95] Ibid., 8.

women;[96] and he discussed the common risk to working women's health in the lacemaking industry, which caused hunched backs, loss of eyesight, emaciation, and pallor.[97] He objected to the entirely unproven claim, made by others, that an 'immoderate use of venereal pleasure' caused uterine cancer, and worried far more about the countless working-class women forced into prostitution by poverty, who languished with tuberculosis in the Paris Pitié hospital where he worked, than about the obesity and hot flushes of the elites.[98] He considered both women and older people less calorific than men and younger people, hence the more common need for warmer clothing and hand-warmers (*chaufferettes*) among older women.[99] But he mainly appeared to consider young women the most at risk of menstrual disorders, with nothing at all to say about their age-related cessation.[100]

Becquerel also authored another treatise on the diseases of the uterus in 1859 in which he said that many of the cancers thought by earlier scholars to be the product of women's older ages had originated in their youth where, if they had been discovered, would never have become lethal.[101] He considered many common gynaecological disorders, such as cervical inflammation and metritis, to result from being excessively sedentary, resolving on their own after the 'critical age'.[102] The one piece of hygienic advice Becquerel provided for women of all ages was this: do some exercise—at least go for walk as often as possible. 'The majority of women do not do enough exercise,' he asserted, 'they barely leave their habitations.' This lack of movement meant they did not consume enough carbon to stimulate their appetite and digestion, causing congestion, plethora, poor circulation, as well as hysteria, other derangements of the uterus, leukorrhea, sterility, miscarriages, producing weak offspring and disposing women to numerous diseases.[103] Despite his general renown in his own time and for long after as an important mid-century medical scholar of public hygiene, contagious diseases, and women's gynaecological disorders, in regard to his views about women's ageing and cessation of menses, Becquerel was part of a minority lineage which rejected all the catastrophising views of the 'critical age' and the long lists of proscriptive and prescriptive 'laws of hygiene' directed towards the elites by which such accounts were generally accompanied. That it was nonetheless possible to draw such conclusions from within a mainstream nineteenth-century medical world-view is important to recognise: other doctors were not passive vectors of a pervasive conceptual ambiance over which they had no control, but rather were active agents in the generation of ideas about women's greater morbidity in ageing

[96] Ibid., 635, 575. [97] Ibid., 631. [98] Ibid., 585.
[99] Ibid., 322. [100] Ibid., 125.
[101] Louis Alfred Becquerel, *Traité clinique des maladies de l'utérus et de ses annexes* (Paris: G. Baillière, 1859).
[102] Ibid., 324. [103] Becquerel, *Traité élémentaire d'hygiène*, 504.

and with the cessation of menses, embellishing an existing French tradition of seeing women as almost a species apart from men.

An important development after 1840 enabled an increasing number of doctors to accept both that the cessation of menses was not necessarily a time of 'incidents', and that it was not the uterus determining all of women's physiology: this was the post-mortem examination of numerous women of all ages, hence also those around the age of 50, who had died of tuberculosis. The Paris gynaecologist Charles Négrier (1792–1862), in his 1840 work on the anatomy and physiology of the human ovary, thus described the non-pathological scarred and shrunken ovaries of numerous women, which he had removed after their untimely deaths a few years after the cessation of their menses, and who had suffered no resulting 'incidents'. He focused in detail on two examples, one from a 50-year-old 'virgin', and another from a several-times mother who died at the age of 48, both victims of tuberculosis, with lithographic anatomical illustrations of their ovaries.[104] Prior to this time, ovaries of very elderly women had indeed been examined and described as shrunken or atrophied, but this was the first thoroughly documented account of the normal recently post-menopausal ovary without accompanying gynaecological disease, permitted by the abundance of corpses resulting from the contagious diseases that killed so many in all ages of life in mid-nineteenth-century France. The ovaries of these women, Négrier said, never contained any vesicular organs, nor any remnant of them recently burst: 'Everything about them announces, on the contrary, a complete cessation of work, dating at least from the time of the last menstrual haemorrhage.'[105] Another 80-year-old tiny, thin Corsican woman he treated had mothered several children, reported having ceased to menstruate at the age of 45, and he could not even find her right ovary after her death, with nothing of the left ovary remaining but a string.[106] He thus joined the growing chorus of views found in the work of numerous anatomists and physicians of the diseases of women who were now converging on the view that the ovary, not the uterus, was the central governing organ of women's reproductive physiology.[107] This turn may have provided the opportunity to shed many of the inherited and unevidenced discourses about women's hysteria, propensity to nervous diseases, and complete revolutions of economy in every moment of uterine change. But the new ovarian account of menstruation appears largely to have simply been seamlessly absorbed into the existing pathological hygienic view of the cessation of menses which had previously accused the uterus of being

[104] Charles N. Négrier, *Recherches anatomiques et physiologiques sur les ovaires dans l'espèce humaine, considérés spécialement sous le rapport de leur influence dans la menstruation* (Paris: Béchet Je. et Labé, 1840).

[105] Ibid., 54. [106] Ibid., 54.

[107] Ibid., 61. For instance, Marie Anne Victoire Boivin, *Traité pratique des maladies de l'utérus et de ses annexes, accompagné d'un atlas de 41 planches in-fol. gravées et coloriées, représentant les principales altérations morbides des organes génitaux de la femme* (Paris: J.-B. Baillière, 1833).

the organ of decline and now instead simply shifted emphasis to the ovaries. Négrier himself accepted the standard account of the cessation of menses as commonly entailing numerous miserable symptoms: he too thus considered the epithet of the 'critical age' appropriate, 'whatever one might say'.[108]

The Need for Hygiene in the Critical Age of the Cessation of Menses

The integration of women's final cessation of menses into the concerns of Montpellier hygienists on the cusp of the eighteenth to early nineteenth century was contemporaneous with the very first French specialist doctoral works on the topic; but it was the Montpellier scholars who did much of the early work of legitimising the idea that women around the cessation of menses needed special hygienic care—the idea that was thereafter repeated in countless medical theses throughout the nineteenth century. The Montpellier candidate Jérémie-André Pingault was the first to write a specific French thesis on the final cessation of menses in 1799, citing Roussel's account of sex differences in ageing and of cultural differences in pubertal development and menstruation observed across global anthropology.[109] He also referred to the lectures on the diseases of women by Joseph-Marie-Joachim Vigarous (1759–1826) given at the Montpellier faculty in the 1790s.[110] Importantly, Pingault misapplied Vigarous's ideas about menstrual suppression in cycling women to those whose menses had definitively ceased due to age—Vigarous had specifically excluded older women from his remarks about the potential negative effects of menstrual suppression,[111] and while he thought that the suppression of menses could cause cancerous tumours to grow, he considered these to affect women of all ages.[112] From Vigarous Pingault derived a mechanistic account of the illnesses emerging with the suppression of menses due to the sympathetic effect on the nervous system of the loss of uterine activity, with resultant plethora, leading to cancers of the breast, uterus, or ovaries, as well as hysteria, breathing problems, palpitations, swollen lungs, coughing of blood, and consumption.[113] Unlike Vigarous, though, he referred to these specifically as symptoms of the final cessation of menses, saying they could be avoided through diet and would be aggravated by alcohol abuse, inactivity, and either the excess or privation of sexual activity.[114] More specific

[108] Négrier, *Recherches anatomiques et physiologiques sur les ovaires*, 61.

[109] Jérémie-André Pingault, *De la cessation des règles* (Montpellier: Tournel, 1799), 4–5. Joseph-Marie-Joachim Vigarous, *Cours élémentaire de maladies des femmes, ou Essai sur une nouvelle méthode pour étudier et pour classer les maladies de ce sexe*, 2 vols (Paris: Deterville, 1801).

[110] Pingault, *De la cessation des règles*, 16.

[111] Vigarous, *Cours élémentaire de maladies des femmes*, vol. 1, 355.

[112] Ibid., 307.

[113] Pingault, *De la cessation des règles*, 13–15.

[114] Ibid., 9.

recommendations were temperament based: sanguine women must avoid dark meats, spirits, coffee, and wine, while pituitary or lymphatic women should eat succulent foods and drink tonic remedies and copious aged wines, taking frequent exercise in the country air.[115] Pingault warned against both blood-letting, which aggravated the nerves of women at this time of life and could cause haemorrhagic bleeding, and the overuse of purgative medications such the aloe-based *pillules de Rufus*.[116] Clearly, none of the mechanistic or hygienic content of Pingault's work derived from Roussel, whose speculations about sex differences in ageing included no such discussion. But his construction of the final cessation of menses as disease-prone and requiring its own hygienic protocol cannot be attributed to Vigarous either.

The second Montpellier candidate to focus on the topic, Joseph Gagnebé in 1801, was entirely non-hygienic and non-mechanistic, and appears to have come to the topic from an entirely different pathway altogether—that of surgery—noting reports of breast and uterine cancer in women after the cessation of menses, citing both Chambon de Montaux and the surgeon Gilles Le Vacher's Besançon dissertation on breast cancer from 1740.[117] Here perhaps is an important clue as to how the Montpellier candidates pieced together a view of the final cessation of menses as pathological. Montpellier medical training in the late eighteenth century permitted a combined specialisation in medicine and surgery and Montpellier graduates were thus more often exposed to that minor current of surgical thought (discussed in Chapter 3) which referred to women's higher risk of breast cancer in their forties and early fifties. Gagnebé leaned most towards surgical recommendation, especially oophorectomy as a treatment for older women's cancers, which was not yet a common practice in France, though it was becoming so in England at this time.[118] But surgery was not the focus in other Montpellier theses around this time, such as that of Antoine Leyral in 1806, which focused entirely on prophylactic hygiene measures for women approaching the cessation of menses.[119] Leyral provided a complex system of hygienic measures for each temperament and for numerous specific complaints of the cessation of menses, too many to describe fully here. For example, to avoid pain, inflammation, haemorrhages, pruritis, or prolapse of the uterus, one should consume a 'humectant and refreshing' vegetal diet with milk, avoiding salted meats and spices, and he recommended baths and genital cleanliness for all.[120] Rheumatic

[115] Ibid., 18. [116] Ibid., 19–20.

[117] Joseph Gagnebé, *Exposition de quelques maladies qui attaquent les femmes à la cessation des règles*. Thèse (Montpellier: Imprimerie de Tournel, 1801), 12; Gilles Le Vacher, *Dissertation sur le cancer des mamelles* (Besançon: J.-B. Charmet, 1740).

[118] Gagnebé, *Exposition de quelques maladies*, 15.

[119] Antoine Leyral, *Essai sur la prophylactique des femmes parvenues à l'époque de la cessation des règles*. Thèse (Montpellier: Imprimerie Auguste Ricard, 1806).

[120] Ibid., 17.

pain could be avoided with mucilaginous broths, lettuce, endives, purslane, chard, the mucosal part of young animals, whey, and lightly purgative mineral waters.[121]

Montpellier theses throughout the early nineteenth century thereafter remained heavily committed to hygienic approaches and prescribed richly from the *materia medica* of herbal remedies known to university pharmacology, an inheritance of the eighteenth-century pride of place given to this aspect of medicine in the training of doctors at the Montpellier faculty.[122] This was true even for those scholars more orientated towards surgery. Jean-Antoine-Placide Jaumes in 1816, even while focusing his thesis mostly on the gynaecological disorders of older women, insisted that the melancholic temperament which he associated with the worst health problems in the *âge de retour*, could be acquired through poor nutrition, breathing humid air, excessive intellectual work, and sedentary living 'like one sees among women in the big towns'.[123] He provided a range of hygienic prescriptions for avoiding gynaecological disorders in the *âge de retour*: fatty, milky, or floury foods should be avoided along with spirits, excessive wine or vinegar, and other acidic substances. But the biggest problem with women's ageing in urban life was inactivity, he affirmed: 'The bodies of women, like those of men, are better formed by work than rest; they degenerate in inactivity and are debased by idleness.'[124] He also recommended warm baths with emollient herbs such as orange-blossom and linden, and dilute, refreshing drinks made of couch grass (*chiendents*), barley, nettle (*parétaire*), chard (*poirée*), and marshmallow, or whey, to prevent haemorrhagic bleeding and other irritations of the uterus.[125] Ultra-salty thermal baths were also advisable for everyone, though in the event of cancer, more unpleasant remedies such as leeches on the vulva might be needed.[126] Sucrion Ramondenc in 1820 similarly affirmed that 'the rules that hygiene prescribes are of the greatest importance and often suffice to prevent afflictions', adding that 'they must be employed with a knowledge of the causes'.[127] Diet should follow according to temperament, and while blood-letting and leeches could be useful among plethoric women, they would be useless, even dangerous in the case of hysteria. He noted the English physician John Fothergill's warnings about purgatives but nuanced the claim by adding that it was mainly pituitary women who needed to avoid these.[128]

However, some of the Montpellier candidates clearly also absorbed the old conceptual layer of anti-pathological naturalisation of women's reproductive ageing of the kind found in the work of the eighteenth-century Montpellier scholar

[121] Ibid., 17–20. [122] Williams, *A Cultural History of Medical Vitalism*, 61.

[123] Jean-Antoine-Placide Jaumes, *Aperçu sur diverses maladies qui peuvent affecter les femmes à l'âge du retour* (Montpellier: Jean Martel aîné, 1816), 9.

[124] Ibid., 10. [125] Ibid., 11. [126] Ibid., 13–14.

[127] Sucrion Ramondenc, *Considérations sur l'état de la femme à l'époque de la cessation des règles*. Thèse (Montpellier: Jean Martel, 1820), 11.

[128] Ibid., 12–14.

of the diseases of women, Jean Astruc (1684-1766), whom we considered in Chapter 1, and which provided little inspiration for hygienic prescriptions. This layer persisted too throughout the nineteenth century, as an important minority position, where it unsettled and diluted the attempts by doctors to subject older women to elaborate regimes of self-management. This naturalisation discourse was even accommodated alongside other catastrophising views of women's ageing, as in the 1822 thesis of Joseph-Lazare-Jacques Coural, who argued, citing Astruc, that once women stopped menstruating, they actually became healthier, slimmer, and appeared to 'become adorned with a new grace', which was the true meaning of the designation *âge de retour*—it was a renewal.[129] Nonetheless, he thought women's old age to be particularly miserable—commonly defined by the loss of capacity for reason, memory, judgement, and sensorial impressions, as well as by oedema, spasms, and cancers of the breast and uterus.[130] This was precisely the kind of collapsing of all the possible diseases of ageing into an account of the effects of the cessation of menses to which the Paris hygienist Claude Lachaise objected in his 1825 book.

One candidate, Nicolas Broye, who was a Swiss candidate from Fribourg at the Montpellier faculty in 1813, even conveyed something of the eighteenth-century German conflation of the temporary menstrual stoppage with the final cessation of menses, accounting for both as problems of plethora.[131] He began his thesis with a quotation from the eighteenth-century German biologist Johann Georg Zimmerman which described why more attention should be paid by doctors to the diseases of woman (even though Zimmerman said very little about these himself): 'Her fate is more troubled, nay sadder, than the fate of men' ('ihr Schiksal is unstreitig weit trauriger als das Schiksal der Männer').[132] Broye said that the cessation of menses was a particularly 'critical' time for 'city women' ('citadines'), and especially for those who had not followed 'the wish of nature', or who had suffered long illnesses in the past, difficult childbirths, a 'frantic life' ('vie effrénée') of debilitating passions, or lived in a low, humid place.[133] But he also—citing the Montpellier professor Vigarous, whose lectures he would have attended—said that once the uterus ceased its activity, 'the mass of forces of the other organs' became more energised: 'Women seem then to acquire a font of inexhaustible life; the time of peril has passed; they are no longer subject to the particular problems of their sex; they acquire the constitution of a man.' This both made them more reasonable, firm, and constant in their tastes, their demeanour

[129] Joseph-Lazare-Jacques Coural, *Considérations générales sur les phénomènes physiologique et pathologique de la femme aux divers âges de la vie*. Thèse (Montpellier: Jean Martel, 1822), 36.

[130] Ibid., 38–40.

[131] Nicolas Broye, *Considérations sur la cessation des règles*. Thèse (Montpellier: Jean Martel Aîné, 1813).

[132] Ibid., 1; Johann Georg Zimmerman, *Von der Erfahrung un der Arzneikunst* (Orell: Füßli, 1787), 605.

[133] Broye, *Considérations sur la cessation des règles*, 7.

more noble and majestic, their passions more decisive, but it also made their voice lower and their seductive charms diminish. Here he referred to Roussel's view of women's disfigurement with ageing caused both by the loss of plumpness of their bodies and the growth of hairs on their chin.[134]

He also leaned upon the Prussian royal physician and Berlin professor of pathology Christoph Wilhelm Hufeland, who had observed that women after the cessation of menses were more prone to cancers as well as a range of other dangerous diseases.[135] Lymphatic women were those who particularly needed to be concerned about cancer, Broye said. Following Hufeland, he thought the best way to prevent breast cancer from developing was by 'combatting local plethora' of the uterus that occurred once the menses ended,[136] primarily through the use of blood-letting, cauterisation, purgatives, and 'diverse surgical means'.[137] Broye was not the last French scholar to refer to Hufeland, whose 1797 book on the *Art of Prolonging Life* appeared in multiple French and English translations throughout the nineteenth century in the growing field of longevity medicine.[138] Nonetheless, among the menopause scholars mostly focused on hygienic measures specific to women around the time of cessation of menses, Hufeland's work had little to offer. He was even one of those who had failed to notice that more men than women died in their fifties, as we saw in Chapter 2.

Women's 'critical age', following Gardanne's thesis in 1812, also became assimilated in the first decades of the nineteenth century into theses on the different ages of women's lifespan in ways that suggest Roussel remained an important influence for those not pursuing the hygiene stream. The candidate Bonafous (who was from the Lot in the south of France but chose Paris for his studies) in 1817 thus included *l'époque critique* as one of the four 'ages of woman', when women could expect to lose their beauty, grow fatter, develop a more masculine sounding voice, and become unhappy because they saw their charms vanishing.[139] In the same year, the Montpellier candidate Gilbert Guyot wrote a similar thesis about the different periods of a woman's life, which had described the cessation of menses as 'the death of sex' and the moment of accelerated ageing, while also accommodating the demographic recognition of women's greater

[134] Ibid., 9–10.

[135] Ibid., 13. Christoph Wilhlem Hufeland, *Enchiridion medicum oder Anleitung zur medizinischen Praxis: Vermächtniss einer fünfzigjährigen Erfahrung* (Berlin: Jonas, 1836), 593.

[136] Broye, *Considérations sur la cessation des règles*, 13–14.

[137] Ibid., 16–17.

[138] Christoph Wilhlem Hufeland, *Die Kunst das menschliche Leben zu verlängern*, 2 vols (Jena: Franz Haas, 1797); Christoph Wilhlem Hufeland, *La Macrobiotique, ou L'Art de prolonger la vie de l'homme, suivi de Conseils sur l'éducation physique des enfants*, trad. A.-J.-L. Jourdan (Paris: J.-B. Baillière, 1836); Christoph Wilhlem Hufeland, *Hufeland's Art of Prolonging Life*, ed. Erasmus Wilson (London: J. Churchill, 1853). On the late nineteenth- and early twentieth-century German history of the longevity movement, see Heiko Stoff, *Ewige Jugend: Konzepte der Verjungung vom spaten 19. Jahrhundert bis ins Dritte Reich* (Cologne: Bohlau, 2004).

[139] J .B .H. Bonafous, *Considérations physiologiques et générales sur les diverses époques de la vie de la femme* (Paris: Didot Jeune, 1817).

longevity.[140] Neither of these works suggested any hygienic measures that might permit women to manage this terrible fact of nature, which they both suggested was a product of the peculiar pattern of women's growth. Guyot echoed the Montpellier hygienist Étienne Tourtelle's account of women youth's being 'shorter and more brilliant' than that of men.[141]

The idea that women became almost or effectively men after the cessation of menses was often also bound up with the catastrophising, non-hygienic accounts of their ageing, but also sometimes implied a flattering development in older women's resemblance to men. Anglade in 1812 had described a woman becoming both physically and psychologically more masculine with the cessation of menses:

> her sensibility becomes blunted (*s'est emoussée*) she becomes firmer and more constant in her will and in her tastes; she no longer has the same avoidance of difficult exercise, she gives over to it without complaint; she develops a taste for tobacco and strong odours, takes pleasure in the use of wine and spirit beverages; in a word, one could say that a woman who no longer menstruates and who remains in good health is almost a man.[142]

Rural versus Urban Menopause as the Model for the Hygiene of Women's Ageing

The idea that negative symptoms associated with the cessation of menses was a feature only of urban elite women and not of peasant women was central to all the hygienic prescriptions provided for this time of life appearing from the first Paris specialist works and in almost every specialist work on menopause thereafter throughout the nineteenth century. It had also been, as we have seen, a central theme in the vapours texts of the eighteenth century, which characterised nervous pathology as a product of the negative effects of civilisation and urban life on women's delicate nerves. Jeannet des Longrois had drawn this distinction in his 1787 *Advice to Women of Forty Years*, noting a huge difference 'between the women of the countryside and those of the big towns, especially Paris'.[143] This difference was due to the clean air and frugality of peasant women's lives. On the other hand, he said, countless dangers menaced those women who lived in humid and stagnant air, abusing fine foods, perfumes, fermented liqueurs and

[140] Gilbert Joseph Magdeleine Guyot, *Quelques propositions sur la femme considérée dans les différentes périodes de la vie* (Montpellier: Jean Martel, 1817), 19–21.

[141] Ibid., 18.

[142] Jean Baptiste Anglade, *Considérations sur les effets que peut produire la cessation des règles.* Thèse (Montpellier: Jean Martel, 1812), 11.

[143] Jeannet des Longrois, *Conseils aux femmes de quarante ans*, 5.

voluptuous pleasures.[144] Similarly, the first Paris thesis on the critical age or cessation of menses by Pierre Béclard in 1802 emphasised it as a time of necessary hygienic intervention, reflecting also the hygienic inclinations of the Paris professors Pinel, Hallé, and Cabanis who all taught at the Paris faculty at this time.[145] Béclard emphasised individual differences between women's experience of the cessation of menses due to constitutional type, history of past illnesses, and how they had lived, as well as their life circumstances and proposed that it was, for many women actually a time of new vigour because of the demise of the influence of the uterus, which made them more like men.[146] But this could also mean that, though relieved of hysteria, older women were now more likely to develop hypochondria like men.[147] Béclard explicitly proposed peasant women as models for other women of how to avoid illness with the cessation of menses since they were 'the least distanced from natural mores':

> The life they lead, shared between work and rest taken in the time assigned by nature, supported by simple nourishment which does not exceed need, conserves them always in the most favourable disposition in the free and easy exercise of all their functions.[148]

The most important things for women to avoid with the cessation of menses were alcohol, aromatic substances, the pleasures of love, and laziness.[149]

It might be expected that the Montpellier scholars would be more attuned to peasant lifeways than those in Paris. The Paris psychiatrist Charles Lasègue in 1884 surveyed the parental backgrounds of recent Paris medical graduates, finding that they were mostly from the middle-class families of small business owners and professionals, especially the sons of pharmacists and other doctors, which he said was generally the case throughout European capital cities.[150] But as Elizabeth Williams has shown, late eighteenth-century Montpellier doctors were generally more exposed to rural populations by virtue of the town being so abundant in medical practitioners, such that the only way they could guarantee a consistent clientele was to travel out to rural hamlets and to see all classes of society, in contrast to most Parisian doctors who served largely the urban elites in the affluent neighbourhoods.[151] The first Montpellier theses on the cessation of menses, while richly hygienic and filled with constitution-specific advice about diet, beverages, exercise, sleep, bathing, and sexual activity, did not portray the ideal as specifically peasant or rural. It may be that precisely because so many of the patients of

[144] Ibid., 6.
[145] Pierre A. Béclard, *Essai sur les maladies auxquelles les femmes sont le plus fréquemment exposées à l'époque de la cessation des menstrues*. Thèse (Paris: Pancoucke, 1802).
[146] Ibid., 4. [147] Ibid., 65. [148] Ibid., 10. [149] Ibid., 17–18.
[150] Charles Lasègue, *Études médicales*, vol. 1 (Paris: Asselin, 1884), 449, 253.
[151] Williams, *A Cultural History of Medical Vitalism*, 23, 31–39.

Montpellier doctors were themselves rural, it would have been nonsensical to lecture to them about living like peasants, in the way the Parisian doctors could with their urban elite patients. It may have been also less appealing to romanticise peasant lifeways for Montpellier doctors who saw plenty of illness among the peasantry. Parisian doctors too sometimes came across women from the countryside of neighbouring regions who had travelled to the outskirts of the capital in search of clinical medical care unavailable near their farmlands, and this may have informed their comparisons of such women with the majority of their patients who were from the urban elites.

But it is also clear that the specific discourse of peasant women as models of health for the corrupt, indolent, and indulgent elites had been established much earlier in the eighteenth century with reference to the vapours. Imported from the vapours into menopause hygiene, the ideal peasant model remained one of the recurrent themes in many of the Paris medical works published throughout the nineteenth century. L. J. S. Jallon from Orléans, who defended one of the very earliest French medical theses on the 'critical age' in women, at the Paris faculty in 1805, claimed to have personally consulted a great number of women in villages in the countryside, who all told him they had no notable health problems following the end of their menstruation.[152] He attributed their lack of difficulty to being 'women who lived according to nature' defined as both having had children and living 'an active and laborious life'. City women, by contrast:

> ... develop these worrying, anomalous afflictions ... that bring so much strain to their thoughts, so much bizarreness to their tastes, so much weakness to their spirit, so much pusillanimity to their soul, so much capriciousness and inconstance to their actions, which sometimes condemns the remainder of their existence to suffering and tears.[153]

The main culprit, in Jallon's view was 'sedentary life'.[154] Peasant women were accustomed to the rigours of heat and cold, strengthened by hard work, eating only what restored their force, and sleeping only when their bodies were fatigued. For these reasons, their end of menses was without symptoms and barely noticeable. Urban women, by contrast, remained trapped inside their apartments, at most working in petty occupations that only ever exercised their fingers; or sleeping in each day until the sun was high in the sky, 'barely daring to take the occasional stroll'. Hence, they were punished by a critical age full of limpness (*la mollesse*) and apathy.[155]

Charles Gardanne's thesis of 1812 had also recommended mimicry of peasant diets for the management of menopausal symptoms, since rural women rarely

[152] L. J. S. Jallon, *Essai sur l'âge critique des femmes*. Thèse (Paris: Didot Jeune, 1805), 13.
[153] Ibid., 12–13. [154] Ibid., 36. [155] Ibid., 36.

appeared troubled by the cessation of menstruation. He considered the problems of urban women's menopause to result from 'foods that were too rich and heating, as well as the excitatory, opiate or purgative medications', and instead recommended 'light foods, taken as much as possible from the vegetables, ripe fruits, citrus and berries' as well as moderate fish and white-fleshed meat.[156] But in the 1816 expansion of his doctoral work into a book, Gardanne elaborated a much more complex system of temperament-specific hygienic advice, requiring not just peasant mimicry, but a detailed set of regimes and abstentions.[157] This was no longer at all about educating women to care for their own bodies such that they would have no need to consult a doctor; on the contrary, it was about a highly prescriptive and proscriptive system following each of Hallé's hygienic divisions: *Circumfusa* (temperature, air, and odour), *Applicata* (baths, clothing, and make-up), *Ingesta* (food and beverages), *Excreta* (bowel function, enemas, purgatives, cupping, cauterisation, and blood-letting), *Gesta* (sleep, movement, and work), and *Percepta* (entertainment, music, reading, the passions, sex, and gambling).[158] Women must undertake a complete change of lifestyle once their menses ceased and 'observe a regular behaviour, in order not to disturb the work of the uterus'. Hygiene in the critical age was a matter of following a complex system of laws of conduct and it was now the doctor's responsibility to 'dictate the laws and to exhort women' to follow them.[159] The perceived importance of Gardanne's approach is indicated by its second edition appearing in 1821 with a different Parisian publisher.[160]

Not deterred by Gardanne's attempt to style himself as the primary expert on menopause, the Paris candidate Albert Assegond ignored the neologism still in his 1821 thesis which reiterated the idea that women were generally more prone to illness than men on account of their delicate tissues, which erupted in even more diseases in the critical age since this was a moment when 'nature puts itself into insurrection'.[161] He too admitted that for some women, the critical age was when 'they seem to receive a new life' because they became more intellectual and ceased 'to live in the manner of their sex', defined as bearing and caring for children.[162] Nonetheless, it was important to take multiple hygienic precautions: avoid balls and spectacles that might 'feed the passions', avoid cold air which

[156] Charles-Pierre-Louis de Gardanne, *Dissertation sur les avis à donner aux femmes qui entrent dans l'âge critique*. Thèse (Paris: Didot Jeune, 1812), 28–29.

[157] Charles-Pierre-Louis de Gardanne, *Avis aux femmes qui entrent dans l'âge critique* (Paris: Gabon, 1816).

[158] Ibid., 97–236. [159] Ibid., 95.

[160] Charles-Pierre-Louis de Gardanne, *De la ménopause ou de l'âge critique des femmes* (Paris: Méquignon-Marvis, 1821).

[161] Albert Assegond, *De la femme, considérée à l'âge critique: Changements physiologiques qui s'opèrent dans on etat physiques et moral, et de l'application des règles de l'hygiène à cette principale époque de la vie*. Thèse (Paris: Didot Jeune, 1821), 8.

[162] Ibid., 12–14.

might stir the internal fluids of the body and cause inflammation, avoid tight undergarments that caused congestions of the genital organs, and engage in exercise and beverage consumption as appropriate for one's constitution—lymphatic women, for instance, needed only light exercise and moderate amounts of wine and coffee.[163] Enemas were recommended, as were purgatives in moderation, and blood-letting from the arm or leeches in the event of haemorrhages.[164]

For other scholars around this same time though, the peasant theme did not disappear, and the 1821 candidate Duplessis declared that one rarely sees the cessation of menses troubling 'a healthy and well-preserved woman'. The most important thing was to avoid strong emotions, wear comfortable clothing, and not become too excited.[165] In 1824 N. N. Firmin Lemoyne insisted emphatically on the need for an active rural-style life to avoid the ravages of the cessation of menses:

> The exercised and laborious life of the villagers, compared to the life of the inhabitants of the big towns, demonstrates that the former, fortified by work, are strangers to all these petty bothers that cause anxiety and torment among the latter. Women of the city thus should, as much as possible, resemble the way of life led by those in the countryside, and replace this state of inertia and indolence that dominates them and which is so contrary to their health, with moderate exercise and innocent distractions.'[166]

Simon's 1831 Paris thesis *Essay sur les crises* referred to a case observation of a country woman patient in her sixties being treated for a swollen knee and fever, whom he described as being of unusual strength and vigour having endured twelve pregnancies over fifteen years, ceasing menstruating at the age of 50 without any incident.[167] He made a point of remarking that her cessation of menses, the 'stormy period' ('époque orageuse') had not been in any way troublesome, as one might expect.[168] Lafontaine-Margariteau's doctoral thesis of 1835 drew a radical distinction between healthy, robust, hard-working peasant women, and *les femmes des villes* who were in general 'feeble, raised for the most part in limpness and in bad habits'; 'their food almost always bad, their habitations even more defective' especially on account of living in 'low and humid places'.[169] Louis

[163] Ibid., 19–22. [164] Ibid., 26–29.

[165] E. Duplessis, *De l'âge critique et des soins hygiéniques que réclament les femmes à cette époque.* Thèse (Paris: Didot Le Jeune, 1821), 8.

[166] N. N. Firmin Lemoyne, *Considérations générales sur les phénomènes qui se manifestent à la cessation du flux menstruel et sur le régime que doivent adopter les femmes pour franchir heureusement cette époque.* Thèse (Paris: Didot Jeune, 1824), 20.

[167] François Simon, *Essai sur les crises.* Thèse (Paris: Didot le Jeune, 1831), 18. [168] Ibid., 21.

[169] Louis-Marie Lafontaine-Margariteau, *Conseils hygiéniques aux femmes depuis leur naissance jusqu'à l'âge critique, ayant pour but principal de les préserver de la leucorrhée flueurs blanches), ou de la diminuer si elle existe.* Thèse (Paris: Didot le Jeune, 1835), 6–7.

Chandelux in 1850 contrasted peasant with urban middle-class lifeways, similarly situating them along binary axis of active versus inactive, chaste versus libertine, sober versus intemperate, poor versus rich, the fresh outdoor air of the paddock versus the stagnant indoor air of the salons and attics. All these factors, he thought, 'exerted a far too obvious influence over the important function of menstruation for them not to matter in its duration'.[170]

While some of the Paris candidates focused their theses largely on a physiological description of the changes that occurred with the cessation of menstruation, most included a substantial section filled with hygienic advice, often with reference to the idea that by following the lifestyle of the rural peasantry, or at least, observing a broad regime of hygienic interventions, the illnesses otherwise incumbent upon women at this time of life might be avoided. It certainly did not appear to occur to any of these writers that someone not following any particular hygienic prescription—let alone someone who enjoyed a critical age filled with wine, salty meats, balls, and copious debauchery—might nonetheless also experience a healthy menopause. Nor did they consider that women pursuing the healthy peasant model might nonetheless develop dangerous gynaecological cancers. In fact, most of the Paris theses in the 1820s and 1830s referred to hygienic advice in the titles of their works. There were 'precautions to take to prevent and combat the incidents and diseases' of the critical epoch;[171] there were 'therapeutic, hygienic and prophylactic' means to know about;[172] and there was 'hygienic advice' to follow.[173]

By the 1820s, the Montpellier candidates too began reproducing the 'peasants do it better' motif with the incorporation of increasingly proscriptive advice of how women should live following the cessation of menses. Jacques-Philippe Labarraque's 1827 thesis on menstruation argued that menopause was generally without danger 'among women who had fulfilled nature's wishes, who did some form of exercise and who lived without recourse to excesses', as was usually the case among women of the countryside. On the other hand: 'rich city women' ('les riches citadines'), whose lifestyles were lazy and inactive, who breathed unhealthy air, and whose health was destroyed by 'the fire and turmoil of passion, the profusion of delicacies, the abuse of perfumes and the use of liquor' could expect

[170] Chandelux, *L'Âge critique de la femme (ménopause)* (Paris: Irgnoux, imprimeur de la Faculté de Médecine, 1850).

[171] Claude-Martial Bardout, *Considérations générales sur la cessation du flux menstruel, et sur les précautions à prendre pour en prévenir les accidens ou les maladies* (Paris: Didot Jeune, 1816); C. L. Junod, *De l'époque critique chez les femmes et des précautions à prendre pour en prévenir et combattre quelques accidens ou maladies*. Thèse (Paris: Didot Jeune, 1822).

[172] Pierre-Jean-Baptiste Bertrand, *Dissertation sur l'aménorrhée définitive ou âge critique des femmes sur les accidents auxquels elles sont exposées à cette époque, et sur les moyens thérapeutiques, hygiéniques et prophylactiques les plus appropriés à leur situation* (Paris: Didot le Jeune, 1824).

[173] Lafontaine-Margariteau, *Conseils hygiéniques aux femmes*.

to have a terrible *époque critique*, filled with emotional suffering and illness.[174] Joseph-Hortense Houlès's Montpellier thesis of 1843 focused on menopause 'from a hygienic point of view', integrating the new statistical realisation of women's lower mortality in every age bracket after 35 years, with the sex-differentiated vitalist account of women's faster rate of ageing, noting the paradox this twin perspective produced: it must be that while women aged faster to begin with, their rate slowed down dramatically in the second half of life, he reasoned. This thesis expressed a higher degree of contempt for older women than most others of its kind: Women's menopause made them lose all their beauty, their figure, they became wrinkled, developed facial hair and deeper voices, and generally became men.[175] Both men and women suffered an *âge de retour* but men retained their full, characteristic energy long after women had lost theirs.[176] Houlès recommended three broad strategies for the hygienic management of menopause which consisted in avoiding the use of medicaments aimed at resuming the menses (the idea attributed to the English doctor John Fothergill's 1776 warning about purgative remedies); preventing the common disorders of menopause which were white vaginal discharge (*fleurs blanches*), haemorrhoids, intermittent fevers, and diaphoresis (sweating); and dealing with any existing illnesses not specific to the critical age but which might recur during it.[177] Menopausal women must avoid anything that might 'excite their imaginations', particularly anything that aroused or perpetuated erotic tendencies.[178]

Indeed, the idea that a hygienic approach to menopause entailed avoidance of anything stimulating on the grounds that women's nerves in the critical age were particularly sensitive produced its own kind of plethora of proscriptive advice. In 1848 the Paris thesis of Jean-Baptiste Nosely proposed that women in the critical age avoid any kind of extreme pleasure or joy, though it was permitted still to enjoy mild emotions and moderate sex.[179] Gustave-Adolphe Plihon in 1859 warned that women should not be complacent in the critical age and should recognise the importance of hygiene at this time of life, even if it was not a particularly dangerous time from the point of view of mortality.[180] Pure country air was recommended, along with increased activity and low, humid places should be avoided. Women should not stay up late, nor sleep for too long; their homes should be bright with natural light and aerated, and corsets were bad for the

[174] Jacques-Philippe Labarraque, *Aperçu physiologico-pathologique sur la menstruation en général, et quelques conseils d'hygiène pour l'âge critique en particulier*. Thèse (Montpellier: Martel aîné, 1827), 13–14.

[175] Joseph-Hortense Houlès, *De la ménopause considérée au point de vue de l'hygiène*. Thèse (Montpellier: Isadore Tournel, 1843), 13–14.

[176] Ibid., 6–7. [177] Ibid., 24. [178] Ibid., 26.

[179] Jean-Baptiste Nosely, *Dissertation sur l'âge critique*. Thèse (Paris: Rignoux, Imprimeur de la Faculté de Médecine, 1848), 27.

[180] Gustave-Adolphe Plihon, *De la ménopause (âge critique)*. Thèse (Paris: Rignoux, Imprimeur de la Faculté de Médecine, 1859), 5–6, 21.

organs and should be avoided.[181] Among those discussing women's ageing or the critical age, by far the most common theme was the idea, already developed in the vapours scholarship of the eighteenth century, that urban, decadent, and elite lifeways were corrupting, accelerated ageing, and caused multiple diseases, while simple women who lived on the land in the regions of France were the pinnacle of health and vitality even into advanced age, as suggested in the drawing (Image 5.1) produced in the 1850s by the Toulousain lithographer and painter Marie-Alexandre Alophe, provocatively entitled 'Woman from the Pyrenees, arriving at 90 without any infirmity'. To survive and thrive in their critical age and beyond, urban women must simply mimic the way of life of the peasantry and eschew all that modernity had to offer them.

By the mid-nineteenth century, the peasant ideal was clearly also instrumentalised to focus medical disapproval of the increased possibilities for women in relation to sociability, entertainment, and consumerism. It is not hard to find examples of clearly moralistic views about urban elite women expressed by the twenty-something men passing through their university training, who now construed menopausal symptoms as merited punishment for those who had enjoyed too much of life's pleasures. The 1850 Paris candidate Louis Chandelux summarised this idea by intoning, 'beaucoup payent alors les anciennes passions'—'past passions cost dearly then'.[182] The features of urban life medical students claimed aggravated menopause symptoms included the wearing of tight corsets which were common among the bourgeoisie and aristocracy but rare among urban working-class and peasant women. Medical works on menopause often railed at length against corsets as one of the major causes of women's pelvic symptoms in the critical age.[183] Joseph-François Garnier in 1820 claimed that corsets caused the digestive disorders of which many women complained in menopause, explaining that the restriction of the viscera produced by them inhibited all the main functions of these organs.[184] Jacques-Philippe Labarraque in 1827 recommended women in menopause to engage in light exercise, avoiding crowds, and to wear loose clothing without a corset.[185] Louis-Marie Lafontaine-Margariteau in 1835 claimed that corsets caused leukorrhea, which in turn caused many of the other symptoms of menopause.[186] Gustave-Adolphe Plihon in 1859 said that corsets inhibited the function of the organs and hence were contraindicated for women approaching menopause.[187] Dr Castan, a urologist from Béziers as late as

[181] Ibid., 30–31. [182] Chandelux, *L'Âge critique de la femme*, 18–19.

[183] <Labarraque, *Aperçu physiologico-pathologique sur la menstruation*, 18–19; Dr André Castan, *Hygiène de l'âge de retour* (Paris: J. B. Baillière et Fils, 1901), 48–49; Mme A. Gensse. *Les Quatres Âges de la femme au point de vue physiologique*, 5th ed. (Paris: Éd. Crété. Corbeil, 1899), 112–121.

[184] Garnier, *Considérations sur l'âge critique*, 20–24.

[185] Labarraque, *Aperçu physiologico-pathologique sur la menstruation*, 18–19.

[186] Lafontaine-Margariteau, *Conseils hygiéniques aux femmes*, 15.

[187] Plihon, *De la Ménopause (âge critique)*, 22–30; Prosper-Louis Sauvé, *Réflexions sur l'âge critique, et particulièrement sur le régime le plus convenable pour préserver les femmes des accidens qui ont*

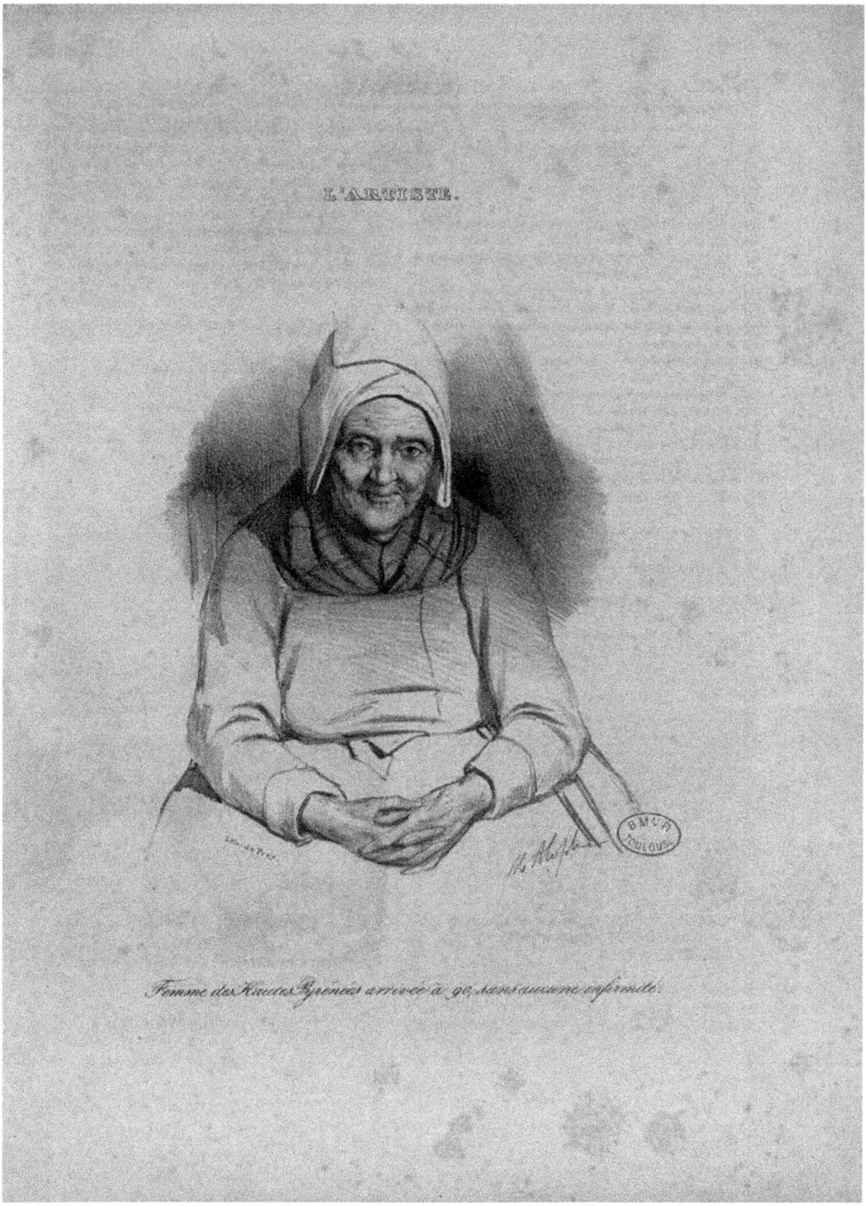

Image 5.1 Marie-Alexandre Alophe, *Femme des Hautes Pyrénées arrivée à 90 ans, sans aucune infirmité,* 1850s. Courtesy of the Bibliothèque Nationale de France.

the turn of the twentieth century attributed all pelvic pain in menopause to the wearing of corsets.[188] But the most vociferous opponent of corsets was the unusual woman who was an expert-writer on women's physiology at the *fin de siècle*, Mme A. Gensse, about whom little is known. Her 1899 book on the *Four Ages of Woman* cited a vast medical literature on the negative effects of corsets on the function of women's organs, detailing which types of stays were the worst culprits in restricting blood flow, crushing the intestines, and promoting the atrophy of the abdominal musculature.[189] Gensse considered gastro-intestinal disorders to be among the primary complaints of women in the critical age, which might explain the special place she gave to the condemnation of corset-wearing among menopausal women.[190] By this time though, as we consider in Chapter 8, she was not the only woman in France publishing expert advice on women's ageing.

Many nineteenth-century doctors also considered alcoholic consumption to be a major aggravating factor in women's menopause symptomology. It appeared among the list of things to avoid in menopause in the works of Gardanne, Labarraque, Nicaise, and Genest.[191] Guimbail remarked that the dyspeptic symptoms many women were reporting in menopause were entirely a product of their common abuse of alcoholic beverages for the alleviation of physical ailments, and that they were often even prescribed such beverages by their physicians.[192] Indeed, Gustave-Adolphe Plihon's doctoral thesis of 1859 recommended that anaemic women eat a rich diet with meats and alcoholic liqueurs.[193] As the social historian Thomas Brenner showed, the development of railways in the nineteenth century resulted in tremendous growth in wine distribution throughout France, with official tax records indicating a threefold increase in wine consumption between the 1830s and 1890s. New forms of more potent alcohol appeared in this period too—France had long produced concentrated spirits for export but historically had low patterns of consumption of these, and they were confined mainly to medicinal use. But in the nineteenth-century, spirit beverages became popular recreationally among the elites, often distilled from grain or beets.[194] As Brenner noted, much of what is known about the history of French alcohol consumption concerns urban populations, and there were probably significant local

coutume de survenir cette époque de leur vie. Thèse (Strasbourg: F. G. Levrault, 1826); Castan, *Hygiène de l'âge de retour*; Emile-Joseph-Amédée Valleteau de Moulliac, *Contribution à l'étude de l'âge critique chez l'homme (Troubles nerveux et psychiques)*. (Bordeaux: A. Destout ainé, 1907), 31.

[188] Castan, *Hygiène de l'âge de retour*, 48–49.

[189] Gensse. *Les Quatres Âges de la femme*, 112–121. [190] Ibid., 104–105.

[191] Gardanne, *Dissertation sur les avis à donner aux femmes*, 27; Labarraque, *Aperçu physiologico-pathologique sur la menstruation*, 14, 18; Auguste Nicaise, *Essai sur l'âge de retour chez la femme*. Thèse (Paris: Rignoux et Cie, 1838), 20; Louis Genest, *Comment prévenir et guérir les maladies du retour d'âge. Hygiène préventive; les ins spéciaux; les meilleurs remèdes* (Paris: M. Drouin, *c.*1920), 152.

[192] Henri Guimbail, *De la folie à la ménopause*. Thèse (Paris: A. Delahaye, 1884), 63.

[193] Plihon, *De la ménopause (âge critique)*, 31.

[194] Thomas Brenner, 'Toward the Cultural History of Alcohol in France', *Journal of Social History*, 23/1 (1989): 71–92 [73–74].

variations according to the differing prevalence of viticulture across regions. An 1850 survey cited by Eugen Weber indicated that most peasants drank no wine at all though some occasionally drank spirits.[195] In any case, the doctors who wrote about menopause noted no objectionable alcoholic consumption among peasant women, whereas they had much to say about urban women's damaging habits in menopause.

The theme of ideal peasant women's health has been remarked upon by most of the historians and feminist researchers who have considered French medical discourses about menopause. The anthropologist Joel Wilbush (one of the first scholars to begin historicising French menopause) described it as a product of the romanticised views of agrarian life that emerged in the early nineteenth century, following Rousseau's model of ideal natural humanity.[196] The demographic historian Christine Théré considers it a reflection of male doctors' negative suspicion of the relative liberties for cultural entertainment, intoxication, exotic consumer goods, as well as opportunities for sociability and public life enjoyed increasingly by elite women in nineteenth-century urban centres.[197] Gender historian Mary Lynn Stewart assimilates it to the late nineteenth-century declining birth rate that preoccupied political elites, resulting in hygienist celebration of mothers of numerous children.[198] In her book on the history of the relation between racial ideas of the French nation and reproductive medicine, Elsa Dorlin dates the emergence of the ideal of peasant women as models of health from the late eighteenth-century context of medical concern about low population growth, which she proposes stimulated the modern overturning of earlier ideas associating pregnancy with illness, such as can be found in the late seventeenth-century obstetrics of François Mauriceau. Pronatalist visions required a new hopeful image of healthy pregnancy to encourage births and the simple peasant ideal epitomised this value.[199] Dorlin attributes the first articulation of this idea to work of the royal physician Joseph Raulin (1708-1784) who wrote throughout the mid-eighteenth century on matters of women's health, nervous diseases, and the health of infants.[200] As we saw in the previous chapter, Raulin was also an important scholar in the elaboration of vapours as a disease of modern civilisation, and

[195] Ibid., 77; Eugen Weber, *Peasants into Frenchmen: The Modernization of Rural France, 1870–1914* (Stanford, Calif.: Stanford University Press, 1976), 144–146.

[196] Joel Wilbush, 'Menorrhagia and Menopause: A Historical Review', *Maturitas*, 10 (1988): 5–26 [8].

[197] Christine Théré, 'Âge de retour et retour d'âge: L'Asymétrie entre les sexes dans les discours médicaux en France (1770–1836)', [Life Change and Change of Life: Asymmetrical Attitudes towards the Sexes in Medical Discourse in France (1770–1836)] *CLIO: Femmes, Genre, Histoire*, 42 (2015): 54–75 [54–55].

[198] Mary Lynn Stewart, *For Health and Beauty: Physical Culture for Frenchwomen 1880s-1930* (Baltimore: Johns Hopkins University Press, 2000), 132–133.

[199] Elsa Dorlin, *La Matrice de la race: Généologie sexuelle et coloniale de la nation française* [2006] 2nd ed.s (Paris: La Découverte/Poche, 2009), 97–103.

[200] Ibid., 99.

indeed the ideal of peasant women's health was applied from the 1750s onwards as a model for elite urban women to avoid nervous disorders. It was seamlessly incorporated into the earliest specialist works on the hygiene of menopause via the engagement with texts about the vapours. However, as we will show in Chapter 7, the idea of pregnancy as an illness-prone time did not vanish from medical thought in the nineteenth century either: all times of uterine change, including puberty, menstruation, pregnancy, childbirth, lactation, and menopause, were proposed in Parisian alienist thought throughout the nineteenth century as a reason for women's greater susceptibility to hysteria, hypochondria, and erotomania at all ages. However, one place where changing medical ideas about the healthiness of childbearing identified by Dorlin were particularly elaborated, was in the growing medical insistence on childbearing as a necessary precondition for women's later ageing health, which was found in many works about the final cessation of menses, critical age, or menopause. As Elizabeth Williams remarks, the Montpellier vitalist account of sex differences underlay many such claims about women's sexual and childbearing functions as the 'only activities consonant with the character of the female vital force'.[201] This was expressed in the monotonously recurrent iterations of the command to 'follow the wishes of nature' which numerous menopause scholars espoused.

On the other hand, it is of course also possible that doctors were, in some respects, reflecting observation of differences in women's reported accounts of ageing at this time, which resulted from important changes in the experience of bodies moving from agrarian to urban (especially sedentary) lifeways. The influx of rural populations into the urban centres of France from the 1830s on, and the burgeoning of both the industrial working classes and of the leisurely middle classes in this period, made new forms of sedentary work habits the norm for larger numbers of people than ever before.[202] Undoubtedly, many of the massive changes in the lifeways of bodies disproportionately impacted women: as gender historian Susan Foley has noted, ideals of women's labour as appropriate only for sedentary pursuits along with the use of corsets among nineteenth-century elites meant that many women were more than ever subject to intense bodily restrictions of movement.[203] These developments may indeed have contributed to a range of novel physiological experiences and detriments in ageing. Recent biomedical research has continued to name both hypercaloric and low-fibre diets, lack of exercise, and obesity as implicated in menopausal symptoms and in increased biomarkers of ageing.[204] Chronic sleep deprivation has been found to

[201] Williams, *A Cultural History of Medical Vitalism*, 229.

[202] Harrison, *The Bourgeois Citizen in Nineteenth-Century France*, 135, 168.

[203] Susan Foley, *Women in France Since 1789: The Meanings of Difference* (Basingstoke: Palgrave, 2004), 31.

[204] Sharon Dormire & Chularat Howharn, 'The Effect of Dietary Intake on Hot Flashes in Menopausal Women', *Journal of Obstetrics, Gynecology and Neonatal Nursing*, 36/3 (2007): 255–262

have a profound impact on inflammatory biomarkers, obesity, hormonal regulation, and mental health.[205] And a growing body of research has shown improvements in the health and subjective experience of sedentary women in menopausal transition with the introduction of regular exercise alone.[206] Chronic sedentary behaviours have been found to compromise metabolic and cardiovascular health in general, which is now considered one of the major culprits of accelerated ageing in people whose work entails all-day sitting (this book, by the way, was written working at a treadmill desk!).[207] All these bodies of recent medical research have important conceptual inheritances from nineteenth-century medicine, but they are also based on statistically powerful data drawn from diverse human populations, and many of the pressures of modernity such studies now identify were indeed coming into force during the nineteenth century, particularly among urban populations.

French doctors and doctoral students at the beginning of the nineteenth century were undoubtedly often influenced by normative ideas about appropriate gender behaviour and a morally conservative suspicion of novel forms of consumption and feminine independence. But they may also have been witness to a relatively sudden shift in the corporeal lifeways of women in the development of urban intensification and middle-class work patterns. Those doctors who remarked that their elite patients spent all their time in the home and barely moving were largely clustered in Paris, where the patient clientele was heavily dominated by sedentary bourgeois and aristocratic women among whom obesity was becoming more common, in contrast to the much wider demography of the Montpellier patients. The Paris doctors' and hygienists' emphatic insistence that

[255]; Anna Brończyk-Puzoń, Dariusz Piecha, Justyna Nowak, Aneta Koszowska, Karolina KulikKupka, Anna Dittfield, & Barbara Zubelewicz-Szodzińska, 'Guidelines for Dietary Management of Menopausal Women with Simple Obesity', *Przeglad Menopauzalny*, 14/1 (2015): 48–52 [48]. Doi: 10.5114/pm.2015.48678.

[205] Rachel Leproult & Eve Cauter, 'Role of Sleep Loss in Hormonal Release and Metabolism', *Endocrine Development*, 17 (2017): 11–21. Doi: 10.1159/000262524.

[206] H. L. Gao, H. X. Gao, & L. Zhang, 'Effects of Walking on Body Composition in Perimenopausal and Postmenopausal Women', Menopause, 23/8 (2016): 928–934. Doi: 10.1097/GME.0000000000000627; Y. Wang, W. Shan, Q. Li, & W. Shan, 'Tai Chi Exercise for Quality of Life in a Perimenopausal Women Organization', *Worldviews Evidence Based Nursing*, 14/4 (2017): 294–305. Doi: 10.1111/wvn.12234; F. F. Conti, O. Brito Jde, N. Bernardes, S. Dias Dda, C. Malfitano, M. Morris, S. F. Llesuy, M. C. Irigoyen, & K. De Angelis. 'Positive Effect of Combined Exercise Training in a Model of Metabolic Syndrome and Menopause: Autonomic, Inflammatory, and Oxidative Stress Evaluations', *American Journal of Physiology*, 309/12 (2015): R1532-9. Doi: 10.1152/ajpregu.00076.2015.

[207] P. T. Katzmarzyk, T. S. Church, C. L. Craig, & C. Bouchard, 'Sitting Time and Mortality from All Causes, Cardiovascular Disease, and Cancer', *Medicine and Science in Sports and Exercise*, 41/5 (2009): 998–1005. Doi: 10.1249/MSS.0b013e3181930355; C.L. Edwardson, T. Gorely, M. J. Davies, L .J. Gray, K. Khunti, E. G. Wilmot, T. Yates, & S. J. Biddle, 'Association of Sedentary Behaviour with Metabolic Syndrome: A Metananalysis', *PLos One*, 7/4 (2012): e34916. Doi: 10.1371/journal.pone.0034916; M. T. Hamilton D. G. Hamilton, & T. W. Zderic, 'Sedentary Behaviour as a Mediator of Type 2 Diabetes', *Medicine and Sports Science*, 60 (2014): 11–26. Doi: 10.1159/000357332; E. Füzéki, L. Vogt, & W. Banzer, 'Sedentary Behaviour and Health', *Gesundheitswesen*, 77/3 (2015): 148–160. Doi: 10.1055/s-0034-1370951.

women needed to move more most likely was a response to profoundly sedentary behaviour among elite women in this time. Medical ideas about ideal peasant lifeways should thus not globally be taken as examples of 'le stupide dix-neuvième siècle', as the royalist writer Léon Daudet characterised his early twentieth-century colleagues' hubris relative to earlier generations.[208] Nor should we assume that the new menopause symptomology was purely a 'constructed' medical imaginary with no contribution from patient physiological experience. In developing menopause as a combination of ill-defined patient-reported symptoms along with the top-down mechanistic theories we have traced in this book, French medical ideas about reproductive ageing may instead indicate to us something of the nexus of the vitalist and materialist concepts elaborated by doctoral candidates and faculty professors, in their interface with the novel inflammatory experiences of nineteenth-century bodies in early urban industrial modernity. The nineteenth century, after all, was a dramatic time both for the elaboration of new medical concepts like menopause, but also for significant changes in the corporeal lives of urban French women. But while the latter were also occurring already in England, and to a lesser degree in other parts of Europe and the USA, none of these other cultures had the elaborate intellectual tradition of describing women's nature as radically apart from men's, which became so prominent in French thought in the second half of the eighteenth century.

The South African/Canadian medical anthropologist Joel Wilbush, who conducted both French historical and cross-cultural research on menopause in the 1970s and 1980s, remarked that 'climacteric disturbances are almost entirely confined to Western societies'.[209] That claim has since been complicated by more recent anthropological studies on non-western women's reports of ageing, and by the spread of western medical concepts globally.[210] As anthropologist Lynnette Leidy Sievert has emphasised, we should not underestimate 'the extent to which the meaning of menopause... varies across populations'.[211] And indeed, anthropological studies on menopause in Japan, Thailand, North Africa, and Pakistan indicate a wide variety of ways that women appear to experience life after the cessation of menstruation and childbearing.[212] Nonetheless, menopausal symptoms being widely reported only in contexts of urbanisation, industrialisation, and the

[208] Léon Daudet, *Le Stupide dix-neuvième siècle: Exposé des insanités meurtrières qui se sont abattues sur la France depuis 130 ans, 1789–1919* (Paris: Nouvelle Librairie Nationale, 1922).

[209] Joel Wilbush, '*La Ménespausie*: The Birth of a Syndrome', *Maturitas*, 1 (1979): 145–151 [145].

[210] Mwenza Blell, 'Menopausal Symptoms Among British Pakistani Women: A Critique of the Standard Checklist Approach', *Menopause*, 22/1 (2015): 79–87.

[211] Lynette Leidy Sievert, 'Menopause Across Cultures: Clinical Considerations', *Menopause*, 21/4 (2014): 421–423 [421].

[212] Emma K. Jones, Janelle R. Jurgenson, Judith M. Katzenellenbogen, & Sandra C. Thompson, 'Menopause and the Influence of Culture: Another Gap for Indigenous Australian Women?' *BMC Women's Health*, 12/43 (2012): 12–43. Doi: 10.1186/1472-6874-12-43.

biomedical definition of the cessation of menses as 'menopause' remains consistent with anthropological comparisons.[213]

Wilbush too drew attention to the likely changes in both biological and cultural contexts of bodily experience in late eighteenth- and early nineteenth-century France that may have caused women to feel differently about their ageing and report symptoms to their doctors in new terms. He noted that most of the nineteenth-century French medical writing on menopause revolved around the definition of a symptomology, rather than being based on clinical observation or the production of anatomical evidence about coherent biological mechanisms. He considered symptoms, by definition, to represent something of the complaints of the patient; and while he acknowledged that doctors' own reportage of patients' symptoms was not a simple reflection of what they had been told, he nonetheless considered the medical description of symptoms to represent patient-doctor communication.[214] While doctors' descriptions of their patients cannot be read unproblematically as reflecting women's experiences, he argued, they also cannot be ignored as possible sources of evidence of the impact of industrial modernity on women's bodies. On the other hand, the symptomatology referred to a vast range of conditions that were also found in men and in young women, and which could not be explained as due to anything specific about the cessation of menstruation, ranging from constipation, abdominal bloating, leukorrhea, and oedema to melancholy, madness, gout, fatigue, back-aches, and gastric reflux.[215]

As Wilbush noted, one of the recurrent 'incidents' (*accidents*) of the critical age which many nineteenth-century medical works described was uterine haemorrhages, which became less common in medical descriptions later in the nineteenth century, and which were notably rare among the reported complaints of menopausal women throughout the twentieth century.[216] He proposed that these may have been a product of the use of purgative medications that were so popular among the European elites from the end of the eighteenth century and into the first decades of the nineteenth, but which went relatively out of vogue after this time.[217] As we have seen, physicians from Jean Astruc to John Fothergill, and countless others after them, indeed blamed these medications for most of the complaints of women around the cessation of menstruation.[218] Gardanne, in his doctoral thesis of 1812, also warned against the use of purgative medications such

[213] Margaret M. Lock, *Encounters with Ageing: Mythologies of Menopause in Japan and North America* (Berkeley: University of California Press, 1993),105; F. Flint, 'Sociology and Anthropology of the Menopause', in P.A. van Keep, D.M. Serr, & R.B. Greenblatt, eds, *Female and Male Climacteric: Current Opinion 1978* (Lancaster: MIT Press, 1979), 1–9 [4–5].

[214] Joel Wilbush, 'What's in a Name? Some Linguistic Aspects of the Climacteric', *Maturitas*, 3 (1981): 1–9 [5].

[215] Eg. Nicaise, *Essai sur l'âge de retour chez la femme*, 8.

[216] Wilbush, '*La Ménespausie*', 147.

[217] Wilbush, 'Menorrhagia and Menopause', 5.

[218] John Fothergill, 'On the Management Proper at the Cessation of the Menses' [1774], *Medical Observations and Inquiries*, V (London: Cadell, 1776): 160–186.

as *les pillules de Rufus*.[219] Here then is one plausible physiological reason for the emergence of novel symptomatic experiences among menopausal women, to which doctors were explicitly responding.

The anthropological psychiatrist Daniel Delanoë has suggested another biological cause for the sudden emergence of menopausal complaints among women in the nineteenth century, remarking in his 2006 book *Sexe, croyances et menopause* that these may have been due to the lower number of children typically born among the French elites due to the popularisation of coitus interruptus. Fewer births are thought by some current gynaecologists to raise the likelihood of uterine fibroid growth, which in turn can produce haemorrhagic bleeding and abdominal pain.[220] This might be a credible speculation, except that most French women at the beginning of the twenty-first century tend to have even fewer children than they did in the nineteenth century, with fibroid formation affecting around 30–50 per cent of women by the time they reach menopause, and yet the specific complaints of haemorrhagic bleeding and abdominal pain in menopause are less common today than they appear to have been 150 years ago. Fibroids may be entirely asymptomatic and need not result in abnormal bleeding. They are common too among women of mid-reproductive age, not merely those close to menopause, and current scientific consensus about what causes them remains divided among numerous hypotheses, which include indeed low number of pregnancies (less than six being the crucial number!), but also genetics, infection-history, early menarche, stress, metabolic disease, cadmium bioaccumulation, as well as caffeine and alcohol intake.[221]

Undoubtedly, many French urban women in this time indeed lived far more indoors than outdoors, engaged in far less physical activity than peasant women; and, among the elites, consumed more food in general, with less fresh produce and a greater proportion of their calories deriving from refined carbohydrates as well as alcoholic beverages.[222] In 1825 the gastronomist Jean Anthelme Brillat-Savarin described the emerging problem of the over-consumption of flour and starch-based foods, particularly sweets and pastries, among the elites, noting that 'obesity is never found among savages nor in the classes of society where one works to eat and where one only eats to live'.[223] Numerous doctors writing on

[219] Gardanne, *Dissertation sur les avis à donner aux femmes*, 30–31.

[220] Daniel Delanoë, *Sexe, croyances et ménopause* (Paris: Hachette Littératures, 2007), 28.

[221] Aamir Khan, Manjeet Shehmar, & Janesh K. Gupta, 'Uterine Fibroids: Current Perspectives', *International Journal of Women's Health*, 6 (2014): 95–114 [95–96].

[222] Peter Stearns, *Fat History: Bodies and Beauty in the Modern West* (New York: New York University Press, 1997), 153–154; James F. Macmillan, *France and Women 1789–1914: Gender, Society and Politics* (London/New York: Routledge, 2000), 27; Jim Chevalier, 'The Queen's Coffee and Casanova's Chocolate: The Early Modern Breakfast in France', in Tamara S. Wagner & Narin Hassan, eds, *Consuming Culture in the Long Nineteenth Century: Narratives of Consumption, 1700–1900* (Lanham, Md: Lexington Books, 2007), 191–208.

[223] Jean Anthelme Brillat-Savarin, *Physiologie du goût, Avec une notice sur l'auteur par Émile de Labédollière* (Paris: G. Barba, 1851), 44.

menopause, particularly in the late nineteenth and early twentieth century, described it as a period of increased obesity, noting the tendency for sedentary women to thicken around the waist in the critical age.[224] It also certainly is possible that many bourgeois women were compromising their sleep quality increasingly due to the introduction of street lighting in urban centres, nightlife activities among the bourgeoisie (balls, banquets, restaurants), and the use of electric lamps in the final decades of the nineteenth century. The renowned and very successful Parisian clinician Sébastien Guyétant writing in 1870 considered 'worldly women' ('les femmes du monde') to be suffering from greater emotional stress and physical discomfort in menopause than 'simple peasant women' ('les simples paysannes') largely as a result of their greater time spent awake at late night and consequent loss of quality sleep.[225] Nineteenth-century doctors' concerns relating to diet, exercise, and sleep quality in ageing are not terribly different from many of the recommendations of major medical bodies and popular health movements in the twenty-first century, although these now tend to be made relative to all bodies, not only those of older women.

Menopausal Hygiene of Sexual Desire

One of the recurrent themes that menopausal women were often thought to need to manage hygienically, which is, however, not at all assimilable to our own scientific views about healthy ageing, was sexual desire. Thus Jeannet des Longrois in his 1787 *Advice to Women of Forty Years*, worried:

> What a mass of dangers menaces these women . . . in whom the fire, the tumult of the passions has constantly stirred the blood through the profusions of delicacies, the abuse of perfumes, fermented liqueurs and the relishing in a thousand pleasures.

The more women had enjoyed themselves in their youth, he claimed, the more their 'mature age leads entirely to a suite of pains to be feared, of regrets forming, of necessary care that must be taken, and of privations that must be imposed'.[226] While the earliest Montpellier and Paris theses took little interest in such themes, by 1805 the Paris doctoral thesis of L. J. S. Jallon was claiming that many of the

[224] Genest, *Comment prévenir et guérir les maladies du retour d'âge*, 104–112; Le Docteur Charles Menville, *Conseils aux femmes à l'époque de l'âge de retour, ou de l'âge critique, et de moyens de combattre et prévenir les maladies qui peuvent survenir à cette époque de la vie* (Paris: Germer Baillière, 1839), 14–15; Le Dr Victor Pauchet. *L'Automne de la vie; L'Homme et la femme à l'âge critique*, préface de M. Brieux de l'Académie Française (Paris: Editions J. Oliven, 1932), 29.

[225] Sébastien Guyétant. *L'Âge de retour et la vieillesse; conseils au gens du monde* (Paris: P. Brunet, 1870), 217–218.

[226] Jeannet des Longrois, *Conseils aux femmes de quarante ans*, 6.

diseases that emerged in women during the 'critical age' were a product of both the abuse of, or the abstinence from, sexual pleasure—both were problematic, he said, though he appeared more concerned about abstinence than excess, remarking, 'I merely add that the celibate life is, more than we imagine, the source of serious pain that afflicts women in their critical age.'[227] P. N. Glinel in 1818 warned that more lascivious women should especially avoid past lovers, as well as erotic paintings, books, or conversations.[228] By 1827, the Montpellier candidate Jacques-Philippe Labarraque began leaning slightly more towards dire concern about excess. He too considered that both 'the abuse or the deprivation of sexual pleasure' could trouble a menopausal woman's physiology, along with 'les chagrins' and tumultuous passion.[229] But he devoted much longer discussion to the problem of 'debauchery':[230]

> Love can bring the greatest disturbance to the nervous system; the practice of coitus which follows from it cannot be too moderated at this time of life; and if there is illness, it must be scrupulously prohibited... Women who are born with a temperament inclined toward lasciviousness, should avoid all thoughts and conversations on these themes, avoid rude paintings and books, and especially avoid men with whom they have had intimate ties.[231]

Paris candidate Auguste Nicaise reiterated a mechanistic account of how sex could be nefarious for women via the uterus's sympathy with the nerves in menopause in his thesis of 1838, claiming that even erotic thoughts could be a source of 'disorders of the nervous system'.[232] Jean-Baptiste Nosely's Paris thesis of 1848 recommended that women in *l'âge critique* avoid both abstinence from sex and also excess, enjoying only 'untroubled pleasures, emotion without convulsion, activity without bother'.[233] Louis Chandelux in 1850 alarmingly advised that menopausal women 'abstain as much as possible from the pleasures of love' since 'repeated coitus, at this age, is considered a cause of cancer'.[234] The 1865 book about *The Dangers of Love, Luxury and Libertinage*, by the mature Paris clinician Laurent Martin, reiterated a similar theme.[235] He described how dangerous sex was generally for ageing bodies, remarking that the medical record was filled with examples of stroke, paralysis, sudden death, and numerous other calamities that resulted from violent emotion and passion in older people. He also strongly

227 Jallon, *Essai sur l'âge critique des femmes*, 37–38.

228 P. N. Glinel, *Sur l'âge critique des femmes: Dissertation médico-physiologique* (Paris: Didot Jeune, 1818), 17.

229 Labarraque, *Aperçu physiologico-pathologique sur la menstruation*, 15.

230 Ibid., 16.

231 Ibid., 21.

232 Nicaise, *Essai sur l'âge de retour chez la femme*, 21.

233 Nosely, *Dissertation sur l'âge critique*, 27.

234 Chandelux, *L'Âge critique de la femme*, 27.

235 Laurent Martin, *Les Dangers de l'amour, de la luxure et du libertinage pour l'homme, pour la femme, pendant la jeunesse, pendant l'âge mûr, pendant la vieillesse* (Paris: Lebigre-Duquesne Frères, 1865).

discouraged women from wearing corsets, dyeing their hair, or otherwise attempting to look attractive in old age.[236] A more moderate tone was adopted by the mature clinician Alex Mayer in 1875. He denied that women lost their capacity for love as they aged but considered that they must become less 'carnal'. He advised women approaching menopause to avoid sex because of its capacity to irritate the nervous system, but added that once the menses had definitively stopped, it was safe to resume moderate activity. Nonetheless, it was most 'important to establish limits' on coitus 'so as not to permit any pretext for its abuse through a derangement of the senses'.[237] These ideas had striking durability, and we find a similar proscriptive view proposed even in a popularised pseudo-medical work on *Menstruation in the Critical Age* of 1909 by a doctor Rhazis (one of the many pseudonyms of infamous pornographer Jean Fauconney).[238] After making a series of hygienic recommendations to women approaching menopause, which included having 'the courage to renounce coitus', Rhazis remarked that it would all, in any case, be useless if a woman had up until that time lived a life of libertinage.[239]

In Chapter 7, we consider how ideas about sexuality and women's critical age converged in the emergence of French alienism, resulting in the invention of new definitions of perversity and madness that menopausal women were thought to suffer. In this way, ideas about hygiene, initially focused on women caring for their own bodies in ageing, developed into ideas about the need for older women to be monitored, pathologised, and institutionalised. Théophile Auber's 1864 work of hygiene aimed at nervous women's various critical ages connected these two different forms of approach.[240] Auber (1804-1873) was a pharmacist at the Val-de-Grâce military hospital and author of many works throughout the 1850s and 1860s about such diverse topics as the Hippocratic philosophy of medicine, the physiology of death, puerperal fever, and the treatment of syphilis.

Conclusion

This chapter has focused mostly on the emergence of hygienic advice to women in the critical age from the birth of doctoral scholarship on the topic until the 1860s, tracing the transformation from its origin in eighteenth-century visions of

[236] Ibid., 380–381.

[237] Alex Mayer, *Conseils aux femmes sur l'âge de retour; médecine et hygiène* (Paris: J. B. Baillière et Fils, 1875), 254.

[238] Peter Cryle & Alison Moore, *Frigidity: An Intellectual History* (Basingstoke: Palgrave Macmillan, 2011), 111.

[239] Docteur Rhazis, *La Menstruation et l'âge critique; causes des règles—complications. La ménopause. Début et caractère* (Paris: De Porter, 1909), 87–88.

[240] Théophile-Charles-Emmanuel-Édouard Auber, *Hygiène des femmes nerveuses ou Conseils aux femmes pour les époques critiques de leur vie* (Paris: Germer Baillière, 1864).

hygiene as preventive medicine and in the Montpellier vitalist tradition, towards the moralist, prescriptive regimes on which a growing number of doctors, particularly in Paris, began insisting after the 1820s. Works by mature clinicians and medical professors published between the 1840 and 1870s reiterated similar views to those espoused in the doctoral works about the need for special hygienic management of women in menopause or the critical age.[241] Hygiene for women in the critical age had become entirely mainstream now in Paris medicine, as indicated by major works such as Théophile Auber's 1864 advice manual for the critical age being published by the eminent medical press Baillière, and by both Dr Émile Bertin's and Dr Ernest Barié's books on the hygiene of menopause of 1866 and 1877 respectively being published by another reputable Paris press, Adrien Delaye.[242] Other works of medical hygiene, published both in Paris and other regional cities between 1869 and 1901, and written 'for both sexes' in old age, for the rich, or for women of all ages, now included chapters on women's critical age or menopause and the hygienic laws that one must follow to be well at this time of life.[243] There were still doctoral works focused on hygienic prescription in both the Paris and Montpellier faculties as late as the 1850s and 1860s, after which time it seems, its pedagogic novelty or utility became exhausted.[244] The demise of this pedagogic insistence on critical age hygiene after the 1860s probably reflected the discourse becoming eclipsed by the growth of new medical specialisms concerned with menopause—as specifically a time of nervous and mental illness in the growth of Paris alienism (the focus of Chapter 7), and as a time of uterine pathologies that required surgical procedures such as hysterectomy and oophorectomy (the focus of Chapter 10).

[241] Charles Menville, *De l'âge critique chez les femmes, des maladies qui peuvent survenir à cette époque de la vie et des moyens de les combattre et de les prévenir* (Paris: Imprimerie de Bourgogne et Martinet, 1840); Mayer, *Conseils aux femmes sur l'âge de retour*; Ernest Barié, *Étude sur la ménopause* (Paris: V. Adrien Delahaye, 1877).

[242] Auber, *Hygiène des femmes nerveuses*; Émile Bertin, *De la ménopause considérée principalement au point de vue de l'hygiène* (Montpellier: C. Coulet/Paris: Adrien Delahaye, 1866); Barié, *Étude sur la ménopause*.

[243] Jean Baptiste Debourge, *L'Hygiène de la vieillesse et les conseils pour la longévité, causeries du dimanche* (Montdidier: Mérot, 1869); F. Cros, *Du Rhumatisme coïncidant avec l'âge critique et de son traitement par les eaux de Lamalou-l'Ancien* (Nice: V.-E. Gauthier, 1884); Alexis Clerc, *Hygiène et médecine des deux sexes; suivies d'un dictionnaire d'hygiène et de médecine*, 2 vols (Paris: Jules Rouff et Cie, 1885); Marcellin Camboulives, *L'Homme et la femme à tous les âges de la vie: Etude hygiénique, médicale, physiologique, sociale et morale* (Paris: E. Flammarion, 1890); Ernest Monin, *L'Hygiène des riches* (Paris: A. Silvestre, 1891); Dr F. Bontemps, *De l'hygiène des âges extrêmes et de la nécessité des services d'enfants dans les hôpitaux, conférence aux femmes de France* (Saumur: L. Picard, 1892); Dr Charles Barbaud & Dr A. Rouillard, *Histoire clinico-thermale de la femme aux trois grandes périodes de sa vie: Puberté, union sexuelle, ménopause. Troubles et accidents de la ménopause (âge critique de la femme), traitement thermal aux eaux de Luxeuil* (Paris: Jouvet, 1895); Dr André Castan, *Hygiène de l'âge de retour* (Paris: J. B. Baillière et Fils, 1901).

[244] Marie-Gustave Léopold Chéneaux, *De la menstruation et de la ménopause, au point de vue de la physiologie et de l'hygiène*. Thèse (Paris: Rignoux, 1859); Jacques Laugier, *De la ménopause (âge critique)*. Thèse (Montpellier: Jean Martel ainé, 1861).

By 1888, Paris professors were proudly declaring the death of the older vitalist concept of hygiene as a field of preventive health, announcing that hygiene now 'had rid itself of dogmatism of the past, of metaphysical influences' and was instead operating 'with notions more and more detached from all empiricism'; it had 'become capable, in the example of medicine, to direct... the individual and the state in the most useful fashion'.[245] Nonetheless, when it came to writing manuals directed to the wider public, Paris doctors remained happy to approach the topic of ageing, especially that of women, in the same fashion as earlier hygienic accounts. Popular health manuals too now prescribed hygienic regimes for women in the critical age.[246] Even well into the twentieth century, while many new medical works on menopause focused on specific gynaecological disorders or on the use of ovarian replacement opotherapy, the idea that women around the time of menopause required special hygienic regimes also continued. Even as late as 1920 there was the mature Paris clinician Louis Genest publishing a hygienic manual for avoidance of the diseases of the *âge de retour*.[247] While his definition of menopause as a condition of 'ovarian insufficiency' and discussion of the physiology of ovulation was recognisably twentieth-century, his hygienic prescriptions were entirely consistent with the trend begun at the end of the eighteenth century which sought to counteract the corrupting forces of civilisation on the delicate constitutions of ageing women. Every new layer added to French menopause, it seems, remained embedded, densifying and complexifying the concept, even as new models moved to the forefront.

[245] Dr Martin, 'L'Enseignement de l'hygiène dans les établissements d'enseignement supérieur', *Revue internationale de l'enseignement*, 16 (1888): 1–22 [1].

[246] Anon., *Les Âges critiques de la femme: Puberté—Ménopause. Guides des mères de famille, des maîtresses de pension et des directrices d'établissements religieux* (Paris: V. Goupy et Jourdan, 1878); Anon., *Accidents du retour d'âge et maladies du système véneux; varices et ulcères variqueux; hémorroïdes, varicocèle; phlébites, œdèmes chroniques; congestions; hérmorrhages, etc.; Leur traitement par l'Elixir de Virginie* (Paris: Moride, 1894).

[247] Genest, *Comment prévenir et guérir les maladies du retour d'âge.*

6

Instrumentalising the Ancient Past and Folk Traditions

Hippocrates, Charlatans, and Purgatives in the Invention of Menopause

French doctors in the nineteenth century were exquisitely conscious of themselves as modern subjects in the history of medicine, and told a variety of historical stories about their place in the development of science. One reason that menopause became a popular thesis topic at the universities of Montpellier and Paris from the turn of the nineteenth century until its end was undoubtedly because of the pedagogic value it offered in cohering a story about French medicine's inheritance of ancient wisdom, along with its triumph over myth, religion, folk traditions, and charlatans, through the embrace of recent physiological science and medical specialisation. This narrative informing new professional identities in nineteenth-century medicine and had acquired special poignancy in the aftermath of the French Revolution, when medical institutions were dissolved and doctors faced criticism of being associated with the Old Regime.[1] But the narrative had been emerging since the 1770s and flourished well into the Directorate and Bourbon restoration periods, where it underpinned the emerging disciplines that addressed women's ageing: hygiene, gynaecology, and alienism/psychiatry. In developing a symptomatology of menopause, French doctors claimed to be resisting traditional popular assumptions—arguing against the view of it as pathological which they said was implicit in the notion of the 'critical age'—while at the same time introducing a novel reductionist account of women's entire physiology as dominated by the uterus, which they characterised as traditionally Hippocratic. They oscillated in several respects between opposing conceptual poles: there were invocations of continuity with past medical traditions and claims to modern scientific rupture; critiques of pathological views of menopause and support for the hygienic insistence that women should actively manage this time of life through a series of medical interventions and habitual abstentions; accounts of menopause as a climacteric revolution in the bodily economy because of the uterus's inherent

[1] John E. Lesch, *Science and Medicine in France: The Emergence of Experimental Physiology, 1790–1855* (Cambridge, Mass.: Harvard University Press, 1984), 12–49; George Weisz, 'The Emergence of Specialism in the Nineteenth Century', *Bulletin of the History of Medicine*, 77 (2003): 536–575.

The French Invention of Menopause and the Medicalisation of Women's Ageing: A History. Alison M. Downham Moore, Oxford University Press. © Alison M. Downham Moore 2022. DOI: 10.1093/oso/9780192842916.003.0007

power to dominate women's physiology; and persistent suggestions that men's critical age was just as important as women's. There was no single prevalent discourse in French medicine about the matter. But copious discourse there certainly was.

To appreciate how our current concepts of menopause still today retain their ability to connote so much more than the simple cessation of menstruation and conceptive capacity, we must take account of the conceptual layering that has been embedded in the term throughout its history. It was modern medicine that made menopause a critical age, not ancient or early modern scholars. And rather than displacing the notion of it as a period of crisis and morbidity, nineteenth-century menopause doctors instead promoted those very meanings through a complex extension and misreading of the past, creating a substantively new concern with women's reproductive ageing that persists in current medical and healthcare models. To accurately identify the historical origin of the medicalisation of menopause, we need to resist believing the self-serving narratives about the medical past told by nineteenth-century doctors for their own purposes, in fashioning their professional identity. Their accounts of folk medicine, and of both continuity and rupture with the 'ancients' and with early modern medicine, misattributed ideas to these concurrent and earlier traditions in order variously to lean upon them, or to posture against them.

The first half of this chapter considers doctors' use of the ancient and early modern medical past in formulating ideas about menopause. The second part focuses on doctors' claims about folk healers, empirics, charlatans, midwives, and *commères* (older women consulted as sources of healing advice), who were believed to be giving purgative remedies to women as a treatment for menopause, here considering the available evidence that such forms of unofficial medical treatment occurred. The folk treatment of menopause was patently a confection of nineteenth-century doctors' self-fashioning, which necessitated someone on whom to pin the chimera of 'traditional myth'. It would be tempting to read their strident insistences about it as indicating that some folk practitioners must really have been targeting the final cessation of menses as a treatable disease, but we have only official doctors' own assertions about this, and there are good reasons to doubt the veracity of their claims. At the same time, there was no clear line between official and popular medicine, and many of the same pharmacological remedies sold by charlatans and empirics were also available in the most respectable pharmacies in the rue de la Médecine in Paris, and were prescribed by official doctors all the time. Many of the arguments they made about folk healers and charlatans were thus also implicit attacks on other kinds of competing forces, including *officiers de santé*, pharmacists, drug traders, and even other institutionally legitimated doctors with whom they diverged in opinion about menstrual physiology, physical or chemical treatment, and the value of purgatives and other medical interventions. The imaginary of charlatan purgative prescription to menopausal women thus performed many roles for nineteenth-century doctors. Solidist followers of François Broussais and his favoured mechanical therapy of phlebotomy (blood-letting) counterpoised their approach to the iatrochemical remedies of both empirics and pharmacies; but folk practioners were target too for also university-trained doctors who struggled to find enough patients in the highly competitive and diverse nineteenth-century medical market. Claiming Hippocrates as an ally was another part of the elitist identity through which Latin-quoting doctors marked themselves as the only legitimate clinicians properly qualified to treat older (especially elite) women. As we saw in Chapter 3, the realisation of the higher ratio of women to men in older age groups was itself part of the stimulus both for the emergence of menopause diagnostics and for the theoretical splitting of morbidity from mortality. The concept of menopause turned older women into a new patient market—not one wrested from folk traditions or transformed from an existing early modern or ancient precedent, but an entirely new cohort of subjects defined for the purposes of elaborate medical description, pedagogy, and long-term clinical treatment.

Menopause and the Invention of Hippocratic Tradition

Almost all nineteenth-century French medical theses on questions of women's health reproduced, on their final page, a list of aphorisms taken from the same source: Galen's first-century CE collation of the fifth-century BCE works of Hippocrates and his followers, revised in the sixteenth century and known as the Hippocratic corpus. Doctoral candidates on matters of women's health ubiquitously cited aphorisms in the opening remarks of their theses, and invariably this always included one particular aphorism which they falsely claimed was from Hippocrates: 'Propter uterum mulier tota morbus est' ('the uterus is the source of all women's diseases').[2] There is in fact no Hippocratic aphorism quite like this, and none of the seventeenth- and eighteenth-century collections of Hippocratic aphorisms list any that clearly resemble it.[3] The closest, Section V, Part 57 of the *Aphorisms*, is the phrase to which some nineteenth-century French medical scholars specifically pointed, and from which recent scholars have considered the nineteenth-century version must have derived: 'katamēniōn genomenōn pleionōn, nousoi xumbainousi, kai, mē ginomenōn, apo tēs husterēs ginontai nousoi' ('When the menses are excessive, diseases take place, and when the

[2] Or with the alternative sentence structure 'Mulier propter uterum tota morbus est': e.g. C. Leblanc, *Essai sur la métrite aiguë de la matrice ou inflammation* (Paris: Didot le Jeune, 1823), title page.

[3] Jacqueline Vons, 'Tota mulier in utero: Introduction'. Centre Montaigne, 4 May 2021: <https://centre-montaigne.huma-num.fr/tota-mulier-in-utero.html#_ftn2> (viewed 19 October 2021).

menses are stopped, diseases from the uterus take place').[4] A 1640 Latin translation from the Greek by the Venetian physician Ioannis Manelphi had suggested an interpretation that highlighted the early modern concern with both menstrual disorders and with suppressed menses in women of cycling age: 'Menstruis largius fluentibus morbi eueniunt: Non fluentibus autem ex utero morbi contingent' ('Diseases occur more broadly during menstruation: when there is no menstrual flow, the uterus causes disease').[5]

Hippocratic aphorism V.57 might have been taken either to naturalise the final cessation of menses (since menstruation no longer threatened women with so many diseases), or to extend concern about amenorrhea to women after the cessation of menses as well; and as we saw in Chapter 1, early modern scholars variously held both of these views, without the question ever being a major focus of medical inquiry. Nonetheless, despite its potential to justify either a pathological or an anti-pathological view of the final cessation of menses, accurate translations of aphorism V.57 were never cited in nineteenth-century French scholarship invoking Hippocrates to justify the medicalisation of menopause. Instead, what doctors cited was one of two variations of a fabricated aphorism attributed to Hippocrates: either one of the *propter uterum* versions, sometimes also attributed to the eighteenth-century German physician Friedrich Hoffmann, but never cited from a specific work of his; or another similar version, proposed by the seventeenth-century Flemish chemist, physician, and Paracelsian Jan Baptista van Helmont (1579–1644), who developed his own unique readings of Hippocrates using rediscovered texts that had been preserved in Arabic translation.[6] Van Helmont's Latin aphorism also differed markedly enough from Hippocratic aphorism V.57 to place it in the category of a substantial exegesis of Hippocrates, rather than a translation: 'Propter solum uterum, mulier est id quod est' ('the uterus alone makes woman what she is').[7] By way of example, van Helmont had noted the fact that a beard did not appear in females at puberty as it did in men, that women had a more 'moist' temperament and an earlier age of puberty, but said nothing of them having distinct patterns of ageing beyond puberty, nor about the final cessation of menses. It seems likely that this was the aphorism from which other *propter uterum* versions were later drawn, either because it was

[4] Hippocrates, *Œuvres complètes d'Hippocrate*, trans. Adolf M. Hakkert (Amsterdam: A. Littre, 1961), via <http://www.perseus.tufts.edu/>; Hippocrates, *The Genuine Works of Hippocrates*, trans. Francis Adams, 2 vols (London: Sydenham Society, 1849), vol. 2, 748.

[5] Ioannis Manelphi, *Hippocratis Aphorismi Nicolao Leoniceno Vincentino interprete, una cum annotationibus* (self-published, 1640), 109.

[6] Jole Shackelford, 'The Chemical Hippocrates: Paracelsian and Hippocratic Theory in Petrus Severinus' Medical Philosophy', in David Cantor, ed., *Reinventing Hippocrates* (Abingdon: Routledge, 2016), [59–88], 60–61.

[7] Jan Baptista van Helmont, *Ortus medicinæ* (London: Elzevirium, 1652), 270; Michael Stolberg, 'A Woman Down to Her Bones: The Anatomy of Sex Difference in the Sixteenth and Early Seventeenth Centuries', *Isis*, 94/2 (2003), [274–299], 289.

misremembered by a scholar who had heard it cited in an oral lecture, or because the first scholars to invoke the *propter uterum* formulations found it either neater grammatically or less controversial in its claims about the uterus than van Helmont's rendition.

Many nineteenth-century scholars nonetheless took van Helmont's rendition as preferable, for what it suggestively offered for their new theories of women's physiology. It could be read as extending the influence of the uterus beyond all women's diseases and into the complete being of womanhood, thus helping to justify the growth of gynaecology as a comprehensive discipline beyond obstetrics, while also stimulating emerging alienist ideas about women's mental/nervous pathologies at all times of uterine change, including menopause. This was an extension of the idea, made popular by Roussel and others in the last decades of the eighteenth century, that women were utterly unlike men, were the more nervous and sickly sex, and were determined by their reproductive physiology. This yielded the view of the final cessation of menses as the catastrophic loss of the very thing that made women distinct, but also the view that women, unlike men, needed to 'manage' their ageing hygienically to avoid diseases of the uterus as well as those thought to be caused by this or their other reproductive organs, such as hysteria. The radical repurposing of Hippocrates had dramatic consequences for the tone of much of the medical discourse of menopause throughout the nineteenth century—a tone that has continued into the era of hormone replacement which, in turn, has often been proposed to save women from a disastrous and sudden ageing, morbidity, and loss of femininity.[8]

Notably neither Hippocratic aphorism V.57 nor the *propter uterum* fake-Hippocrates aphorism, nor van Helmont's aphorism were cited by French scholars of women's health before the early nineteenth century. Even those eighteenth-century scholars who considered the uterus to cause vapours or hysteria do not appear to have engaged with any of these aphorisms at all. Even François Mauriceau—that rare exception in the history of early modern French medicine who believed that women were only healthy if they menstruated regularly and that the final cessation of menses caused high rates of death in women—did not refer to the 'Hippocratic' aphorism, even though it could easily have been made to speak to his concerns. Mauriceau cited Hippocrates in support of the view that pregnant women could suffer many of the same diseases as non-pregnant women.[9] But in his own 1694 work of aphorisms about pregnancy and the diseases of women, he included one which certainly could have inspired the *propter uterum* aphorism that circulated in the nineteenth century: 'Le dérèglement des

[8] Elizabeth Siegel Watkins, *The Estrogen Elixir: A History of Hormone Replacement Therapy in America* (Baltimore: Johns Hopkins University Press, 2009), 69–92.

[9] François Mauriceau, *Observations sur la grossesse et l'accouchement des femmes, et sur leurs maladies & celles des enfans nouveau-nez. En chacune desquelles les causes & les raisons des principaux évenemens sont décrites & expliquées* (Paris: Chez l'auteur, 1694), 251.

fonctions de la matrice est cause de la plus grande partie des maladies des femmes' ('Most of the diseases seen in women are caused by dysregulation of the functions of the womb').[10] This was a somewhat less absolute statement even than the *proper uterum* version, referring to not all the diseases but merely most of them, and was certainly less encompassing of women's entire nature than van Helmont's aphorism. Notably, Mauriceau did not lean on Hippocrates to legitimate his own assertion but claimed the aphorism as entirely his own. Hippocratic aphorisms certainly were cited by early modern medical scholars, including many that referred to the uterus, menstruation, or the diseases of women. The Belgian surgeon Paul de Sorbait, for example, cited several both from Hippocrates and from Galen in his 1672 compendium of *Treatments of All Diseases of Men, Women and Children*.[11] But among them there was no mention of aphorism V.57, nor of any other statements about women's diseases or nature all deriving from the uterus.

The Montpellier anatomy and physiology professor Charles-Louis Dumas (1765–1813) appears to have been the first to cite van Helmont's 1652 aphorism in a published work, his 1800 *Principes de physiologie*, and to provide the rationale for its application to the new theories of women's nature:

> The power of the womb is familiar to us. One knows with how much energy it reacts to the whole body...One knows what extraordinary disturbance it can excite in the whole machine, and how much the whole system of physical and psychological affections seems to be modified by its perpetual influence. The activity of the womb has been taken for the source of the distinctive qualities of woman, and all the natural and physical conditions that make her what she is: *Propter solum uterum mulier est id quod est.*[12]

But the other great Montpellier professor Joseph-Marie-Joachim Vigarous also cited van Helmont's aphorism in his 1801 published lectures on the diseases of women, which were based on the lectures that he gave at the university throughout the 1780s and 1790s—a time during which Dumas was a student at Montpellier (defending his thesis in 1790).[13] So it seems likely that Dumas learnt the van Helmont aphorism from Vigarous, who had clearly read van Helmont's

[10] François Mauriceau, *Aphorismes touchant la grossesse, l'accouchement, les maladies, et autres dispositions des femmes* (Paris: L. d'Houry, 1694), 6.

[11] Paul de Sorbait, *Insitutionum medicarum et anatomicarum, methodus medendi, cum controversiis, annexa sylva medica. Diende sequuntur: Curationes omnium morborum, virorum, mulierum et puerorum. A capite ad calcem, nec non cura morbi venerei, et tractatus de febribus, peste et venenis* (Nuremberg: Michael & Johan Friderici, 1672), 465.

[12] Charles-Louis Dumas, *Principes de physiologie, ou Introduction à la science expérimentale, philosophique et médicale de l'homme vivant*, 2 vols (Paris: Crapelet, 1800), 1, 418–419.

[13] Joseph-Marie-Joachim Vigarous, *Cours élémentaire de maladies des femmes, ou Essai sur une nouvelle méthode pour étudier et pour classer les maladies de ce sexe*, 2 vols (Paris: Deterville, 1801), vol. 1, 44; Charles Louis Dumas, *Questiones medicinae duodecim* (Montpellier: J.-F. Tournel, 1790).

Ortus medicinæ, while Dumas himself had no reference for the quotation, further suggesting he may have heard and transcribed it from Vigarous's lectures. Notably, Vigarous appeared to doubt the view that the uterus had so great an influence over women's entire physiology, but said that van Helmont's aphorism was 'in accord with Hippocrates', who had described in *De locis in homine* (Places in Man) how others viewed all women's diseases as deriving from the uterus, citing from a Latin version of Hippocrates: 'morborum omnium qui muliebres vocantur uteri in causâ sint' ('all the diseases of women are said to be caused by the uterus').[14] This quotation did not attribute to Hippocrates himself the view of the uterus as the source of all women's diseases, but rather indicated that it was what Hippocrates had heard others say and which he was merely reporting. But Vigarous also related the remark to another ancient source, Democritus' letter to Hippocrates (letter 23) which referred to there being 'six hundred' (meaning 'countless') uterine diseases—again not Hippocrates' express view, but something said to him by someone else.[15] It thus seems to have been Vigarous who introduced the practice of evoking van Helmont's aphorism about the importance of the uterus for women's health. But his careful attribution of who said what, with specific citations of named ancient works, was not repeated in any of the numerous nineteenth-century medical works that thereafter cited one or other supposedly Hippocratic aphorism in support of the view that menopause, as a time of drastic uterine change, necessarily required medical treatment and hygienic management.

Jean-Louis Alibert (1768–1837), a Paris professor of medicine (though a native of the region east of Toulouse) and royal doctor to both Louis XVIII and Charles X, appears to have been the first to cite the *propter uterum* saying in his 1804 three-volume *New Elements of Therapy and of the Materia Medica*.[16] He was a protégé of Cabanis and a friend of Pierre Roussel, writing a eulogy to him for the 1803 third edition of the *Système physique et moral de la femme*, in which Alibert praised Roussel as having 'unveiled the organism' of woman 'with such finesse and so much penetration', and as having 'proved his long commerce with antiquity' in engaging with Hippocrates and Galen.[17] In the 1804 work on the *materia medica*, Alibert included a series of rules for the differentiation of people in medical treatment by sex, age, temperament, climate, and season, as well as individual

[14] This is found in Hippocrates, *De Locis in Homine*, in *Magni Hippocratis Opera Omnia*, Greek–Latin dual edition, ed. Carolus Gottlob Kühn (Leipzig: Cnobloch, 1826), 149 [101–153].

[15] Vigarous, *Cours élémentaire de maladies des femmes*, vol. 1, 44–45.

[16] Jean-Louis Alibert, *Nouveaux élémens de thérapeutique et de matière médicale, suivis d'un nouvel essai sur l'art de formuler*, 3 vols (Paris: Crapart, Caillet et Ravier, 1804), vol. 2, 661.

[17] Jean-Louis Alibert, 'Éloge historique de Pierre Roussel', in Pierre Roussel, *Système physique et moral de la femme, ou Tableau philosophique de la constitution, de l'état organique du tempérament, des mœurs et des fonctions propres au sexe*, 3rd ed. [1775] (Paris: Crapart, Caillet et Ravier, 1803), 7, 36 [1–52].

idiosyncrasies, appetites, and habits.[18] Alibert's first rule was that before medicating, a doctor should always consider whether treatment was even needed at all, citing Sydenham in the view that some diseases simply resolved by themselves.[19] Alibert invoked one of the versions of the *propter uterum* aphorism (*Mulier propter uterum tota morbus est*), claiming it was from Hippocrates. It appeared as the final sentence (the cherry on top) of his twentieth rule 'With regard to sex', which followed from the nineteenth rule 'With regard to age'. In the age rule, he had said that 'the two extremities of life resemble one another more than is commonly believed', and that only from puberty until sometime in ageing were men and women distinct from one another. The twentieth rule specified:

> Woman is altogether more sensitive and more mobile than man.... The particular disposition of the uterus, moreover, requires continual modifications in the prescription of medicines, according to the state of pregnancy, menstruation, etc. Never forget Hippocrates' physiological insight: *Mulier propter uterum tota morbus est.*[20]

The seed of ancient misattribution was now planted, along with the suggestion that all of women's reproductive life stages must now be considered in relation to this new 'Hippocratic' aphorism.

The Hippocratic aphorisms were patently in vogue in the decades after the revolution in French medicine, offering a means to mediate between the need for medical professors to distance themselves from all that was associated with the Old Regime, while still paying homage to both the Enlightenment and ancient tradition, and acting as a shorthand for the new physiological medicine that integrated surgery, pharmacy, and the nosology of diseases—of which both Pinel and Cabanis were visionaries.[21] A new French translation of the aphorisms by the Paris medical professor François Christophe Florimond de Chevalier de Mercy appeared in 1801, published in Toulouse.[22] Cabanis had been scheduled to give a new series of lectures on the Hippocratic aphorisms in 1797 (though he does not appear to have delivered them),[23] and a new translation of the Hippocratic aphorisms appearing in 1817 was riddled with quotations from him.[24] The renowned

[18] Alibert, *Nouveaux Élémens de thérapeutique et de matière médicale*, vol. 2, 645–662.

[19] Ibid., 645. [20] Ibid., 661.

[21] John E. Lesch, *Science and Medicine in France: The Emergence of Experimental Physiology, 1790–1855* (Cambridge, Mass.: Harvard University Press, 1984), 33–34.

[22] François Christophe Florimond de Chevalier de Mercy, *Traduction des œuvres médicales d'Hippocrate, sur le texte grec, d'après l'édition de Foës*, 4 vols (Toulouse: Fagès, Meilhace et Comp., 1801).

[23] Martin Staum, *Cabanis: Enlightenment and Medical Philosophy in the French Revolution* (Princeton: Princeton University Press, 1980), 267.

[24] François Christophe Florimond de Chevalier de Mercy, *Nouvelle Traduction des aphorismes d'Hippocrate, conférés sur l'édition grecque publiée en 1811, ou l'on trouve les variantes des manuscrits de*

Paris obstetrician Claude Gardien in his 1807 treatise on the diseases of women cited a Hippocratic aphorism from Section VI, Part 29: 'Mulier podagra non laborat, nisi menstrua defecerint' ('A woman does not suffer from gout unless her menstrual periods have failed'), which Gardien anachronistically read as being about the symptoms of menopause.[25] In 1840, the Paris clinician Charles François Menville referred to this same aphorism too, and also assumed it to refer to menopause, but—'without accusing Hippocrates of error'—graciously pointed out that gout was not particularly common in older women at all.[26] Menville also ridiculed many scholars for citing both the *propter uterum* and Van Helmot's aphorisms in their depiction of menopause as a time of morbidity and as the start of women's decrepitude.[27] By 1840, it had already become a ubiquitous convention in works on menopause and on the diseases of women to invoke either van Helmont's aphorism or some version of the fake-Hippocratic *propter uterum* aphorism.

Neither van Helmont's scholarship nor Paracelsian thought generally was widely taken up in French medicine of the nineteenth century (although there was more history of doing so at Montpellier than at Paris). And yet this particular aphorism was at least as widely cited as the *propter uterum* aphorism in texts dealing with menopause. Van Helmont's alleged rendition of Hippocrates appealed to many doctors of menopause in all French medical faculties because it proposed an even more radical insistence, not only on the importance of uterine disorders (helping to justify the growth of gynaecology as a discipline), but also on the idea that reproductive capacity was the single defining feature of womanhood, making the cessation of menstruation a truly 'critical age' which it was in doctors' ambit to treat—even as they insisted that it was not a disease. But even the *propter uterum* aphorism was widely read as extending to all aspects of women's health and behaviour, not merely to diseases. Several scholars attributed the aphorism not to Hippocrates but to Hoffmann. In 1847, the Lyon professor of pathology Jean-Louis Brachet asked in his treatise on hysteria, 'Is it true that, according to Hoffmann, *mulier propter solum uterum tota morbus est* (the uterus is the source of all women's disease)?'[28] The Paris doctoral candidate Tual had

la Bibliothèque du Roi et des commentaires spécialement applicables à l'étude de la médecine pratique (Paris: Adrien Égron, 1817).

[25] Claude Martin Gardien, *Traité complet d'accouchemens et des maladies des filles, des femmes et des enfans*, 4 vols (Paris: Crochard, 1807), vol. 1, 405.

[26] Charles François Menville, *De l'âge critique chez les femmes, des maladies qui peuvent survenir à cette époque de la vie et des moyens de les combattre et de les prévenir* (Paris: Imprimerie de Bourgogne et Martinet, 1840), 509.

[27] Charles François Menville, *Conseils aux femmes à l'époque de l'âge de retour, ou de l'âge critique, et de moyens de combattre et prévenir les maladies qui peuvent survenir à cette époque de la vie* (Paris: Germer Baillière, 1839), 16.

[28] Jean-Louis Brachet, *Traité de l'hystérie* (Paris: Baillière, 1847), 209.

attributed the aphorism to both Hoffmann and Hippocrates in his 1838 thesis on diverse questions.[29] But the phrase is not found in Hoffmann's complete works.[30]

Many eminent and student doctors claimed to be representatives of a more authentic 'Hippocratic' tradition. Engagements with, and distortions of, the Hippocratic corpus were tremendously important for the formulation of nineteenth-century medical ideas about women's health. As Helen King remarks, the claim to hysteria being a traditional Hippocratic concept was central to its investment with authority in late nineteenth-century thought.[31] As King and other medical history scholars have noted, eighteenth- and nineteenth-century forms of citation of Hippocratic 'tradition' in fact always produced new interpretations of the ancient texts, even as they claimed to be authentic to them. Every era had its own Hippocrates (misconstrued as a single author), moulded to fit the prerogatives of each contemporary conceptual formation.[32] Nowhere was this more apparent than in the myth of menopause as something that ancient medicine had conceived, albeit falsely considering it a disease, which only modern French medicine had now corrected. It seems they even invented their very own unique 'Hippocratic' aphorism to decorate this myth.

Hippocratic ideas about the uterus and diseases of women were radically reinterpreted, revised, and modified by many nineteenth-century doctors of women's health. These reinterpretations made the ancient physician into an ally in the specific modern insistence on women's reproductive capacity as the defining feature of their being and provided support to the novel claim that women's mental health was entirely controlled by their reproductive organs, variously yielding the concepts of hysteria, nymphomania and the nervous symptomatology of menopause. Both the *propter uterum* aphorism falsely attributed to Hippocrates and van Helmont's aphorism were taken to provide this kind of legitimation. Prosper-Louis Sauvé's 1826 Strasbourg thesis on the 'critical age' had used van Helmont's version of the expression, adding that the uterus had such a great influence on women's constitution, 'even in health, and modified so much their way of seeing and feeling, that one can quite rightly consider it the engine and agent of all their actions'.[33] The 1827 Paris thesis of N. M. Verdé de Lisle on inflammation of the uterus also chose the van Helmont version in support of the view that there was a heightened sensitivity resulting from the sympathy of the uterus with other

[29] C.-F.-M. Tual, *Questions sur diverse branches des sciences médicales.* Thèse (Paris: Rignoux et Cie, 1838), 12.

[30] Friedrich Hoffmann, *Opera omnia physica-medica*, 6 vols. (Geneva: Fratres de Tournes, 1748).

[31] Helen King, *Hippocrates' Woman: Reading the Female Body in Ancient Greece* (London: Routledge, 1998), 206.

[32] David Cantor, 'Introduction: The Uses and Meanings of Hippocrates', in David Cantor, ed., *Reinventing Hippocrates* (Abingdon: Routledge, 2016), [1–22], 2–3.

[33] Prosper-Louis Sauvé, *Réflexions sur l'âge critique, et particulièrement sur le régime le plus convenable pour préserver les femmes des accidens qui ont coutume de survenir à cette époque de leur vie* (Strasbourg: F. G. Levrault, 1826), 2.

organs 'that we find as the cause of numerous diseases' of women.[34] Another 1827 Paris doctoral candidate, Pierre-Ulysse Meige, hedged his bets, citing both the *propter uterum* aphorism and van Helmont's version in his thesis on chronic and acute metritis.[35] Given the popularity of Vigarous's published lectures on the diseases of women, it is not surprising that his van Helmont citation was the one to stimulate so many of the early doctoral candidates writing about menopause. But it is striking that the practice was not found in the early specialist Montpellier theses of Pingault, Gagnebé, Anglade, and Broyes, suggesting Vigarous himself and those he trained may have discouraged this use of it to conceptualise the final cessation of menses.[36]

This pattern was repeated in numerous other Parisian works of the nineteenth century whenever a medical scholar wished to insist that women were prone to specific mental or physical diseases around the time of the final cessation of menses, in puberty, pregnancy, or around the time of childbirth.[37] Pierre Vialenc, in his 1816 Paris thesis on amenorrhea, invoked '*Propter uterum*...' to support his statement about women's entire lives being dominated by suffering on account of the uterus, even though there are several far more specific Hippocratic aphorisms referring to absent menses that he might have cited instead.[38] Henri Muret too chose the *propter uterum* aphorism as the first sentence of his 1826 Paris doctoral thesis on the diseases of menstruation.[39] Henri-Louis Bayard opted for this aphorism on the title page of his 1836 Paris thesis about hysteria which he called 'uteromania'—a disease he considered to occur in women of various critical ages, including those in their forties and who had recently ceased menstruating.[40] Auguste Mouton's 1834 Paris thesis on *The Influence of the Uterus on the Physical and Moral System of Woman* cited the *propter uterum* aphorism in a section devoted to 'expiring menstruation' in older women. Here Mouton affirmed that

[34] N. M. Verdé de Lisle, *Dissertation sur la métrite aiguë, ou inflammation aiguë de la matrice*. Thèse (Paris: Didot le Jeune, 1827), 5.

[35] Pierre Ulysses Meige, *Dissertation sur la métrite, considérée dans son état aigu et chronique* (Paris: Didot le Jeune, 1827), 5.

[36] Jérémie-André Pingault, *De la cessation des règles* (Montpellier: Tournel, 1799); Joseph Gagnebé, *Exposition de quelques maladies qui attaquent les femmes à la cessation des règles*. Thèse (Montpellier: Imprimerie de Tournel, 1801); Jean Baptiste Anglade, *Considérations sur les effets que peut produire la cessation des règles*. Thèse (Montpellier: Jean Martel, 1812); Nicolas Broye, *Considérations sur la cessation des règles*. Thèse (Montpellier: Jean Martel Aîné, 1813).

[37] Aimé Schwob, *Contribution à l'étude des psychoses menstruelles considérées surtout au point de vue médico-légal*. Thèse (Lyon: Storck, 1893), 17, 28–29. F.-A.-Hippolyte Liébeaux, *Dissertation sur la ménaphanie: La Non-apparition des menstrues chez les filles pubères*. Thèse (Paris: Didot le Jeune, 1830), 9; J. A. Macé, *Essai sur les hémorrhagies utérines après la délivrance*. Thèse (Paris: Didot le Jeune, 1814).

[38] Pierre Vialenc, *Dissertation sur l'aménorrhée ou suppression des règles* (Paris: Didot jeaune, 1816), v.

[39] Henri Muret, *Essai sur le traitement des principaux dérangements des menstrues, considérées dans les différents âges de la femme* (Paris: Didot Jeune, 1826), 5.

[40] Henri Lois Bayard, *Essai médico-légal sur l'utéromanie (nymphomanie)*. Thèse (Paris: Didot le Jeune, 1836), title page, 26, 27, 37, 64.

the declining function of the uterus in menopause made women less governed by it, and hence less distinctive and feminine. He also reiterated the pathological state of the uterus at this time of life if a woman had lived dissolutely and failed to observe the 'rules of hygiene'. Though the *âge de retour* passed commonly without disturbance, it could also 'see the development of the most diverse and dreadful diseases', which he suggested the supposedly Hippocratic expression would predict.[41] The renowned Paris doctor and hygienist Marc Colombat de l'Isère (1797–1851) in 1838 cited van Helmont's version in his highly successful *Treatise on the Diseases of Women*, after describing all the diseases of women he thought must be caused by the final cessation of menses, since they were found more often in older women.[42]

By mid-century, the pattern had begun to spread to other medical cultures too. The English physician Edward Tilt copied the habit from the Paris scholars with whom he had studied in the 1830s, citing both the *propter uterum* aphorism and the van Helmont version in his 1850 book *On the Disease of Menstruation and Ovarian Inflammation*, though not in his other major work on the 'change of life'.[43] By 1874, the two aphorisms had been combined into a single quotation by the Belgian doctor D'Hooghe in his Anvers medical society prize-winning essay 'On the Influence of the Zygomatic Diseases of Pregnancy, Parturition and After', without reference to the translator/modifier at all.[44] Hippocrates was now held singularly responsible for all the recently invented modern and early modern ideas about women's physiology and ageing, projected back onto the ancient past. But one or the other of the aphorisms could also still be cited in isolation: in 1876, the Paris gynaecology professor Antoine Jozan reverted singularly to the *propter uterum* aphorism, managing to cite it no less than three times in the 1894 thirteenth edition of his highly successful *Complete Practical Treatise of the Diseases of Women*.[45] It mattered little that there was no such phrase in any of Hippocrates' works. The aphorism now had a power all its own.

Inventing Ancient Traditions of Menopause Pathology

Menopause itself, then, served a function for French doctors in providing a terrain on which to negotiate their relationship between modern scientific methods and

[41] Auguste Mouton, *Influence de l'utérus sur le système physique et moral de la femme.* Thèse (Paris: Didot le Jeune, 1834), 38–39.

[42] Marc Colombat de l'Isère, *Traité des maladies des femmes et de l'hygiène spéciale de leur sexe*, 3 vols (Paris: Librairie médicale de Labé, 1838–1843), vol. 1, 48–49.

[43] Edward John Tilt, *On Diseases of Menstruation and Ovarian Inflammation, in Connection with Sterility, Pelvic Tumours, and Affections of the Womb* (London: John Churchill, 1850), xxiii.

[44] Dr D'Hooghe, 'De l'influence des maladies zygomatiques sur la grossesse, la parturition et ses suites', *Annales de la Société de Médecine d'Anvers*, 36 (1874), 70 [70–86].

[45] Antoine Émile Jozan, *Traité pratique complet des maladies des femmes* [1776], 13th ed. (Paris: Garnier Frères, 1894), 8, 181, 390.

the authority of ancient medical traditions. Almost all French medical works on menopause published in the nineteenth century recounted a story of a supposedly 'traditional' view of menopause that their own scientific approach claimed to overturn. According to this 'traditional' myth, menstruation was a means for a woman's body to rid itself of disease elements, producing both the mythical view of menstrual blood as venomous, and a popular conception of menopause as a dangerous time, or 'critical age', because the cessation of menstruation would result in the accumulation of the blood and its disease elements inside the menopausal woman's body. The claim appeared in books and theses on menopause from the late eighteenth century, and thereafter became a staple trope in writing about it into the first decades of the twentieth. The Parisian hygienist Claude Lachaise, whom we met in both Chapters 3 and 5, had objected in 1825 to the emerging trend in menopause scholarship of using the medical past to make claims of overturning traditional myths.[46] In his book on the hygienic physiology of women he referred to the poisonous view of menstrual blood—accurately attributing it to the Roman naturalist Pliny the Elder (23–79 CE), but also suggesting that it was transmitted through early modern medicine via Reinier de Graaf, Jean Fernel, and countless others.[47] As we saw in Chapter 1, some early modern scholars did sometimes repeat Pliny's claims, but usually to dismiss them, and the notion of toxic blood was not ever proposed as an explicit rationale for the medical treatment of women after the final cessation of menses. But Lachaise fiercely criticised the uterine reductionist perspective attributed to both Hippocrates and van Helmont, identifying it with the problem of most of his contemporaries being fixated on the doctrine of 'the uterus as a thinking organ, susceptible to passions and alone impressing upon women all the characteristics of her sex'; and of seeing the majority of nervous diseases as caused by 'venereal appetite', or the abuse of pleasures that have perturbed women's sensibility.[48]

> Arriving at the critical age, woman does not lose the tastes of her sex, as one reads in the majority of treatises of physiology; that ridiculous error again comes from the influence accorded freely to the uterus on the production of woman's intellectual attributes.[49]

However, Lachaise did not manage to deter numerous doctoral candidates and mature clinicians from repeating the idea that modern medicine was the first tradition to break with an ancient and perennial view of menopause as a dangerous 'critical time', and to see it instead as a natural process that was nonetheless a complete revolution of women's physiological economy, requiring medical and

[46] Claude Lachaise, *Hygiène physiologique de la femme, ou de la femme considérée dans son système physique et moral* (Paris: Mequignon Marvis, 1825).
[47] Ibid., 408. [48] Ibid., xxii–xxiii. [49] Ibid., 405.

hygienic attention. The 1827 Montpellier medical thesis of Jacques-Philippe Labarraque blamed 'the ancients' for the ubiquitous premodern view of menopause as dangerous, adding that according to his mentor Desormeaux, only Aristotle and Hippocrates were exempt from the error.[50] The 1848 Paris thesis of Jean-Baptiste Nosely, after quoting the *propter uterum* aphorism, added too that the critical age was a period of transition in which 'the woman loses the attributes of her sex'.[51] He vaguely attributed to 'the ancients' in general the notions of menstrual blood as toxic, of its excretion helping to purify the economy of the body, and of the nefariousness of all forms of failure to menstruate in women.[52]

The Paris clinician Charles Menville revived Lachaise's scepticism in response to these new reductionist claims in 1839 advice manual, even more emphatically rejecting all this fashionable nonsense in no uncertain terms:

> Arriving at the critical age, woman does not lose all the fineness of her sex, as one often hears repeated by those who would freely accord a great influence of the uterus on a woman's intellectual attributes. Any sane study of the vital functions would show these ideas to be foolishly exaggerated. The uterus, like all the important organs, has numerous correspondences with the brain, the lungs, the stomach; but it does not have a preeminent action over all other organs, and does not constitute woman herself, as one ridiculously pretends (*Propter uterum solum mulier est id quod est*).[53]

Nonetheless, Menville reiterated in similarly vague terms the contours of the 'traditional' myth 'that the ancients formed for themselves about the nature of menstrual blood . . . which made them think that the critical age was necessarily fateful for women'.[54] Louis Chandelux, in his Paris thesis of 1850, cited the *propter uterum* aphorism in support of the view that the uterus has a remarkable influence on both the physiological and moral habits of women, adding that 'this influence is incontestable; it did not escape the ancient observers', and was alone responsible for the 'marked differences' between the sexes, including their unique patterns of ageing.[55] Gustave-Adolphe Plihon, in his doctoral thesis of 1859, agreed: 'The uterus dominates the physiology of women, it is an incontestable fact,' supporting the focus of his thesis on menopause.[56] At the same time as the supposedly ancient reduction of women's entire physiology to the governing role of the uterus was constantly leaned upon to legitimate the treatment of menopause

[50] Jacques-Philippe Labarraque, *Aperçu physiologico-pathologique sur la menstruation en général, et quelques conseils d'hygiène pour l'âge critique en particulier* (Montpellier: Jean Martel aîné, 1827), 8.
[51] Jean-Baptiste Nosely, *Dissertation sur l'âge critique.* Thèse (Paris: Rignoux, 1848), 7.
[52] Ibid., 6. [53] Menville, *Conseils aux femmes à l'époque de l'âge de retour*, 16.
[54] Ibid., 10.
[55] Louis Chandelux, *L'Âge critique de la femme (ménopause)* (Paris: Irgnoux, 1850), 6.
[56] Gustave-Adolphe Plihon, *De la ménopause (âge critique).* Thèse (Paris: Rignoux, 1859), 5.

as a topic of special medical concern, both ancient and eighteenth-century doctors were blamed for misunderstanding menopause as the time when toxic menstrual blood accumulated in women's bodies causing disease. Jacques Laugier's Montpellier thesis of 1861 attributed this idea variously to Hippocrates, Fothergill, Pinel, and Tissot, apparently without checking to see whether the notion did indeed appear in their work.[57]

Engagement with ancient medicine appears to have been particularly important in French doctors' accounts of menopause, demonstrating their modern scientific enlightenment. Another Paris clinician, Ernest Barié, in 1877 noted ambiguously that Hippocrates' expression was 'exceeded' by van Helmont's rendition of it, implying a mistranslation that contributed to the erroneous views about 'the malignancy of menopause' that he claimed had prevailed through early modern medical history.[58] But Barié did not appear to criticise van Helmont for reducing women to their reproductive capacity. In fact, he too reiterated precisely such reductive views of female anatomy. Van Helmont was probably a target here because of his association with the esoteric-alchemical medicine of Paracelsus, which diverged from the dominant Galenic/Hippocratic model in the late sixteenth and early seventeenth centuries.[59] In criticising van Helmont, then, and affirming the correctness of the Galenic/Hippocratic accounts of menstruation, Barié was re-instantiating these medical traditions over the more marginal Paracelsian strand, while also positioning French medicine against religious prejudice in evoking the menstrual taboos of the Hebrew scriptures, and, finally, conflating these two forms of 'error' as the one bulwark of 'tradition'. This was a delicate mediation between, on the one hand, notions of inheritance of the 'good' medical tradition, entailing rejection of all folk and esoteric medical alternatives, and, on the other hand, the claim to a modern scientific rupture from the nonrational past and from folk traditions viewed as perennial.

Barié specifically noted that neither Hippocrates nor Galen held the view of menstrual blood as containing disease elements, and recounted Hippocrates' testimony of having compared a sample of menstrual blood to the blood collected from the slit throat of a murder victim. Of Galen and Hippocrates, he remarked that 'their opinion was the correct one and modern studies have but confirmed it'.[60] Nonetheless, he too claimed that the menopause myth was of ancient origin, albeit not Hippocratic. He accurately identified the Roman natural philosopher Pliny the Elder as the source of the claim that the presence of a menstruating woman could turn liquors into vinegar, and attributed to Palladius' fifth-century CE treatise on agriculture the idea that a menstruating woman could kill all the

[57] Jacques Laugier, *De la ménopause (âge critique)* (Montpellier: Jean Martel ainé, 1861), 9.

[58] Ernest Barié, *Étude sur la ménopause* (Paris: V. Adrien Delahaye, 1877), 11.

[59] Jole Shackelford, *A Philosophical Path for Paracelsian Medicine: The Ideas, Intellectual Context, and Influence of Petrus Severinus (1540–1602)* (Copenhagen: Museum Tusculanum Press, 2004).

[60] Laugier, *De la ménopause*, 13.

insects in a garden just by walking through it.[61] He related these presumptions further to the seventeenth-century Dutch anatomist Reinier de Graaf's view of menstrual blood as having 'moribund and morbid qualities'.[62] But despite his use of quotation marks here, these were Barié's terms, not de Graaf's. De Graaf had little to say about the properties of menstrual blood per se, and made no specific reference to the final cessation of menses. He described menstruation as a fermentation and leakage, not a ridding of the body of disease elements.[63] Nonetheless, Barié appeared determined to make de Graaf an inheritor of the Roman view of poisonous menstrual blood. It is striking also that he could find no intermediary examples between the fifth and the seventeenth centuries, if indeed the myth was as perennial as he implied. In fact, in the chapter where Barié claimed to provide a historical account of the view that menstruation rids the body of disease and hence that menopause is dangerous and must be medicated, we find no quotations from the thinkers he named as espousing this view, and instead only Roman and religious expressions of the idea of menstrual blood itself as impure or poisonous, without any mention of the final cessation of menses in ageing.[64]

Further in this same chapter, Barié referred at length to Hebrew scripture as a source of such views about menstruation as impure, citing the book of Moses.[65] This appears consistent with a common theme in nineteenth-century French medicine, in which the clinician's scientific identity was now often associated with overturning religious mythology and non-rational belief.[66] But none of the cited forms of past insistence on menstrual blood as impure generated any specific ideas about the meaning of its cessation; nor did they make the argument, which Barié and others claimed was 'traditional', that the cessation of menses was dangerous because disease elements now remained trapped within a woman's body, meaning purgation or blood-letting was needed to replace the usual route of exit of the menstrual flow. This would be a specific extension of the mythology of menstrual blood as catharsis into a theory of women's reproductive ageing, which none of the ancient or early modern sources cited by Barié, either medical or religious, appeared to have made. As medical historian Michael Stolberg has shown, and as we considered in Chapter 1, some early eighteenth-century Latin sources did briefly evoke the notion of the end of menses as producing plethora in women's bodies, for which the treatment was either phlebotomy or purgation. But these same sources also considered plethora to be a disease of ageing in men and of menstrual disorders in young women, who were commonly prescribed

[61] Ibid., 12. [62] Ibid., 12.

[63] Reinier de Graaf, *A New Treatise Concerning the Generative Organs of Women* [1668], trans. H. D. Jocelyn and B. P. Setchell, *Journal of Reproduction and Fertility*, 17 (1972): [1–222], 131–135.

[64] Barié, *Étude sur la ménopause*, 10–13. [65] Ibid., 12.

[66] Jacques Léonard, *La Médecine entre les pouvoirs et les savoirs: Histoire intellectuelle et politique de la médecine française au XIXe siècle* (Paris: Editions Aubier, 1992).

blood-letting and purgative medications as well.[67] In any case, though, neither Barié and nor any of the others had apparently read these sources, so it is unclear how they might have been exposed to such an idea through historical precedents.

Androgynous Ageing

The reduction of women to the uterus both in sickness and in health, both in physiology and in behaviour, went far beyond Hippocrates, and had important implications for the ways that menopause was conceived. But even as it formed the basis for assertions of radically sex-differentiated ageing, it also resulted in statements about the sexes becoming alike in old age. The Montpellier professor Joseph Vigarous, in his published lectures of 1801, near his explanation of the origins of ideas about the role of the uterus attributed to Hippocrates, said that between that ages of 40 and 50 years women's bodies became less influenced by the uterus and hence less nervous and sensitive. He viewed this as largely a positive development: 'women seem to acquire an inexhaustible font of life' and were 'no longer subject to the particular pains of their sex'. He said they began to acquire 'the constitution of man' at the very age when men in turn began to lose their masculine constitution.[68] The sexes in ageing became less distinct from each other. Vigarous's positive take on the loss of sex distinction in ageing was sometimes reiterated by later doctors and medical students writing about menopause, but often too such works proposed a considerably less flattering take on the question. The notion that because the uterus so defined women, its cessation of function in menopause meant that they were no longer truly women at all, could be leveraged towards various accounts of the value and possibilities of older feminine roles, both positive and negative.

Many of the specialist works published on menopause referred to it as a drastic loss of femininity, using one or another version of the Hippocratic expression in support of this claim. Louis-Josef Windrif, in his 1811 Strasbourg thesis on women's 'critical age', remarked that 'woman', having lost her generative capacity along with the menstrual flow and 'ceasing to live in the manner of her sex... is assimilated to man, from whom she now differs only in form'.[69] In 1822, the Montpellier candidate Joseph Coural had insisted that once women stopped menstruating, they actually became healthier, lost weight, and appeared 'beautified by new graces'. He thought the term 'âge de retour' referred to the rejuven-

[67] Michael Stolberg, 'A Woman's Hell? Medical Perceptions of Menopause in Preindustrial Europe', *Bulletin of the History of Medicine*, 73/3 (1999): [404–428], 406–407; David Titius, *De fine mensium initiis morborum variorum opportuno: Dissertatio inauguralis medica* (Halle: Henckelii, 1710).

[68] Vigarous, *Cours élémentaire de maladies des femmes*, vol. 1, 47.

[69] Louis-Joseph Windrif, *Essai sur les phénomènes de l'âge critique chez la femme; sur les principaux accidens que l'on remarque à cette époque, et sur les moyens de les prévenir.* (Strasbourg: Levrault, 1811), 2.

ation which he considered menopause could produce.[70] The Paris candidate Albert Assegond in 1821 claimed that women became like men in menopause and lost their distinctive character as well as their charm.[71] But he also said that they acquired a new form of beauty at this time and that, 'arriving at their critical epoch, they seem to receive a new life and appear rejuvenated just as they approach their winter'.[72] Although he thought menopause caused both sexual and aesthetic losses, he also considered that women 'whose minds are cultivated conserve quite powerful means of seduction'.[73] Joseph-Pierre-Éléonor Pétrequin's Paris doctoral thesis of 1836 on the topic of menstruation described its cessation as the moment when 'woman ceases, so to speak, being a woman'.[74]

Dr Ernest Barié reiterated the androgyny claim in 1877, adding that 'little by little, the menopausal woman . . . approaches the habitus of a man'. He said that in her climacteric years, the Enlightenment patron of the arts Marquise du Deffand had once quipped, of her own youthful past, 'Autrefois quand j'étais femme!' ('In the past, when I was a woman!')[75] It seems likely that he borrowed this purported quotation from the English physician Edward Tilt, who cited it in 1857 in the first major English work on the 'change of life' in women (following his doctoral studies in France in the 1830s); or from the Belgian physician Charles Van Leynseele, who also cited it in 1860 in his book on the hygiene of women.[76] But the quotation had also appeared in the 1846 Louis-Julien Larcher book *Woman Judged by the Great Writers of Both Sexes*, which in turn attributed it to the journalist Nestor Roqueplan.[77] It was repeatedly quoted in a wide range of genres as a witticism about older women throughout the nineteenth century. The idea suggests that nineteenth-century medical visions of sex were in fact more mutable than would be predicted by the 'two-sex' model of male–female differentiation that historian Thomas Laqueur claims was dominant at the time.

Many medical scholars also described a kind of distress experienced by nineteenth-century menopausal women in the view that this was the beginning of the decline both of their beauty and their worth to society. The emphasis placed on women looking pretty and being valuable primarily for their youthful beauty

[70] Joseph-Lazare-Jacques Coural, *Considérations générales sur les phénomènes physiologiques et pathologiques de la femme aux divers âges de la vie.* Thèse (Montpellier: Jean Martel, 1822), 36.

[71] Albert Assegond, *De la femme, considérée à l'âge critique. Changements physiologiques qui s'opèrent dans son état physiqus et moral, et de l'application des règles de l'hygiène à cette principale époque de sa vie.* Thèse (Paris: Didot Jeune, 1821), 11.

[72] Ibid., 12. [73] Ibid., 13.

[74] Joseph-Pierre-Éléonor Pétrequin, *Recherches sur la menstruation* (Paris: Didot le jeune, 1836), 11.

[75] Barié, *Étude sur la ménopause*, 50.

[76] Edward John Tilt, *The Change of Life in Health and Disease: A Practical Treatise on the Nervous and Other Affections Incidental to Women at the Decline of Life* (London: J. Churchill, 1857), 27; Charles Van Leynseele, *Hygiène de la femme, ou l'art de conserver la santé et de prolonger la vie, depuis la naissance jusqu'à l'extrême vieillesse*, 2 vols (Gand: H. Hoste, 1860), vol. 2, 267.

[77] Louis-Julien Larcher, *La Femme jugée par les grands écrivains des deux sexes; ou, La femme devant Dieu, devant la nature, devant la loi et devant la société: riche et précieuse mosaïque de toutes les opinions émises sur la femme* [1846], 3rd ed. (Paris: Garnier Frères, 1854), 294.

in bourgeois sociability, along with the denial to them of numerous other social, professional, and political roles, as well as educational opportunities, undoubtedly placed new pressures on elite women to catastrophise their ageing. Unsurprisingly then, many may indeed have found the idea of growing older deeply worrying. Medical writers themselves were fully complicit in the generation of a negative set of ideas about the relationship between menopause and feminine beauty, often emphasising it as 'the decline' or 'the death of sex', and drawing attention to the loss variously of firmness, prettiness, and desirability in terms of which they characterised women's (but never men's) ageing. Skipping instantly ahead to the appearance of extreme old age, they described menopause as the moment of commencement of this state, implying that women immediately lost desirability upon the end of their regular menstrual cycle. This was part of the heritage of the vitalist view of women's physiology, and of the confluence of old temporal layers referring to crisis and climacteric ages that were embedded in the concept of menopause. The cessation of menses was not just the end of one aspect of women's countless lifetime capabilities; it was a revolution of their entire vital economy, which was utterly dominated by the uterus. In losing the capacity to reproduce, women were thought to have lost a great part of their vitality, their singular distinction from men, and their purpose in the world. Menopause was the fateful moment when their ageing decline began.

While the drifting of the sexes towards a middle ground often flattered older women by suggesting that only now were they, like the Marquise du Deffand, worthy company for men and truly able to function intellectually and morally like them, in other cases the suggestion of masculinisation was coupled with a view of the post-menopausal body as grotesque and unattractive because it now lacked the desirable youthful femininity which had marked women as radically different from men. The use of particularly derogatory language to describe women's ageing was a feature of many of the medical works on menopause during the nineteenth century. This lent the message of such texts a certain cruel irony. While denying that menopause was a disease that required medicating or more broadly that it was something that women needed to worry about, they elaborated on it as a potential cause for fear, dread, and self-disparagement. Louis Gardanne's Paris thesis of 1812 described the cessation of menstruation thus:

> The facial traits weaken, the vital movements fall into languor... The skin loses its tone, softness and elasticity, becomes wrinkled and acquires a sombre tint... The hair loses volume and colour, the voice is altered, the breasts sag—in fact, the entire body falls into disrepair.[78]

[78] Charles-Pierre-Louis de Gardanne, *Dissertation sur les avis à donner aux femmes qui entrent dans l'âge critique*. Thèse (Paris: Didot Jeune, 1812), 17–18.

In 1818 another young Paris doctoral student, P. N. Glinel, formulated his take on women's ageing in similar terms. As soon as the regular menstrual cycle ended, a woman could rapidly expect to become fat (or emaciated), develop sagging (or swollen) breasts, lose timbre and strength in her voice and colour and softness in her skin, and generally, 'old age is imminent'.[79] In 1848 Jean-Baptiste Nosely described the critical age as the moment when 'woman loses the features of her sex'.[80] The uterine reductionist model, then, claimed as ancient and Hippocratic, but also often justified according to vitalist reasoning that viewed reproductive potency as the measure of vitality, had profound consequences for the tone of much French medical writing about older women in the nineteenth century. When we turn our attention to women writers (medical and literary) who responded to such discourses in Chapter 8, it will be clear just how unhelpful they were for even the most intelligent women facing ageing in the late nineteenth and early twentieth centuries.

Charlatans, Empirics, Midwives, and *Commères* in the Medical Reclamation of Women's Health

Few doctors and doctoral students writing about attitudes to menopause specifically blamed anyone in particular for the 'traditional' view about menstruation as toxic which they claimed to debunk. But some did attempt to group all other competing forms of medicine with the now-discredited practices of the medical past. This was a tricky business, though, because, as we have seen, French doctors of the nineteenth century represented themselves as simultaneously both revolutionary new scientific clinicians and inheritors of ancient wisdom. Who, then, could be held responsible for the 'traditional' folly about menopause to which they counterpoised their own approach? As Matthew Ramsey has described, nineteenth-century biomedicine did not simply evolve seamlessly from early modern medicine: it emerged in fierce competition with numerous other health practitioners who, throughout the eighteenth—and even much of the nineteenth—century, were far more numerous than official doctors. This is particularly clear if we count not only the numerous folk healers, empirics, charlatans, and *commères* who were already more common than doctors, but also surgeons, *officiers de santé*, *sages-femmes*, drug traders, and pharmacists.[81] Doctors of women's health were particularly so embattled: they had to compete not only with all these other kinds of official practitioners, but with the vast field

[79] P. N. Glinel, *Dissertation médico-physiologique sur l'âge critique des femmes*. Thèse (Paris: Didot Jeune, 1818), 12.

[80] Nosely, *Dissertation sur l'âge critique*, 7.

[81] Matthew Ramsey, *Professional and Popular Medicine in France, 1779–1830* (Cambridge: Cambridge University Press, 1988), 18.

of unofficial midwives and *accoucheurs* who remained the primary deliverers of babies in rural France throughout the nineteenth century, despite the important shift towards regulation of the industry that had been occurring since the mid-eighteenth century.

Menopause was a concept that emerged entangled in the formation of gynaecology as separate from obstetrics. By the 1890s, when older French women first became targets for the surgical removal of reproductive organs in combination with organotherapy ovarian-extract supplementation, as we consider in the final chapter of this book, it was fully assimilated to these specialist disciplines. But it was in the eighteenth century that both gynaecology and obstetrics initiated the modernisation and medicalisation of women's healthcare—a process in which France played a leading role among the swathe of European nation undertaking a similar renovation. Childbirth was increasingly medicalised in France following on the gradual improvement of forceps delivery over the seventeenth and eighteenth centuries, and was progressively re-situated as part of the expertise of university surgeons. Midwives were increasingly pressured to conform to modern biomedical models, as indicated in the 1750 ordinance that mandated a two-year theoretical education for them, followed by an additional two-year supervised apprenticeship, subject to examination by a board of surgeons.[82] In 1882 the Paris hospital system created a new branch of surgical care that employed specialist maternity-delivery doctors (*médecins-accoucheurs des maternités*).[83] Midwives were clearly not the primary culprits for the generation of the 'traditional' ideas about menopause that French doctors criticised; but the continuing competition between them and the emergent fields of obstetrics and gynaecology possibly contributed to the justification of doctors themselves as scientific correctors both of the past and of popular medicine, and as the uniquely educated authorities on matters of women's health.[84] Occasionally, too, they were named as responsible for long-term effects on women's bodies that only later manifested as disease in menopause. The first Paris medical thesis on the final cessation of menses, defended by Jean-Baptiste Chouffe in 1802, had thus suggested that uterine disorders of this time resulted from earlier childbirth injuries caused by midwives, whom he characterised as 'ignorant women.'[85]

Such accusations were not the most common, as *sages-femmes* were increasingly assimilated to biomedicine and subject to hospital doctors' training and

[82] Jürgen Schlumbohm, 'Comment l'obstétrique est devenue une science: La Maternité de l'université de Göttingen, 1751–1830', *Actes de la recherche en sciences sociales*, 143 (2002), 18–30.

[83] Robert Vial, *Histoire de l'enseignement des Hôpitaux de Paris: Les Blouses blanches en formation initiale et continue* (Paris: L'Harmattan, 1999), 107.

[84] On the large numbers of folk healers in the Maine-et-Loire region during the nineteenth century, see Sylvain Sionneau, *Les Hors-la-loi de la médecine au XIXe siècle en Maine-et-Loire* (La Crèche: Geste, 2015).

[85] Jean-Baptiste-P. Chouffe, *Des accidents et des maladies qui surviennent à la cessation de la menstruation*. Thèse (Paris: Croullebois & Gabon, 1802), 8.

surveillance. It was not easy, then, to pin 'popular myth' and malpractice claims on them. But there were many other competing health practitioners circulating throughout France during the nineteenth century, some itinerant and highly specialised in particular diseases, others settled on the edges of large towns and more generalist, as several historians have described.[86] Folk healers (*guérisseurs*), *empiriques* (so called because their knowledge was purely empirical or practical but not officially learned), *charlatans*, and *commères* (crones), but also pharmacists and traders of medical products, were of considerable concern to nineteenth-century doctors of women's health, since their combined economic power vastly outnumbered that of the university-trained clinicians who invented the concept of menopause, by a factor of as much as 5:1 throughout the eighteenth and early nineteenth centuries.[87] While biomedicine grew massively throughout the nineteenth century, considerably reducing this unfavourable ratio (from the doctors' perspective), competition for patients remained fierce in all but the largest urban centres throughout the nineteenth century.[88] There were also the *officiers de santé*, a lower tier of legitimate health practitioners formalised in 1803 and phased out after 1892. All such alternative practitioners remained an important form of competition to university-trained doctors, particularly throughout rural France, over the period of our study. This was especially so before 1848, when the first advisory institution on public health was created to regulate medical practice nationally.[89]

As Elizabeth Williams remarks in her monograph on Montpellier vitalism in the eighteenth century, doctors in that small southern city, renowned for its medical faculty since the late Middle Ages, were in much greater competition with other kinds of medical practitioners than were doctors in Paris or other parts of France, on account of the relatively high ratio of medical clinicians to the general population: roughly 14.3 doctors and 16.6 surgeons per 10,000 habitants in the 1780s. This made it difficult for Montpellier clinicians to find enough patients to generate a comfortable middle-class living for themselves.[90] Throughout the eighteenth and nineteenth centuries, folk healers of various kinds were also far more common in the southern provinces, particularly in rural areas, than in Paris or in many of the northern provinces.[91] Paris in the early nineteenth century,

[86] Michel Vernus, *Médecine populaire en Franche-Comté: Petites et grandes histoires des faiseurs de secrets et autres rebouteux* (Pontarlier: Éditions du Belvédère, 2013); Sionneau, *Les Hors-la-loi de la médecine*; Ramsey, *Professional and Popular Medicine in France.*

[87] Vernus, *Médecine populaire en Franche-Comté*, 58–62; Sionneau, *Les Hors-la-loi de la médecine*, 13–37.

[88] George, D. Suusman, 'The Glut of Doctors in Mid-Nineteenth-Century France', *Comparative Studies in Society and History*, 19/3 (1977): 287–304.

[89] Ramsey, *Professional and Popular Medicine in France*, 105.

[90] Elizabeth A. Williams, *A Cultural History of Medical Vitalism in Enlightenment Montpellier* (London: Routledge, 2003), 35–50.

[91] Ramsey, *Professional and Popular Medicine in France*, 235.

where, according to Matthew Ramsey's estimate, there were a total of 10.5 physicians and surgeons combined per 10,000 inhabitants, was already among the most medicalised centres of Europe at this time.[92] There was thus a strong temptation for doctors both to promote the benefits of clinical medicine for conditions that might not seem obviously in need of treatment, and to discredit practitioners of folk medicine, referred to as empirics, *commères*, or sometimes simply *bonnes femmes*, many of whom were themselves older women with little sense of women's ageing as something that, per se, required treatment. With women constituting more than double the population of men on account of their greater survival in the older ages, older women clearly constituted a crucial demographic for medical services.[93] Menopause was a modern scientific concept of a condition that no traditional practitioner treated, and it could therefore be presented as a diagnosis with a hygienic solution, addressing the many mysterious symptoms of relative ill health that could occur in ageing.

Many of the nineteenth-century medical hygiene texts produced by doctors in the south of France thus made strident claims about their authority to treat older women's bodies, and warned against trusting traditional remedies. The Montpellier-trained physician and viscount Louis-Charles-Édouard de Lapasse, in a book in 1861 about the hygiene of longevity, railed against the remedies of empirics and women folk healers ('remèdes d'empirique ou de bonne femme'), in which the local population still had too much faith for his liking.[94] In alarmist tones, he warned of the 'tempting demon' who attends to older women suffering vapours and migraines, 'personified by the maid with a stitched bonnet and...a loose tongue' promising, 'Oh yes! If madame were to believe in me, she would soon be cured without need to speak of it to monsieur.'[95] Such practitioners also served as a useful alibi for doctors whose own remedies were frequently ineffective—Lapasse remarked 'that he [the doctor] is not always well informed, and that often too, he is called too late', only after the remedies of charlatans and *commères* had already been tried.[96] Lapasse was hardly an entirely orthodox biomedical doctor himself, as a supporter of magnetism and other treatments not accepted in the university-medical mainstream, such as the use of oxygen to cure migraines.[97] Menopause stood precisely at the crux of biomedicine's claims to authority to treat a new patent cohort that had not previously been identified by any earlier or competing health tradition as in need of special care.

Renowned medical scholars had more broadly been denouncing the pharmacological practices of empirics, charlatans, and folk healers repeatedly in major works from the end of the eighteenth century, often with reference to the

[92] Ibid., 59–61. [93] Ibid., 226.

[94] Louis-Charles-Edouard Lapasse, *Hygiène de longévité, guérison des migraines, maux d'estomac, maux de nerfs et vapeurs* (Paris: Victor Masson/Garnier Frères, 1861).

[95] Ibid., 151. [96] Ibid., 149. [97] Ibid., 24–28.

treatment of women. In his 1789 book on the physical and mental diseases of women, the Paris professor Pierre Boyveau-Laffecteur claimed to be defending women from the 'crowd of Empirics who arrive, from the moment of puberty, to lay siege to their understanding, leading them through error upon error into painful disease and death'.[98] In the Paris professor Jean-Louis Alibert's highly influential three-volume 1803 work of general chemical medicine, published in nine editions up to 1829, he recounted numerous tales of empirics mistreating various conditions, remarking that the empiric practitioner was 'justifiably compared to a blind man armed with a stick: he strikes haphazardly and indiscriminately at both the disease and the sick person'.[99] The empirics' employment of pharmacological substances was 'irrational' ('peu rationnel').[100] Alibert counterpoised it with the way a proper doctor proceeds with these very same substances, evoking an approach that was systematic but nonetheless vague in its distinguishing criteria: 'The doctor prepares, places and directs the subjects; he oversees the regime, removes obstacles, and neglects nothing that can assure the success of his treatments.'[101] However, in this same work, he acknowledged in a footnote that empirics sometimes, by chance, managed to treat women's diseases successfully.[102]

Another influential scholar to blame charlatans, drug traders, and folk healers for the mistreatment of women's diseases in particular was the Paris professor of hygiene and medicine Gabriel Jouard, whom we met in the preceding chapter. In his 1804 book comparing women's and men's physiology, he discussed charlatans treating gynaecological disorders with high doses of drastic remedies, expressing amazement that more damage to women was not done via such treatments.[103] He accused charlatans, empirics, *commères*, and all kinds of drug traders of being singularly focused on their income at the expense of patient care, listing all the conditions they pretended to treat—but women's critical age was not among them. Nonetheless, he also accused 'methodical medicine' of excessive reticence—even of being 'pusillanimous'—in seeking to treat the diseases of women, implying that official doctors might benefit from imitating something of the rashness of popular healers and hawkers of remedies.[104]

Concerns about unofficial medical practitioners and folk remedies were clearly part of other French doctors' thoughts on menopause more specifically too. The Paris luminary of Montpellier origin, Philippe Pinel, in 1809 criticised empirics and women health practitioners (*bonnes femmes*) who claimed to heal women's

[98] Pierre Boyveau-Laffecteur, *Essai sur les maladies physiques et morales des femmes* (Paris: Chez l'auteur, 1789), 4.
[99] Alibert, *Nouveaux Élémens de thérapeutique et de matière médicale*, vol. 2, 662. This repeated in vol. 3, 110. See also vol. 1, 346, 516.
[100] Ibid., vol. 3, 479. [101] Ibid., 429. [102] Ibid., vol. 2, 370, footnote 1.
[103] Gabriel Jouard, *Nouvel Essai sur la femme considérée comparativement à l'homme principalement sous les rapports moral, physique, philosophique, etc.* (Paris: Chez Crochard, 1804), 88.
[104] Ibid., 89–91.

uterine and nervous diseases, invariably failing, but in the process attempting multiple 'futile treatment plans'. Women with 'hypochondriac symptoms' were particularly susceptible to being preyed upon by such individuals, he said.[105] Both volumes of his 1797 *Nosographie philosophique* were full of warnings against polypharmacy, and specifically the ill-conceived treatments that he said women in the final cessation of menses often used when they developed hypochondria or hysteria, before turning to a proper doctor.[106] Notably though, he also accused English physicians of 'jealousy and intrigue, on the part of the most accredited doctors, towards one who is habitually and disdainfully called an empiric'.[107]

Treating women in the critical age was not a simple matter, Pinel suggested. He described a complex case example of an elite woman from Caen who suffered heavy menstruation between the ages of 42 and 50 years and then developed symptoms of diabetes.[108] Like the English physician Fothergill, Pinel considered that the abuse of aromatics, spirits, and emetic remedies could all in themselves cause haemorrhagic bleeding in older women.[109] Pinel's own nosography was precisely about rejecting the 'emphatic promises of charlatanism, which purports to cure all diseases', even those which it was 'dangerous to attempt' or were 'beyond the feeble resources' of official medicine of the time.[110] He thus warned against the use of aphrodisiacs, not because he viewed them as ineffective, but rather because he said that while they worked in the short term, they did so at the cost of accelerating ageing.[111] Nonetheless, women's final cessation of menses was hardly a major theme in Pinel's work, and the elaboration of how charlatans and empirics could not be trusted to medicate the final cessation of menses was undertaken largely by the specialist candidates whose theses focused on the treatment of older people or of women in the critical age.

The Montpellier candidate Antoine Leyral applied the broader critiques of unofficial medical practitioners to the question of treating older women in his 1806 thesis on the prophylactic measures necessary for managing 'the epoch of the cessation of the periods'.[112] Leyral claimed that both charlatans and *officiers de santé* gave inappropriate and dangerous treatments to women in the critical age in

[105] Philippe Pinel, *Traité medico-philosophique sur l'aliénation mentale* [1800], 2nd ed. (Paris, J. A. Brosson, 1809), 24.

[106] Philippe Pinel, *Nosographie philosophique, ou la méthode de l'analyse appliquée à la médecine*, 2 vols (Paris: Maradon, 1797), vol. 1, 826–827; vol. 2, 110, 542; Philippe Pinel, *Traité médico-philosophique sur l'aliénation mentale* [1800], 4th ed. (Paris: 1809), ix, xv, 400, 380, 508.

[107] Pinel, *Traité médico-philosophique*, 388.

[108] Philippe Pinel, *Nosographie philosophique, ou la méthode de l'analyse appliquée à la médecine*, 3 vols (Paris: J. A. Brosson, 1810), vol. 3, 589.

[109] Pinel, *Nosographie philosophique* [1797], vol. 1, 280.

[110] Philippe Pinel, *La Médecine clinique rendue plus précise et plus exacte par l'application de l'analyse, ou Recueil et résultat d'observations sur les maladies aiguës, faites à la Salpêtrière* (Paris: Brosson, Gabon et Cie, 1802), x–xi.

[111] Pinel, *Nosographie philosophique* [1797], vol. 2, 113.

[112] Antoine Leyral, *Essai sur la prophylactique des femmes parvenues à l'époque de la cessation des règles*. Thèse (Montpellier: Imprimerie Auguste Ricard, 1806).

the effort to resume their menses, citing a case example in which a 40-year-old woman had been prescribed aloe pills by a health officer to restimulate her missing menses, but which instead brought her 'to the edge of the grave'.[113] He claimed that a charlatan in the village of Mindigour (in the lower Limousin) had treated another woman, aged 46 years, who had hysteria—as indicated by an ulcer that appeared on her left leg every time she menstruated. The charlatan prescribed cauterisation, which merely aggravated her symptoms. Leyral described the woman patient as 'the dupe of this modern Thessalus' (referring to the mysterious son of Hippocrates mentioned by Galen). She should instead have trusted a qualified doctor, and had she done so, she would have been prescribed blood-letting to relieve her plethora instead. This was something that could only be determined after properly assessing whether a woman's symptoms were a result of 'sympathy' of the uterus with other parts of the body, or of plethora.[114] He said misuse of pharmacy was problematic for women around the 'critical epoch', who should be particularly wary of unqualified practitioners because it was a time of life in which cancerous degeneration of the uterus became more frequent. He warned especially against the use of hemlock (*la ciguë*), which he said could cause deadly haemorrhages in the critical age.[115]

Louis Gardanne (the inventor of the neologism *la ménopause*) complained in his first book of 1816 (the revised version of his 1812 Paris doctoral thesis) that some women 'have more confidence in the medications of old crones (*des vieilles commères*), the doctor's most formidable obstacle, than they do in the benefits of hygiene.'[116] In 1812, the same year in which Gardanne defended his thesis on menopause, another Paris candidate, Joseph Capuron, railed against the abuse of purgatives, blood-letting, and cauterisation, which he said charlatans and *commères* hawked to women in the critical age.[117] This was because, he said, in popular belief, 'menstrual blood is destined to purge the body of some sort of virus or impure ferment, and consequently, the sudden or premature cessation of this flow must be very dangerous'.[118] Consequently, many women turned to enemas, baths, purgatives, blood-letting, cauterisation, and blistering plasters or ointments (*vésicatoires*) in the misguided view that the menses must be made to resume, instead provoking the very ailments they looked to avoid—here citing Fothergill as an authority.[119] Prosper-Louis Sauvé's 1826 Strasbourg thesis on menopause complained that 'it is unfortunate that women have more confidence in any number of absurd and complicated recipes that are sold by *commères* and charlatans than in the well-meaning assistance offered by hygiene, especially if it is well

[113] Ibid., 21. [114] Ibid., 21–22. [115] Ibid., 23.
[116] Gardanne, *Avis aux femmes qui entrent dans l'âge critique*, 96.
[117] Joseph Capuron, *Traité des maladies des femmes, depuis la puberté jusqu'à l'âge critique inclusivement*. Thèse (Paris: Croullebois, 1812), 126.
[118] Ibid., 230. [119] Ibid., 230, 240–241.

regulated'.[120] Older men too were sometimes included among those considered susceptible to the claims of empirics and charlatans to cure the ills of ageing. The Montpellier candidate F.-Hyacinthe Teysset in 1825 mocked the standard person who wants to live as long as possible and so consumes 'all the elixirs, health granules, powders, all the specifics that charlatanism and incompetence prescribe as if to give one's days an unlimited duration'.[121] But in general, these kinds of remarks were overwhelmingly confined to discussing women's specific ageing.

Complaints about charlatans, empirics, folk healers, and *commères* became a common refrain in general works on women's health and obstetrics from the early nineteenth century too. Claude Gardien's widely cited *Traité complet d'accouchements* of 1807, in providing advice on breastfeeding, warned against the 'supposedly specific remedies of *commères*' which he said were 'useless and expose the breasts to chills'.[122] He also described a popular narcotic solution devised by the eighteenth-century surgeon Gilles-Joseph Decourcelle, called the 'American elixir', which was used to stimulate breast milk and which Gardien considered of some use in women with weak temperaments whose menses were slow to resume after childbirth.[123] Nonetheless, he warned against its overuse given that it could cause violent colic or aggravate a cough, again accusing *commères* of indiscriminately prescribing it.[124]

Paris professors of the mid-nineteenth century often reiterated earlier denigrations of troublesome charlatans, *commères*, empirics, and drug merchants, as well as other kinds of discredited healing practitioners, particularly in relation to the diseases of women and in relation to women's ageing. Marc Colombat de l'Isère complained in his 1838 treatise that women often became discouraged in their treatments, resorting in despair instead to 'bizarre remedies' and turning to '*commères*, charlatans, magnetists or homeopaths, who…promise them a prompt and radical cure, but most often only hasten the fatal term'.[125] He said there were many 'empiric methods' for treating ovarian inflammation in which women trusted since they occasionally, albeit rarely, managed to cure someone.[126] He claimed that charlatans were preying upon older women's fear of losing their beauty by offering skin products that promised rejuvenation.[127] His principal advice to women in the critical age was to 'avoid all the drugs to which are attached the most pompous names: *health pills, longevity elixir* or proprietary formula…all the

[120] Sauvé, *Réflexions sur l'âge critique*, 8.
[121] F.-Hyacinthe Teysset, *Quelques généralités sur l'hygiène des vieillards.* Thèse (Montpellier: Jean Martel, 1825), 3.
[122] Gardien, *Traité complet d'accouchemens et des maladies des filles*, vol. 3, 294.
[123] Gilles-Joseph de Courcelle & Étienne Chardon de Courcelles, *Élixir américain, approuvé par le gouvernement* (Vitry: Chez Seneuze, 1792).
[124] Gardien, *Traité complet d'accouchemens et des maladies des filles*, vol. 3, 392.
[125] Colombat de l'Isère, *Traité des maladies des femmes*, vol. 2, 658–659.
[126] Ibid., 846.
[127] Colombat de l'Isère, *Traité des maladies des femmes*, vol. 3, 1111.

recipes offered out of ignorance, charlatanism or crones' gossip *commérage*' which were sold purely for profit to older women, promising them 'miraculous cures'.[128] Colombat de l'Isère's 1838 treatise on the diseases of women, published in four French editions, was also translated into English in 1850, helping to spread the French concept of menopause as a topic worthy of medical specialisation and as a condition requiring hygienic care to the UK and North America.[129] Louis Becquerel, too, in 1859 complained of a 'multitude of charlatans and industrialists who, to give themselves a scientific veneer, created a speciality of exploiting uterine diseases'.[130] He said there was 'a multitude of empiric medicaments' that had been proposed for the treatment of sterility, but that as none were of any clinical value, it was pointless even to list them.[131]

Hygienists too joined in the exercise of pouring scorn on folk-medical practices, since they were clearly different from their own comprehensive lifestyle advice. The Paris professor of hygiene Michel Lévy railed against the 'purgatives, evacuants, laxatives ('désobstruants') that charlatanism proposes, that ignorance accepts, that prejudice popularises'. He said that hypochondriacs were the primary market for such drugs because they were too 'disturbed' ('déréglés') to persevere with more effective dietary and other hygienic means. Only with diet could a 'durable modification of the functional rhythm' of the organs be assured.[132] He reserved particular scorn for the empiric practice of giving the same remedy to many different people, citing the example of one practitioner who sold a toothpaste which—outrageously for Lévy—was prescribed to all and sundry without any individual diagnosis.[133] The critical ages were particularly delicate times, during which only the best medical care could be trusted. Nonetheless, he rejected the claim made by the Montpellier doctor Dominique Raymond in 1757 that leukorrhea (now commonly listed as a symptom of women's critical age) was one of the diseases that it was dangerous to try to cure.[134] Lévy attributed to Roussel the realisation that menstruation was the 'sign and measure of women's health'. For good measure, he attached to this another Hippocratic aphorism, III.28, which referred to diseases of childhood that more often become chronic in women after puberty, but which he interpreted as indicating that the key to a symptomless menopause lay in the prophylactic treatment of any diseases to

[128] Ibid., 1096–1097.

[129] Marc Colombat de l'Isère, *A Treatise on the Diseases of Women and Special Hygiene of Females*, trans. Charles D. Meigs (Philadelphia, Lean & Blanchard, 1850).

[130] Louis Alfred Becquerel, *Traité clinique des maladies de l'utérus et de ses annexes*, 2 vols (Paris: G. Baillière, 1859), vol. 1, 14.

[131] Becquerel, *Traité clinique des maladies de l'utérus*, vol. 2, 455.

[132] Michel Lévy, *Traité d'hygiène publique et privée*, 2 vols (Paris: J.-B. Baillière et fils, 1844–1845), vol. 2, 242.

[133] Ibid., 237.

[134] Ibid., vol. 1, 106, 191. Dominique Raymond, *Traité des maladies qu'il est dangereux de guérir*, 2 vols (Avignon: F. B. Merande, 1757), vol. 1, 359.

which a woman had previously been prone.[135] The ancients, after all, could be made to say just about anything that nineteenth-century doctors wanted them to, while empirics and *commères* could be criticised for providing much the same remedies as official doctors, minus the elaborate theory and rationale.

The term *commère*, which could refer not only to a 'gossip' but also to a 'godmother', was used in eighteenth- and nineteenth-century medical works to describe lay women empirics/folk healers who prescribed and sold medicinal remedies. In some cases, they did so by offering highly specialist treatments for particular diseases as itinerant practitioners travelling throughout a region; in others, in a more generalist capacity in settled practices on the outskirts of large towns and cities. A definition of the term appears in Jean-Pierre Gallais's gossipy 1817 work *Mœurs et caractères du dix-neuvième siècle* (Habits and Characters of the Nineteenth Century), though it gives little indication of its more specific use in medical descriptions, except to convey that it had a distinctly negative connotation: '*Commères* is a word used to refer to women of low condition who want to know all the latest news of the neighbourhood and who speak indiscreetly of all and sundry,' Gallais said.[136] When used in the medical context, the term conveyed something of the same negative meaning of a know-it-all woman who, in this case, provided medical advice, performed surgeries, or prescribed or made pharmacological remedies, but who, according to the official doctor criticising her, actually knew too little to be doing so. It is not clear whether such practitioners themselves ever used the term as a self-description, as was the case for those labelled both *charlatans* and *guérisseurs* (healers).[137] In the 1723 theatrical musical *Les Trois Commères* by Alain-René Lesage, the characters thus called are effectively midwives, but also make medical remedies and even poisons with which they malevolently threaten the other characters. The three women are mocked as together constituting three-quarters of the worth of an official male doctor, in a song which includes the line: 'J'ai bien l'habit de Médecin, Mais non pas les prérogatives' ('I do have the garments of a doctor but not the prerogatives').[138] Four *commères* also appear briefly in the fourth book of Victor Hugo's 1862 *Les Misérables*, where they are likened to the three witches of Shakespeare's *Macbeth*, except that here it is Napoleon Bonaparte's fateful reign that they predict.[139]

The word *commère* or *coumère* was a term of affection or parentage in old French and in medieval Provençale and retained that spectrum of meanings into

[135] Lévy, *Traité d'hygiène publique et privée*, vol. 1, 191.

[136] Jean-Pierre Gallais, *Mœurs et caractères du dix-neuvième siècle*, 2 vols (Paris: Belin-le-prieur, 1817), vol. 1, 206–207.

[137] Ramsey, *Professional and Popular Medicine in France*, 133.

[138] Alain René Le Sage, *Les Trois Commères; pièce en trois actes* [1723] (Paris: Chez la veuve Duchesne, 1784), 57–58.

[139] Victor Hugo, *Les Misérables IV—L'Idylle rue Plumet et l'épopée rue Saint-Denis*, II: *Gavroche en marche* [1862]; *Œuvres complètes de Victor Hugo*, vol. 5 (Paris: Imprimerie nationale, 1909), 250.

the early twentieth century. But it seems only to have been used from the early eighteenth until the late nineteenth century in the sense of a woman who provided unofficial medical treatments. Even throughout the nineteenth century, the word held various meanings, mostly negative, but also sometimes admiring. In romantic fiction of the 1830s it could evoke a striking, confident, and intimidating mature woman, as in Jules Barbey d'Aurevilly's memoirs, which described a boy's mother as a superb Amazon with 'a head magnificently positioned on shoulders that have an air of indomitable resolution. Proud *commère*!'[140] One rare source to mention *commères* in the medical sense after the nineteenth century was a satirical opinion piece by a 'Dr Ravarit' from Poitiers in the *Chronique médicale* in 1908 protesting that *commères* should not be treated with disdain in the manner that had become customary among urban doctors, because, he said, their remedies were sometimes effective, as 'our rural colleagues' knew all too well. He cited the example of one such practitioner with whom he was acquainted who had experimentally trialled her medicinal formulas on rabbits before giving them to women. Nonetheless, the article as a whole also mocked the persistence of credence in folk remedies, telling stories of fever treated by covering the patient's feet with a cataplasm of chopped onions, of immolated pigeon used to cure meningitis, of a head-cold cured by a handkerchief soaked in urine, and closed with a comparison to 'the savages of central Africa and their sorcerers with their gris-gris and their amulets'.[141]

The term was not generally used to refer to midwives (*sages-femmes*), though in practice some individuals operated as both unofficial *accoucheurs* and folk healers, offering advice and remedies to women about conception and pregnancy, including menstrual problems and infant health. An 1813 letter to the *Journal de médecine, chirurgie, pharmacie, etc.*, complaining of a bungled surgical operation performed on an infant with a reported birth deformity of the hand, referred to the unofficial practitioners responsible for the injury as *commères*.[142] As Matthew Ramsey has noted, the fluidity of popular medical practices in this period makes it problematic to speak of discrete types of practitioners within a fixed typology.[143] By the second half of the nineteenth century the medical individuals to whom the term *commères* referred appear to have been largely subsumed under the broader, non-gender-specific, and increasingly derogatory designation of *charlatans*. An 1857 brochure by the successful doctor Sébastien Guyétant, who, like Gardanne and Sauvé, wrote on both menopause and women's reproductive health, warned against the alternative remedies of healers who were not medical doctors, in

[140] Jules Barbey d'Aurevilly, *Premier Memorandum: 1836–1828* (Paris: Alphonse Lemerre, 1900), 268.

[141] Dr Ravarit, 'Remèdes de commères au XXe siècle'. *La Chronique médicale*, 16 (1908), 239–240.

[142] Anon., 'Variétés', *Journal de médecine, chirurgie, pharmacie, etc.*, 26 (1813), 422–429 [423].

[143] Ramsey, *Professional and Popular Medicine in France*, 177.

whom too many menopausal women placed their faith; but he referred to these people simply as *charlatans*.[144]

As Ramsey has also shown, the sale of pharmacological remedies represented up to half of the revenue of non-official practitioners of all kinds throughout the first half of the nineteenth century.[145] Numerous such practitioners evidently provided elixirs and pills that claimed to treat a wide variety of conditions in both sexes, among which were included 'women's complaints'—generally very vaguely defined. Some offered remedies that claimed to be able to stimulate menses in women who had never had them or who had suppressed menstruation, as well as curing leukorrhea (*les blanches*), uterine pain, and tumours. One such remedy was the 'Turkish balm' sold by a German folk practitioner, Albertina Dränkler, who set up a practice in Strasbourg in 1801.[146] This same balm was also listed in the personal apothecary of Marie-Gabrielle de Sinety, Duchess of Gramont, in the Vaucluse department, in the first half of the nineteenth century, along with numerous other medicinal products, including an *élixir de longue vie*.[147] Another *élixir de longue vie* made by a proprietor named Perret in the rue du Vieux Colombier in Paris was sent to the Commission des Remèdes Secrets (Commission for Secret Remedies) in 1827, seeking approval for legal sale, but it was rejected by a commissioner named Guéneau de Mussy—probably François (1774–1853), who became doctor to the restoration monarch Charles X. His nephew Noël (1813–1885), who was the grandson of the Paris professor of hygiene Jean Noël Hallé, later wrote about menopause erotomania, as we consider in the next chapter.[148] Perret's elixir too was claimed to stimulate the menses (though for whom it did not specify), among many different revitalising benefits.[149] Products targeting longevity were already commonly described among the wares of 'charlatans' even in the early eighteenth century, as indicated in a 1704 Latin–French dictionary which connected the two.[150]

[144] Guyétant, *Conseils au femmes*, v.

[145] Ramsey, *Professional and Popular Medicine in France*, 113.

[146] AD Bas-Rhin 5 M22, no. 6, cited in Ramsey, *Professional and Popular Medicine in France*, 138–139.

[147] Remèdes et recettes à l'usage de la famille de Gramont et particulièrement de Marie-Gabrielle de Sinety, duchesse de Gramont (s.d., XVIIIe s-vers 1850): *Archives du duché de Caderousse (1008–XIXe siècle)*, Papiers personnels et familiaux Maison de Gramont: 2 E 9/165.

[148] Noël Guéneau de Mussy, 'L'Érotisme de la ménopause', *Gazette hebdomadaire de médecine et de chirurgie*, 37 (13 October 1871): 591–595.

[149] Guéneau de Mussy, 'Remèdes secrèts: Séance du 11 Novembre 1827, Académie royale de médecine', *Archives générales de médecine*, 18 (Paris: Béchet jeune, 1828), 583 [581–585]; discussed also by Mathew Ramsey, 'Academic Medicine and Medical Industrialism', in Ann La Berge and Mordechai Feingold, eds, *French Medical Culture in the Nineteenth Century* (Amsterdam: Rodopi, 1994), 335 [25–78].

[150] Anon., 'Baume turc', *Dictionnaire universel françois et latin, contenant la signification et la définition tant des mots de l'une et l'autre langue, avec leurs différents usages, que des termes propres de chaque estat et de chaque profession; la description de toutes les choses naturelles et artificielles; l'explication de tout ce que renferment les sciences et les arts; avec des remarques d'érudition et de critique*, 3 vols (Paris: Estienne Ganeau, 1704), vol. 1, 227.

Nonetheless, the claims about stimulating menses included in the long lists of varied effects of many such remedies did not appear to focus on older women at all until late in the nineteenth century (as discussed further in this chapter). This suggests that if folk practitioners prescribed them for this purpose, it was only after getting the idea from official medical accounts of menopause as a symptomatic condition. The widely read 1817 book of 'curative' and purgative medicine by the royal surgeon Louis Leroy only mentioned stimulating menstruation as a specific aim of such remedies in relation to young women and pubescent girls.[151] Leroy did discuss the *retour d'âge*, but only to say that the cessation of menses was 'a natural event' ('un évènement naturel'), not itself requiring medication, and that men were just as much at risk of death and disease after the age of 50 as women. The cessation of menses around this age was not the sign of a woman's 'decrepitude', nor a state of dryness, nor was it truly 'a suppression that she experiences': it was simply the end of women's 'aptitude of the second degree'. But Leroy did admit that if a woman around this time suffered 'incidents' (*accidents*), such as leukorrhea, haemorrhagic bleeding, and abdominal pains, then purgation would be appropriate, as in other ages and sexes—but only 'if she is sick'.[152] This book was by far the most read work on purgation throughout the nineteenth century, and was published in another twenty French editions up to 1856, as well as being translated into Spanish, Dutch, and Italian. It seems hard to imagine that, if purgatives had ever been a major product either prescribed to or sought by menopausal women, there would not be more discussion of this practice here.

It is not clear how many women (either young or old) were ever drawn to use purgatives or emmenagogues to self-medicate against the loss of menses either in youth or in ageing. There are several other possible reasons why women might wish to use such remedies that are entirely unrelated to menopause. Firstly, folk healers, empirics, charlatans, and apothecaries often sold abortifacients, but were vulnerable to prosecution if they explicitly declared this illegal aim. The description of a remedy as being able to 'resume the menses' may often have functioned as a coded indication of its abortifacient properties. Emmenagogic herbs had been listed as having both of these uses in Dioscorides' ancient *Materia medica*, and were widely known among early modern and nineteenth-century doctors to cause both abortion in pregnant women and menstruation in some women suffering suppression of menses.[153] The eminent professor of legal medicine at Paris Ambroise Tardieu complained in 1864 of the many abortive remedies sold by a variety of alternative medical practitioners throughout France. He said that in a

[151] Louis Leroy, *La Médecine curative, ou la purgation dirigée contre la cause des maladies* [1817], 14th ed. (Paris: Chez l'Auteur, 1827), 233–236.

[152] Ibid., 234, 240–242.

[153] Pedanius Dioscorides of Anazarbus, *De materia medica*, trans. Lily Y. Beck (Hildesheim: Georg Olms Verlag, 2017), 179, 234; John M. Riddle, *Contraception and Abortion from the Ancient World to the Renaissance* (Cambridge, Mass./London: Harvard University Press, 1992), 29–32, 50, 89, 103–104.

group of seventy-five people prosecuted for this crime between 1846 and 1850, there were thirty-seven midwives (*sages-femmes*), nine doctors, one herbalist-pharmacist, two charlatans, and two 'matrons' (*matrones*). Three-quarters of those accused were women.[154] He identified purgatives, emmenagogues, diuretics, and sudorific remedies as the most common drugs used for abortion by 'empirics, matrons and charlatans', adding:

> I would be at a loss to enumerate all the countless recipes that have been composed and administered with the aim of procuring an abortion, and whose use is especially widespread in the countryside and far from the large population centres.[155]

Secondly, as we considered in Chapter 1, although there was no clear medical consensus about the need for young women to menstruate regularly to be fertile or well, many official medical scholars throughout the eighteenth century had referred to the stoppage of menses in young women as indicating both infertility and general poor health, a view that became more dominant towards the end of the eighteenth century. In the first half of the nineteenth century, many (though again, not all) major works on menstruation insisted on the importance of regular menstruation both as a proxy for women's general good health and as necessary for fertility. This was based on the emerging mechanistic physiological understanding of the phases of ovulation, which defined menstruation as the final shedding of the uterine lining after unsuccessful fertilisation of the egg.[156] By this account, menstruation must occur to allow renewed uterine preparation for conception.[157] Popular forms of folk medicine, which often drew from the work of university medical scholars, may therefore also have treated missing menses during the reproductive years with a view to enhancing general health, or in the aim of enabling conception.

Might older women too have tried to take such remedies with a view to resuming their menstrual cycles and bearing more children after the age of 40 or 50? We have no compelling evidence of this. Given both the limited medical understanding and the relative poverty of many healers and hawkers of remedies, it seems possible that some may have encouraged the use of such substances to resume

[154] Ambroise Tardieu, *Étude médico-légale sur l'avortement, suivie d'observations et de recherches pour servir à l'histoire médico-légale des grossesses fausses et simulées* (Paris: J. B. Baillière, 1864), 22.

[155] Ibid., 30.

[156] Maurice Chaslon, *Essai sur la menstruation* (Paris: Didot Jeune, 1803), 17; Adam Raciborksi, *Du rôle de la menstruation dans la pathologie et la thérapeutique* (Paris: J. B. Baillière, 1856), 2.

[157] Charles N. Négrier, *Recherches anatomiques et physiologiques sur les ovaires dans l'espèce humaine, considérés spécialement sous le rapport de leur influence dans la menstruation* (Paris: Béchet Je. et Labé, 1840); Félix-Archimède Pouchet, *Théorie positive de l'ovulation spontanée et de la fécondation des mammifères et de l'espèce humaine, basée sur l'observation de toute la série animale* (Paris: J. B. Baillière, 1847).

menstruation in older women simply in order to expand the market for their products. Indeed, implicit in the French medicalisation of menopause is the sense that official doctors, too, needed older women for much the same reason. It is also worth considering that peasant women in many rural areas may not have had a clear sense of a specific age when their menstruation could be expected to cease, nor would they have experienced menstruation as a regular occurrence during their reproductive years. This is especially likely if their lifespan had been filled with either repeated pregnancies, infectious diseases, or chronic undernutrition, such as anthropologists of menopause have observed in multiple recent contexts.[158] Such conditions were likely prevalent among European peasant women from ancient times until the nineteenth century, as Helen King has suggested.[159] Moreover, not all peasant peoples of the Hexagon in the nineteenth century had records of their birth easily at hand that allowed them to track their age throughout their lifetime, although parish priests held birth and baptism records which could be consulted for particular official purposes. We take it for granted that knowing our age in numeric years is a core feature of identity in modern times, but nineteenth-century peasants did not often understand themselves in this way, and probably even less understood life after menstruation as something that needed medicating. France in the nineteenth century was also not the French society of the early twenty-first century, where women have increasingly delayed childbearing in their youth due to competing priorities of self-fulfilment, travel, higher education, and careers, and where IVF programmes for women in their forties have consequently flourished.[160] Even with the relative popularity of simple contraceptive measures (withdrawal before ejaculation) among French elites of the eighteenth and nineteenth centuries, most women in this period still bore several children well before the age of 40 years, and would have been less likely than women today to have sought further conception after this time.

Until the 1890s, presentations of popular remedies in relation to women's complaints, or with the effect of resuming menses listed among their benefits, had not referred specifically to menopause or to women's critical age at all. But in 1894 an anonymous brochure extolling the virtues of a product called *l'élixir de Virginie*, complete with testimonials, indeed claimed to alleviate symptoms of the *retour d'âge—a* term that referred still both to menopause and to men's midlife

[158] Beverly I. Strassmann, 'The Biology of Menstruation in Homo Sapiens: Total Lifetime Menses, Fecundity, and Nonsynchrony in a Natural-Fertility Population', *Current Anthropology*, 38/1 (1997): 123–129; Thomas C. T. Buckley & Alma Gottlieb, eds, *Blood Magic: The Anthropology of Menstruation* (Berkeley: University of California Press, 1988), 44–45.

[159] Helen King, *Hippocrates' Woman: Reading the Female Body in Ancient Greece* (London/New York: Routledge, 1998), 27.

[160] A. P. Ferraretti et al., 'Trends over 15 years in ART in Europe: An Analysis of 6 Million Cycles', *Human Reproduction*, 2017/2 (2017): hox012. Doi:10.1093/hropen/hox012; Elise de la Rochebrochard, 'One in Thirty Children in France Conceived Through Assisted Reproductive Technology', *Population & Societies*, 556 (2018): Hal-01990070. <https://hal.archives-ouvertes.fr/hal-01990070/document>.

complaints. This brochure seems likely to have understood the term in a largely non-gender-specific way, since it was not claimed to influence anything unique to women in any other respect. In fact, this elixir appears to have been broadly marketed by chemists for the vitality of middle-aged people, without any uptake of the now-popular idea among doctors that women had a particular form of *retour d'âge* called 'menopause'. The remedy promised to cure a wide variety of complaints of the sanguine humoral type, which included haemorrhoids, varicose veins, oedema, and hot flushes—the last of these was becoming a widely listed symptom of menopause (though still less so than it is understood to be in our own time). The Virginia elixir was produced by the Pharmacie Moride in the rue de la Tacherie in the Marais, not far from the *École de Médecine*, and so was certainly at least semi-respectable.[161] The brochure was also republished in several editions into the 1920s, suggesting the remedy must have had a certain popularity to be sold for as long as thirty years.[162]

Purgatives, Empirics, and Menopause

Another dimension of the discourse of menopause doctors about folk remedies and the supposedly 'traditional' mistreatment of women in the critical age was displayed in the ubiquitous French quotation of the English physician John Fothergill's short 1774 pamphlet arguing that the final cessation of menses should not be medicated with purgatives, which could instead stimulate uterine haemorrhaging.[163] Translated into French in 1778, this pamphlet was cited thereafter by most of the French scholars writing about menopause throughout the nineteenth century, even though, as we discussed in Chapter 1, its central piece of advice not to medicate the final cessation of menses had already been offered by other French and English physicians long before Fothergill.[164] The critique of the widespread use of purgatives for all sorts of medical conditions in general had long been a subject of debate in French medicine, beginning with an oft-cited, scathing Latin book about the question as early as 1714 by the Reims physician Philippe Hecquet, who had been Dean of the Paris faculty of Medicine in the early

[161] Pierre Guincêtre and Pierre Julien, 'La Publicité médico-pharmaceutique de l'Astrologue Normand en 1904', *Revue d'histoire de la pharmacie*, 78 (1990): [390–397], 396.

[162] Anon., *Accidents du retour de l'âge et maladies du système véneux; varices et ulcères variqueux; hémorroïdes, varicocèle; phlébites, œdèmes chroniques; congestions; hérmorrhages, etc.; Leur traitement par l'élixir de Virginie* (Paris: Moride & Cie, 1894). The Bibliothèque Nationale de France holds editions from both 1894 and 1923.

[163] John Fothergill, 'On the Management Proper at the Cessation of the Menses' [1774], *Medical Observations and Inquiries*, vol. 5 (London: Cadell, 1776): 160–186.

[164] John Fothergill, *Conseils pour les femmes de quarante-cinq à cinquante ans, ou conduite à tenir lors de la cessation des règles* [1778] (Paris: Briand, 1778).

eighteenth century.[165] They had also been made the subject of suspicion in gynaecological works from as early as the late seventeenth century: François Mauriceau had remarked in his 1695 treatise on pregnancy that 'purgatives ordinarily cause more harm than they do relief', and described a 45-year-old woman who had developed a fatal uterine cancer after being treated with copious blood-letting and purgative remedies.[166]

Purgative medications of many varieties had long been used in French and other medical traditions, in the view that they could correct imbalances of the humours, and they remained a central therapy of folk practitioners and drug traders throughout the nineteenth century.[167] Royal surgeon Louis Leroy's multi-edition book celebrating their many uses is just one indication of their ubiquity in pharmacological practice, though it was also a tool of self-promotion for the product made by his son-in-law and from which the family had long profited.[168] But there was increased opposition to such chemical remedies in official medicine, in part because they were associated with charlatans and empirics.[169] Secret remedies had been brought under state scrutiny precisely in order to police the production of unofficial medical products since the introduction of the law of 21 Germinal, Year XI (11 April 1803) which prohibited their sale, followed by the establishment of an Imperial Commission in 1811 which assessed petitions from manufacturers for authorisation of their remedies.[170] Indeed, Leroy had complained that scholars writing about and producing 'specifics' (such as himself) had 'often been treated as charlatans', which he said was unfair because charlatans never showed the understanding of the causes of diseases that made his own approach legitimate.[171] Strong chemical purgation could also be dangerous, and deaths were sometimes recorded from its use.[172] The opposition to purgatives and other chemical remedies throughout the eighteenth century had often followed the lines of solidist and iatromechanical views of physiology in their rejection of

[165] Philippe Hecquet, *De purgandâ medicinâ a curarum sordibus* (Paris: Chavelier, 1714); Anthelme Balhasar Baron Richerand, *Nouveaux éléments de physiologie*, 4 vols (Paris: Richard, Caille et Ravier, 1812), vol. 1, 325.

[166] François Mauriceau, *Observations sur la grossesse et l'accouchement des femmes, et sur leurs maladies & celles des enfans nouveau-nez: En chacune desquelles les causes & les raisons des principaux évenemens sont décrites & expliquées* (Paris: Chez l'auteur, 1695), 312, 314.

[167] Robert Weston, *Medical Consulting by Letter in France, 1665–1789* (Abingdon: Routledge, 2016), 190–192.

[168] Louis Leroy, *La Médecine naturelle et curative, ou la Purgation dirigée contre la cause des maladies*, 4e édition (Paris: chez l'auteur, 1817);; Matthew Ramsey, 'Academic Medicine and Medical Industrialism: The Regulation of Secret Remedies in Nineteenth-Century France', in Ann La Berge & Mordechai Feingold, eds, *French Medical Culture in the Nineteenth Century* (Amsterdam: Rodopi, 1994), 42–43 [25–78].

[169] F. J. Lebout, *La Vrai Médecine aux prises avec le charlatanisme, ou Examen critique de plusieurs doctrines médicales très dangereuses pour le peuple, et particulièrement de la médecine, dite curative, de M. Leroy* (Paris: Béthune et Plon, 1837).

[170] Ramsey, 'Academic Medicine and Medical Industrialism', 27–28.

[171] Leroy, *La Médicine naturelle et curative*, 50–51.

[172] Ramsey, 'Academic Medicine and Medical Industrialism', 44.

iatrochemical humoralism, associated with Galen, but also with Paracelsus and van Helmont. The menopause doctors' championing of Hippocrates may have been convenient for this reason too: it allowed a distancing from Galenism (while still claiming an ancient inheritance), and aligned better with the new fields of hygiene, gynaecology, and alienism, all of which emphasised women's nervous sensitivity in menopause. Seventeenth- and eighteenth-century iatromechanists, such as Philippe Hecquet, Giorgio Baglivi, and Hermann Boerhaave, had favoured therapies such as phlebotomy, leeches, and cauterisation over chemical means. By the beginning of the nineteenth century, there were few scholars interested in pursuing such a dichotomous and narrow view of therapies, although phlebotomy did see a resurgence in the early nineteenth century via the influence of François Broussais (1772–1838) and his followers, adding new fuel to the anti-chemical current.[173] Mechanical therapies had their vociferous opponents, most often among those favouring chemical or hygienic medicine, such as the Paris doctor Joseph-Marie Audin-Rouvière, who campaigned his whole career against both phlebotomy and leeches.[174] But none of this stopped chemical and mechanical remedies from being prescribed to women in the critical age, and specialist works on menopause often referred to both in addition to elaborating regimes of hygiene and medical care.

Nineteenth-century works on women's health sometimes recommended purgatives, but also sometimes warned against them. Jean-Louis Alibert's 1803 book on the *materia medica* described multiple legitimate medical purposes of such substances, but also remarked that 'purgatives have been so widely abused' that it was necessary to confine them to a precise set of indications for their use.[175] The Paris candidate Leblanc, writing his thesis on metritis (inflammation of the uterus) in 1823, claimed that the use of purgatives in the treatment of this disorder could cause cancer, implying that this was a matter of medical consensus in the long history of gynaecology.[176] In 1803 a work focused specifically on the use of purgatives in the critical age by the Paris candidate J. N. Guilbert had connected the earlier discussions of the chemical and hydraulic effects of purgatives

[173] François-Joseph-Victor Broussais, *Histoire des phlegmasies ou inflammations chroniques, fondée sur de nouvelles observations de clinique et d'anatomie pathologique: Ouvrage présentant un tableau raisonné des variétés et des combinaisons diverses de ces maladies, avec leurs différentes méthodes de traitement*, 2 vols (Paris: Gabon, 1808); L. W. B. Brockliss, 'Before the Clinic: French Medical Teaching in the Eighteenth Century', in Caroline Hannaway and Ann la Berge, eds, *Constructing Paris Medicine* (Amsterdam: Rodopi, 1998), 76–77 [71–115].

[174] Joseph-Marie Audin-Rouvière, *La Médecine sans médecin, ou Manuel de santé* (Paris: Chez l'auteur, 1825); Joseph-Marie Audin-Rouvière, *Plus de sangsues!* (Paris/Brussels: Berthot, 1827); Ramsey, 'Academic Medicine and Medical Industrialism', 29–30.

[175] Alibert, *Nouveaux Élémens de thérapeutique et de matière médicale*, vol. 1, 271.

[176] Leblanc, *Essai sur la métrite aiguë*, 14.

with Fothergill's warning against their use in women around the cessation of menses.[177] Guilbert complained:

> One sees still a certain type of practitioner who knows only how to use pharmaceutical means, and who, among these, essentially employs the purgatives—that is, who abuses this means of healing.[178]

The Paris professor Moreau de la Sarthe also discussed Fothergill's book in 1803.[179] He was followed by the Paris obstetrician Claude Martin Gardien in 1820, who leveraged it against the 1787 work of Jeannet des Longrois which, Gardien noted, had conflated the suppression of menses in cycling women with the final cessation due to age, thus mistakenly extending all the possible diseases of menstrual suppression to the critical age.[180] Discussing purgatives, Gardien remarked that 'Fothergill objected with good reason to this practice' on which so many earlier physicians had insisted (notably Jeannet des Longrois); and which, he said, 'women themselves sought out with avidity, and abused' based on the belief that a toxic accumulation would result from not menstruating, unless the body could be induced pharmacologically to purge blood or other substances.[181] Gardien also took the opportunity to acknowledge four particular Paris students who had focused on the final cessation of menses with better results than either Fothergill, Jeannet des Longrois, or the earlier Montpellier physician Jean Astruc: Chouffe, Béclard, Lamaze, and Jallon. He ignored Gardanne and his neologism, as well as all seven Montpellier students and the two Strasbourg students who had by this time also written specifically about the age-related final cessation of menses.[182] So Fothergill not only served as a weapon for mechanist physicians to mount an assault on chemical therapies, empirics, and folk healers, but also as a measure for Gardien to sort his most favoured students from the rest at the Paris faculty, and as a weapon against rival faculties—particularly Montpellier, which continued to pose a competitive threat to Paris claims of ownership over the topic of menopause advice, hygiene, and treatment. Several of the first doctoral theses in French on the final cessation of menses had also referred to Fothergill's text, embracing the English physician's anti-iatrogenic and hygienic approach, beginning with the Montpellier candidate Jérémie-André Pingault in 1799.[183] Most of

[177] J. N. Guilbert, *Des purgatifs à la cessation des menstrues*. Thèse (Paris: Imprimerie de la Bibliothèque Médicale, 1803), 5.

[178] Ibid., 3.

[179] Jacques Louis Moreau (de la Sarthe), *Histoire naturelle de la femme, suivie d'un traité d'hygiène appliqué à son régime physique et moral aux différentes époques de la vie*, 3 vols (Paris: L. Duprat, 1803), vol. 1, 410–411.

[180] Gardien, *Traité complet d'accouchemens et des maladies des filles*, vol. 1, 368–369.

[181] Ibid., 374. [182] Ibid., 369.

[183] Jérémie-André Pingault, Jérémie-André, *De la cessation des règles* (Montpellier: Tournel, 1799), 11, 18, 21.

the early specialist books and theses on the final cessation of menses up to 1816 also cited it; although notably Jean-Baptiste Chouffe, who was the first Paris student to do so and one of those approved by Gardien, was actually somewhat critical of Fothergill's overgeneralisation about purgatives being bad for all women at this time of life.[184]

In 1805 there was a new translation of Fothergill's tract by Charles-François-Simon Giraudy (1770–1848), a doctor and, later, alienist at the Charenton asylum.[185] In the introduction to his translation, Giraudy took the opportunity to connect Fothergill's disapproval of purgative treatment for women in the critical age with the anti-mechanist agenda among French doctors of his generation, expressed in a similar disapproval of blood-letting as a treatment for older adults.[186] Giraudy went so far as to reproach Fothergill for failing to mention this other equally overprescribed treatment for women in the critical age, which he proposed was even more problematic than purgatives, since it caused hysteria, hypochondria, and other nervous disorders to which women at this time of life were already prone.[187] Fothergill was thus not only useful as a reinforcement against the folk practitioners using pharmaceutical means and the Montpellier doctors whose approach often retained a more nuanced use of herbal remedies, but also in the struggle to displace existing established medical practices and make room for the new disciplines of hygiene, gynaecology, and alienism. Menopausal and, more broadly, ageing women were potential targets for them all.

Despite Fothergill's warning and the wide embrace of his anti-iatrogenic approach to the final cessation of menses, and despite the long struggle by some doctors against the use of purgatives and phlebotomy for women in menopause, these kinds of interventions nonetheless remained part of treatment practices well into the early twentieth century.[188] In 1821, the Paris candidate Albert Assegond cited Fothergill's warning,[189] but also listed 'pharmaceutical means' such as purgatives for constipation, as well as blood-letting, cupping, foot baths,

[184] Chouffe, *Des accidents et des maladies*, 42, 51; I. A. Labretoigne-Lavalette, *Réfléxions sur les maladies qui surviennent aux femmes à l'époque de la cessation des règles*. Thèse (Montpellier: Imprimerie Auguste Ricard, 1805), 28; C. A. M. Peloux, *Essai sur l'époque critique et sur les moyens propres à prévenir les accidents et les maladies qui en dépendent* (Paris: Didot Jeune, 1812), 10, 15, 24; Jean-Antoine Poussié, *Réflexions sur l'hygiène qui convient aux femmes arrivées à l'âge de retour*. Thèse (Montpellier: Jean Martel aîné, 1813), 6, 14–15; Claude-Martial Bardout, *Considérations générales sur la cessation du flux menstruel, et sur les précautions à prendre pour en prévenir les accidens ou les maladies*. Thèse (Paris: Didot Jeune, 1816), 40–41; Gardanne, *Avis aux femmes qui entrent dans l'âge critique*, 50–51, 63, 127, 154, 195.

[185] John Fothergill, *Conseils aux femmes sur les moyens de prévenir ou d'arrêter les suites facheuses de leur temps critique*, trans. Charles François Simon Giraudy (Paris: Crochard, 1805).

[186] Charles François Simon Giraudy, 'Introduction du traducteur' in Fothergill, *Conseils aux femmes sur les moyens*, [vii–xxiv], xiv.

[187] Ibid., xxi–xxiii.

[188] Their use is described still in Adolphe Charreire, *Myomes et ménopause, atrophie, dégénérescences malignes, indication*. Thèse (Montpellier: G. Firmin, Montane & Sicardi, 1907), 43–44.

[189] Assegond, *De la femme, considérée à l'âge critique*, 22.

and leeches, noting that all of these could be helpful for uterine haemorrhages in menopause, as long as they were used in moderation.[190] In 1828, the Paris candidate Duplessis recommended gentle purgatives to relieve the constipation he considered common in menopause, and noted the wide variety of such medications sold by pharmacies, such as 'Rufus's pills' (a mild purgative containing aloe, saffron, and myrrh), and other proprietary elixirs.[191] But he too enlisted Fothergill in his own disapproval of the habitual morning herbal drink of *vulnéraire* (woundwort or kidney vetch) for this purpose, which he said many women abused.[192] In 1837, the Paris candidate Charles-Victor Harreaux included purgatives as one of the crucial remedies for constipation in hypochondriac women in the critical age too.[193]

On the other hand, in 1824, N. N. Firmin Lemoyne, a Paris candidate who was a native of Montpellier, sided clearly with Fothergill in seeing purgatives as one of the very causes of women's complaints in the critical age, along with sudden temperature changes, defective foods, having damp feet, living in low, humid dwellings, consuming too much tea, coffee, or alcohol, or having too many enemas.[194] Here, as was often the case among menopause scholars, Fothergill was taken as support for a fundamentally hygienic approach (the topic of our next chapter). Constant Saucerotte, one of the Paris champions of the statistical evidence of women's greater longevity and of the anti-pathological view of women's ageing, in 1828 criticised Fothergill for exaggerating the ailments of menopause,[195] but agreed with him that purgatives, as well as most laxatives, were generally a bad idea.[196] The Montpellier candidate Jacques-Philippe Labarraque in 1827 discussed purgatives as a drug of abuse along with opiates, alcohol, and debauchery, all of which he said were pernicious to women in the critical age.[197]

Such questions also formed part of the contestation of the meaning of menstruation that was occurring in the early to mid-nineteenth century. In 1856, the renowned Parisian doctor Adam Raciborski placed the blame for erroneous treatments of menstrual disorders squarely on the shoulders of clinicians who categorised menstruation as a state of sanguine plethora, in which harmful elements

[190] Ibid., 26–27.

[191] E. Duplessis, *De l'âge critique et des soins hygiéniques que réclament les femmes à cette époque* (Paris: Didot Jeune, 1828), 15.

[192] Ibid., 16.

[193] Charles-Victor Harreaux, *Essai sur une variété d'hypocondrie particulière aux femmes de l'âge critique*. Thèse (Paris: Imprimerie et fonderie de Rignoux et Cie, 1837), 24.

[194] N. N. Firmin Lemoyne, *Considérations générales sur les phénomènes qui se manifestent à la cessation du flux menstruel et sur le régime que doivent adopter les femmes pour franchir heureusement cette époque*. Thèse (Paris: Didot Jeune, 1824), 12–13.

[195] Constant Saucerotte, *Nouveaux conseils aux femmes sur l'âge prétendu critique, ou conduite à tenir lors de la cessation des règles* (Paris: Madame Auger-Méquinon, 1828), 5.

[196] Ibid., 28.

[197] Jacques-Philippe Labarraque, *Aperçu physiologico-pathologique sur la menstruation en général, et quelques conseils d'hygiène pour l'âge critique en particulier*. Thèse (Montpellier: Chez Jean Martel aîné, 1827), 16.

were thought to need flushing out of the body through the use of emetic, purgative, and drastic remedies. This erroneous view of the mechanism of menstruation, he claimed, resulted both in the belief that diseases in young women could be cured simply by provoking menstruation, and in the mistaken avoidance of potentially valuable remedies which had the side effect of suppressing menstruation.[198] Notably, Raciborski here specified that the erroneous treatments he was referring to were those relating to young women, not older ones; and he attacked neither the ancient medical past, religious customs, nor folk healers, but indeed his very own contemporaries who continued to espouse the plethora view of menstruation.

The tone of Fothergill's tract, taken along with the assertions of Gardien, Labarraque, and others about the patient demand for purgatives, certainly seem to suggest that by the late eighteenth century at least some doctors, and perhaps some charlatans, folk healers, or women themselves were attempting to medicate away the final cessation of menses through the extension of common medical practices intended for younger women with 'untimely stoppage', which was associated with both hysteria/vapours and infertility. From the early modern sources discussed in Chapter 1, however, it seems that no physician actually advocated in writing trying to bring back the menses in women after their final cessation. Indeed, others before Fothergill (Freind, Duncan, and Astruc) had previously specifically excluded it, insisting that the age-related cessation of menses was part of the natural life course (or God's will) that should not be interfered with. Nonetheless, French doctors writing about menopause throughout the nineteenth century, particularly those trained in Paris, ubiquitously cited Fothergill in support of the view that the iatrogenic medication of menopause was part of an ancient and folk chemical tradition that had only recently been debunked by scientific, modern medicine. Fothergill was thus enlisted in French doctors' own anti-pathological insistences, making his anti-chemical stance a central theme of both pedagogic induction and professional identity.

Fothergill's contribution to medical thought about the cessation of menses is widely cited as one of the most important publications by most scholars who have worked on the comparative history of menopause.[199] However, the impact of his work in France was certainly not immediate, and it is clear from the earlier writings of Duncan and Astruc, and the contemporaneous work of Goubelly and Chambon de Montaux, that the French did not require Fothergill to give them the

[198] Adam Raciborski, *Du rôle de la menstruation dans la pathologie et la thérapeutique* [1844] (Paris: J.-B. Baillière, 1856), 3.

[199] Christine Théré, 'Âge de retour et retour d'âge: L'Asymétrie entre les sexes dans les discours médicaux en France (1770–1836)', *CLIO: Femmes, genre, histoire*, 42 (2015): 54–75; Louise Foxcroft, *Hot Flushes, Cold Science: A History of the Modern Menopause* (London: Granta Books, 2011), 92–120; Annick Tillier, 'Un âge critique: La Ménopause sous le regard des médecins des XVIIIe et XIXe siècles', *CLIO: Femmes, genre, histoire*, 21 (2005): 268–280. Doi: 10.4000/clio.1471; Michael Stolberg, 'Von den "Stufenjahren" zur "Menopause": Das Klimakterium im Wandel der Zeit', *Wurzburger Medizinhistorische Mitteilungen*, 24 (2005): 41–50; Wilbush, 'Menorraghia and Menopause'.

idea of describing women at this life stage. Clearly, many of the doctoral candidates and clinicians citing Fothergill viewed him as an important external verifier of the otherwise entirely French-dominated claim that women themselves worried too much about the cessation of menses and that the role of doctors was to set them straight on the matter. He provided discursive reinforcement for their self-important posturing as much as for their embrace of hygienic advice in the educational insistence on to the new role of doctors treating older elite women. But it also seems likely that Fothergill was so popular in French medicine because his pamphlet served internal arguments and was generative for the new theorisation of women's reproductive ageing, in multiple ways: for those displaying contempt for vitalist approaches to older women's health based on the model of humoral constitutions; for vitalists attempting to discredit mechanistic views of menstruation as the release of sanguinary plethora and of all menopausal women therefore needing phlebotomy; but also for alienists wishing to claim menopausal women among their own patient cohort by emphasising the damage that could be done to their nerves through common medical practices aimed at uterine health. The last purpose certainly underlay Giraudy's 1805 comments in his new translation of Fothergill. By focusing on Fothergill's version of the purgative objection, the new specialist scholars writing about women's critical age at both Montpellier and Paris could sustain the rejection of earlier figures such as Jeannet des Longrois, with his expansive list of diseases of older women to be treated with purgatives and blood-letting, now unfashionable in the new hygiene circles; or Duncan because he gave both Catholic religious and iatrochemical grounds for his analysis of women's physiology and denied all purpose for the treatment of the final cessation of menses; or Astruc because he was a mechanist with a hydraulic view of menstruation of the kind that vitalist medicine now eschewed, and because he too failed to provide a rationale for the exciting new medicalisation of menopause. As Elizabeth Williams notes, 'to young progressives Astruc came to represent what was hated and must be repudiated in medicine'.[200] But Jeannet des Longrois, with his typically eighteenth-century conflation of amenorrhea and the final cessation of menses and his listing of every possible disease of ageing as a direct consequence of it, was by far the biggest statue to be pulled down to make room for the new generation of menopause experts.

Claims about modern medical treatment of menopause breaking with erroneous 'traditional myths' clearly also derived from the competitive relations between different medical faculties of French universities in the late eighteenth and early nineteenth centuries—particularly between the two largest and most reputable faculties of Paris and Montpellier. Following the revolutionary changes in French medical institutions of 1790s, scholars in both schools writing about women's

[200] Williams, *A Cultural History of Medical Vitalism*, 120.

critical age or menopause made strident assertions of their modernity and scientific method, but important differences underlay their approaches to disease according to their greater or lesser orientation towards mechanistic, iatrochemical, vitalist, and organicist views of physiology. French doctors writing on menopause, then, in their critiques of 'traditional' attitudes, were probably more concerned with current competitive conflicts and with their own professional identity than with the medical past per se, despite their historical claims to enlightenment. Invocations of 'tradition' could refer to popular medicine which was assumed to be frozen in time—a relic of the past in which the follies of yesteryear were unwisely preserved. But it also referred to earlier generations of luminary figures in the history of French medicine, and to esteemed older professors attached to outmoded therapeutic methods, who could not be directly attacked and whose approaches were thus subsumed under the vague designation of traditions and myths. Although there is little evidence that folk practitioners and pharmacists ever specifically sought to medicate women's ageing with their remedies, it suited doctors to blame them for the supposedly 'traditional' purgative treatment of menopause and the toxic view of the bodies of women who were no longer menstruating. These practitioners could be safely denigrated and ridiculed in published scholarship and it certainly served doctors' competitive and professional interest to do so.

7

Menopause, Erotomania, and Degeneration in French Psychiatry

'La femme est la partie nerveuse du genre humain.'
('Woman is the nervous part of the human race.')
Pierre Berthier, *Médecine mentale*, 1857.[1]

'Les dégénérés, d'où ils viennent, sont, comme les monstres, susceptibles d'une classification scientifique.'
('Wherever they come from, degenerates, like monsters, are amenable to scientific classification.')
Charles Féré, *La Famille névropathique*, 1898.[2]

Few scholars of the history of psychiatric degenerationism in the nineteenth century appear to have noticed that menopausal women were consistently included among the list of 'misfits' of *fin-de-siècle* France, and were even sometimes the object of specialist works focused entirely on their unique mental or nervous pathologies.[3] Several major historical studies of nineteenth-century psychiatry or of European degenerationism make no mention of it whatsoever.[4] To be sure, menopause was not the most prominent topic in French degenerationist

[1] Pierre Berthier, *Médecine mentale* [1857], 2nd ed. (Paris: V. Masson, 1860), 38.

[2] Charles Féré, *La Famille névropathique: Théorie tératologique de l'hérédité et de la prédisposition morbides et de la dégénérescence*, 2nd ed. (Paris: F. Alcan, 1898), 230–1.

[3] On the other hand, numerous scholars have noted (in a single sentence each) that in the nineteenth century menopause was one of the things thought to cause hysteria or madness, including: Jessie Hewitt, *Institutionalizing Gender: Madness, the Family, and Psychiatric Power in Nineteenth-Century France* (Ithaca, NY/London: Cornell University Press, 2020), 24; Susan A. Ashley, *'Misfits' of Fin-de-Siècle France and Italy: Anatomies of Difference* (London: Bloomsbury, 2017), 176; Annick Tillier, 'Un âge critique: La Ménopause sous le regard des médecins des XVIIIe et XIXe siècles', *CLIO: Femmes, genre, histoire*, 21 (2005): 268–280; Christopher Crenner, *Private Practice: In the Early Twentieth-Century Office of Dr. Richard Cabot* (Baltimore: Johns Hopkins University Press, 2005), 120; Kelly Hurley, *The Gothic Body: Sexuality, Materialism, and Degeneration at the Fin de Siècle* (Cambridge: Cambridge University Press, 1996), 120; Mark S. Micale, *Approaching Hysteria: Disease and Its Interpretations* (Princeton: Princeton University Press, 1995), 39; German E. Berrios & Roy Porter, *A History of Clinical Psychiatry: The Origin and History of Psychiatric Disorders* (London: Athlone, 1995), 579.

[4] Daniel Pick, *Faces of Degeneration: A European Disorder, c.1848–c.1918* (Cambridge: Cambridge University Press, 1993); Ian Dowbiggin, *Inheriting Madness, Professionalization and Psychiatric Knowledge in Nineteenth-Century France* (Berkeley: University of California Press, 1991); Robert A. Nye, *Masculinity and Male Codes of Honor in Modern France* (New York/Oxford: Oxford University Press, 1993); Jean-Christophe Coffin, *La Transmission de la folie* (Paris: Harmattan, 2003);

The French Invention of Menopause and the Medicalisation of Women's Ageing: A History. Alison M. Downham Moore, Oxford University Press. © Alison M. Downham Moore 2022. DOI: 10.1093/oso/9780192842916.003.0008

Darwinian reproductive fitness that coloured later conceptions.[9] Another difference was that for Millot, entire nations of certain historic eras degenerated *en masse*, rather than specific strata or subgroups of the nation which thus became objects of persecution or denigration. Nonetheless, Millot clearly also blamed immoral behaviours and lifeways, imagining these could influence the inheritance of traits in the offspring—an idea suggested too in 1772 by the Paris naturalist Antoine Léonard Thomas in his historical survey of women's declining morals over recent centuries.[10] Modern French people had 'considerably abused those things necessary to our existence, especially our regenerative faculties, and by depravity of morals' had caused men 'to degenerate', Millot said, as reflected in the population decline France had begun to manifest.[11] The French nation was 'degenerating a great deal in the large towns and the neighbouring villages...' because people '...give themselves over too frequently to sensual love for it not to greatly damage their health, even their vitality'. Concupiscence was among the most dangerous threats to the health of the nation, Millot thought, namely all forms of it that did not result in conception.[12]

Millot's doctoral thesis, defended in Latin at the Paris faculty in 1771, had focused on uterine prolapse in women after childbirth and in old age.[13] He became best known for publishing a book in 1800 on the biological mechanism of sexual reproduction, followed shortly by another work on *The Art of Improving and Perfecting the Human Generations*, which advised couples how to have perfect children through sex-differentiated hygienic regimes of breastfeeding, avoidance of constipation, diet, exercise, and sleep, as well as discipline, religious induction, and education.[14] To be clear, Millot did not write anything specifically about menopause, but he is considered here because he provided a crucial bridge for two different ways of talking about degeneration in relation to reproductive medicine. The first was to describe the decline of peoples through a loss of hereditary vigour, as indicated by non-reproductive sexual behaviours; the second to describe the decline of the body's reproductive physiology in the process of ageing.[15] The idea that ageing badly in sexually moral terms caused the decline and decadence of nations was not well developed in Millot's work, despite his evocation of both forms of the word. But in the late nineteenth century several medical scholars did explicitly propose such a relationship between the loose morals,

[9] Petteri Pietikäinen, *Madness: A History* (London/New York: Routledge, 2015), 127–128.

[10] Antoine-Léonard Thomas, *Essai sur le caractère, les mœurs et l'esprit des femmes dans les différens siècles* (Paris: Moutard, 1772).

[11] Millot, *La Gérocomanie*, 55. [12] Ibid., 287.

[13] Jacques-André Millot, *De Uteri prolapsu: Theses anatomicae et chirurgicae* (Paris: P. A. le Prieur, 1771).

[14] Jacques-André Millot, *L'Art de procréer les sexes à volonté, ou histoire physiologique de la génération humaine* (Paris: Migneret, 1807); Jacques-André Millot, *L'Art d'améliorer et perfectionner les générations humaines*, 2 vols (Paris: Migneret, 1801).

[15] Millot, *La Gérocomanie*, 111.

perversions, and nervous pathologies of menopausal women and the degeneration of nations and races.

Between Millot's two forms of degeneration, and the late nineteenth-century view of menopausal erotomania as a sign of national decline, sat the development from 1812 to 1920 of medical ideas about the nervous and mental pathologies of women in the 'critical age'. As Robert Nye has considered, medical ideas about sexual variations were very often thought through the lens of degeneration precisely because of the link between sex and reproduction.[16] But it may seem odd that medical ideas about menopause would have raised the spectre of degeneration, given that older women who were no longer menstruating would presumably be unlikely to reproduce, thus contributing to humanity's inheritance of degenerate traits. Certainly, menopausal women did not constitute a major object of concern within the vast sea of writing about degeneration. Nonetheless, doctors writing about mental nervous pathologies increasingly included menopause as a causative factor, often drawing explicit parallels between perversion, degeneration, and women's reproductive ageing.

Degeneration in nineteenth-century French medicine was thought dangerous not only because sick traits could be passed on directly from one generation to the next through sexual reproduction (as in both Lamarckian and Darwinian-inspired forms of the idea), but also because degeneration was thought to be transmissible through cultural contagion, which could affect other humans in ways that could then be passed on through *their* offspring. This idea was not logically consistent with understandings of biological inheritance of the time, and sociological scholars of the *fin de siècle* sceptically questioned the mechanisms of such supposed transmissions between biology and culture that were so often proposed by doctors, psychiatrists, criminologists, and hygienists on these mysterious grounds.[17] The sexual drive was generally considered dysfunctional insofar as it was not purely oriented towards conception: non-reproductive 'perversions' (e.g. homosexuality, fetishism, sadism, masochism) like older women's sexual encounters, which all held little risk of conception, were therefore specifically those considered the most 'degenerate'. According to an oft-cited reductive view of the purpose of sex as purely for reproduction, women after the cessation of menses were thought to be no longer fit for sexual relations of any kind.[18] The menopausal erotic maniac, like the non-reproductive sexual pervert, was thus very much a threat to the health of the nation, even if she was not now likely to bear children of her own.

[16] Nye, *Masculinity and Male Codes of Honor in Modern France*, 71.

[17] Jean Demoor, Jean Massart, & Émile Vandervelde, *Évolution régressive en biologie et sociologie* (Paris: Félix Alcan, 1897).

[18] Auguste Debay, *Histoire naturelle de l'homme et de la femme* (Paris: E. Dentu, 1862), 445. Cited by Tillier, 'Un âge critique', 275.

Degenerationism no doubt expressed this peculiar culturalist form of anxiety in French medicine because of the influence of the eighteenth-century Parisian evolutionist Jean-Baptiste Lamarck (1744–1829), whose concept of the inheritance of acquired characteristics inspired medical speculations about the impact of culture on human evolution of which Lamarck himself would probably not have approved.[19] The Austrian/French psychiatrist Bénédicte-Augustin Morel (1809–1873) helped to legitimate the concept of degenerationism in Lamarckian terms in Parisian alienist circles following the publication of his 1857 *Traité des dégénérescences*.[20] Other early and mid-century scholars such as Jean-Étienne Dominique Esquirol (1772–1840), Alexandre Brierre de Boismont (1897–1881), and Noël Guéneau de Mussy (1813–1885) developed the theme of uterine changes, including menopause, causing erotic mania through the 'sympathetic' relation of the uterus or ovaries to women's nervous system. The next two generations of French psychiatrists, which included Benjamin Ball (1833–1893) and Valentin Magnan (1835–1916), followed by Paul Legrain (1860–1939), Émmanuel Régis (1855–1918), but also the prison doctor Émile Laurent (1861–1904), then expanded on these concepts. They presented them in relation to sexual behaviours they claimed were signs of degeneration, such as homosexuality and fetishistic perversions, but also menopausal eros, in part through their engagement with Austrian and Italian scholars such as Richard von Krafft-Ebing, Emil Kraepelin, and Cesare Lombroso, who also now included menopausal sexual perversion in their accounts of female deviancy.[21] According to the idea that became widely cited in psychiatry of the 1880s and 1890s, aberrant sexual behaviours, mental and nervous pathologies, and a wide spectrum of inherited diseases were signs of retrograde evolution, in which humans devolved to earlier, less perfect forms which would ultimately cause the extinction of the human race—or the defeat of modern nation-states by more robust European enemies.[22] The presence of such individuals in society was thought to be damaging not only because they might reproduce and make other degenerates like themselves, but also because they seduced others sexually, spread their degenerate ideas, engaged in political revolutions, produced corrupting works of art, literature, music, and scholarship, and generally participated in the cultural life of the nation to ill effect.[23] French

[19] Ernst Mayr, *The Growth of Biological Thought: Diversity, Evolution, and Inheritance* (Cambridge, Mass.: Harvard University Press, 1982), 108.

[20] Bénédicte Augustin Morel, *Traité des dégénérescences* (Paris: J. B. Balliere, 1857).

[21] Carolyn Warman, 'From Lamarck to Aberration: Nature, Hierarchies, and Gender', *Journal of the History of Sexuality*, 18/1 (2009): 8–25; Michel Coddens, 'La Théorie de l'hérédité-dégénérescence: Morel, Lombroso, Magnan et les autres', *L'En-je lacanien*, 27/2 (2016): 123–149.

[22] Pick, *Faces of Degeneration*, 40.

[23] Sylvie Chaperon, *Les Origines de la sexologie 1850–1900* (Paris: Louis Audibert, 2007), 66–69; Leslie Choquette, 'Degenerate or Degendered? Images of Prostitution and Homosexuality in the French Third Republic', *Historical Reflections/Réflexions historiques*, 23/2 (1997): 205–228; Robert A. Nye, 'Sexuality, Sex Difference and the Cult of Modern Love in the French Third Republic', *Historical Reflections/Réflexions historiques*, 20/1 (1994): 57–76.

psychiatry was a major vector of such ideas between the 1850s and the 1890s. Jessie Hewitt's 2020 monograph *Institutionalizing Gender* demonstrates the many French psychiatric characterisations of political radicals and feminists as degenerate and deranged subjects throughout the nineteenth century, and there is little doubt that the revolutionary uprisings of both 1848 and 1870 renewed French alienists'/psychiatrists' pessimism about the evolutionary health of the population.[24]

Still, degenerationist ideas of this kind infused medical and political writing about sexual and cultural matters throughout Europe in the late nineteenth century, not only in France.[25] The infamous 1892 tirade of the Austrian Zionist Max Nordau against decadent theatre, literature, art, and music implied a similar model of degeneration of the human species through cultural and behavioural influence.[26] The eminent Viennese psychiatrist Richard von Krafft-Ebing was also known for statements about sexual pathologies caused by genetic taint, which might take the form of having an alcoholic parent, or a family history of nervousness.[27] He too included erotically manic women (and men) around the *Klimakterium* among his examples of degenerates, as did the renowned Italian criminologists Cesare Lombroso and Guglielmo Ferrero.[28] The acquired-trait view of inheritance was categorically rejected in the 1890s by late nineteenth-century biologists such as the renowned Freiburg evolutionist August Weismann (1834–1914).[29] Darwinian evolutionary biologists of the twentieth century typically thereafter denied absolutely that genes could be altered by the actions of particular generations (although later epigenetic science has more recently refocused attention on environmental changes to gene expression, if not to the genome itself).[30] The modern biological model of genomic fixity emerging between the 1890s and 1940s no doubt helped to (eventually) seal the fate of neo-Lamarckian speculations about degenerate traits;[31] but this was not immediately accommodated in French medical ideas about ageing, nervous pathology, and sexuality between the 1880s and the 1920s. It was thus possible for respectable doctors to

[24] Jessie Hewitt, *Institutionalizing Gender: Madness, the Family, and Psychiatric Power in Nineteenth-Century France* (Ithaca, NY/London: Cornell University Press, 2020), 152–164.

[25] Pick, *Faces of Degeneration.*

[26] Max Nordau, *Entartung* [1892], 3rd ed. (Berlin: Carl Dunder, 1896).

[27] Richard von Krafft-Ebing, *Psychopathia Sexualis, mit besonderer Berücksichtung der konträren Sexualempfindung: Eine medizinisch-gerichtliche Studie für Ärzte und Juristen* [1886], 2nd ed. (Stuttgart: Verlag von Ferdinand Enke,1903), 80–99; Cesare Lombroso & Guglielmo Ferrero, *La donna delinquente: la prostituta e la donna normale* (Turin: L. Roux, 1893), 42; see Alison M. Moore, *Sexual Myths of Modernity: Sadism, Masochism, and Historical Teleology* (New York: Lexington Books, 2016), 23–54.

[28] Richard von Krafft-Ebing, *Lehrbuch der Psychiatrie: Auf Klinischer Grundlage für Praktische Ärzte und Studirende* [1879], 5th ed. (Stuttgart: F. Enke, 1893), 122, 158–159.

[29] August Weismann, *Das Keimplasma: Eine Theorie der Vererbung* (Jena: Fischer, 1892).

[30] Eva Jablonka and Marion J. Lamb, *Evolution in Four Dimensions: Genetic, Epigenetic, Behavioral, and Symbolic Variation in the History of Life*, rev. ed. (Cambridge, Mass.: MIT Press, 2014), 457–458.

[31] Mayr, *The Growth of Biological Thought*, 108.

make claims about menopausal nervous illness and erotic mania as signs of degeneration well into the 1920s.

As we saw in the previous chapter, after the 1770s and throughout the nineteenth century, women's 'critical age' or menopause was commonly cited as one of the vulnerable periods for the emergence of nervous pathologies, such as hysteria, hypochondria, or the vapours, though this idea was also sometimes contested. Parallel to these developments was the emergence of specialist French writing on madness (*la folie*), which overlapped with the designation of nervous pathology. Here too, beginning in the 1820s, women's 'critical age' or menopause began to be listed as one of the causes. The influential Paris alienist Étienne-Jean Georget (1795–1828), a student of Pinel, referred to it in all his major works on both mental and nervous pathologies, and no doubt would have joined the growing chorus of opinion on the matter had he not died suddenly at 33.[32] He said that the 'critical time' was one in which 'the vital equilibrium is easily disturbed'.[33] In the 1840s and 1850s the idea attracted renewed interest among scholars writing on the new concept of hereditary mental and nervous diseases, though some influential works in this genre still frequently ignored menopause.[34] Many of those who did now refer to menopause as a time of mental pathology also referred to it as a time of heightened sexual excess and perversion. Nineteenth-century doctors' accounts of sexual desires and acts in women in or after menopause as aberrant, perverse, or degenerate derived from the degenerationist view that held all non-reproductive sex in suspicion as a mark of retrograde evolution, since lust should emanate directly from the reproductive drives. This contained an element of a very old conceptual layer derived from medieval Catholic theology,[35] though extended in the newer biomedical mechanistic model that had been emerging throughout the eighteenth century that held the uterus (later the ovaries) to be the determining organ of women's sexual impulses, as well as both menstruation and ovulation. Without the latter functions and with the atrophy of these organs after menopause, there was no reason to expect an older woman either to want sex or to be capable of pleasure. In his 1838 treatise on the diseases of women, the Paris doctor Sébastien-Didier l'Héritier remarked—as if were a complete

[32] Étienne-Jean Georget, *De la folie, considérations sur cette maladie, suivies de recherches cadavériques* (Paris: Crevot, 1820), 148–154, 334; 184–185; Étienne-Jean Georget, *De la physiologie du système nerveux et spécialement du cerveau, recherches sur les maladies nerveuses en général et en particulier sur le siège, la nature et le traitement de l'hystérie, de l'hypochondrie, de l'épilepsie et de l'asthme convulsif*, 2 vols (Paris: J.-B. Baillière, 1821), vol. 1, 184–185; 196–197; Étienne-Jean Georget, *De la folie ou aliénation mentale* (Paris: Rignoux, 1823), 9–10, 88.

[33] Georget, *De la folie*, 153.

[34] For instance, Prosper Lucas, *Traité philosophique et physiologique de l'hérédité naturelle dans les états de santé et de maladie*, 2 vols (Paris: J. B. Baillière, 1850).

[35] Jessica E. Godfrey, *Attitudes to Post-Menopausal Women in the High and Late Middle Ages, 1100–1400* (Jessica E. Godfrey, 2011), 30–32; Ruth Formanek, 'Continuity and Change and the "Change of Life": Premodern Views of the Menopause', in Ruth Formanek, ed., *The Meanings of Menopause: Historical, Medical, and Clinical Perspectives* (Hillsdale, NJ: Analytic Press, 1990), 3–41.

paradox—that 'at the time of the cessation of periods... it can happen that women sometimes experience the desire for sexual relations'.[36] The conflation of sexual desire with fertility was found just as much in French literary engagements with medicine: Honoré de Balzac's 1838 *Physiologie de l'amour*, for example, described the 'critical age' beginning around the age of 40 as signalling the loss of women's capacity for 'passions'.[37] In 1868, the Paris gynaecologist Adam Raciborski naturalised the connection in asserting that 'the females of mammals also have their puberty and their critical age' in the sense that

> they are only apt for reproduction quite some time after birth, and at a certain age, once they begin to grow old, they no longer display manifestations of rut and they become completely sterile.[38]

Raciborski (following Jean-Étienne Esquirol) cited the case of a woman of 50 years who had ceased menstruating one year previously but resumed regular menstruation again for several years following 'an amorous passion' that 'troubled her rest'.[39] Not only should sexual impulses be expected to cease with the end of menstruation, but the finished menses in turn could be aberrantly reawakened by sexual stimulus.

If the post-menopausal state was widely agreed to be a normatively sexless time, then expressions of it after menopause could be taken automatically as signs of pathology. Many doctors also argued that the transitional state that was the *âge critique, temps critique, âge de retour*, or simply *la ménopause*, before the menses had definitively ended, could be a time of heightened and aberrant eroticism. One idea appearing from early in the nineteenth century was that menopause was essentially a circular repetition of puberty, particularly mimicking the pre-menstrual state of pubescent girls. This meant that women in the critical age could display a resurgence of heightened sexual desire, even 'erotic mania', similar to that supposedly observed in puberty. Jacques Devers's Paris thesis on menstrual suppression and cessation of 1822, for instance, began by evoking the parallels between 'the first appearance of menses' and 'their cessation'.[40] Nervous disorders such as hysteria, hypochondria, melancholy, mania, convulsions, apoplexy, and paralysis were to be expected at both times of life.[41] The Paris alienist Alexandre Brierre de Boismont (1879–1881) played a major role in developing this concept when he included several chapters on the 'critical age' in his large

[36] Sébastien-Didier l'Héritier, *Traité complet des maladies de la femme, étudiées sous les rapports physiologique, nosographique et thérapeutique* (Paris: Bulletin du Bureau Clinique, 1838), 149–150.

[37] Honoré de Balzac, *Physiologie de l'amour* (Paris: Chapentier, 1828), 21.

[38] Adam Raciborski, *Traité de la menstruation, ses rapports avec l'ovulation, la fécondation, l'hygiène de la puberté et de l'âge critique* (Paris: J. B. Baillière, 1868), 43.

[39] Ibid., 255.

[40] Jacques Devers, *Essai sur la cessation des règles*. Thèse (Paris: Didot le Jeune, 1822), 5.

[41] Ibid., 11.

1842 work on the pathologies of menstruation.[42] Brierre de Boismont's patient case studies exemplified the 'plethoric' issues of uterine tumours and haemorrhages, which he emphasised were not accompanied by any mental symptoms.[43] Nonetheless, he insisted that 'disorders of the nervous system' were also 'very pronounced' among women during the critical age.[44] These took the form of 'exhausting dreams, insomnia, bizarre sensations and desires, spasms, sadness, anger, melancholy, changes of character and states of exaltation'.[45] But there were also 'a certain number of women' whose pathology manifested in the 'organs of generation', producing an 'excitement that becomes the source of strong, impetuous desires', which if satisfied, resulted in haemorrhages or even cancer.[46]

Brierre de Boismont's 1851 article in the *Annales medico-psychologiques* on the role of menstruation in mental pathology was also widely cited by most other scholars writing thereafter about degenerate mental pathologies in menopause.[47] He discussed many case examples of other doctors that referred to mental illness in menstruating women and women whose menses were suppressed, including Esquirol, as well as the eighteenth-century Dutch scholars Gerard van Swieten and Herman Boerhaave, who wrote about hysteria; he added that he himself had also observed mental illness in women in the *temps critique*.[48] Brierre de Boismont was thus a crucial link in drawing earlier ideas about menstrual hysteria into the new elaboration of mental pathology in menopause. This was not an obvious step, as we saw in the previous chapter—many doctors in the first half of the nineteenth century frankly doubted that hysteria applied to women in the critical age at all, given that the uterus was no longer exerting its control of the organism, and cited case examples of women whose nervousness appeared to be cured by the final cessation of menses. Brierre de Boismont insisted that hysteria, hypochondria, and other serious mental pathologies were all common in menopause precisely because they were features of young women prior to menstruation, which tended to improve once the menses flowed. The pattern was that all forms of irregular or missing menses deranged the nervous system. He conceded some mystery about whether it was menstruation and disturbances thereof (including menopause) that caused mental illness, or whether mental illness caused perturbations to the menses. He said he had observed both patterns, with many women cured once their menses resumed.[49] Either way, there was no doubting the intimate relationship of the uterus to women's nervous systems.

[42] Alexandre F. Brierre de Boismont, *De la menstruation, considérée dans ses rapports physiologiques et pathologiques* (Paris: Germer Baillière, 1842).

[43] Ibid., 234. [44] Ibid., 236. [45] Ibid., 237. [46] Ibid., 238.

[47] Alexandre F. Brierre de Boismont, 'Recherches bibliographiques et cliniques sur la folie puerpérale, précédées d'un aperçu sur les rapports de la menstruation et de l'aliénation mentale', *Annales médico-psychologiques* (1851): 574–610.

[48] Ibid., 593. [49] Ibid., 594–595.

He devoted an entire section of the paper to the *temps critique*, with eleven case examples of women aged between 42 and 55 years whose menses had either ended or become irregular (both of which Brierre de Boismont took to be a sure sign of approaching menopause in anyone over 40, despite observing irregular and suppressed menses in women of all ages).[50] The approach of the *âge de retour* was 'often the point of departure for madness'.[51] He considered menopause to be one of the peak times when hysteria in particular could be expected, citing Hoffmann as his authority on the matter, but he also credited the Paris professor Pierre Béclard with the observation of hypochondria in this period of women's lives.[52] Two common features of menopausal madness were desire for alcohol and orgasms of 'an extreme intensity'.[53]

One 45-year-old woman of 'high birth' (Observation XVIII) trailed the streets of Paris at night propositioning men 'of the lowest class' for sex, leading to her being brought to an asylum. The only problem was that there appeared to be nothing wrong with her: 'Nothing in her words, her actions appeared in line with this perversion of the sexual instinct [*l'instinct génésique*].' Brierre de Boismont said the clinicians spent hours chatting with her on several occasions and pressing her for answers, during which she treated them with a 'cold and contemptuous air', but they still could not agree what her pathology was.[54] She appears to have been kept in various asylums for many years, becoming increasingly frustrated and hostile to treatment and thus to be seen as a troublesome patient. Boismont pronounced flatly: 'This woman died insane.'[55] Similarly, Mademoiselle C. (Observation XXI) was a tall, strong 44-year-old woman with brown hair, a 'developed and cultivated intellect', an 'imperious character', and a strong will (*d'une grande force de volonté*) who became 'delirious' during her menstrual period after a personal disappointment. On arrival at the clinic, she refused to wear clothes at all and so was placed in a straitjacket. She returned to sanity after her menses ceased, and provided interesting conversation to the doctors by virtue of her 'varied knowledge'.[56] But the pattern apparently kept recurring with each menstrual cycle, leading her family to seek her 'interdiction', for fear that she would compromise the family reputation and fortune. The magistrates interviewed her during one of her lucid phases and so adjourned the case, seeing no cause for her incarceration. Only after Brierre de Boismont wrote to the magistrates reporting a relapse was a provisional administrator of her affairs appointed.[57]

These stories appear to confirm the potential for the menopausal erotic pathology hypothesis to result in women being treated as mad and subject to confinement in asylums purely on account of their unusual sexual behaviours and

[50] Ibid., 599–610. [51] Ibid., 601. [52] Ibid., 599. [53] Ibid., 599.
[54] Ibid., 600. [55] Ibid., 601. [56] Ibid., 603. [57] Ibid., 604.

corporeal habits. Jessie Hewitt's case studies of individuals' involuntary psychiatric confinement by their families in nineteenth-century France similarly identified unconventional life choices as having made people from upper middle-class and aristocratic families vulnerable to this form of control.[58] Article 18 of the new 1838 law, known as *la loi Esquirol*, enabled this kind of collusion of psychiatry with parental control over sons and daughters.[59] It authorised the Paris police prefect to place in asylums all those 'whose state of madness compromised public order or the security of persons', contributing to the doubling of the asylum population between 1838 and 1848, and its continued growth throughout the period from 1849 to 1939 from 20,000 to 110, 000.[60] Since under Napoleonic law, women were the legal property of their fathers while unmarried, and their husbands once married, the 1838 law created conditions for the radical denial of their liberty by families and by psychiatrists purely in relation to their sexual conduct. Brierre de Boismont's case examples suggest this was certainly happening to women in their forties and fifties on the grounds that they suffered menopausal erotic mania or hysteria.

One reason menopause was of interest to French psychiatrists as a possible cause of mental pathologies and a sign of degeneration, from this time until after the First World War, is that it appeared to offer one of those rare examples of something material that explained nervous disease, otherwise noted to be so often without detectable lesions. Ian Dowbiggin's work on the history of French psychiatry has drawn attention to the struggles of clinicians and researchers in this period to locate physiological mechanisms of madness that aligned to the new dominant materialist insistence of modern biomedicine.[61] As Robert Nye notes, degeneration appealed to alienists in the generation orbiting the Paris physiology professor Claude Bernard (1813–1878), offering the hope that it would lead to the discovery of the organic, material causes of hereditary diseases as well as mental and nervous pathologies.[62] Menopause was not clearly mechanistically defined, but the cessation of menses was nonetheless now widely recognised as entailing distinct physiological changes to the internal reproductive organs, which appeared to be a universal condition of women's reproductive life cycle—comparable to puberty and pregnancy. As such it appeared to provide a solid example of physiological causation that supported the agenda of claiming hysteria, hypochondria, melancholy, and mania as nervous disorders for which the lesions simply had not yet been located. Degeneration too was viewed as a

[58] Hewitt, *Institutionalizing Gender*, 92–116.

[59] Dowbiggin, *Inheriting Madness*, 95–100.

[60] Aude Fauvel, 'Avant-propos', *Romantisme*, 141 (2008): 3–9 [6]; Thierry Haugsten, 'Les Évolutions institutionnelles et théoriques de la psychiatrie française entre 1838 et 1914', *Annales médico-psychologiques, revue psychiatrique*, 172/1 (2014): 45–51.

[61] Dowbiggin, *Inheriting Madness*, 44, 149.

[62] Nye, *Masculinity and Male Codes of Honor*, 72.

physiological mechanism, albeit inexplicably projected onto a wide variety of decadent cultural expressions and perverse sexual fantasies. Continuing ideas about hysteria played their role here too. As Mark Micale notes, after the 1890s the search for identifiable lesions underlying hysteria, associated with Charcot's work, was increasingly viewed by both neurologists and psychiatrists in Europe as a failed enterprise.[63] Nonetheless, by this time, the view of menopausal women as degenerate, manic, and hypersexual had already been reiterated many times in major French psychiatric works, even as a few dissenters had also managed to hold their ground.

In 1848, Michel-Victor Barbier defended his Paris thesis on the influence of menstruation on mental illness.[64] He said that, from his own clinical observations at the Charenton asylum, those with regular menstruation displayed no signs of influence of their approaching or current menstruation on their mental health, whereas those with irregular menstruation did.[65] He also noted large numbers of women whose menses were suppressed, with mental pathologies seeming to emerge around the same time, including numerous case observations. One woman aged 40 became melancholic, started having religious hallucinations, and began frenetically masturbating, all around the time when her menses abruptly ceased. She made a complete recovery only when her menses returned several months later.[66] Barbier included an entire chapter on the 'Influence of menopause on mental illnesses' which disagreed with Esquirol's suggestion that many women with a lifelong history of nervous diseases were relieved of them by the cessation of menses in ageing.[67] He claimed that, of 170 women he had treated at the Charenton asylum, 39 had gone mad at the time of their menopause. Of these 39, he estimated that 12 were also due to a hereditary cause, 9 appeared to have no other cause than menopause itself, 11 also had 'moral' causes, and 5 had other physiological causes.[68] But he cited only one case observation here, Mme D. (age not recorded), whose menstruation had ceased one year earlier. She had always enjoyed good health and had experienced no negative events that could explain her mental illness other than menopause. She began having abdominal pains, feeling weak, trembling, and wanting to cry all the time, and complained of smelling bad odours constantly. She was 'tormented' by worries about her son and husband, and reproached herself for being incapacitated. As a treatment, she was repeatedly cauterised on the leg, 'perhaps as a means of supplementing the menstrual flow which had ceased to take place', Barbier speculated. After one month of this she was apparently cured.[69]

[63] Mark Micale, *Approaching Hysteria: Disease and Its Interpretations* (Princeton: Princeton University Press, 1995), 26, 278.

[64] Michel-Victor Barbier, *De l'influence de la menstruation sur les maladies mentales.* Thèse (Paris: Rignoux, 1848).

[65] Ibid., 6–7. [66] Ibid., 10–11. [67] Ibid., 31–2.

[68] Ibid., 30. [69] Ibid., 31–32.

The Absorption of Women's Ageing into French Degenerationist Psychiatry

The erotic-mania/puberty view of menopause was the central claim of another Paris thesis by Henri-Eugène Rocque in 1858.[70] He claimed that menopausal women, like teenage girls before their period, develop 'bizarre tastes, changes of character…become irascible, morose and prone to emotions'. Others were tormented by headaches, migraines, insomnia, exhausting dreams, vertigo, dizzy spells, hot flushes, palpitations, heavy sweating, digestive problems, flatulence, troubled breathing, and often had sore and swollen breasts, just as they did in puberty.[71] The puberty/menopause parallel was not intuitive, the author acknowledged:

> Although the final result must precisely be the inverse, that is, in the first case, complete development; in the second case, the atrophy of the organ; the preparatory work for both seems absolutely identical.[72]

Rocque claimed that he had the opportunity to observe in insane asylums that these two ages of puberty and menopause were when *la manie érotique* was most common, arguing that these distinct ages for the 'maximum development of the passions' had been observed by all the great minds who had probed the mysteries of the human heart. He attempted to attribute the idea to a long list of other (both eminent and obscure) medical scholars that 'love is never so close to fury as when it begins to form and when it is close to being finished'.[73] However while some of those he cited by way of support—including Béclard, Beau, Pinel, Vigarous, Hardy and Béhier, Grisolle, and Hoffmann—indeed drew parallels between puberty and menopause, or between menstruation and hysteria, nonetheless they made no explicit claims about menopausal women being erotic maniacs, with the exception of Brierre de Boismont. Rocque cited a substantial body of case histories of women aged 40–50 years whom he had treated or observed in his clinical training; most, however, referred not to mental illness in particular but to headaches, nose-bleeds, backaches, and heavy uterine bleeding, and are listed under the headings of 'plethoric affections' and 'haemorrhages'.[74] Only those case histories listed in the final section of his thesis, on 'nervous affections', seem to reflect anything like his account of menopausal mania or hysteria. But on closer inspection, these all describe women over 50, some as old as 65, who were, by his own account, suffering epileptic seizures.[75] Could the absence of any specific case

[70] Henri-Eugène Rocque, *Essai sur la physiologie et la pathologie de la ménopause*. Thèse (Paris: Rignoux, 1858).
[71] Ibid., 25. [72] Ibid., 26. [73] Ibid., 28–29.
[74] Ibid., 31–45. [75] Ibid., 46–50.

examples of the sexually manic menopausal patient that Rocque claimed was common reflect a degree of fantasy in this student-doctor's perceptions?

The year before, in 1857, the first major specialist work on menopause was published in English by the gynaecologist Edward Tilt (1815–1893). It too had a lot to say about erotomania in the climacteric, which he considered to be a 'mental affection' caused by 'morbid ovarian influence, by uterine affections, and by the various kinds of pudendal disease'.[76] Tilt had completed his doctoral studies at the University of Paris in the 1830s, and it was clearly this experience that informed his uptake of the French medical concepts of menopausal nervous pathologies.[77] He had already broached the subject of women's 'critical ages' in another 1851 book full of very French-sounding hygienic advice.[78] Although Tilt's work was heavily derivative of existing French scholarship, he was immediately reviewed by Brierre de Boismont, and cited by numerous other French scholars too who took his English language publications as confirmation of the universal importance of their discovery of menopausal mental pathologies.[79] Numerous historians have cited Tilt's ideas about menopausal nymphomania, without apparent awareness of the significant corpus of French works that clearly influenced the Englishman's account.[80] But he was above all an important vector for the spread of French medical concepts of women's ageing into the English-speaking world.

Another curious contributor to the development of the menopausal degenerate madness idea was the Montpellier-trained alienist and inspector of Paris asylums Pierre Berthier (1830–1877), who had worked in the 1850s and 1860s at the asylums of Auxerre and of la Madeleine in Bourg-en-Bresse. Berthier's 1857 general manual of mental medicine referred to 'periodicity' as one of the defining features of madness—it was not constant and recurred whenever the nervous system was perturbed.[81] One way this could happen was through 'venereal excesses' which weakened the nerves; other ways included though lactation, pregnancy, and due to inheritance.[82] Other behavioural (*morales*) predispositions could also

[76] Edward John Tilt, *The Change of Life in Health and Disease: A Practical Treatise on the Nervous and Other Affections Incidental to Women at the Decline of Life* (London: J. Churchill, 1857), 239.

[77] Edward John Tilt, *Questions sur diverses branches des sciences médicales*. Thèse (Paris: Rignoux, 1839).

[78] Edward John Tilt, *On the Preservation of the Health of Women at the Critical Periods of Life* (London: John Churchill, 1851).

[79] Alexandre Brierre de Boismont, 'Bibliographie: The Change of Life in Health and Disease. A practical Treatise on the Nervous and other Affections incidental to Women at the Decline of Life. By Dr. Edward John Tilt, London, 1857', *Annales médico-psychologiques: Revue psychiatrique; Bulletin officiel de la Société Médico-Psychologique*, vol. 16 (Paris: Victor Masson, 1858), 480–482.

[80] Susan P. Matterns, *The Slow Moon Climbs: The Science, History and Meaning of Menopause* (Princeton: Princeton University Press, 2019), 279; Louise Foxcroft, *Hot Flushes, Cold Science: A History of the Modern Menopause* (London: Granta Books, 2011), no page numbers; Elaine Showalter, *The Female Malady: Women, Madness, and English Culture, 1830–1980* (London: Penguin, 1985), 129.

[81] Berthier, *Médecine mentale*, 26. [82] Ibid., 27–30.

contribute, such as drinking alcohol, being an artist or intellectual, having been brought up too strictly as a child, and religious excess.[83] Women passed on madness to their children more often than men, and more often to daughters than sons.[84] Mixing of the races, too, resulted in mental alienation, explaining its high prevalence among the English and French aristocracies, which for centuries had formed too many conjugal alliances.[85] 'Woman is the nervous part of humanity,' he announced, explaining that women's periodic changes, such as puberty and menopause, were thus also periods of susceptibility to madness, due to the pathological sympathy of the uterus and the brain.[86] Menopause should be a period of 'sexual neutrality', but the disturbance of equilibrium created by the cessation of the menstrual flow caused *hypérémie* (accumulation of blood) in the brain, making it phlegmatic and soft.[87] Citing the English doctor Tilt, he claimed women in the critical age became morose but also coquettish, or else highly religious.[88] But he also drew from Hoffmann and Stahl in his account of melancholic hypochondria, which was provoked in women of all ages by the absence of menstruation.[89]

In his 1874 book on mental pathologies of menstrual origin, Berthier, like Brierre de Boismont, raised the idea that it was mental pathology that disturbed the menses, rather than the other way around.[90] Whatever the direction of influence, the uterus and brain existed in a special sympathetic relation.[91] His many case examples referred mostly to young women, but several referred to women in the 'critical age' or *âge de retour*, whose symptoms would clearly not today be classed as indicating mental pathologies. One, the case of a woman aged 51 who suffered 'cerebral congestion' with a sudden loss of motor control of one side of her body and face and abrupt incapacity to work, resulting in her death within three years, reads much like what twenty-first-century medicine might identify as a stroke rather than a menopausal mental pathology.[92] He described another patient he had seen who was 48 years old and a nun, who had developed migraines (which he considered to be a nervous symptom) coinciding with the cessation of her menses. He prescribed cauterisation on her leg as form of 'artificial fluxion' to substitute for her absent monthly flow.[93] Another two patients, one 46 and the other 53, in the asylum of Madeleine de Bourg, had also developed migraines and intermittent fevers (another supposedly nervous symptom) following their cessation of menses. Their fevers passed, but they remained insane, he said.[94] Another woman aged 41 had ceased menstruating and developed a heart condition and vertigo, dying within a year. Berthier conceded that her critical age could not entirely explain this, but affirmed that it must surely nonetheless have

[83] Ibid., 40–46. [84] Ibid., 31–32. [85] Ibid., 35.
[86] Ibid., 38. [87] Ibid., 50–60. [88] Ibid., 61. [89] Ibid., 63.
[90] Pierre Berthier, *Des névroses menstruelles, ou La Menstruation dans ses rapports avec les maladies nerveuses et mentales* (Paris: Delahaye, 1874), 5–6.
[91] Ibid., 9. [92] Ibid., 91. [93] Ibid., 25. [94] Ibid., 28.

contributed.[95] He concluded that for some women neurosis (*la névrose*) was the 'obligatory consequence of menstruation' but that the cessation of menses often simply brought 'a different neuropathy'.[96] Several cases are described of 'erotomania', including one in a woman aged 52 who had not menstruated in ten years, but entered marked 'erotic delirium' after her menses returned spontaneously.[97] He cited the example of Barthez's patient, discussed in the previous chapter, who had developed headaches, hot flushes, and tingling in her extremities as she was 'nearing the time when one might expect her periods to finish' ('approche du temps où l'on a lieu de croire que les règles finiront'). This was known to be caused by the exhaustion of heavy bleeding, which in turn was caused by 'hysterical orgasm'.[98]

Berthier too provided a curious bridge between the eighteenth-century vitalist and mechanistic accounts of hysteria and vapours that conflated menstrual suppression with the final cessation of menses, and the nineteenth-century (mostly Parisian) alienist view of all of women's reproductive changes, especially menopause, as the cause of mental and nervous pathologies in degenerate patients. Consequently, in rehearsing the standard Montpellier hygiene statement about how clean country living according to the 'wishes of nature' ('le vœu de la nature') results in an easier menopause, while a life of debauched, urban, gluttonous laziness made it troublesome for the nerves, he added to the list of aggravating factors carrying 'the weight of a hereditary burden' ('le poids d'une charge héréditaire').[99] Nonetheless, his work was also full of qualifying statements, notation of exceptions, and concessions to opposing viewpoints. He soberly admitted that nymphomania was extremely rare at any age.[100] And he conceded that some women in menopause were cured of mental pathologies associated with their periods.[101] His own patient data clearly indicated far more diagnoses of hysteria and nervousness in young women than in midlife, leading him to conclude that the critical age was overall a less aggravating state than menstruation.[102]

In the 1860s and 1870s, general psychiatric textbooks reiterated the new account of menopause as a time of mental and nervous pathology. The eminent Strasbourg professor Henri Dagonet mentioned repeatedly in his influential 1862 *Traité élémentaire et pratique des maladies mentales* that both puberty and the 'critical age' were periods of life which exerted an 'incontestable' pathogenic influence on the mental state of women and girls.[103] The Paris professor Eugène Bouchut, in his 1877 book of lectures on the acute and chronic nervous disorders, also flagged the critical age as a time of new, prolonged 'nervousness'

[95] Ibid., 39–40. [96] Ibid., 50. [97] Ibid., 142.
[98] Ibid., 64. [99] Berthier, *Des névroses menstruelles*, 238–239.
[100] Ibid., 178. [101] Ibid., 156. [102] Ibid., 244.
[103] Henri Dagonet, *Traité élémentaire et pratique des maladies mentales, suivi de considérations pratiques sur l'administration des asiles d'aliénés* (Paris: J. B. Baillière et fils, 1862), 194, 238, 258, 398, 411.

('nervosisme'), particularly for upper-class women.[104] Another 1862 *Practical Treatise of Mental Diseases* by the Paris professor Louis-Victor Marcé likewise cited the critical age as one of the causes of madness in women.[105] There were also several new books and theses which advanced the discourse of menopausal mental pathologies and nervous disorders, with a focus on erotic mania. The Paris graduate and faculty professor Noël Guéneau de Mussy (1813–1885) sparked considerable interest in the notion that menopausal women were sexually excessive with an article in the Parisian *Gazette hebdomadaire de médecine et de chirurgie* (Weekly Gazette of Medicine and Surgery) in 1871, subsequently cited by many other scholars.[106] This doctor was writing to report numerous cases of what he described as 'erotism, or female satyriasis' ('érotisme, ou satyriasis féminin') in his observation of women in the *âge critique*, who up until this time had 'moderate erotic instincts', but who now found themselves 'tormented by intolerable, violent, genital/sexual excitation ('excitations génésiques'), which, he remarked, was often aggravated by bedrest, adding 'these erotic crises may be very short and can repeat themselves several times in a day; they can also endure for hours'.[107]

Guéneau de Mussy also reported on several case examples of women he had treated. The first in 1870 was a 45-year-old woman visiting Paris from somewhere outside 'the continent', though he did not say from where. She was 'of an austere demeanour', had very seldom had sexual relations, and was the mother of six children, the last of whom was born when she was 39 years old, after which she had no further 'conjugal relations'.[108] She was still menstruating, but Guéneau de Mussy considered her to be now 'approaching menopause' based on what she reported, which he classified as a 'vésanie génitale' ('genital vesania' (madness)).[109] She complained of swollen, painful, sensitive breasts and abdominal bloating for five to six days prior to each menstrual period; and told him that, having always been quite 'cold' sexually, she now found herself very responsive to her husband, experiencing a 'violent excitation' when he came to caress her without performing 'the conjugal act', after which she was exhausted, with trembling, weak legs, and sensitivity and pain in the right iliac region, for several days. She had trouble sleeping because her 'imagination constantly brought memories of conjugal scenes back to her that had caused her much less emotion when they occurred'. Her clitoris and mons pubis were affected by 'pruritus' (itching) and she was driven to scratch herself furiously.[110] Another patient of a similar age he described as suffering 'very painful challenges' ('épreuves très-pénibles') of a similar kind; nonetheless, she enjoyed 'an appearance of radiant health' ('jouissait d'une santé

[104] Eugène Bouchut, *Du nervosisme aigu et chronique et des maladies nerveuses* (Paris: J. B. Baillière et fils, 1877), 27–28.

[105] Louis-Victor Marcé, *Traité pratique des maladies mentales* (Paris: Baillière, 1862), 142–143, 388.

[106] Noël Guéneau de Mussy, 'Érotisme de la ménopause', *Gazette hebdomadaire de médecine et de chirurgie*, 37 (13 October 1871): 591–595.

[107] Ibid., 593. [108] Ibid., 591. [109] Ibid., 593. [110] Ibid., 591.

en apparence florissante').[111] Her family life became troubled, and she developed heavy haemorrhagic bleeding with a uterine fibroid, becoming anaemic and suffering uterine prolapse. Guéneau de Mussy prescribed a supportive belt for the prolapse, and (sedative) potassium bromide, warm baths with sodium arsenate, along with suppositories of belladonna, camphor, and hemlock ('cigüe'). He heard from this patient again several years later when she was 50 years old, reporting good health and only minor recurrences of her symptoms, which she was able to manage with doses of bromide or arsenic and hydrotherapy treatments once or twice a year.[112]

In the late 1870s, another three Paris doctoral candidates produced theses on mental and nervous pathology in menopause: Louis-Antoine Pagès in 1876, Théodore Willette in 1877, and Henri Ricard in 1879.[113] The convergence of this swathe of candidates on menopausal madness was most likely on the advice of the professor of clinical training in mental pathology of the Paris faculty, Benjamin Ball. Along with his colleague Charcot, Ball was one of the most influential scholars of French mental and nervous pathologies in the late 1870s. Pagès was from the south of France (Lot) and graduated from the rapidly growing faculty of Nancy within the distinctly psychiatric camp, but claimed the 'nervous' symptoms of menopause under his remit as well. He acknowledged that the view of menopause as a time of disturbances was controversial in nineteenth-century French medicine beyond psychiatry, with many doctors attributing to it every single affliction seen in older women, while others 'react too strongly against this tendency' in considering menopause an innocuous natural process.[114] He admitted that the naturalising view (which he attributed to Raciborski) was 'seductive', but nonetheless he was not persuaded by it because, he said, in practice things proved otherwise ('pratiquement, les choses sont loin de se passer de la sorte').[115] He expressed frustration at the constraints of sexual modesty ('la pudeur') that made it difficult to extract certain kinds of information from menopausal women.[116] He cited the erotomania claims of other scholars, namely Brierre de Boismont: with the atrophy of the genital organs in menopause, 'the woman feels a reawakening of erotic tendencies which are sometimes dispiriting'.[117] He was not prepared to say that only women who had indulged in 'venereal vice' in their youth were prone to menopausal erotomania, since he considered all women at risk of such pathologies; but he did consider those who had 'greatly indulged in the pleasures [of bodily life]' to be particularly susceptible since their nervous

[111] Ibid., 592. [112] Ibid., 593.

[113] Louis-Antoine Pagès, *De la ménopause et de son influence dans la production de l'aliénation mentale.* Thèse (Nancy: A. Parent, 1876); Théodore Willette, *Étude sur les accidents nerveux de la ménopause.* Thèse (Paris: A. Parent, 1877); Henri Ricard, *Étude sur les troubles de la sensibilité génésique à l'époque de la ménopause.* Thèse (Paris: A. Derenne, 1879).

[114] Pagès, *De la ménopause et de son influence*, 6.

[115] Ibid., 22. [116] Ibid., 6–7. [117] Ibid., 19.

system had been excessively excited, 'acquiring a sort of hyperaesthesia' in the critical age.[118]

Henri Ricard (1849–1910), who later entered politics and became a senator from the Côte d'Or under the Third Republic, wrote his doctoral thesis in 1879 *On Disturbances of Genital Sensitivity in Menopause*, describing patients he had treated as an intern at the Sainte-Anne asylum.[119] Like others before him, he posed as a paradox the idea that a woman whose ovaries were ceasing to function in menopause should experience abnormally great genital excitation.[120] He appeared to resolve the paradox by arguing that there were two distinct phases of menopause: the first in which the periods became irregular, which was characterised by 'a considerable perturbation of equilibrium in the economy of the woman', resulting in a 'resurgence of ovarian function'. This was the 'veritable pathological era of menopause', during which numerous different disorders of genital sensitivity and nervous pathology could abound. But he also considered the second phase, after which the menses had definitely ceased, as a time of heightened susceptibility to nervous troubles, though he was not prepared to define at what point in a woman's ageing she could finally be said to be no longer menopausal and hence free of the dangers of hysteria, which he also called 'lypemania', 'hypochondria', and '*vésanies*'.[121] He cited Raciborski's concept of nervous plethora as the proximate cause of women's madness around menopause, after carefully considering whether genital symptoms had any place in the development of their mental pathologies. The cessation of the catamenial flow caused sanguinary plethora, as in premenstrual women, but with the ovarian failure of menopause, he said, the nerves too became plethoric.[122]

Ricard also cited twenty case observations of women ranging in age from 41 to 56 at the Sainte-Anne clinic in the late 1870s, which provide important clues to the sorts of conditions he and the other Paris scholars were now classifying as menopausal nervous pathology. He described many of them as suffering genital itching, burning, electrical sensations, and sexual arousal, as well as paranoid and persecutory delusions. When no gynaecological lesions were found on inspection, they were diagnosed with nervous pathology. Common to them too, as in other case observations of 'mad' menopausal women in late nineteenth-century French asylums, was anaemia, general poor health, or other major diseases such as tuberculosis (cases III, VII, VIII, XII), chronic insomnia (cases XII, XIV, XVI, XVIII), grief from deceased children or miscarriages (cases III, XVIII), being victims of sexual or domestic violence (cases III, XV), chronic alcoholism (cases XVI, XVII), as well as, in some cases, previous histories of serious mental

[118] Ibid., 24. [119] Ricard, *Étude sur les troubles de la sensibilité génésique*.
[120] Ibid., 7. [121] Ibid., 8–9, 13–14. [122] Ibid., 41.

pathology dating from well before their cessation of menses (cases IV, XV).[123] But none of these other salient factors appears to have deterred Ricard from stridently concluding that menopause was the primary cause of their delusional states: 'The perturbation occasioned in the economy of women by the cessation or the irregularity of the menstrual flux is sufficient alone to provoke these troubles'.[124] Masturbation was a proximate cause too of their delusions, which could take the form of aberrant 'erotism'.[125] Here too he cited Guéneau de Mussy's case example of a menopausal woman who began seeking sex from random strangers when her periods ceased.[126] Strikingly, almost all of Ricard's case observations are described as having paranoid delusions to the effect that some person or some supernatural force was causing both their abnormal genital sensations and their cessation of menstruation, deliberately tormenting them out of malice. It is not clear if this marked consistency was a product of clinical suggestion on the part of Ricard or the other doctors at the Sainte-Anne clinic—certainly this particular delusional narrative is not reported in other case observations around the same time in other clinics.

The candidate Théodore Willette (1854–1936), defending at the Paris faculty, addressed menopausal neuropathy (*névropathie*) primarily, but also referred to his patients as 'mad' (*aliénées*) and their pathology as madness (*la folie*).[127] Clearly the disciplinary boundaries between the emerging disciplines of neurology and psychiatry were still far from settled either pedagogically or clinically, and menopause now sat precisely in the contested zone that might be claimed by all kinds of doctors, neurologists, psychiatrists, hygienists, gynaecologists, and general physicians. Willette too insisted that women 'very rarely escape' nervous symptoms in menopause, sometimes even succumbing to extremely grave ones, such as 'hysteria, epilepsy, hemiplegia, paraplegia, troubles of the sense organs, and madness in all its forms, principally lypemania [melancholy]'.[128] By including as symptoms of this 'proteiform neuropathy' the broad spectrum of things associated with menopause (hot flushes, blushing, heart palpitations, vertigo, migraines, and other 'benign' complaints), as well as most forms of mental and nervous pathology, Willette was able to designate most menopausal women as in need of neurological or psychiatric treatment.[129] His thesis showed statistics indicating lower numbers of asylum patients in several datasets in the 40–45 and 45–50 age ranges than among younger women, and cited numerous case studies of other doctors whose nervous and mad patients were apparently cured by their menopause.[130] And yet curiously Willette still concluded that menopause mostly initiates new mental pathologies, only occasionally curing existing ones.[131]

[123] Ibid., 14–15. [124] Ibid., 44. [125] Ibid., 27–28, 31–32, 37. [126] Ibid., 28, 38.
[127] Willette, *Étude sur les accidents nerveux de la ménopause*, 15–18.
[128] Ibid., 5, 7, 9. [129] Ibid., 6. [130] Ibid., 16–19. [131] Ibid., 26.

As the topic of menopause continued to appear in increasingly diverse forms of medical and medically inspired forms of writing, it was also now commonly cited as a cause of madness or nervous disorders. Many of the new works of popular medical advice published in the final decades of the nineteenth century continued to supply the standard accounts found in the Montpellier scholarship and much of the Parisian hygiene scholarship on menopause, with a focus on purely physiological symptoms (weight gain, hot flushes, sleep disturbance, gout, skin conditions, or the more serious cancerous growths), while emphasising the need for hygienic self-care with regard to diet, sleep, exercise, alcohol, and avoiding sexual relations. The brief account of menopause found in Apollinaire Bouchardat's mammoth hygiene treaty of 1881 (published in four editions up to 1891) was typical in this regard too—not a whiff of hysteria or hypochondria, just the standard 'critical age' symptomatology to be tempered through correct lifestyle choices.[132] Bouchardat was a chemist by training, having completed his Paris doctoral work in 1832 on treatments for cholera, and held the chair of hygiene in the Paris medical faculty under the Second Empire. His perspective was thus both less specialised and more holistic, but also very unlike the psychiatric writers with their need to name physiological causes for mental pathologies, and their motivation to assimilate menopause to this agenda.

But many such works now also added warnings about the danger of mental illness in menopause to their prescriptive hygiene advice. The 1878 anonymous manual on the *Critical Ages of Woman* directed at mothers, boarding-house mistresses, and convent directors included a discussion of the nervous pathologies and mental illnesses of menopause that it said were the result of 'nervous plethora' (citing Raciborski's term).[133] This manual appears to have been produced by a Parisian manufacturer of the proprietary *Aloe natalensis* elixir called 'Nataloïne' invented by the Swiss chemist Friedrich August Flückiger. It promoted Nataloïne heavily as a remedy for plethora in menopause, and thus may have had its own commercial reasons to latch onto the circulating medical idea of the nervous dangers of women's critical age.[134]

[132] Apollinaire Bouchardat, *Traité d'hygiène publique et privée basée sur l'étiologie* [1881], 3rd ed. (Paris: Félix Alcan, 1887), 444, 637, 999–1002.

[133] Anon., *Les Âges critiques de la femme. Puberté—ménopause: Guide des mères de famille, des maîtresses de pension, et des directrices d'établissements religieux* (Paris: V Goupy et Jourdan, 1878), 9–10.

[134] Ibid., 14–16; Émile-Clément Jungfleisch, 'Sur la constitution des aloïnes de l'Aloès du Natal', in *Comptes rendus hebdomadaires des séances de l'Académie des sciences*, vol. 155 (Paris: Gauthiers-Villard, 1912), 172–175.

Menopausal Erotomania and Degeneration

Degenerationist psychiatric works increasingly converged on the new menopausal mental pathology concept, now not only in France but also in Germany and the Austro-Hungarian empire. The first major German-language specialist work on menopause appeared in 1874, by the Prague gynaecologist Enoch Kisch.[135] He included a whole section on 'mental ailments' ('psychische Leiden') citing a number of French works (Gardanne, Dubois d'Amiens, Brierre de Boismont). He also raised the spectre 'of excessive feelings of lust' ('des excessiven Wollustgefühles') in women at this time of life.[136] Two specialist German theses appeared on the theme of mental pathologies in menopause in the 1880s too, one by Siegfried Kracauer on *The Melancholy of Women After the Climacteric*, defended at the German university in Breslau in 1882, and the other by Julius Brühl *On the Mental Disturbances of the Climacteric*, defended in 1887 at the University of Augsburg in Bavaria.[137]

Menopausal madness was no longer a purely French fascination, but a fascination in France it remained nonetheless. Charcot's protégé Charles Féré (1852–1907), who was chief medical officer of the Bicêtre hospice in the late 1880s and throughout the 1890s, situated menopause among the 'diverse conditions that commonly provoke hereditary illness', along with puberty, menstrual troubles, fatigue, infections, intoxication, auto-intoxication, and either physical or emotional (*moraux*) shocks.[138] Féré's account of heritable diseases in the highly influential *La Famille névropathique* (The Neuropathic Family) of 1884 emphasised only hereditary dispositions towards contracting certain diseases, with nothing determined absolutely (as in the current medical model of the relationship of diseases to gene polymorphisms). In it he expressed sympathy for the teratological view that many dysfunctions were also determined in the course of ageing and development.[139] It was in synthesising the notions of inheritance with the teratological perspective that Féré elaborated his view of degeneration, or what he alternatively called 'devolution'. But he also subscribed to the view that this degeneration or devolution, manifesting as all those diseases deemed hereditary (including menopausal nervous disorders), profoundly impacted the health of society:

[135] Enoch Heinrich Kisch, *Das klimakterische Alter der Frauen in physiologischer und pathologischer Beziehung* (Erlangen: Ferdinand Enke, 1874).

[136] Ibid., 137.

[137] Julius Brühl, *Über die psychischen Störungen des Klimakteriums*. Dissertation (Würzburg: A. Memminger, 1887); Siegfried Kracauer, *Die Melancholie der Frauen nach dem Climacterium*. Dissertation (Breslau: F. Jungfer, 1882).

[138] Féré, *La Famille névropathique*, 225.

[139] Ibid., 228.

> If malformation is the most important condition for morbid predispositions in the individual, then malformed individuals in the national organism constitute the most favourable terrain for the development of social ills [*maladies sociales*]…Modern societies groan under the weight of their unproductive or destructive members, the basis of whose impotence, exhaustibility, irritability, impulses is malformation…[140]

In his 1899 work on the sexual instinct, Féré remarked that menopause, entailing 'the atrophy of the entire genital system', often marked the end of women's sexual instinct, but adding that the 'frequent exceptions' noted by others could hardly be considered 'normal manifestations'. Bizarrely, he cited here the ribald erotic memoirs of the sixteenth-century aristocrat Pierre de Bourdeille, seigneur de Brantôme (1540–1614), which were published as *Vie des dames galantes* in no less than thirty editions between 1800 and 1899.[141] Both menopause and the surgical castration of men could 'leave the sexual needs intact, and sometimes even exaggerate them'. But this was due to an 'involutional degeneration of the sexual organs', comparable to the phantom limb experiences of amputees.[142] Sexual excess could occur during any of the periods of 'physiological crisis', Féré asserted, which included during puberty in both sexes, during menstruation, in the euphoria of consumption (tuberculosis) and in women's menopause, though people of nervous disposition were the most prone to it. It could generally be accommodated within 'normal relations', but sometimes developed a 'morbid character' when associated with onanism, bestiality, or homosexuality.[143] Féré considered menopausal sexual desire of any kind abnormal and degenerate, so it too fell automatically under the category of morbid excess. In such a framework, it is not surprising to find older women's expressions of sexuality alone being taken as signs of a nervous or mental pathology, which from reading the case examples of many alienists/psychiatrists of the 1860s–1890s certainly appears to have been the case at least some of the time. Féré considered morbid sexual jealousy a feature of menopausal women too. He said it was one of the most common causes of women's admission to insane asylums, and was often linked to 'nervous debility' and hypochondria, with the most obsessive forms found in 'degenerates'.[144]

Not all the major psychiatric works of the late nineteenth century insisted on the significance of menopause in relation to women's madness, however. In 1888 the Paris professor of psychiatry Benjamin Ball published a specialist book on what he described as 'erotic madness', which focused largely on men and partly on women. In it he presented some fascinating case examples of women he

[140] Ibid., 229.

[141] Pierre de Bourdeille seigneur de Brantôme, *Vies des dames galantes* (*c.*1666) (Paris: Victor Bunel, 1880).

[142] Charles Féré, *L'Instinct sexuel: Évolution et dissolution* (Paris: Félix Alcan, 1899), 241.

[143] Ibid., 112. [144] Ibid., 119.

diagnosed as erotically mad, but with no mention of either menstruation or menopause as causative.[145] Ball considered women's ovaries to be often the cause of nymphomania, which he insisted was not a mental illness at all, but a purely physiological dysfunction in which the genital organs became hypertrophic or tumorous, inflaming the brain.[146] Ball, the son of an English father and a Swiss mother, was born in Naples and trained in Paris. He completed his doctoral work on pulmonary embolism in 1862, before working with both Jacques-Joseph Moreau de Tours and Charcot at the Salpêtrière.[147] He described a 70-year-old female patient who had been treated there, who was demure, eloquent, and polite, always immaculately groomed, with a lifelong history since adolescence of very abundant and promiscuous sexual appetite. He could find nothing wrong with her physically, and she displayed no signs of madness that he could identify other than being entirely unconventional in her consistent pursuit of regular sex with random strangers including minors, even well into her senior years, which had caused her to be brought to the Salpêtrière. This was not nymphomania, Ball insisted, since the patient was perfectly healthy and was satisfied after each of her sexual encounters, unlike nymphomaniacs who were always insatiable, had constant clitoral erections, elevated heart-rate, and after autopsy were found to have ovarian abnormalities and meningitis.[148] Ball classed this patient instead as displaying sexual 'excitability' of the 'aphrodisiac' variety, but he also referred to her as 'this debased woman, this monster' ('cette femme avilie, ce monstre').[149] He presented her story as a cautionary one for those who assumed that women's sexual drives should naturally become tempered by ageing.[150] Clearly this was not always the case. But there was no mention of her menopause, nor of her ageing exacerbating her erotic impulses.

The influential Sainte-Anne asylum psychiatrist Valentin Magnan, a rival of Ball who had received his training at Montpellier, similarly ignored menopause altogether in his 1885 work on the perversions.[151] But his 1895 work with his student Paul Legrain on 'degenerates' mentioned it several times, citing it as one of the physiological 'moments' that could cause 'cerebral disturbance', along with puberty, pregnancy, and menstruation.[152] Magnan and Legrain here also took menopause as a case example to explain how mental pathologies could remain latent during youth, only to surface later in life under the pressure of 'momentous' physiological life changes: 'We have seen how vividly the degenerate reacts in the

[145] Benjamin Ball, *La Folie érotique* (Paris: J. B. Baillière, 1888).

[146] Ibid., 90–102.

[147] Benjamin Ball, *Des Embolies pulmonaires*. Thèse (Paris: Rignoux, 1862); Obituaries: Benjamin Ball, *British Medical Journal*, 18 March (1893), 613–614.

[148] Ball, *La Folie érotique*, 90. [149] Ibid., 76. [150] Ibid., 74.

[151] Valentin Magnan, *Des anomalies, des aberrations et des perversions sexuelles* (Paris: A. Delahaye & E. Lecrosnier, 1885).

[152] Valentin Magnan & Paul Maurice Legrain, *Les Dégénérés: État et syndromes épisodiques* (Paris: Rueff, 1895), 61, 133, 220.

face of all those physiological moments: puberty, the appearance of the period, pregnancy, childbirth, menopause, etc.'[153] Degenerates were recognisable by their inability to remain stable through the changes of life; and women's physiology made them especially unable to maintain stability due to the many changes their bodies invariably underwent. Senility was their only hope: 'degenerates appear less susceptible to descend into madness' once old, because they would then experience a 'diminution of the integrity of the very cerebral activity which is necessary for the confection of a delirium'.[154] Magnan and Legrain did not say at what age this diminution was common, but menopausal women were clearly still too young to benefit from it.

Nonconformists like Ball notwithstanding, throughout the 1880s and 1890s, most works in the blossoming genre of French degenerationist psychiatric writing about sexual 'perversions', 'anomalies', and 'aberrations' that attracted the diagnosis of mental pathology now made mention of menopause, at least briefly. Some even wrote entire theses on it—including Ball's own students. One such was Henri Guimbail, who was an intern at the Roche-sur-Yon asylum in the Vendée, and who defended his Paris thesis in 1884 on the topic of *La Folie à la ménopause*.[155] Curiously, Guimbail remarked that statistical data had demonstrated that the two age bands most represented among the mentally insane were those aged between 15 and 30 and between 30 and 45. He considered this to suggest that, particularly for women, both puberty and especially menopause must be responsible—not appearing to realise that, by contemporary accounts, most girls reached puberty before the age of 15 and most women did not reach menopause until between the ages of 45 and 50 years or older.[156] For women, he claimed that it had 'already been demonstrated' that 'the period most favourable for the development of aberrations of the mind is that long stage of life that starts with puberty only to end around the age of 50'.[157] Menopause was such a stormy time for women that its 'disastrous effect' on the mind could only be compared in men to the effects of general paralysis and alcoholism.[158] He complained that alienists had failed to address the matter adequately in merely asserting that menopause 'was a serious cause of mental alienation' but without detailing its forms or explaining the mechanism of its action.[159] Leaning on the work of the English physician Edward Tilt, he distinguished between, on the one hand, the *temps des écarts* (gap period) in which menstruation became irregular, and, on the other

[153] Ibid., 229. [154] Ibid., 133.

[155] Henri Guimbail, *De la folie à la ménopause*. Thèse (Paris: A. Delahaye, 1884).

[156] Ibid., 7–8. See, for instance, the much cited and multiple-edition general work of pathology: Augustin Grisolle, *Traité de pathologie interne* [1844], 8th ed., 2 vols (Paris V. Masson et fils, 1862), vol. 2, 961; also the specialist gynaecological works, both student and senior: Joseph-Pierre-Éléonor Pétrequin, *Recherches sur la menstruation*. Thèse (Paris: Didot le Jeune, 1836), 12; and Amédée Courty, *Traité pratique des maladies de l'utérus et de ses annexes* [1866] (Paris: P. Asselin, 1872), 353.

[157] Guimbail, *De la folie à la ménopause*, 13.

[158] Ibid., 14. [159] Ibid., 9.

hand, menopause proper, in which no more menstruation occurred. The first period was the one in which the 'apparatus revolted' and was thus the dangerous moment for mental pathology:[160]

> The ganglionic system, being accustomed for so many years to presiding over the important function of ovulation, does not adjust easily to the partial inaction into which it will be plunged. It also revolts and this final combat result for the woman in a state of hyperexcitation of the general nervous system...[161]

Many of the psychiatric writers discussing this topic insisted on the role of degeneration in the development of menopausal madness. Jules-Bernard Luys (1828–1897) had defended his Paris thesis on hereditary illnesses (published as a book in 1863) and worked at the Charité hospital before becoming a colleague of Charcot at the Salpêtrière.[162] In his 1881 *Clinical and Practical Treatise of Mental Illnesses* he asserted that 'The influence of sex...and of the uterine functions is destined to play a very important role in the appearance and evolution of mental illnesses',[163] and that there were 'certain forms of lypemania' that were particular to women 'at the moment of the critical period'.[164] One 'particular' form of women's pathology in the *âge de retour* was characterised by 'depression of the mental faculties' and sadness, interspersed with episodes of anxiousness and agitation.[165] Women's madness was more often hereditary, he said, and though they were less often than men mad due to alcoholism in France, they were more prone to alcoholism during menopause.[166] In his 1893 treatment manual, he referred to the 'latent degenerates' who tended towards intellectual or artistic activities and must be monitored in the spirit of preventive care. Intellectual work must be limited to the bare necessities and emotional stimulation avoided absolutely.[167] Such women were of particular concern and their menstruation, pregnancy, and menopause were all 'worrying stages' that could give rise to 'the most acute mental disturbances', requiring special vigilance on the part of the family and their doctor.[168]

The Paris neurology professor Jules Dejerine (1849–1917) explained, in his 1886 book on the hereditary nervous diseases, that degenerate, eccentric individuals could often pass through life without ever 'presenting pathological problems, properly speaking'. Nonetheless, all of the periods of transition would be baneful

160 Ibid., 16–17. Tilt, *The Change of Life in Health and Disease.*

161 Guimbail, *De la folie à la ménopause*, 17–18.

162 Jules-Bernard Luys, *Des maladies héréditaires* (Paris: Baillière, 1863); Jules-Bernard Luys, *Hôpital de la Charité: Leçons cliniques sur les principaux phénomènes de l'hypnotisme, dans leurs rapports avec la pathologie mentale* (Paris: G. Carré, 1890).

163 Jules-Bernard Luys, *Traité clinique et pratique des maladies mentales* (Paris: A. Delahaye & E. Lecrosnier, 1881), 238.

164 Ibid., 234. 165 Ibid., 496. 166 Ibid., 255. 167 Ibid., 172–176.

168 Jules-Bernard Luys, *Le Traitement de la folie* (Paris, 1893), 175–177.

(*funestes*) for them, and it was these individuals who supplied the most cases of 'la folie de la ménopause' and senile dementia.[169] The Sainte-Anne psychiatrist Paul Legrain (1860–1939), in his 1886 Paris thesis about degenerate delirium supervised by Valentin Magnan (which was published as a book), listed menopause among the states of vulnerability that created a 'morbid opportunity' for delirium, which he considered to be exacerbated in general by 'advanced age'.[170] He announced that the true cause of delirium was 'hereditary predisposition' in degenerate bodies, since degenerates were defined by the sensitivity of their nervous systems, to which he gave a fancy-sounding Latin name: 'locus minoris resistentiœ' ('site of minimal resistance').[171] He noted that the concept of women's genital organs having a 'reflexive action' on the nervous system had given rise to the creation of several new categories of madness, such as 'menstrual madness', 'puerperal madness', and 'menopausal madness', which were all forms of nervous 'vésanies' ('madness'). He thus considered all such ideas of 'sympathetic madness' to be 'very right and very generative' ('très juste et très fécond').[172] Another 1886 work on hereditary forms of madness was by Honoré Saury, also one of Magnan's students who had worked at the Sainte-Anne asylum in the 1880s and who later worked at the Suresne asylum near the Bois de Boulogne.[173] Like Legrain, Saury noted with satisfaction the growing number of physiological conditions recently identified in the medical literature to be associated with nervous and mental pathologies—among them 'la ménopause'.[174]

By the 1880s, these ideas had begun spreading to other medical cultures too. In 1882, Siegfried Kracauer defended the first specialist German psychiatry thesis on women's mental pathologies in the *Climacterium* (as it was also sometimes spelt in German).[175] The University of Brussels professor of legal medicine Jules Dallemagne mentioned in his 1895 work on degeneration that 'sex plays a role in the aetiology of morbid emotions', with women being more prone to these on account of menstruation, pregnancy, childbirth, lactation, and menopause, which were all known to disturb the nervous system.[176] Nor was the idea of menopausal madness limited only to university professors and asylum doctors: the Paris prisons hospital doctor Émile Laurent mentioned briefly in his posthumously published 1905 work on 'erotomania' that this disorder was 'not rare' in women

[169] Jules Dejerine, *L'Hérédité dans les maladies du système nerveux* (Paris: Asselin et Houzeau, 1886), 82–83.

[170] Paul Maurice Legrain, *Du Délire chez les dégénérés: Observations prises à l'asile Sainte-Anne, 1885–1886* (Paris: A. Delahaye et E. Lecrosnier, 1886), 237–238.

[171] Ibid., 238. [172] Ibid., 258–259.

[173] Honoré Saury, *Étude clinique su la folie héréditaire* (Paris: Delahaye, 1886).

[174] Ibid., 4.

[175] Siegfried Kracauer, *Die Melancholie der Frauen nach dem Climacterium*. Dissertation (Breslau: F. Jungfer, 1882).

[176] Jules Dallemagne, *Dégénérés et déséquilibrés* (Bruxelles: H. Lamertin, 1895), 603.

during menopause.[177] Some of these mentions were brief, but they became increasingly ubiquitous. This certainly helped to encourage a few highly motivated psychiatrists to run with the idea that menopause was a calamitous time for women's nervous systems, activating even the most hidden and latent taints of degeneration. In 1910 the first Swiss work in German appeared on the theme of menopausal psychosis too, written by an immigrant student from the Crimea named Sorokina who had studied at the University of Bern between 1903 and 1907.[178] This work too insisted on the role of hereditary alienation in the development of melancholic symptoms in some women during menopause (using the novel German word *die Menopause*) or what Sorokina called the 'degenerative age' (*der Rückbildungsalter*)—here implying two senses of the concept of degeneration, as both hereditary devolution and involution with ageing.[179] This work referred to mostly German sources about hereditary psychosis and sexual perversions (especially Emil Kraepelin and Richard von Krafft-Ebing), triangulating these with French journal publications on menopause.[180]

The idea of menopausal mental pathology also spilled over into more general works of medical hygiene aimed at non-medical readerships. The Parisian doctor, hygienist, and medical journalist Ernest Monin stoked the fire of old ideas about the relationship between the genital organs and mental illness with his popular 1890 book on the topic. In it he had much to say about menopause, indicating the new medical concept's definitive entry into the public realm.[181] He said that menstruation caused mania in women, while epilepsy appeared with the first menstruation, thereafter recurring every time a girl menstruated; but that mania could also arise when suppressed menses caused mental disturbances and when menopause disrupted 'the nervous equilibrium', resulting in women becoming 'sad and capricious'.[182] The troubles of menopause were a sort of 'tribute to neurosis' that nearly all women must pay as they aged, Monin declared, with few remaining free of symptoms.[183] Menopausal women were 'seized by genital excitations', feared damnation, and became prone to insomnia, morbid jealousy, phantom pregnancies, melancholy, neuralgias coinciding with genital pruritus (itching), nervous dyspepsia, vertigo, and tendencies towards drug abuse and suicide. All this was caused by the 'ovarian hypofunction' that characterised the 'critical age'.[184] All women and girls could fall prey to a sort of sexual anxiousness known as 'Venus inimica' (legitimised by its novel Latin name which he said was inspired by the Roman physician Aulus Cornelius Celsus, who was known for describing love as war). This was an 'anxious form of neurosis' which was usually

[177] Émile Laurent, *Fétichistes et érotomanes* (Paris: Vigot Frères, 1905), 206, 241.
[178] M. Sorokina, *Über die Psychosen des Climacteriums.* Dissertation (Bern: Gottfried Iseli, 1910).
[179] Ibid., 26. [180] Ibid., 5–6.
[181] Ernest Monin, *Les Troubles nerveux de cause sexuelle* (Paris: O. Doin, 1890), 11.
[182] Ibid., 39–42. [183] Ibid., 45. [184] Ibid., 43–44.

caused by being exposed to sexual conversations, readings, or engravings. Widows and menopausal women often had this kind of 'exaggeration of the genital sense', sometimes taking the form of 'erotic hallucinations'.[185] Monin was very much a deliberate medical populariser—he worked as a scientific journalist for Parisian literary periodical *Le Gils Blas*, was known as a regular of the Montmartre Bohemian nightclub Le Chat Noir in Paris, and gave speeches about the mission of medical popularisation and hygiene.[186] Parts of his work read as decidedly lowbrow in their titillation factor. Nonetheless, he was published by a reputable press in the Place de l'Odéon and displayed detailed technical comprehension of the most recent scientific research papers.

Monin cited a Belgian doctor named Keiffer (albeit misspelling his name), whose curious theory of menstrual auto-intoxication around this time also received a brief flurry of attention in numerous European and North American medical gazettes.[187] The theory was that either the foetus during pregnancy, or the menstrual blood suppressed in amenorrhea, could send toxic substances into the bloodstream of a woman, causing mental derangement. Menopausal women were included here among the victims of 'ménorrhémie'.[188] Numerous recent medical historians have claimed that the early modern doctors writing about menstruation subscribed to the view that all forms of missing menses, including menopause, caused women to be poisoned by their own toxic blood—although, as we saw in Chapter 1, such a view was rarely implied by the first German or French scholars to consider the effects of either amenorrhea or the final cessation of menses. On the other hand, here suddenly was precisely such a view in clear form at the *fin de siècle*, no doubt inspired by the recent craze in medical thought for the notion of intestinal autointoxication, believed to result from constipation.[189] Yet despite worrying about women's reproductive organs poisoning their brains, Monin sided with the anti-hysterectomy camp in the debate that divided gynaecological surgeons around this time, arguing that 'castrated women' (those whose ovaries had been removed) suffered phantom pain where their ovaries had been, leading frequently to a generalised hysteria.[190]

[185] Ibid., 55–56.

[186] Evanghélia Stead, '*Musa Medicinalis*: Variations sur la médecine et les lettres au tournant du siècle dernier', *Romantisme*, 94 (1996): 111–124; Ernest Monin, *La Vulgarisation médicale* (Paris: Réunion amicale de la presse scientifique, 1893).

[187] Monin, *Les Troubles nerveux de cause sexuelle*, 46; J. H. Keiffer, 'La Menstruation dans ses rapports avec la pathologie générale', *L'Obstétrique*, 4 (15 July 1897): 492104; Dr Schwab, 'Revue critique: De l'auto-intoxication gravidique et ses conséquences', *Archives générales de médecine* 8/1 (1897): 720–738 [725–731]; Antoine Porot, *Les Syndromes mentaux* (Paris: Doin & Cie, 1928), 221; Suzanne Marchand, 'Cachez ce sang que je ne saurais voir: Les Menstruations au Québec (1900–1950)', *Rabaska: Revue d'ethnologie de l'Amérique française*, 10 (2012): 69–80.

[188] Monin, *Les Troubles nerveux de cause sexuelle*, 45–46.

[189] Micaela Sullivan-Fowler, 'Doubtful Theories, Drastic Therapies: Autointoxication and Faddism in the Late Nineteenth Century and Early Twentieth Centuries', *Journal of the History of Medicine and Allied Sciences*, 50 (1995): 364–390.

[190] Monin, *Les Troubles nerveux de cause sexuelle*, 53.

He recommended water and air cures, tonic remedies, gymnastic exercises, massages, and galvanisation, all of which he considered far more reliable than the ovarian opotherapy extracts and surgeries now being promoted to menopausal women, particularly those who had received hysterectomy and/or oophorectomy (the focus of our final chapter).[191]

Parisian medical pedagogy, too, continued in its development of the menopausal psychosis hypothesis. Despite the well-known rivalry between Valentin Magnan and Benjamin Ball,[192] and despite Ball's own failure to blame menopause in his own account of older women's sexual perversion, both he and Magnan trained students who wrote similar specialist works on menopause madness between 1888 and 1902. One of Ball's and Charcot's students, Paul Bruant, wrote his Paris thesis in 1888 on *The Melancholy which Arises During Menopause*, providing a fairly unoriginal account of menopause as the loss of women's 'physiological function' and their femininity, as if this automatically explained why they would become depressed.[193] He also reproduced the idea of menopause causing new 'erotic impulses', referring to Brierre de Boismont's stories of high-society ladies seducing young working-class men and adolescents.[194] He considered menopause to radically change a woman's personality: 'a hitherto virtuous person neglects her duties as a mother and allows herself to be drawn into debauchery'.[195] He cited numerous case examples, of which the following three are representative. The first is described as aged 49, a 'worker' (*ouvrière*), literate, melancholic with hallucinations, insomnia, and hypochondriac fears, who became depressed one year after her final menstruation. Another, aged 51, *une lingère* (laundry worker), who suffered heavy uterine haemorrhage, was melancholic with hallucinations and persecution fears. She had a family history of mental alienation, was married at 33, and had a child who died. A third was 59 years old, unemployed, illiterate, had five children of which one died in an accident, and had had two miscarriages. She caught smallpox and recovered, after which her menses never returned. Her husband said she had always been taciturn. She had suffered delirium since her menopause.[196] Unlike his fellow student Paul Garat (see below), Bruant's cases were at least an appropriate age, though again it is striking how much painful life experience of bereavement and infectious diseases pepper the accounts of these supposedly mad women apparently tormented by their menopause.

Paul Garat, another student of Ball and Charcot, defended his Paris thesis in 1898 on *The Influence of Menopause on the Development of Madness*, providing substantial statistical data and case examples that make his doctoral work

[191] Ibid., 49.

[192] Jean Garrabé, 'Les Chaires de clinique des maladies mentales et des maladies nerveuses à Paris', *L'Information psychiatrique*, 88/7 (2012): 549–557.

[193] Paul Bruant, *De la mélancholie survenant à la ménopause*. Thèse (Paris: Henri Jouve, 1888), 9.

[194] Ibid., 11. [195] Ibid., 14. [196] Ibid., 36–43.

particularly noteworthy.[197] In working under Ball's supervision at the Sainte-Anne asylum the previous three years, he had been struck by the number of women admitted around the 'so-called critical' age.[198] He acknowledged that the view he was espousing, of menopause as 'producing a profound perturbation of the economy' of women, which he considered to reflect 'popular common sense', had become a minority view in general medicine amid the mass of medical hygiene books and doctoral theses full of anti-pathological insistences and self-care advice to women. He pointed here in particular to the widely cited Montpellier gynaecology professor Amédée Courty.[199] Garat attributed the medical non-consensus about menopause to the division between gynaecology, which was concerned only with physiological questions, and psychology, which dealt with the mental.[200] He appeared not to consider that the division may also have been due to the different patient cohorts experienced by each: in his case, working only with those already committed to insane asylums, and in the case of gynaecologists, working with the general female population in women's hospitals and clinics. He leaned on the descriptions of critical age nervousness in the work of both Pinel and Esquirol, before citing Brierre de Boismont's paper of 1851, Morel's treaty of 1860, and his mentor Ball's lessons on mental illnesses. Via Cabanis, he even evoked the pre-menopause view of physiological crises associated with the age of 49 in both sexes (the seventh septenary), in support of his account of menopause as such a critical time of nervous perturbation.[201] Some conceptual layers can indeed persist long after their peak moment of credibility.

Garat claimed that there was an absence of rigorous statistical data demonstrating the correlation between menopause and mental illness only because the age of the mentally ill was not always recorded. He cited the data from the asylums of the *département* of the Seine which did include age, as well as Esquirol's data from the Salpêtrière, but in both cases, the larger cohorts are not women between the ages of 45 and 55, but those in their twenties, thirties, and early forties. Esquirol in fact attributed more disorders to menstruation than to menopause,[202] and the biggest group of patients in the Sainte-Anne data were melancholiacs with an average age of 42—a bit early for menopause by most nineteenth-century accounts, which tended to situate it most commonly between ages 45 and 50. The next biggest group were maniacs, with an average age of 38;

[197] Paul Garat, *Influence de la ménopause sur le développement de la folie*. Thèse (Paris: G. Steinheil, 1892).

[198] Ibid., 3.

[199] Ibid., 5; Amédée Courty, *Traité pratique des maladies de l'utérus et de ses annexes* [1866] (Paris: P. Asselin, 1872).

[200] Garat, *Influence de la ménopause sur le développement de la folie*, 7.

[201] Ibid., 8–10.

[202] Étienne D. Esquirol, *Des maladies mentales considérées sous les rapports médical, hygiénique et médico-légal*, 2 vols (Paris: J. B. Baillière, 1838), vol. 1, 59.

hysterics and epileptics had an average age of 26.[203] It is not exactly compelling data to support Garat's claims about menopause causing mental illness, and he offered no explanation for the disparity. He also included data on criminal convictions published by the penitentiary administration of the Ministry for the Interior during the period 1883–1886. But here again, the largest group of women was that between the ages of 30 and 40.[204] Possibly Garat was unaware that menopause did not commonly occur at such young ages.

Like others, Garat subscribed to the *folie érotique* theory of menopausal nervous pathology, but unusually cited specific case examples of this in women he had helped to treat. Here the age ranges at least seemed more appropriate. One was a 48-year-old English mother of eight who had suffered a gynaecological illness some years earlier and now no longer had a regular menstrual cycle. (Though Garat makes no mention of it, it is possible that she was given a hysterectomy and/or oophorectomy in her gynaecological treatment since, as we will see in the following chapter, these surgeries were becoming increasingly common in Paris hospitals around this time for a wide variety of gynaecological disorders). Since separating from her husband she had 'erotic spasms that repeated themselves several times a day', though we are not told whether this is the terminology used by the patient herself. Garat claimed to have witnessed precisely one of these spasms when the woman entered the examination room, adopted a fixed gaze and shuddered, after which a liquid secretion squirted out from under her skirt and onto the floor.[205] We are neither told of what this secretion consisted, from which orifice it emitted, nor what about the episode indicated the erotic nature of the episode. It seems likely that Garat himself had no answers to these questions or he would have volunteered this information. But he nonetheless presumed, firstly, that the secretion was vaginal, not urinary or excremental; secondly, that it was related to sexual arousal rather than to vaginal or uterine discharge: and thirdly, that her sensations were erotic rather than painful, hesitant, or embarrassed.

Another case referred to a 52-year-old woman with facial asymmetry, who was small and slightly chubby. At 18 she had contracted typhoid fever and experienced hallucinations, after which she always seemed to need to move a lot. She married at 25 and had eight children before the age of 34. She had been known to have uncontrolled bouts of eating. Her husband was a drunkard and beat her, so she had left him some years ago and had had no other sexual partners since. One of her sons had died fifteen years earlier, and she had first come to the asylum eight years later 'at the time of her menopause' (when she was 45). Her 'problem' seemed to be that she would have unexplained moments of excited genital sensations, as well as desires to scream and hit something. Garat noted several times in

[203] Garat, *Influence de la ménopause sur le développement de la folie*, 18–19.
[204] Ibid., 75–79. [205] Ibid., 30–31.

his report that she never masturbated ('jamais d'onanisme'), so this could be ruled out as a cause.[206] Another 45-year-old widow, named as Mme M. Élisabeth, is described as having 'mental degeneration' with depression and hypochondria. She had no appetite, had severe insomnia, and complained of injuries which no doctor could verify after five separate medical examinations. Although her menses had recently ceased following the death of her husband, this had caused no problems, by her own account. Nonetheless, Garat considered her 'hypochondria' to be the result of her menopause.[207] Garat's case examples too are revealing for the complexity of external sources of hardship and suffering (bereavement, domestic violence, separation from husbands while caring for numerous children, other forms of serious illness) that these supposedly menopause-mad women reported.

Another of Ball's students who embraced the menopausal madness claim was the Paris-trained psychiatrist Emmanuel Régis. Régis was raised in the south of France and had worked at the Sainte-Anne asylum in Paris with Ball before becoming professor of medicine, then later chair of mental pathology at the University of Bordeaux.[208] Régis published a widely cited *Practical Manual of Mental Medicine* in 1885, and its second edition of 1892 was also published in the USA in English translation in 1894.[209] It devoted a section to the 'Insanity of the Menopause' in a chapter focused on forms of madness associated with specific physiological states such as puberty in both sexes, menstruation, pregnancy, childbirth, with puerperal fever, during lactation, in association with dementia, and during menopause.[210] Régis thought menopause was 'justly called a critical epoch' because for many women it resulted in 'psychic modifications, which may sometimes go so far as to cause insanity'. This was especially a danger for nervous women who were 'thus originally predisposed, but who have been able to keep this tendency latent during all their active life, in spite of all the physical and moral shocks they have endured', but who, at the moment of the cessation of menses, 'become suddenly insane'.[211] Régis admitted that menopausal madness frankly had no 'special clinical physiognomy': it could vary infinitely in its presentation, but was generally characterised by impulsiveness, including a strong attraction to alcohol (dipsomania), the desire to light fires, to commit theft, murder, and especially suicide, and sometimes by 'bizarre sexual hallucinations'.[212]

[206] Ibid., 31–34. [207] Ibid., 58–59.

[208] Sandor Ferenczi, 'Die psychiatrische Schule von Bordeaux über die Psychoanalyse', in Sandor Ferenczi, *Bausteine zur Psychoanalyse*, vol. 4 (Bern: Hans Huber, 1939), 12–24.

[209] Emmanuel Régis, *Manuel pratique de la médecine mentale* (Paris: Octave Doin, 1885). Emmanuel Régis, *A Practical Manual of Mental Medicine* (Philadelphia: Blakiston, 1898).

[210] Régis, *Manuel pratique de la médecine mentale*, 223–237; Régis, *Practical Manual of Mental Medicine*, 331–347.

[211] Régis, *Practical Manual of Mental Medicine*, 234.

[212] Régis, *Manuel pratique de la médecine mentale*, 235.

Régis's 1904 *Précis de psychiatrie* reiterated these claims about 'mental perversions that one observes in the female sex at the time of the climacteric', which included 'irritability', 'mysticism', and 'érotisme'.[213] This major textbook of early twentieth-century psychiatry was published in six editions up to 1923 and accounted exhaustively for all the recent theories of psychiatric aetiology, diagnosis, and causation. Menopause appears throughout this work as one of the possible causes of madness, as well being the focus of a small chapter. The urge to steal was associated with pregnancy, menstruation, menopause, alcoholism, and degeneration.[214] Pregnancy, puberty, menstruation, lactation, and menopause were all characterised by 'genital auto-intoxication'.[215] Régis considered that this auto-intoxication derived from the thyroid gland, and that it should be taken as the new hypothesis to explain menopausal madness, replacing outdated ideas of 'sympathy' of the genital organs and the brain.[216] Melancholic depression was particularly a disease of the menopause.[217] But the mental troubles of menopause could also be found in men, he claimed, who also underwent a 'critical age' around age 50, which he called 'la ménopause virile'.[218] Régis recognised the difficulty of separating 'climacteric psychoses, properly speaking' from psychoses that simply coincidentally appeared around this time of life and were only indirectly influenced by it.[219] Nonetheless he proposed no means to decide which was which, and it seems clear that in practice French psychiatry indeed classified all kinds of people and their troubles (both internal and external) under the category of menopausal mental pathology if they were within as much as even fifteen years on either side of the statistically common age of cessation of menses. Despite his insistence on the role of the thyroid gland rather than the gonads, Régis recommended only one treatment for menopausal psychosis: ovarian extract for women and testicular extract for men.[220]

Régis, in turn, guided his students towards even more specialist studies on menopause nervous pathology. In 1899, Yervant-Vahram Chahinian (from Armenia) became one of a steadily increasing number of immigrant graduates of the Bordeaux medical faculty in this period, defending his thesis on the role of puberty, sexual relations, and menopause in women's 'neurasthenia'—the new term that was becoming fashionable as a substitute for the now unfashionable hysteria, *vésanies*, or vapours.[221] Chahinian gave the same account as Magnan, Legrain, Garat, and Régis of how menopause was one of the eras in women's lifespan when they were susceptible to nervous pathology, along with puberty and pregnancy. The underlying cause was genetic predisposition, which 'puts the

[213] Emmanuel Régis, *Précis de psychiatrie* [1904], 3rd ed. (Paris: Octave Doin, 1906), 537.
[214] Ibid., 142. [215] Ibid., 525. [216] Ibid., 539. [217] Ibid., 161–162.
[218] Ibid., 537–538. [219] Ibid., 538. [220] Ibid., 540.
[221] Yervant-Vahram Chahinian, *Contribution à l'étude de la neurasthénie liée aux trois grandes étapes génitales de la femme, puberté, union sexuelle, ménopause, considérée plus spécialement dans ses rapports avec l'éducation.* Thèse (Bordeaux: J. Pechade, 1899).

organism in a state of receptivity'.[222] He thought that those doing intellectual work were especially susceptible, as well as those living in cities,[223] that masturbation could cause it, as could sexual variations that were 'against nature' (such as those described by Richard von Krafft-Ebing), including even *coitus interruptus*.[224] A short chapter dedicated to *Érotisme de la menopause* cited Guéneau de Mussy at length as well as Brierre de Boismont, but Chahinian differed from their accounts of menopausal erotic mania in emphasising that social class and cultural pressures were also major factors in its causation. Nervous disorders affected women around the time of menopause because they were treated with cold indifference as they aged, which irritated their nervous systems.[225] Recommended treatments included hypnotherapy, electrotherapy, hydrotherapy, fresh country air, high altitude, and massages.[226] Chahinian also touted the benefits of the new ovarian opotherapy (organotherapy) which was now being prescribed to women for menopause symptoms both natural and artificial (following hysterectomy and oophorectomy), as well as the thyroid opotherapy which was favoured by Régis.[227] Chahinian mentioned an intriguing sanatorium called 'Kikli' in the mountains near Trieste where menopausal women were sent to recover their nervous equilibrium. Situated at an altitude of 800 metres, it offered a simple cure which consisted in patients spending all day outside naked in the sunshine. He noted that this was very popular with southern Germans and Austrians.[228]

Régis for his part, had continued to publish on questions relating to degeneration and mental pathology throughout the 1890s, before turning towards psychoanalysis in the early twentieth century. He contributed a case-study paper to the *Journal de médecine de Bordeaux* in 1893 on madness caused by removal of a women's ovaries, in which he remarked upon the emergence in the USA of oophorectomy as a treatment for insanity.[229] This had never been practised in France, he said, where such surgeries had hitherto not been used for psychiatric purposes, only gynaecological ones. The treatment had recently become controversial among American psychiatrists, with most rejecting its utility, and Régis flagged this dispute to his French colleagues in light of his own and other French colleagues' case observations indicating that oophorectomy could produce new manifestations of psychosis in hitherto sane women. Madame X, 35 years old, Jewish, of average intelligence, and sane but with a family history of mental alienation, had developed a painful ovarian tumour following several miscarriages.[230] Her ovaries and fallopian tubes were removed on 20 October 1892, after which she developed vivid auditory hallucinations and elaborate paranoid ideas, becoming morose and suicidal just eight days later. She was referred to Régis sometime

[222] Ibid., 26. [223] Ibid., 28–29. [224] Ibid., 41–46. [225] Ibid., 60–62.
[226] Ibid., 69–79. [227] Ibid., 77–78. [228] Ibid., 79.
[229] Emmanuel Régis, 'Cas de folie consécutive à une ovarosalpingectomie', *Journal de médecine de Bordeaux*, 37 (10 September 1893): 413–417.
[230] Ibid., 414.

after this, who consulted with a Dr Ferré, professor of experimental medicine at the faculty of Bordeaux. A treatment plan involving injections of ovarian liquid was prescribed, beginning on 5 April 1893, following the opotherapy extraction methods of Brown-Séquard and d'Arsonval (who had treated men for frailty and impotence with testicular extracts). The treatment produced almost immediate improvements in Madame X, who, over several months, became more orderly in her thoughts and stopped being obsessed by her paranoid ideas; the hallucinations faded into the background, she became calmer and affectionate to her loved ones again, but still spoke with 'occasional rather gross invective' about the patients next to her.[231] Régis considered her only partially cured and appeared much less excited about the ovarian treatment than the gynaecological surgeons who were writing about it at the same time (whom we will meet in the final chapter of our book).[232] He cautioned about the dangers of surgical menopause for women's mental health, indicating that psychiatrists should not consider it therapeutic to remove the ovaries, although he reported a moderately helpful opotherapy remedy in those to whom the surgery had already been given for other reasons.

From the 1870s until around 1920, French psychiatric and neurological writers discussing menopause began increasingly to use the term *involution* to describe the tissue changes in the uterus and ovaries following the cessation of menses. Like the words *dégénération* or *dégénérescence*, involution suggested a reversal of progress, and was used in French works to refer to the ageing process in which the sex-specific traits of women after puberty returned to the pre-pubescent state, where menstruation did not occur and conception was not possible. This idea did not only derive from Kraepelin, though certainly his influence contributed to the further development of the menopausal degeneration idea. The notion of retrograde development had long been implicit in the term *âge de retour*, and was repeatedly referred to in specialist works on menopause and on the ageing uterus. In 1879 the Paris doctoral student Louis Bourlet (a student of Ball and Broca) had described the process of uterine atrophy after menopause as a return to the state of a pre-pubescent girl.[233] The 1897 Bordeaux thesis of Henri-Paul-Marie Dupuy on metritis during menopause defined this stage of women's lives as 'a poorly delimited period in which the senile involution of the uterus occurs' ('une période mal délimitée pendant laquelle se fait l'involution sénile de l'utérus').[234] Émile van Peteghem's Paris thesis of 1893 had similarly defined the moment when there are no more periods and ovulation ceases as signalling the 'senile involution' of

[231] Ibid., 415–416. [232] Ibid., 416–417.

[233] Louis Bourlet, *Étude sur la métrite interne chronique après la ménopause* (Paris: A. Parent, 1879), 6.

[234] Henri-Paul-Marie Dupuy, *Métrite hémorrhagique de la ménopause et de la vieillesse.* Thèse (Bordeaux: Imprimerie du Midi, 1897), 10.

the female reproductive system.[235] Henri Guimbail too had referred to the entire age band of 45–60 years in women as *la période d'involution*.[236]

The first decade of the twentieth century saw a flurry of new theses and books on the need for menopausal women to be treated by psychiatrists and neurologists, not only in France but also in Switzerland, England, Italy, and Germany. In 1907 a Paris doctoral student named Émile Vermorel defended a thesis on the thyroid origins of nervous heart palpitations in puberty and in menopause, providing a novel take on the matter which followed Régis's hunch about thyroid function (rather than the reproductive organs) playing a role in this symptom.[237] Another Toulouse doctorate, defended by Alexandre-Jacques-Bernard Gerdessus in 1910 on 'Menopause and its Role in Psychiatry', clarified that menopause was now to be understood not as the time following the final menstruation, but as the *temps de passage* in between the regular cycle and its final cessation.[238] This was necessarily 'a time of organic decadence' which 'in reality' was 'a function of pre-senility' given that women's growth ceased around 30 years of age, after which only decline was possible.[239] Much of Gerdessus's thesis in fact focused mainly on men, who were now to be included in the term *la ménopause*, despite them never having menstruated. This curious development allowed for a continuation of the old unisex use of the terms 'critical age' and 'climacteric', and allowed psychiatrists and neurologists to make a claim for treating an even larger patient cohort of not only all women, but also all men aged between 40 and 60 years.

Gerdessus claimed that menopausal psychosis was most often melancholic, coming in five forms: with delirium, simple, hypochondriac, with stupor, and with persecution complex.[240] He discussed the new experimental surgical treatments that were now being used by gynaecologists which induced artificial menopause, remarking that while it was safe to remove the uterus, removal of the ovaries should be avoided if possible because it caused mental disturbances.[241] He discussed criminality in menopause, which included kleptomania, pyromania, and homicide as well as sadism, nymphomania, erotomania, fetishism, and exhibitionism.[242] His treatment section focused far more than any previous similar works on pharmacological remedies, including ergot, hydrastis (goldenseal), hamamelis, viburnum bark, opium, laxatives, mountain salt, and Ovarine powder—the commercial Merck pharmaceutical sheep-ovary opotherapy

[235] Émile van Peteghem, *Des endométrites de la ménopause*. Thèse (Paris: Ollier-Henry, 1893), 17.

[236] Guimbail, *De la folie à la ménopause*, 7.

[237] Émile Vermorel, *De l'origine thyroïdienne de certaines tachycardies ou palpitations, dites nerveuses, de la puberté et de la ménopause*. Thèse (Paris: Alfred Leclerc, 1907).

[238] Ibid., 9.

[239] Alexandre-Jacques-Bernard Gerdessus, *La Ménopause et son rôle en psychiatrie*. Thèse (Toulouse: Dirion, 1910), 10–11.

[240] Ibid., 40. [241] Ibid., 52. [242] Ibid., 76–81.

product now being used by doctors in France, Switzerland, and Germany and which we discuss in our final chapter.[243]

The erotomania theory did not go away either: the Bordeaux candidate Emile-Joseph-Amédée Valleteau de Moulliac (born 1884) claimed in his 1907 thesis that 'perversion of the sexual appetite' was one of the most important symptoms of menopause.[244] Menopause either extinguished sexual desire altogether, or else resulted in its perverse 'awakening'. He advised that all women should avoid all sex after menopause but noted sympathetically that some 'unfortunate women' ('malheureuses') were compelled to pursue 'voluptuous pleasures with a veritable rage, showing something certainly pathological (*maladif*) in their case'.[245] This was caused by 'the congestive state of the genital channels' ('l'état congestif des voies génitales') which caused erotic impulses during the critical age.[246] He cited both Luys and the Italian degenerationist psychiatrist Angiolella in support of the view that 'the end of the menstrual periods signals the explosion of certain morbid predispositions which until then have remained latent',[247] adding that 'decadence commences at the very moment when reproductive functionality begins to decline', and hence the madness of menopause was an expression of the subject's degeneration ('une expression de la dégénérescence du sujet').[248]

Louis Genest reiterated the claim as late as in 1920, adding that 'erotic delirium' was common in older married, widowed, and celibate women: 'One often sees the sudden irruption of strange ardours in women who up until then had been rather cold and for whom sexual relations had procured only a very limited pleasure.'[249] Genest had an elaborate explanation of how the weakening of reproductive desire produced a kind of frigidity characterised by 'perpetual excitation' or 'an amorous appetite that nothing can surpass, and which is moreover rarely satisfied'.[250] This was a sort of 'erotic spasm' that could lead to no peace. 'Once a woman accepts the end of her amorous life, things go better in every respect since sexual relations after menopause are not without danger.'[251] This view was certainly consistent with other interwar psychiatric writings on women's frigidity which, rather than representing it as an absence of desire, constructed it as another form of perversion in fixating on clitoral pleasure instead of coital receptivity.[252] But it also continued the themes of earlier claims, such as those of Brierre de Boismont and

[243] Ibid., 80–81. Prosper Mossé, *État actuel de l'opothérapie ovarienne: Étude expérimentale et clinique*. Thèse (Paris: J. B. Baillière, 1899).

[244] Emile-Joseph-Amédée Valleteau de Moulliac, *Contribution à l'étude de l'âge critique chez l'homme (troubles nerveux et psychiques)*. Thèse (Bordeaux: A. Destout ainé & Cie, 1907).

[245] Ibid., 21, 27. [246] Ibid., 29. [247] Ibid., 19.

[248] Ibid., 49–50; G. Angiolella, 'Le Psicosi in rapporto alle fasi fisiologiche dell'organismo', *Rivista sperimentale de freniatria*, 31 (1905): 105–154.

[249] Louis Genest, *Comment prévenir et guérir les maladies du retour d'âge. Hygiène préventive; les soins spéciaux; les meilleurs remèdes* (Paris: M. Drouin, *c.*1920).

[250] Ibid., 21. [251] Ibid., 28–29.

[252] Peter Cryle & Alison Moore, *Frigidity: An Intellectual History* (Basingstoke: Palgrave Macmillan, 2011), 232–237.

Noël Guéneau de Mussy, about menopausal erotomania as the final rebellion of the declining ovaries or uterus.

In a 1911 article published in the French psychiatry journal *L'Encéphale*, the neuro-psychiatry researchers Aaron Rémond (from Metz) and Paul Voivenel (from Toulouse) tried, like others, to widen the menopausal mental illness patient cohort by including men under the category.[253] They began thus with the statement: 'We have the intention here to envisage menopause in the extremely enlarged sense, sufficient to allow us to group under the same rubric phenomena that appear in one and the other sex.'[254] They were emboldened to make the claim because hysteria, which had initially only referred to women's mental pathologies, had recently become widely used in French psychiatry to refer to men's madness as well.[255] They cited the Kraepelin-inspired concept of 'pre-senile involution' which had begun reinforcing French degenerationist accounts of mental pathologies in ageing with the 1907 French translation of Kraepelin's 1883 *Compendium der Psychiatrie.*[256] In this work, Kraepelin too had described hereditary 'manic-depressive' psychosis as exploding generally in puberty or in menopause.[257] Rémond and Voivenel explained that menopause was 'the physiological period that tends toward the effacement of the sexes, as opposed to puberty that prepares their differentiation'.[258] This showed that it was effectively retrograde—not in the rejuvenative sense but in the decadent sense—just as degeneration represented the devolution of humanity. Rémond and Voivenel here also cited Kraepelin's case study of a melancholic menopausal woman whom he treated for ten years before she was cured, by way of example of the work to be done by psychiatrists with this still (largely untapped) potential long-term patient cohort. The organs affected were the adrenals, the uterus, and ovaries in women, and the testicles and prostate in men, with the primary symptoms being hypertension, vertigo, buzzing in the ears, frequent headaches, and even the remarkably eighteenth-century-sounding 'vapours', by which here they meant merely the return of menstruation after a long absence. They claimed that menstruation was a kind of detoxification, and that with its cessation, women retained 'a certain number of products' that could not be eliminated, which were the cause of the hot flush symptom that endured until the body adjusted. They rejected the purely ovarian insufficiency-based model of women's menopause, despite it being by now quite broadly accepted in French, German, English, and American gynaecology, noting that the

[253] Antoine Rémond & Paul Voivenel, 'Essai sur le rôle de la ménopause en pathologie mentale', *L'Encéphale: Revue de psychiatrie clinique, biologique et thérapeutique*, 6/2 (1911): 113–126.

[254] Ibid., 113.

[255] See Mark Micale, *Hysterical Men: The Hidden History of Male Nervous Illness* (Cambridge, Mass.: Harvard University Press, 2008).

[256] Emil Kraepelin, *Introduction à la psychiatrie clinique*, traduite sur la 2e édition allemande, par MM. Albert Devaux et Prosper Merklen (Paris: Vigot Frères 1907).

[257] Ibid., 27.

[258] Rémond & Voivenel, 'Essai sur le rôle de la ménopause'. 115.

ovaries could continue to function after the cessation of menses, which was the more significant change, indicating an important role of the uterus.[259] Menopause in both sexes involved atrophy of some parts (ovaries and testicles) and hypertrophy of others (uterus and prostate), as well as 'auto-intoxication' that resulted from 'the accumulation in the organism of substances that cease to be eliminated', along with 'Basedow syndrome', or Graves' disease (hyperthyroidism) in women, bringing nervous and mental pathologies.[260] Crises of mysticism were also a feature of menopause in both sexes, which often ended in dementia if it did not disappear as soon as the critical age had passed.[261]

These scholars too evoked a particular form of menopausal nervous symptom they called 'erotic delirium', citing Guéneau de Mussy, and describing women becoming overwhelmed by novel passions and engaging in uncharacteristic behaviours 'that nothing in their past would have predicted'.[262] They claimed that this same erotic delirium was responsible for the 'morbid jealousy' that was another feature of menopausal nervousness, with its worrisome potential for 'medico-legal consequences'.[263] They claimed that many of the crimes of corrupting minors into debauchery, sexual violence, homosexual acts, and other forms of 'criminal eroticism' were most likely caused by the critical age, following Krafft-Ebing's definition of 'temporary psychopathy'.[264] We arrive now at the peak moment for the association of menopause with the traits most heavily pathologised by French medical culture of the long nineteenth century.

[259] Ibid., 116–117. [260] Ibid., 119, 121. [261] Ibid., 124.
[262] Ibid., 123. [263] Ibid., 123. [264] Ibid., 126.

8
The First Discussions of Menopause in the Work of Women Medical and Health Writers in France

> 'Le symptôme capital de la ménopause est la cessation du flux menstrual.'
>
> ('The principle symptom of menopause is the cessation of the menstrual flux.')
>
> Dr Hélina Gaboriau, *Les Trois Âges de la femme*, 1923.[1]

This chapter considers the earliest accepted women medical researchers and clinicians of the early twentieth century who turned their attention to questions of ageing uterine diseases, but also the even earlier nineteenth-century women who authored gynaecological works while working unofficially as doctors, as well those who authored popular manuals of women's health, including several writers from other cultures whose work was translated into French in the 1890s or the first decade of the twentieth century. Throughout this book, there has been a recurrent thread of how the concept of menopause was assembled from earlier temporal layers and given deliberate, historically self-conscious thrust by medical students and university professors of physiology, psychiatry, and hygiene in the context of emerging competitive pressures that shaped the two largest French medical faculties of the late eighteenth and nineteenth centuries. It seems likely that the exclusion of women from official medical practice throughout the time of the emergence of menopause had important consequences for the tone of much medical writing about it. Midwifery manuals from 1600 to 1870 made no mention of any crisis, climacteric years, madness, rapid ageing, or physical symptoms associated with the final cessation of menses; but the medical and hygienic writing of women in the late nineteenth century, after the official discourse of menopause had begun to circulate publicly, indeed referred to aspects of this new concept. What did they have to say about it? This chapter considers all the women-authored French medical works and advice manuals published throughout

[1] Dr Hélina Gaboriau, *Les Trois Âges de la femme: Puberté, maternité, ménopause* (Paris: Larousse, 1923), 183.

The French Invention of Menopause and the Medicalisation of Women's Ageing: A History. Alison M. Downham Moore, Oxford University Press. © Alison M. Downham Moore 2022. DOI: 10.1093/oso/9780192842916.003.0009

the nineteenth century which mentioned women's 'critical age', as well as a few that did not, situated in relation to the exclusion of women from the title of doctor up until 1875. While these works clearly demonstrate engagement with doctors' books and theses on menopause, mostly they reproduced only a fraction of the elaborate symptomatology, or the hygienic prescriptions given to women in the critical age found ubiquitously in the works authored by men. Only one work, that of Virginie Messager (b. 1805), published in 1859, surpassed even the most pathologising works by medical men about menopause—proposing that it was an even more dangerous time than anyone else thought.[2]

We then consider those research studies conducted by women on the diseases of women's ageing after women were permitted to enter the medical profession. Here too there was a distinctly less catastrophising and generalising tone in the specification of particular disease cohorts that were no longer taken to be representative, along with the wholesale abandonment of both the elaborate schema of hygienic prescription, and the simultaneous claims of historical innovation and ancient inheritance which doctors of the nineteenth century continually crowed about. The early twentieth-century women medical scholars focusing on menopause-related topics, all developed research questions that reached beyond the repetitive clichés of nineteenth-century works on the critical age, *âge de retour*, and menopause, focusing instead on the deadly illnesses that some women genuinely developed in midlife and for which cures were now sought in approximatively structured clinical trials. It might be tempting to consider that it was thus only once women entered the medical profession as doctors in France that more specific and serious investigation of the diseases of women's ageing truly began, but it was also coincidentally around this same time that the experimental standards of medical research throughout the western world were becoming reconstructed and professionalised in ways that made much of what doctors wrote in the nineteenth century look suddenly quite speculative and amateurish—not only when they were talking about menopause. By the 1920s, charlatans and folk healers too now constituted a far smaller and legally constrained proportion of practitioners, so while some doctors may have continued to worry about them, the esteem of biomedicine was far greater than in the nineteenth century, placing alternative health practices largely outside the concerns of the new university-trained physicians and researchers. Some doctors by this time too, as we saw in Chapter 6, had even begun to defend *commères* from the contempt with which they were often held in biomedicine.

Annick Tillier has highlighted that in the early formation of medical ideas about menopause, women themselves were absent from the conversation since

[2] Virginie Messager, *Guide pratique de l'âge critique, ou Conseils aux femmes sur les maladies qui peuvent les attaquer à cette époque de leur vie; suivis de réflexions et d'observations sur les maladies laiteuses* (Paris: chez l'auteur, 1843).

there were no women recognised as doctors in France until 1875, when Madeleine Brès (1842–1921), after more than ten years of study, scholarship, and clinical practice, was finally awarded a medical degree from the University of Paris at the age of 33.[3] In the very year of Brès's graduation, the Paris doctor and journalist Gustave Antoine Richelot collated all his numerous articles published in the conservative thrice-weekly *l'Union médicale* in previous years into a whole book of argument against the aberrant spectre of the *femme-médecin—a* figure he claimed was 'a disease of our time', threatening the whole health of society by distracting women from their true mission, which was to be mothers raising the men of tomorrow.[4] Indeed, even twenty-five years after Brès's *license* graduation, medical journals continued to publish articles about women's incapacity to practice medicine on account of their supposed excess nervousness and lesser capacity for reason—drawing on the very same discourses about women's nature that helped to produce the concept of menopausal morbidity and nervous or mental pathologies. It was on such grounds that a doctor Fiessinger called doctoresses 'one of these weeds that have invaded the flora of modern society' in his 1900 article in the Paris annual journal *La Médecine moderne* (running from 1890 to 1941).[5] Françoise Kern-Coquillat has shown that the topic continued to arouse debate well into the First World War period.[6] But by the first years of the twentieth century, there were also those taking up the fight in favour of women doctors, even historicising the continuity of their de facto roles as such, ever since Graeco-Roman times, as in the enormous and erudite 1900 thesis by the Paris medical candidate and Russian immigrant Mélanie Lipinska.[7]

This context is important, not only because many of the first women doctors wrote about women's health, bringing a fresh perspective on what was by 1875 already a very established medical culture of only men writing about menopause; but also because their acceptance into the academy tended to follow a much longer and more arduous trajectory, even once the possibility of graduation was

[3] Annick Tillier, 'Un Âge critique: La Ménopause sous le regard des médecins des XVIIIe et XIXe siècles', *CLIO: Femmes, genre, histoire*, 21 (2005): 268–280 [279].

[4] Gustave Antoine Richelot, *La Femme-médecin* (Paris: E. Dentu, 1875), 8.

[5] Dr Ch. Fiessinger, 'L'Inaptitude médicale des femmes', *La Médecine moderne: Journal de thérapeutique, de médecine, de chirurgie, d'accouchements et de pharmacologie*, 11/11 (7 February 1900): 81. Cited also by Thomas Bauer, *La Sportive dans la littérature française des Années folles* (Lille: Presses Universitaires de Septentrion, 2011), 61.

[6] Françoise Kern-Coquillat, 'Les Femmes médecins dans le service de santé (1914–1918)', *Deportate, esuli, profughe (DEP): Rivista telematica de studi sulla memoria femminile*, 24 (2014): 48–75. See also Thérèse Planiol, *Herbes folles hier, femmes médecins aujourd'hui* (Anjou: Editions Cheminements, 2000). See also Michèle Le Doeuff, *Le Sexe du savoir* (Paris: Aubier, 1998).

[7] Mélanie Lipinska, *Histoire des femmes médecins depuis l'antiquité jusqu'à nos jours*. Thèse (Paris: Librairie G. Jacques & Cie, 1900); see Jacqueline Fontaine, *Les Étudiantes en médecine à la faculté de Montpellier au cours de la Troisième République* (Paris: L'Harmattan, 2016), 49–75; also Lucie Begert, Izel Demirbas, & Aude Fauvel, 'Terre promise ou terre interdite? La Suisse: l'Eldorado ambigu des premières femmes médecins, 1867–1939 [Promised land or forbidden land? Switzerland, the ambiguous El Dorado of the first women doctors, 1867–1939]', *Revue d'histoire des sciences humaines*, 35 (2019), 59–96.

opened to them in the last decades of the nineteenth century. The first women to graduate were thus older than most of the male graduates writing their theses on women's critical age, meaning both that they had often been exposed to longer clinical apprenticeship, and that they were themselves sometimes of an age to be considered (according to the prevalent discourse) 'menopausal' or even 'old' at the time they wrote their major works on women's health. It is certainly significant that the immense nineteenth-century medicalisation of women's physiology—including the confection of entirely new categories of morbidity such as menopause, as well as the substantial re-elaboration of pre-existing categories such as hysteria, hypochondria, and nymphomania—occurred in the context of the deliberate exclusion of women from practising as doctors. Here it is worth remembering too how frequently menopause doctors disparaged *les vieilles commères* (older women folk healers and midwives) who they viewed as their competitors for older women's healthcare, we considered in Chapter 6. Menopause was, to some degree, thus nested in a new dyadic gender order in which older women were to be the patients more than ever before, while their own capacity to treat patients was denied, increasingly yoked to a hierarchical system in which they could participate only as official *sage-femmes* or as nurses, in both cases lower paid than, and subordinate to, male clinicians. How then did the entrance of women into the medical profession as doctors destabilise this gender order? And with what implications for medical concepts of women's ageing?

When the Paris monthly *Chronique médicale* (founded in 1894) interviewed Madeleine Brès in 1895 about her role as the first woman-doctor recognised in France in 1875, she explained that her earliest inspiration towards the practice of medicine occurred when she was 8 years old and was taken along with her wheelwright father while he worked at a hospital in Nîmes in the south of France, and where she observed the nuns confecting herbal remedies and other potions, which inspired her to imitate them. She thus took it upon herself to interview the patients and develop a concern for their health, playfully administering her own remedies to them made of orange peel and black liquorice. The resident physician, a Dr Pleindou, would often remark what a wonderful little nurse she was, and what a shame it was that she could not become a doctor.[8] As a widow with three children, she completed a *baccalauréat*, then seven years of university study and hospital clinical practice.[9] After eventually receiving her *license*, she then opened a gynaecology practice in the rue de Rivoli in Paris which she ran for forty years, also founding and editing the journal *L'Hygiène de la femme et de*

[8] Actualités médicales, 'La Première Doctoresse française: Conversations avec Mme Madeleine Brès, docteur en médecine', *La Chronique médicale: Revue bi-mensuelle de médecine scientifique, littéraire et anecdotique*, 2/7 (1 April 1895): 190–196 [191].

[9] Planiol, *Herbes folles hier*, 50.

l'enfant 1883–1896.[10] She did not appear to write anything specifically about menopause or the diseases of ageing, but this is noteworthy in itself given she was the first authorised woman gynaecologist in France. She clearly saw menopause as a less significant matter for women's health than the many other conditions impacting women of reproductive ages. This was consistent with the history of midwifery texts authored by women throughout the early modern period and up to this time.

Similarly, the earlier work of Marie Anne Victoire Boivin (1773–1841), a literate *sage-femme* who authored highly esteemed medical books about gynaecology and obstetrics, focused primarily on the physiology and anatomy of gynaecological cancers, pregnancy, and childbirth. Boivin (Image 8.1) was director of both the Hospice de la Maternité in Bordeaux and of the Maison Royal de Santé in the 1820s and 1830s, and the German University of Marburg gave her an honorary medical degree in 1827 in recognition of her scholarship, even as French universities refused to let her obtain one by thesis examination (of which she was clearly capable).[11] The King of Prussia had already awarded her the Order of Civil Merit in 1814, and she had even managed to win a prize from the Société de Médecine de Paris for her 1818 essay on uterine haemorrhages by disguising that she was a woman—using just her initials; though when the ruse was discovered, the faculty refused to award the prize to her.[12] The Paris publishing house Gabon nonetheless published her essay as a book the following year, referring to her competition win in the title.[13] Notably, in 1812 (the same year as the Paris student Louis de Gardanne sought to name menopause), Boivin, aged 39 years, had authored a book of obstetrics, replete with colour illustrations that she herself drew of all the known birthing positions of the foetus, and which included the seventeenth-century obstetric aphorisms of François Mauriceau.[14] But here there was no *Propter-uterum* aphorism of the kind ubiquitously cited by the medical men writing about menopause already by this time. This book was translated into both Italian and German,[15] and became a compulsory textbook for midwifery

[10] Mary R. S. Creese & Thomas M. Creese, *Ladies in the Laboratory II: West European Science, 1800–1900. A Survey of their Contributions to Research* (Lanham, Md/Oxford: Scarecrow Press, 2004), 66–67; Élide Montesi, *Les Filles d'Hippocrate* (Tilly: Éditions Acrodacrolivres, 2015), 33.

[11] Marilyn Bailey Ogilvie, *Women in Science: Antiquity through the Nineteenth Century. A Biographical Dictionary with Annotated Bibliography* (Cambridge, Mass.: MIT Press, 1986), 43.

[12] June K. Burton, *Napoleon and the Woman Question: Discourses of the Other Sex in French Education, Medicine, and Medical Law 1799–1815* (Lubbock: Texas Tech University Press, 2007), 103–106.

[13] Marie Anne Victoire Boivin, *Mémoire sur les hémorragies internes de l'utérus, qui a obtenu le prix d'émulation au concours ouvert (en 1818) par la Société de Médecine de Paris, par Mme veuve Boivin, suivi des Aphorismes d'Andrew Blake sur les hémorragies utérines* (Paris: Gabon, 1819).

[14] Marie Anne Victoire Boivin, *Mémorial de l'art des accouchements, suivi des Aphorismes de Mauriceau* (Paris: Méquignon père, 1812).

[15] Marie Anne Victoire Gillain Boivin, *Dell'Arte di assistere ai parti opera classica della signora Boivin*, trans. Domenico Meli (Milan: Giovanni Silvestri, 1822); Marie-Anne-Victoire Boivin, *Handbuch der Geburtshülfe, nach den Grundsätzen der Entbindungs-Anstalt zu Paris, und denen der*

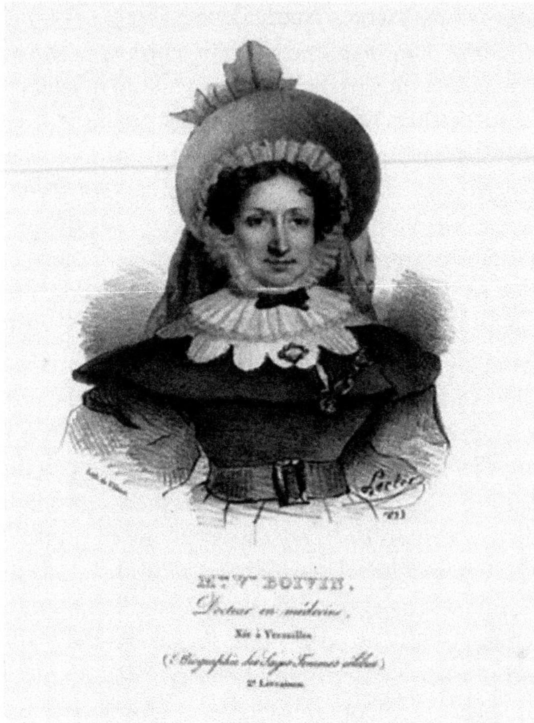

Image 8.1 Auguste Toussaint Leclerc, lithograph of Marie Boivin, 1833. Registration number 1896,0511.248. Courtesy of the British Museum.

and obstetrics students both at the University of Paris and at the School of Maternities in Berlin.[16] It was followed by several French translations that Boivin produced of works of English obstetrics, then by an 1833 work of gynaecological diseases which was rapidly translated into English, written in collaboration with the Montpellier professor of medicine Dr Antoine Louis Dugès (1797–1838).[17] Dugès was the nephew of an *officier de santé* of the same name who was the father

berühmtesten in- und ausländischen Geburtshelfer: Mit 106 lithographirten Abbildungen, welche die Behandlung aller Arten der Entbindung zeigen, 6 synoptischen Tabellen, das Ergebniß von 24,214 Fällen darbietend, und einem Anhange: die Aphorismen von Mauriceau und Orazio Valota enthaltend, trans. Robert Ferdiand, ed. Dietrich Wilhelm Heinrich Busch (Marburg: Johann Christian Krieger, 1829).

16 Nathalie Sage Pranchère, *L'École des sages-femmes: Naissance d'un corps professionnel 1786–1917* (Tours: Presses Universitaires, 2017), 315–318.

17 Marie Anne Victoire Boivin & A. Dugès, *Traité pratique des maladies de l'utérus et de ses annexes, accompagné d'un atlas de 41 planches in-fol. gravées et coloriées, représentant les principales altérations morbides des organes génitaux de la femme*, 2 vols (Paris: J.-B. Baillière, 1833); Marie Boivin & A. Dugès, *A Practical Treatise on the Diseases of the Uterus and its Appendages; translated from the French of Mme. Veuve Boivin, Sage-femme Surveillante en Chef de la Maison de Santé, etc. and A. Dugès, Professeur a la Faculté de Médecine de Montpellier, etc. With Copious Notes, by G. O. Heming, F.L.S. Consulting Accoucheur to the St. Pancras Infirmary, etc* (London: Sherwood, Gilbert & Piper, 1834).

of Boivin's own *sage-femme* mentor, Marie Louise Dugès Lachapelle (1769–1821), whose mother, in turn, had also been a renowned *sage-femme*, Marie Dugès (1730–1797).[18] Boivin was thus partially integrated into official medicine through her international success and her collaborations, while still operating on the margins of medicine, like many other midwives and health officers and indeed all the practitioners discussed in Chapter 6 who were *les hors-la-loi de la médecine* ('the legal outsiders of medicine', as Sylain Sionneau calls them);[19] and like them all, she did not pertain to treat older women as special targets of medical attention. Perhaps it was to her relative pecuniary peril: Mélanie Lipinska's exhaustive research on women doctors in 1900 indicated that Boivin died in poverty at the age of 68, after living for several years in ill health on a miserly state pension.[20]

Boivin is considered here precisely because, although she wrote only a small amount about menopause in general gynaecological reference works, what she did write was singularly dismissive of many of the more fanciful notions about women's physiology to which many doctors remained attached in this time. It is striking that midwives even in Boivin's time, even one so cognisant of the history of gynaecology and whose clinical experience was so vast, even one who specifically studied uterine haemorrhages (a widely reported symptom of menopause in the nineteenth century), still saw no grounds for substantially medicalising women's final cessation of menses. Her heavily referenced 1833 two-volume treatise, co-authored with Dugès when she was 60 years old, referred to numerous other works of gynaecology.[21] The authors mentioned 'the cessation of menses', which they noted was also called both *la ménopause* and *l'âge critique*, describing it as the time of women's lives when they could be susceptible to exhausting uterine haemorrhages (*métrorrhagie*), in between periods of scant or absent menstruation. Most importantly, they emphasised repeatedly, if haemorrhagic bleeding persisted for more than three years, or occurred many years after the final cessation of menses, then there was urgent cause for further investigation to ensure it was not the sign of a deadly uterine disease.[22] They said that statistical data (unspecified) revealed uterine cancers to be more common in women between 40 and 50 years than in any other decade, though less common in women older than 50 than in puberty,[23] and they considered these to have a possible hereditary component since patients presenting with them often reported their own mothers to have suffered them too.[24] Eight of their case examples referred to women between 45 and 55 years old who suffered gynaecological pathologies, especially uterine tumours of different kinds—including one that was clearly lethal, though

[18] Burton, *Napoleon and the Woman Question*, 104–105.

[19] Sylvain Sionneau, *Les Hors-la-loi de la médecine au xixe siècle en Maine-et-Loire* (La Crèche: Geste, 2015).

[20] Lipinska, *Histoire des femmes médecins*, 322.

[21] Boivin & Dugès, *Traité pratique des maladies de l'utérus.*

[22] Ibid., vol. 1, 30–31; vol. 2, 13, 384. [23] Ibid., vol. 2, 9. [24] Ibid., vol. 2, 108.

the vast majority of the more than sixty case examples described in this work referred to much younger women.[25] They noted that medicine's capacity to cure uterine cancers successfully was so low that many of the women who suffered them turned to 'all the litany of remedies of old women (*des vieilles*) and charlatans' out of desperation.[26] While remarks about folk healers, charlatans, empirics, and *commères* were certainly common in nineteenth-century works on the diseases of women (as we saw in Chapter 6), it was unusual to see patients acknowledged as turning to them due to the failures of official medicine.

Boivin and Dugès also described the 'derangements of menstruation' which they considered to play a 'big role in the sanitary state of women' of all ages, such that the period of the final menstrual cessation could also be 'rich in diseases', although more often it was a time that simply worried women for no good reason. Menstrual irregularity could occur for three or four years, they warned, which sometimes alarmed women who were actually in 'perfect health'.[27] Like their unusual contemporary Claude Lachaise and the slightly later Charles Menville, who both criticised the prevalent derogatory and uterine-reductive discourses about menopause,[28] Boivin and Dugès too cited the contemporary demographer Louis-François Benoiston de Châteauneuf in support of the view that the troubles of the critical age had been too often 'exaggerated'.[29] However, they were unique among French medical scholars in the nineteenth century in one other respect, citing a case example of a black African women, aged 49, who had died in a Montpellier hospital of pneumonia, and who was found in the autopsy to have several gynaecological features of note: both a surgically constructed cutaneous canal (*pertuis*) covering her intact clitoris and urethra, designed to channel both menstruation and urination, which they considered must have been created in childhood according to certain (unspecified) African cultural customs; and three large uterine fibroid tumours—the kind that were already understood to be non-cancerous and frequently asymptomatic.[30]

The authors also devoted a substantial chapter to the 'uterine neuroses' (*névroses utérines*), the mechanistic cause of which they noted was the subject of marked medical disagreement.[31] They declared themselves to be abstaining from pronouncing on the topic, before frankly doubting that mental pathologies had

[25] Ibid., vol. 1, 113, 124, 297, 327, 331; vol. 2, 43, 52, 92.

[26] Ibid., vol. 2, 99.

[27] Ibid., vol. 1, 29–30.

[28] Claude Lachaise, *Hygiène physiologique de la femme ou de la femme considérée dans son système physique et moral* (Paris: Mequignon Marvis, 1825); Charles Menville, *De l'âge critique chez les femmes, des maladies qui peuvent survenir à cette époque de la vie et des moyens de les combattre et de les prévenir* (Paris: Imprimerie de Bourgogne et Martinet, 1840).

[29] Boivin & Dugès, *Traité pratique des maladies de l'utérus*, vol. 1, 30; Louis-François Benoiston de Châteauneuf, *Mémoire sur la mortalité des femmes de l'âge de quarante à cinquante ans, lu à l'Académie des sciences, dans la séance du 13 mai 1818* (Paris: Martinet, 1822).

[30] Boivin & Dugès, *Traité pratique des maladies de l'utérus*, vol. 1, 327.

[31] Ibid., vol. 2, 461–503.

anything to do with the genital organs since many of the women who developed them had entirely normal genitalia, while others developed gynaecological disorders not as the cause but as the effect of their *vésanie* ('hysteria'); moreover, married women who had not been at all 'saturated with conjugal pleasures', had also nonetheless been observed to develop mania.[32] They politely corrected the renowned Paris scholar of hysteria, hypochondria, and melancholy, Jean-Baptiste Louyer-Villermay, remarking that it was 'not altogether correct to say' that the womb was the origin of nervous disorders, since nymphomaniacs instead had far more turgescence of the clitoris and ovaries than of the uterus.[33] They also doubted that what was often called nymphomania was really a disease at all, suggesting that 'following a precise logic', it was more appropriate to consider it a 'violent passion'.[34] Pregnancy was singled out as one of the times of susceptibility to hysteria, as was youthful amenorrhea.[35] But in none of this discussion did Boivin and Dugès identify women in menopause as susceptible to nervous disorders or erotomania.

It may seem surprising to see women such as Boivin so integrated in medical clinical work and publication in France despite the continued institutional opposition they faced towards recognition as doctors. Notably, Switzerland provided full equal opportunity to women medical students from as early as 1867, though as Lucie Begert, Izel Demirbas, and Aude Fauvel have shown, many of those women who graduated from the universities of Zurich, Bern, Geneva, Lausanne, and Basel in the second half of the nineteenth century faced multiple career obstructions afterwards.[36] One was Marie de Thilo (b. *c.*1849), a young unmarried and multilingual woman, possibly using a pseudonym, having migrated from Russia or the Baltic region to study medicine at the University of Geneva in the 1870s, and establishing her first clinic in la Chaux-de-Fonds in the Neuchâtel canton near the French border in 1883.[37] In addition to translating works of Dostoyevsky from Russian to English, she also authored several works on the medical hygiene of women in both French and German, including one in 1891 which had separate chapters on both the 'critical age' and 'old age'.[38] She seems to have given a series of seminars based on each of these chapters the following year in her home town, though it is impossible to know how many older women turned up to hear her talk about their ageing.[39]

32 Ibid., vol. 2, 456. 33 Ibid., vol. 2, 457.
34 Ibid., vol. 2, 500. 35 Ibid., vol. 2, 483–496.
36 Begert, Demirbas, & Fauvel, 'Terre promise ou terre interdite?' 37 Ibid., 78.
38 Marie de Thilo, *L'Hygiène de la femme, I. Hygiène générale. II. L'Enfance. III. La Jeune Fille. IV. La Femme mariée. V. L'Âge critique. VI. La Vieillesse* (Paris: Fischbacher, 1891), 85–91; Also Marie de Thilo, *Frauenkrankheiten wie Unterleibs- und Nervenleiden, Blutarmut und Bleichsucht und deren Behandlung* (Stuttgart: Verlag Reform, 1905); Fyodor Dostoyevsky, *Buried Alive, or, Ten Years Penal Servitude in Siberia*, trans. Marie von Thilo (London: Longmans, Green, and Co., 1881).
39 Anon., 'Mlle de Thilo, docteur-médecin spécialiste', *L'Impartial* (Thursday, 18 February 1892), 6.

Thilo placed the critical age as beginning at the age of 40, which was uncommonly early by most medical accounts of the time, which usually placed it between 45 and 50 years, though the late eighteenth-century doctor Jeannet des Longrois held the age of 40 to be a turning point too.[40] Thilo said this age endured for between two and eight years and announced it as: 'the cessation of the sexual life of woman' since 'the reproductive organs no longer function, and atrophy slightly, the svelte and gracious form disappears', warning that for some women it was also a time of dangerous diseases.[41] She listed the symptoms of hot flushes, back pain, constipation, general body aches, bloating, haemorrhages, and melancholy as common, but offered no particular hygienic advice for remedying these.[42] She seemed even less interested in 'old age', for which she recommended merely warm baths, cutting up one's food into small pieces if the teeth were not good, and consuming everything in moderation.[43] Of all the women doctors and medical writers who turned their attention to menopause and women's ageing in this time, Thilo—as remarkable an individual as she clearly was—appeared to absorb more completely than anyone the negative generalisations of the most pathologising men's writing on the topic, but without the elaborate hygienic prescriptions that usually accompanied them.

As Boivin's earlier example shows, women were clearly also able to work as unofficial (albeit underpaid) doctors even in the early nineteenth-century via the Paris midwifery pathway which was increasingly fully integrated into the medical faculty and clinics throughout the nineteenth century. Women in this pathway too began including menopause among the topics of women's health about which they wrote both manuals aimed at the public, and scholarly books. From the late 1850s onwards, there were several midwives at the University of Paris who attended many of the same lectures provided for medical studies, afterwards writing advice manuals on women's reproductive health based on their learning, such as Mesdames Virginie Messager between 1851 and 1859, Wion Pigalle in 1858, and Delestrée in 1875. Virginie Messager (born around 1805) was by far the most prolific mid-century master midwife,[44] self-publishing four books in the 1850s based on what appears to have been a long clinical experience acquired prior to this time, since her works all cited numerous case examples of women she had treated, detailing the medicaments, hygienic prescriptions, and physical therapies she had prescribed them and with what result.[45]

[40] Jean-Baptiste-Claude Jeannet des Longrois, *Conseils aux femmes de quarante ans* (Paris: Méquignon, 1787).

[41] Thilo, *L'Hygiène de la femme*, 85. [42] Ibid., 87–88. [43] Ibid., 90–91.

[44] Otto Henri Lorenz, *Catalogue général de la librairie française: 1840–1865*, vol. 3, I–O (Paris: O. Lorenz, 1869), 457.

[45] Virginie Messager, *Traité pratique des maladies des femmes* (Paris: Chez l'auteur, 1851); Virginie Messager, *Traité pratique des fleurs blanches et des ulcérations de la matrice* (Paris: Chez l'auteur, 1851); Virginie Messager, *Manuel de la jeune mère, ou Conseils aux jeunes femmes sur les soins que demandent... leur santé et celle de leurs enfants en bas âge; suivi d'Une instruction sur les soins de la toilette, ou*

Messager's 1851 *Practical Treatise of Women's Diseases* referred to her as 'Professor of Births and ex-Sage-Femme at the Paris Bureau de Bienfaisance', and said that she now (in 1851) ran 'une maison spéciale' in Paris that was 'one of the most considerable and the most frequented of our time', located at number 4, Place de l'Oratoire opposite the Louvre—the site of the Oratoire Presbyterian temple since 1789.[46] It is not clear if this clinic was in any way associated with the temple or merely rented a section of the building for its operations but given Messager's vague and euphemistic description of it as 'une maison spéciale', it seems possible that it was specifically a medical clinic for Protestant women. It was clearly a private clinic, judging from the many case examples cited in Messager's works: these were almost entirely women of the Paris and provincial urban elites, including the aristocracy, as well as foreign nationals (several Prussian and English, one Mexican, and one West African) who lived in Paris either as immigrants or temporarily due to their husbands' commercial activities or diplomatic postings.[47] It was not purely an obstetric clinic as so many other women's clinics remained in this time, and this is important for appreciating the unique character of Messager's work—in fact she wrote the largest book (415 pages) about women's 'critical age' of any writer in the nineteenth century, albeit long in part due to an added section on lactation. This probably reflected the pattern of Messager's career as a *sage-femme* in which much of her experience was gained in the care of pregnancy, childbirth, and its aftercare while working at the Bureau de Bienfaisance—a free philanthropic service which would have catered mostly to birthing mothers of the Paris working class.[48] Since taking up her role at the Oratoire private clinic, on the other hand, her clientele now shifted to women who were affluent enough to pay for medical care throughout the lifespan, including for very common and relatively minor complaints such as headaches, acne, weight gain, or constipation. As in the work of the medical men on the diseases of menopause discussed throughout this book, many of Messager's case examples are suggestive of a wide range of infectious and chronic diseases which were being clustered under the *âge de retour* by virtue of them occurring in women aged between 35 and 60 years and being accompanied by menstrual stoppage or cessation. This was though a particularly large age range that Messager was prepared to accept in her account of this dangerous 'moment' in women's lives.

Moyens de conserver et de rendre aux diverses parties du corps leur fraîcheur et leur état naturel (Paris: Chez l'auteur, 1852); Messager, *Guide pratique de l'âge critique*. Discussed also by Annick Tillier, 'Un âge critique: La Ménopause sous le regard des médecins des XVIIIe et XIXe siècles', *CLIO: Femmes, genre, histoire*, 21 (2005): 269–280.

[46] Messager, *Traité pratique des maladies des femmes*, title page.

[47] Messager, *Guide pratique de l'âge critique*, 74, 115, 141, 138, 231, 260.

[48] Olivier Faure, 'La Médecine gratuite au XIXe siècle: De la charité à l'assistance', *Histoire, économie & société*, 3–4 (1984): 593–608.

There is minimal physiological mechanistic description in this work and even fewer references to the work of doctors, though many of the concepts on which Messager elaborated in relation to women's physiology were clearly derived from the dominant medical discourse which had been developed in the faculties of Montpellier and Paris over the previous fifty years: the denigration of empirics and folk healers;[49] the idea that women in hot countries had fewer periods and ceased menstruating earlier;[50] women as the nervous and weaker sex, their entire lives traversing from one form of illness to another (puberty, menstruation, pregnancy, childbirth, lactation, and menopause) and in each case, due to the sympathy of the uterus with the entire economy of woman;[51] the dichotomy of decadent urban elites plagued by symptoms of the critical age versus virtuous hard-working peasant who breezed through this time;[52] as well the more recent idea that was taking hold among Paris alienists in the 1850s, that anything more than very minimal sexual pleasure after the *âge de retour* caused both madness or gynaecological diseases.[53] Most of Messager's book consists of case observations, with a long essay (nearly half the entire book) about the diseases of lactation—clearly nothing to do with menopause—which is indicative of Messager's enthusiasm to situate the cessation of menses within the larger medical topic of women's morbidity in all times of reproductive change, as well as perhaps, her relatively greater experience with obstetric and child-rearing care than with older women, who constituted only a small minority of her patients.[54] Nonetheless, it is noteworthy that by the 1850s, some French midwives like Messager now included women around the final cessation of menses among their patients—something not previously evidenced in any midwifery sources prior to this time and still not common throughout the remainder of the nineteenth century.

Messager said that she wrote the book with the intention of avoiding medical jargon so that women themselves might read it and benefit from it by understanding that they needed to act preventively towards all the many diseases of the *âge de retour*, indicating a specific elite market for this book among around 25 per cent (in the early nineteenth century) of literate women in France at this time who also could afford to buy books.[55] Indeed, Messager may have published the book (which would have cost her money to have printed) precisely with a view to attracting more patients from this particularly lucrative class. Unlike the working-class expectant mothers of her early career, the menopause patient cohort were women who not only had money to pay for treatment, but who might be expected to need more frequent, recurrent, and long-term treatment throughout their later ever-increasing lifespan given the higher prevalence of morbidity in ageing

[49] Messager, *Guide pratique de l'âge critique*, 177. [50] Ibid., 24.
[51] Ibid., 7–17. [52] Ibid., 240. [53] Ibid., 72–73. [54] Ibid., 285–400.
[55] Ibid., 20; Martyn Lyons, *Readers and Society in Nineteenth-Century France: Workers, Women, Peasants* (London: Palgrave, 2001), 1–16.

generally among urban, sedentary populations. With an insistent discourse, which Messager's book amply provided, of how the cessation of menses meant all women were at risk of a wide array of dangerous and lethal diseases unless they submitted to preventive medical treatments such as phlebotomy, cauterisation, cutting, cupping, enemas, vaginal douches, baths, as well as prescriptions for diet, herbal teas, and medications, the market for older women patients among the elites could potentially be considerably expanded.[56]

Notably, Messager claimed to be publishing the first proper book dedicated to women's critical age or *âge de retour* associated with the final cessation of menses, which she said doctors were reluctant to treat for fear of demeaning women: 'It is thus a new service that I believe I am providing to women in not hiding from them the ills to which their blitheness (insouciance) and ignorance can expose them.'[57] She was clearly ignorant of the substantial corpus of specialist works already existing on the topic, such as Charles-Pierre-Louis de Gardanne's two books of 1816 and 1821, Charles Menville's two books of 1839 and 1840, as well as the 1857 work of the English physician Edward Tilt (who had trained in France), not to mention the sixty-five medical theses that had been defended on the topic at French universities between 1799 and 1859, to which Messager would though presumably have had little access—midwives, after all, did not usually have library privileges.[58] Menopause was too often normalised, she complained, and women needed to be made more aware of its dangers.[59] But Messager was not all doom and gloom either. The cessation of menses represented a fundamental shift in women's physiology towards nourishing only themselves, producing a stronger pulse, flushed cheeks, firmer bodies, and a sort of rejuvenation—this was the meaning of the term *âge de retour*. She said that although women became less pretty after the end of their menses, they acquired another, more authentic and distinguished form of beauty; although some grew fatter, they also developed more 'supple' and lustrous voices, indicating their 'maturity of intelligence'. They were now less attracted to 'coquettishness' and endowed with 'solid qualities of the mind' and could thus better choose the objects of their affection 'in one or the other sex', also becoming more forgiving of others' foibles and more teacherly towards the young.[60]

[56] Ibid., 246–269. [57] Ibid., 10–12.

[58] Ibid., 11; Charles-Pierre-Louis de Gardanne, *Avis aux femmes qui entrent dans l'âge critique* (Paris: Gabon, 1816); Charles-Pierre-Louis de Gardanne, *De la ménopause ou de l'âge critique des femmes* (Paris: Méquignon-Marvis, 1821); Charles Menville, *Conseils aux femmes à l'époque de l'âge de retour, ou de l'âge critique, et de moyens de combattre et prévenir les maladies qui peuvent survenir à cette époque de la vie* (Paris: Germer Baillière, 1839); Charles Menville, *De l'âge critique chez les femmes, des maladies qui peuvent survenir à cette époque de la vie et des moyens de les combattre et de les prévenir* (Paris: Imprimerie de Bourgogne et Martinet, 1840); Edward John Tilt, *The Change of Life in Health and Disease: A Practical Treatise on the Nervous and Other Affections Incidental to Women at the Decline of Life* (London: J. Churchill, 1857).

[59] Messager, *Guide pratique de l'âge critique*, 11–12. [60] Ibid., 47–48.

Although Messager ignored (or was ignorant of) all the medical writing on menopause to date, she clearly was very aware of the important anti-pathological and naturalising movement among demographers and doctors like Antoine Deparcieux (1746), Benoiston de Châteauneuf (1822), Constant Saucerotte (1828), and Louis Noirot (1850), who had all referred to mortality statistics indicating women's greater survival relative to men in all the ages over 35 years, in arguing against the view that the cessation of menses constituted a 'critical age'.[61] She dedicated a substantial section of her book to dismissing such objections, without herself naming any of those who had made them.[62] She did this in a number of ways. Firstly, by contesting the meaning of the mortality statistics, arguing that if the critical age was not a dangerous time, then there should be many more women surviving this age given they were no longer exposed to death in childbirth;[63] she said more women actually died in their fifties than in their forties, indicating the cessation of menses must be the cause. She said the cessation occurred between 42 and 48 years, with the most common age being 45, here diverging from the standard medical account which emphasised the period of menstrual irregularity leading up to the final cessation as the 'critical' time, and locating this time between 45 and 52 years with the most common age around 48 or 49;[64] Messager instead emphasised that it was only after the final cessation had definitively occurred that women were suddenly at risk of countless diseases for which they should take equally countless precautions.[65] But she did not cite any specific statistical data to support her claim, so it is not clear on what her confidence to assert this was founded. Moreover, her case examples told a very different story—she also seems to have been content to diagnose women in their thirties who had suppressed menses as being in their *âge de retour*, and clearly treated many women in their forties who had irregular menstruation but had not yet ceased definitively.[66] She sometimes also seems to have recommended women against using medical treatments which they sought out of worry that their mild symptoms might indicate serious pathology, indicating that her heavily prescriptive account did not necessarily reflect the way she practised, lending further support perhaps to the view that her insistence on the need for routine medical treatment of menopause was more of a marketing tool than a description of her treatment approach.[67]

[61] Antoine Deparcieux, *Essai sur les probabilités de la durée de la vie humaine, d'où l'on déduit la manière de déterminer les rentes viagères, tant simples qu'en Tontines* (Paris: Frères Guerin, 1746); Louis-François Benoiston de Châteauneuf, *Mémoire sur la mortalité des femmes de l'âge de quarante à cinquante ans, lu à l'Académie des Sciences, dans la séance du 13 mai 1818* (Paris: Martinet, 1822); Constant Saucerotte, *Nouveaux conseils aux femmes sur l'âge prétendu critique, ou conduite à tenir lors de la cessation des règles* (Paris: Madame Auger-Méquinon, 1828); Louis Noirot, *Études statistiques sur la mortalité et la durée de la vie dans la ville et l'arrondissement de Dijon depuis le 19e siècle jusqu'à nos jours* (Paris: J. Baillière, 1850).

[62] Messager, *Guide pratique de l'âge critique*, 14–17, 29–30; 55–57.

[63] Ibid., 15. [64] Ibid., 24. [65] Ibid., 57.

[66] Ibid., 60, 74, 106, 174, 238, 260. [67] Ibid., 33.

The other way Messager rejected the demographic naturalising and anti-pathological view of menopause was to insist on the distinction between mortality and morbidity: it was 'not absolutely necessary for diseases to be always lethal for them rightly to be considered dangerous'.[68] Even if it was true that more women survived in their forties and fifties than in their childbearing years, they only survived 'in langor and suffering' unless they took great care of their health in the form of preventive medications, medical examinations, and hygienic interventions.[69] Also, the true mortality of women's *âge de retour* was never properly estimated, she said, since many of the diseases of old age which only killed women in the later decades after menopause had actually initiated around the time of their final cessation of menses and thus could be assumed to be caused by this fundamental revolution of woman's economy.[70] Her book was about trying to catch those diseases in their early development before they became lethal in later life, through the systematic preventive treatment of any menstrual irregularity or general complaints of women aged anywhere between 35 and 60 years.[71]

She appears to have favoured mechanical treatments, especially phlebotomy of the arm and leeches on the thighs, in the manner of François-Joseph-Victor Broussais, indicating this as her primary treatment for any woman presenting with menstrual irregularity, unless she was 'delicate' and therefore likely to be weakened by the blood loss.[72] This was probably because Messager viewed the cessation of menses as meaning that blood (though not toxic) was nonetheless now trapped inside women's bodies (as in descriptions of plethora—though she avoided this technical term), thus seeking an outlet in some other form, causing chest infections, haemorrhoids, blood in the urine, or other forms of 'inflammation'.[73] Although she said that purgatives were less useful than they were popular, she also did not hesitate to prescribe them if there was any indication of constipation, though she warned against the resinous kind (such as Jalap and aloe).[74] The most common symptoms of the final cessation of menses she described were hot flushes, sleep disturbance with 'painful dreams', abdominal pain, colic, vomiting, pain around the kidneys, swollen breast, a swollen belly that increased over time (due to polyps or to cancer), haemorrhagic bleeding,[75] white discharge,[76] fat gain,[77] palpitations, skin disorders,[78] as well as migraine, hysteria, hypochondria, melancholy, vapours and 'erotomania'—also called 'amorous delirium'.[79]

In fact she devoted considerable space to the matter of nervous pathologies, saying that asylums were full of women in the critical age suffering hysteria,

[68] Ibid., 56. [69] Ibid., 15. [70] Ibid., 11, 14–15. [71] Ibid., 55.

[72] Ibid., 83–85; 246–256; François-Joseph-Victor Broussais, *Cours de pathologies et thérapeutique générales*, 2 vols (Paris: J. B. Baillière, 1834).

[73] Messager, *Guide pratique de l'âge critique*, 58, 63.

[74] Ibid., 257–262. [75] Ibid., 85. [76] Ibid., 37–39.

[77] Ibid., 48. [78] Ibid., 64–66. [79] Ibid., 72–73.

especially childless women who had 'abused everything, those whose imagination has been constantly excited by pleasures, by a life of luxury, or have been raised in affluence then fallen suddenly into abandonment or poverty'.[80] This was because the blood from the uterus that could no longer exit via menstruation was instead diverted to the rest of the body where it created pressure on the nerves, thus increasing women's nervousness.[81] Reading novels, being moved by tender music, or attending 'rousing spectacles' were particularly risky for older women, and childless women who engaged in unusual intellectual or artistic pursuits became particularly prone to madness in the *âge de retour*.[82] Because madness was such a debilitating condition, she advised those who knew eccentric women to monitor them closely during the critical age, making sure they did not stray from their routines.[83] Sexual activity was particularly problematic, she warned, and the error of allowing oneself to be 'dominated by the last fires' of lust in the *âge de retour* could cause abdominal pain and menstrual symptoms even long after the final cessation of menses. 'This foul disposition is often found especially in women of high society (*du grand monde*) whose sensations are constantly excited by luxury and refinement.'[84] She advised married women not to avoid sex but also not to initiate it, since conjugal relations 'can at this moment often cause more suffering than felicity'.[85] The *âge de retour* was a time when one's 'sensations, our impressions need to be managed'.[86] And of course, it was refined city women living in opulence who needed most to change their ways at this time of life, not the 'country women who lead a simple life, dedicated to manual labour'.[87]

Both the faculties of Paris in 1866 and Montpellier in 1868 formally permitted women to attend medical lectures (though not to graduate), but in practice, some women, especially midwives, had begun doing so even before this time.[88] Midwifery training had, in any case, since the start of the century become rigorously biomedical and included training in substantial medical theory and technical mastery (including forceps delivery) of the same kind provided to medical students.[89] Mademe Delestrée, writing in 1875 said she was *Maîtresse Sage-Femme* (Master Midwife) and *Professeur d'accouchement* (Professor of Births), at the Paris faculty, and successor to Amélie Wion Pigalle (1826–1874), who had previously held this same title.[90] Nonetheless, Delestrée appears to have plagiarised (by today's terminology) the work first published by Wion Pigalle in 1858, passing off as her own what was effectively the seventh edition of the latter's work, after

80 Ibid., 77–78. 81 Ibid., 47. 82 Ibid., 52, 72, 242–244. 83 Ibid., 80.
84 Ibid., 51. 85 Ibid., 242. 86 Ibid., 241. 87 Ibid., 30.
88 Fontaine, *Les Étudiantes en médecine à la faculté de Montpellier*, 9–10.
89 Sage Pranchère, *L'École des sages-femmes*, 31–36.
90 Mme Delestrée, *Le Conseiller secret des femmes, ou Conseils sur les moyens de se préserver des maladies qui atteignent spécialement les femmes*, septième édition entièrement refondue (Paris: Chez l'auteur, 1875), title page.

simply rearranging the order of the chapters.[91] Wion Pigalle (sometimes written Vion Pigalle) had also self-published in 1865 a book about the pernicious effect on one's health of fearing cholera, suggesting she was particularly attuned to the ways the medicalisation of society could itself be iatrogenic.[92]

Wion Pigalle, like Marie Boivin, referred to only one symptom she associated with the 'critical age' that required medical attention: uterine haemorrhages, though she specified that these only tended to occur at this time of life if one had danced, ridden horses, taken hot baths, or used *chaufferettes* (foot or hand warmers) 'to excess'.[93] Haemorrhages, when occurring after the cessation of menses, were often a sign of uterine polyps, fibroids, or cancer.[94] She too warned that uterine cancers were most common after the cessation of menses, in the 'critical age', though they were not uncommon at other ages too. She said that once such cancers became painful, it was usually too late to cure them, emphasising that any suspicion of them as signalled by haemorrhages, chronic leukorrhea, or lumbar pain should be investigated, rather than letting modesty stop women from allowing a doctor to inspect their genitalia.[95] On the other hand, neuropathy of the womb and nervous crises were conditions she considered only to affect women from puberty to the age of 40, becoming rare after the cessation of menses.[96] She recommended hygienic measures for those who were suffering the symptoms of an emerging inflammation of the ovaries or uterus, consisting of warm baths with emollient herbs, enemas with mallow and the heads of poppies, gentle purgatives, a bland diet, and use of a light abdominal compression belt.[97]

This manual had specific short chapters for the diseases of breastfeeding, for the problem of sterility, but also a rather chaotically structured one for the 'critical age' caused by the cessation of menses.[98] The most common problems here were swollen inflammation of the articulations, gout-like conditions, rheumatism, skin diseases, oedema, and cancer.[99] But Wion Pigalle also discussed uterine haemorrhages, leukorrhea, polyps, hard tumours (*squirres*), and hysteria, though specifying that constitution played a crucial role, and that, in any case, city women could avoid all such problems by imitating the 'privations' of women of the countryside: a frugal diet, regular exercise, and fresh air were the ways to avoid all disease. Her general hygiene advice to all women around the cessation of menses was to avoid long sessions of gambling, avoid crowds and breathing the air around them, avoid tight corsets and dresses that exposed one's shoulders and chest, avoid soft beds, and if plethoric—avoid staying too long in bed, rising early to take exercise instead. Sad emotions were to be avoided too, as they were bad for one's health,

[91] Amélie Wion Pigalle, *Le Conseiller secret des femmes, ou Conseils sur les moyens de se préserver des maladies qui atteignent spécialement les femmes* [1858], 3rd ed. (Paris: Georges Kugelmann, 1861).

[92] Amélie Wion (Vion) Pigalle, *De la peur du choléra et de l'influence pernicieuse que ce sentiment exerce sur la santé* (Paris: Chez l'auteur, 1865).

[93] Ibid., 14. [94] Ibid., 15. [95] Ibid., 25. [96] Ibid., 27.

[97] Ibid., 32. [98] Ibid., 33–34; 35–36; 37–40. [99] Ibid., 37.

while overly heating diets (*un régime échauffant*) caused haemorrhoids and apoplexy. She warned against the use of purgatives and the excess use of enemas, both of which she said were common remedies to which women turned when worried about their health for any reason.[100]

There was also other constitution-specific advice: nervous women needed a regular sleep pattern and to avoid floury foods which would give them gas; sanguine women suffering heavy periods (obviously prior to the cessation of menses) needed to eat white meats and drink water with a little wine, eat acidic fruits, copious vegetables, and avoid game meats, salted meats, coffee, tea, and most alcohol; lymphatic women were to consume old wine, black coffee in small quantities, practice dry frictions of their skin, and wear flannel clothing. Robust (sanguine) women who did not observe these recommendations would suffer hot flushes, insomnia, tiring dreams, breathing difficulties, vision problems, buzzing in one's ears, inflammatory intestines, and haemorrhoids, while nervous women would be prone to hysteric sensations of strangulation and suffocation.[101]

It is not clear how widely distributed or read were either Virginie Messager's or Amélie Wion Pigalle's manuals, or the repackaged version self-published by Mme Delestrée in 1875. Certainly, no mention of any of these can be found in doctors' works on women's diseases, though it is perhaps unsurprising to find that most doctors simply ignored what midwives had to say on such matters given the limited esteem they had for these rival professionals in the market for elite women patients. Menopause, after all, had been purely a medical man's topic for over forty years. But the integration of the newly defined 'critical age' into midwifery manuals from this time onwards clearly marked the second half of the nineteenth century as an important turning point in the history of such texts, which had previously rarely even mentioned the final cessation of menses, let alone describing it as anything in need of elaborate medical attention. Menopause and the need to manage it was now something that not just men were talking about (Image 8.2).

In 1862 there also appeared a short book by a medical couple writing on chronic metritis—a symptom commonly reported in menopause—the Bouffiers. Prosper Bouffier was a Paris doctor and Madame Bouffier was a 'sage-femme of the first class of the Faculty of Paris', and their book was published by the esteemed Paris scientific press J. B. Baillière, breaking the pattern of earlier works by midwives which most often had to be self-published.[102] They defined the period of women's lives after the 'critical era' as 'post-sexual'.[103] They also reiterated the common account of women's health as dependent upon menstruation, without which it was prone to 'a state of nervous over-excitation', including around the

[100] Ibid., 38–40. [101] Ibid., 39–40.

[102] Prosper Bouffier & Madame Bouffier, *Maladies des femmes: Métrite chronique* (Paris: J. B. Baillière, 1862).

[103] Ibid., 10.

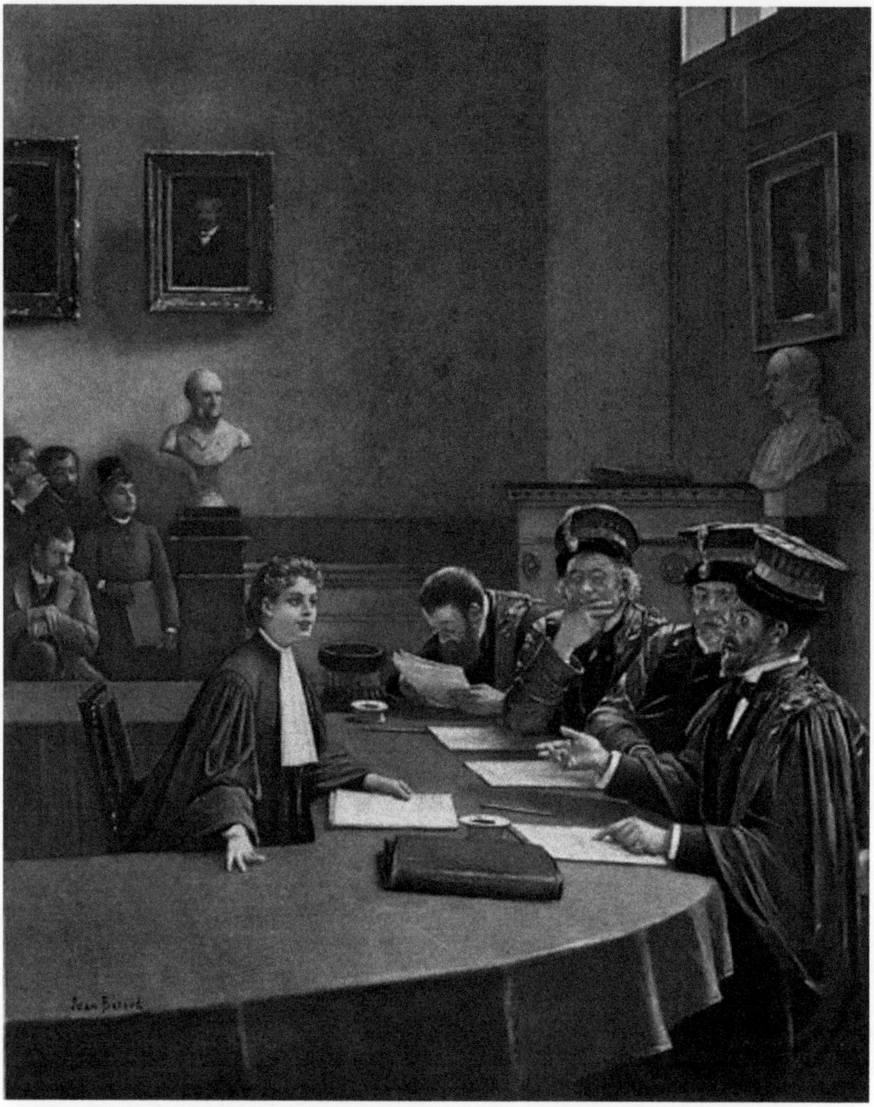

Image 8.2 The struggle of English women to qualify as doctors captured the imagination of French illustrators precisely around the time of the first medical theses by women defended at the University of Paris. This renowned image portrays Elizabeth Garrett Anderson (1836–1917), defending her thesis around 1900. Jean Béraud lithographe, Thèse de Elizabeth Garrett Anderson: *La Première Thèse féminine à la Faculté de Médecine c.*1900. (BIUM Coll. icon. S B/1036.) Courtesy of the Bibliothèque Interuniversitaire de Santé. Courtesy of Wikimedia, Creative Commons Attribution-ShareAlike 4.0 International.

time of the cessation of menses. Unlike Virginie Messager, though, they considered that the critical time only occurred until the menses had definitely ended, after which, the uterus 'returning to rest, ceases to exert its action on the whole organism'.[104] Any kind of sudden stoppage of the menses was inclined to be followed by haemorrhages, they said, though these could also be caused by excessive sexual relations, the overuse of pessaries, by refusing to breastfeed one's own infants, or by fibroid polyps, cancer, or tuberculosis.[105] But metritis was a disease of menstruating women, by their account, and older women only remained vulnerable to it in the final years before the cessation of menses. Curiously though, they did not repeat the warning of earlier midwives such as Boivin, who were keen for women to understand that haemorrhagic bleeding occurring many years after menopause was cause for serious medical concern.[106]

By the *fin de siècle* respectable Paris publishers were clearly becoming more open to the work of midwives. Another *sage-femme*, Madame A. Gensse had more success on her own than earlier midwives writing on matters of women's reproductive health, with a book also published by Baillière et fils in 1894, while a new monthly journal that she launched in 1900 ran for three years was devoted to matters of *La Beauté par l'hygiène* (Beauty via Hygiene).[107] She was also author of a work on *Les Quatre Âges de la femme au point de vue physiologique* (The Four Ages of Woman from the Physiologic Point of View), published in its fifth edition in 1899, though no copies have survived of any earlier editions, suggesting it may initially have been self-published in only a small number, only later being picked up by a press in Corbeil, south of Paris.[108] The title of this book evoked older ideas about lifespan divisions. As we considered in Chapter 2, the Enlightenment fascination with life stages provided one of the conceptual layers towards an account of the *âge de retour* as a distinct new phase proposed for men and women both, in which one was no longer young but also not yet old. But accommodating this intermediate stage between maturity and old age required five or six 'ages', since four, counting childhood (1–12 years) youth (13–20 years), and maturity (20–40 years), left only one (potentially) very large age from the late thirties until death—precisely the problem to which the eighteenth-century Encyclopedists had objected. By reverting to four ages, was Mme Gensse then suggesting that women were already old from the time their fertility began to wane?

Furthermore, the same title, *Les Quatre Âges de la femme* had been used by several illustrators and poets in the early nineteenth century, such as the engraver/

[104] Ibid., 11. [105] Ibid., 21–24.

[106] Boivin & Dugès, *Traité pratique des maladies de l'utérus.*

[107] Mme A. Gensse, *La Femme et la génération* (Paris: J.-B. Baillière et fils, 1894); Mme A. Gensse, ed., *La Beauté par l'hygiène: Journal de la famille: Médecine, littérature, sciences, arts*, premier volume 15 Janvier 1900, mensuel, 28cm.

[108] Mme A. Gensse, *Les Quatre Âges de la femme au point de vue physiologique* [1894], 5th ed. (Corbeil: E. Crété, 1899). Discussed also by Mary Lynn Stewart, *For Health and Beauty: Physical Culture for Frenchwomen 1880s–1930* (Baltimore: Johns Hopkins University Press, 2000), 82, 121.

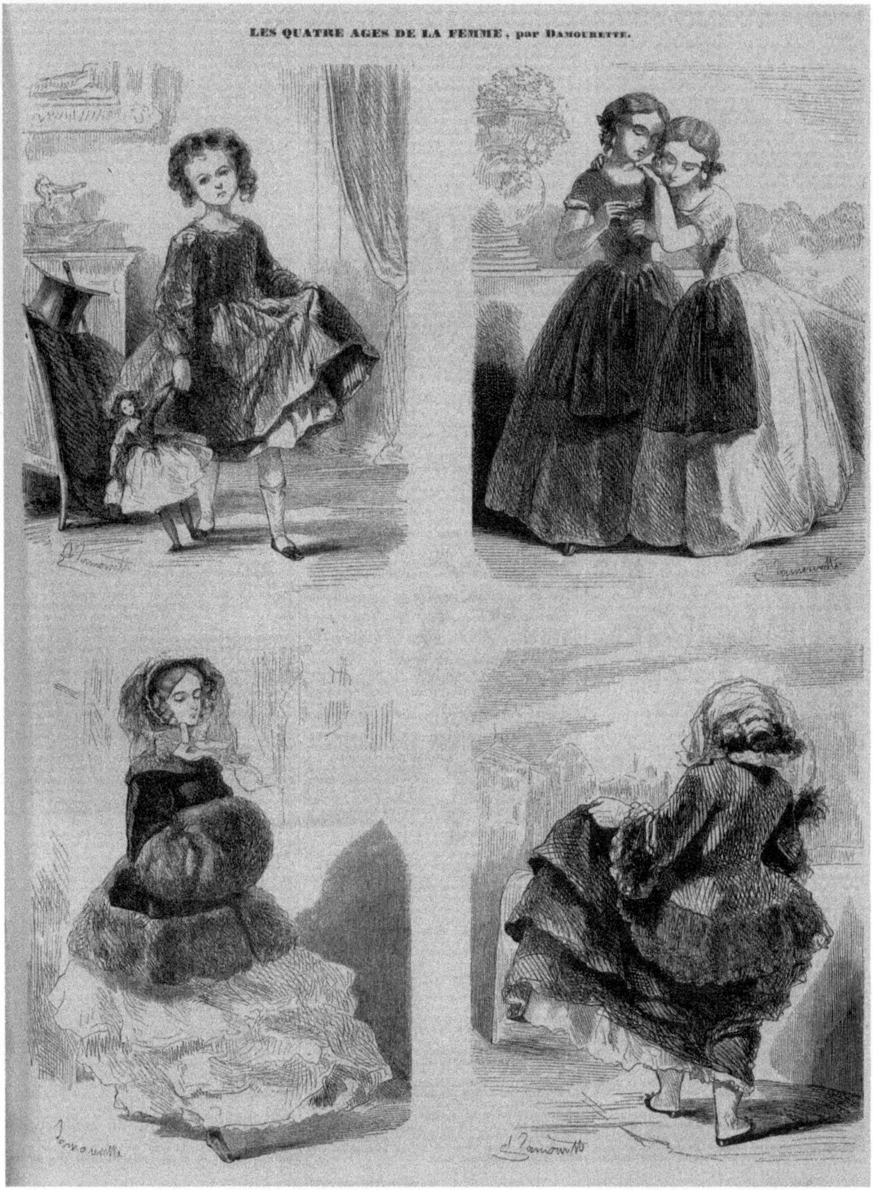

Image 8.3 Abel Damourette, *Les Quatre Âges de la femme*, 1853. Courtesy of Brown University Library.

lithographer Abel Damourette whose 1853 image is produced here (Image 8.3). Here the fourth age of woman is shown with her back turned, satirically playing on the idea that older women's faces were so unattractive as to be unworthy of representation, or perhaps admitting that it was simply impossible to draw someone potentially as young as 40 or as old as 95, such as the grouping of women's lifespan into just four ages would imply. Notably too, the fourth-age woman mirrors the first-age child in playfully lifting her skirt, in contrast to the more demure second and third ages of youth and maturity—referring to the idea that ageing was a 'retour' to the childhood state before sexed distinction occurred, such as had been argued in 1803 by the hygienist Gabriel Jouard.[109] Also bearing this same title was an 1815 Catholic poem by F. Ponchon which was republished twice more up to 1834, and which had entreated women of all ages towards religious morality appropriate for their life stage. Here the fourth-age poem pleaded for women to shun venery (*volupté*) and aspire to 'moral beauty', rather than the 'ridicule of coquettish combat against time', and prepare for death—here too implying that women over 40 belong in the category of old age, defined as inappropriate for sexual relations.[110] It advised women in their fifties 'do not go, in your ambition, to re-educate yourself, nor to research the arts in your later life; it would be to alienate yourself, better to get to know nature'.[111] But most of all it warned against the pursuit of love.[112]

It is not clear if Madame Gensse intended to refer to either of these previous invocations of women's four ages, but something of both their reduction of all older women as belonging in one big life stage, as well as the desexualisation of midlife, was also ambiguously present in her perspective. After the age of the 'mother', there was the age of the 'grandmother' which similarly grouped all post-reproductive women into one category of physiology with much of the chapter focused on the period around the cessation of menses. Gensse made a point of remarking that being a grandmother was not necessarily a sign of old age, since one could indeed become one while still fertile oneself. And despite her book referring to four ages, she also presented an alternative schema which was the eighteenth-century Encyclopedist conceptual layer of Daubenton—with the six ages that included an intermediate *âge de retour* between 45 and 60 years.[113] Nonetheless, she appeared to view the end of menstruation as heralding 'the end of sexual life' in a similar manner to the Ponchon poem with the same title as her book, as doctors and now midwives writing on menopause had sometimes suggested as well.[114] In a similar paradoxical fashion to earlier medical works on menopause, she said that women feared this time of life more than was justified, while also warning of weight gain around the waist, hot flushes, swollen breasts, acne, neuralgias, and sometimes breast or uterine cancer—hardly the stuff of reassurance.[115] The solution was to 'observe oneself attentively', avoid constipation, ensure restful sleep, and see a doctor at the first sign of any abnormal

[109] Gabriel Jouard, *Essai sur quelques points de l'histoire naturelle médicale de la femme, considérés sous les rapports physique, anatomique, physiologique, avec des applications à la pathologie.* Thèse (Paris: S. A. Huguelet, 1803), 22–23.

[110] F. Ponchon, *Eulalie, ou Les Quatre Âges de la femme* (Paris: Rosa, 1815), 164.

[111] Ibid., 176. [112] Ibid., 181–182.

[113] Gensse, *Les Quatre Âges de la femme*, 101.

[114] Ibid., 102. [115] Ibid., 103.

symptoms of the breasts or the uterus. Nonetheless, she devoted the largest sections of this chapter to rheumatism and gout,[116] and another to the perils of tight corsets.[117]

The First French Women Gynaecologists and Menopause

Between 1896 and 1904, there were several Paris medical theses and books by women on questions relating to menopause and they were all very unlike previous works written by men in the nineteenth century. In 1896 Angélina Guillarmou wrote about the use of physiotherapy in the gynaecological treatment of uterine pathologies, including the haemorrhagic bleeding of menopause, following the Swedish physician Thure Brandt (1819–1895), whose methods had been brough to France by the Paris obstetrics professor Horace Stapfer (1848–1913), after his professional mission in Sweden in 1891 (he was Guillarmou's thesis supervisor).[118] Marie Schultz was another unusual candidate at the University of Paris who graduated in 1897 with a thesis on the surgical treatment of croup (laryngotracheobronchitis), before turning to her first and quite successful book in 1902 written in collaboration with the widely published Paris obstetrician-gynaecologist Alfred Auvard (1855–1940), focused on medical hygiene related to women's reproductive health (republished in 1909).[119] Schultz and Auvard published several works together, including another book on women's general hygiene in 1903 which was mostly about diet, sleep, and exercise, with a section on old age which applied as much to men as to women.[120] They were both involved with the theosophical movement in Paris which had formed in the 1880s,[121] and Schultz was sent on a French Ministry of Education mission to India to gather information on Hindu philosophy and its pedagogy, resulting in the report she prepared for the Ministry, which was published by the Paris Theosophical Committee in

[116] Ibid., 105–111. [117] Ibid., 112–121.

[118] Angélina Guillarmou, *Kinésithérapie gynécologique: Valeur hémostatique de certains mouvements musculaires contre les méno et métrorrhagies chroniques (système de Brandt). Etude pratique.* Thèse (Paris: Steinheil, 1896); M. Stapfer, 'La Kinésithérapie gynécologique: Traitement des maladies des femmes par le massage', *Annales de gynécologie* (1892): 81–118; Anders Ottosson, 'The Age of Scientific Gynaecological Masseurs: "Non-Intrusive" Male Hands, Female Intimacy, and Women's Health Around 1900', *Social History of Medicine*, 29/4 (2016): 802–828.

[119] Marie Schultz, *Contribution à l'étude du traitement opératoire du croup écouvillonnage du larynx et dilatation de la glotte (catheterisme temporaire unique et multiple du larynx): Étude basée sur 170 observations du service de diphtérie de l'hôpital Trousseau* (Paris: Steinheil, 1897); Dr Marie Schultz & Dr Alfred Auvart, *Hygiène génitale de la femme, menstruation, fécondation, stérilité, grossesse, accouchement, suites de couches* (Paris: Octave Doin, 1902).

[120] Marie Schultz, *Hygiène générale de la femme, alimentation, vêtements, soins corporels, d'après l'enseignement et la pratique du Dr Auvard* (Paris: O. Doin, 1903).

[121] Marie Schultz & Alfred Auvard, *L'Évoluisme* (Paris: A. Maloine, 1914).

1909.[122] She and Auvard also translated the *Bhagavad Gita* from Sanskrit into French together.[123]

Their 1903 book on general hygiene for women was actually so general that it barely even mentioned anything specific to women, and said nothing about either menstruation or menopause.[124] Their 1902 book on gynaecological hygiene had only a short chapter on menopause in which they provided a very sober and naturalising account of it in the form of answers to commonly asked questions, such as 'Is it appropriate that so many women fear the era of menopause?', to which they answered, 'Under normal conditions, the era of menopause is to be feared no more than puberty.' The authors took care not to deny that the complaints of some women at this time of life were 'real', while also emphasising that they were generally neither serious nor common, and any discomfort women experienced signified 'momentary failures in the efforts of nature to maintain the equilibrium in the function of the organs, despite the modifications impressed upon the entire organism by the suppression of the physiological activity of the genital system.'[125] Sometimes this caused temporary depression, otherwise known as neurasthenia, which in more nervous women translated into hot flushes, vertigo, migraines, neuralgia, nervous asthma, palpitations, sweats, frequent urination, diarrhoea, salivary problems, suppressed appetite, bloating, constipation, buzzing in the ears, fainting, or momentary vision problems.[126] The final cessation of menses signalled a permanent shift towards 'the asexual period' of a woman's life as indicated by the atrophy of the vagina and the sagging of the breasts.[127] Nonetheless, their hygienic recommendations did not include any sexual or moral advice, threats, or severe warnings, or burdensome regimes, only prescriptions of moderation in gastronomy and alcohol consumption, of hydrotherapy, adequate sleep, moderate muscular exercise in the fresh air, enjoyment of non-fatiguing pleasures such as reading, music, travel, visits to the countryside, as well as recommending avoidance of constipation (implying enemas or suppositories), and generally creating a tranquil life for oneself surrounded by family and friends.[128]

In 1904 there was also the Paris thesis of another very idiosyncratic individual, Anne Darcanne-Mouroux (1878–1963), who later published fiction under the name Marthe Bertheaume (discussed in Chapter 9). Her medical thesis focused on the reason why some women permanently ceased menstruating precociously

[122] Marie Schultz, *La Philosophie indoue, rapport adressé à M. le ministre de l'Instruction publique en France, à la suite d'une mission confiée à l'auteur pour étudier, aux Indes, la nature, la valeur et l'enseignement de cette philosophie* (Paris: Comité de publications théosophiques, 1909).

[123] Anon, *Bhagavad Gitā*, ed./trans. Drs A. Auvard & M. Schultz (Paris: A. Maloine et fils, 1919).

[124] Schultz, *Hygiène générale de la femme.*

[125] Schultz & Auvard, *Hygiène génitale de la femme*, 29.

[126] Ibid., 30. [127] Ibid., 31. [128] Ibid., 32.

(before the age of 40).[129] Darcanne-Mouroux hypothesised that this phenomenon was explained by inherited traits—some women had small uteruses which indicated 'super-involution'—a variation on Kraepelin's 'pre-senile involution' cited in French degenerationist views of ageing (discussed in the previous chapter).[130] In eighteenth-century medicine, the final cessation of menses had emerged as a subtopic within a larger conversation about suppressed menses and infertility in young women, resulting at the turn of the century in the separation of the two questions, with the youthful form of absent menstruation designated 'amenorrhea' and the ageing form designated 'menopause'. Doctors had long been citing examples of women who stopped menstruating even as young as in their twenties, never to resume again, so on being presented with a case of a young woman who had not menstruated for several years but was otherwise in good health, it was difficult for anyone to say whether this constituted amenorrhea or menopause, given the mechanisms for such stoppage were not understood. Darcanne-Mouroux grouped such phenomena under menopause, providing a new, quasi-degenerationist take on the matter in evoking the idea of 'involution', implying a teratological disorder. She said the phenomenon ran in families, citing examples among her case observations, which included a Jewish woman who began menstruating at the age of 9 but lost this capacity at the age of 17 when she became obese; another woman from Smyrna got her first period at the age of 13 but lost it again at the age of 20. While no one could say if these women would ever menstruate again, they reported their own mothers to have experienced exactly this.[131]

Darcanne-Mouroux said that although precocious menopause was rare, it was valuable to study since these women suffered all the same negative symptoms as women in the critical age: headaches, nausea, diarrhoea, hot flushes, and cardiac pathologies.[132] And yet in her summary of thirty-eight case observations, she noted that most of the women appeared to be in good health, despite their atrophied wombs and lack of menstruation.[133] This thesis was similar to others around this time which continued to be defended by men studying medicine at the Paris faculty; since the last years of the nineteenth century, these had been becoming more specialised and original too, with the routine rehearsal of much-repeated ideas about the 'critical age' and its heavily prescriptive hygiene no longer seen as a sufficient contribution to knowledge to warrant award of the title of *Docteur.*[134] As Jacqueline Fontaine has shown, in the final decade of the

[129] Anne Darcanne-Mouroux, *Contribution à l'étude clinique de la ménopause précoce*. Thèse (Paris: H. Jouve, 1904). The BNF lists this thesis under Darcanne-Mouroux's later pseudonym, Bertheaume, presumably because she was more famous for her literary than her medical works.

[130] Ibid., 46–50. [131] Ibid., 57, 63, 90–98. [132] Ibid., 8–9. [133] Ibid., 54–56.

[134] Henri-Paul-Marie Dupuy, *Métrite hémorrhagique de la ménopause et de la vieillesse*. Thèse (Bordeaux: Imprimerie du Midi, 1897); Raoul Stopin, *Essai sur les métrorrhagies de la menopause* (Paris: Henri Jouve, 1898); Hyacinthe Le Barzic, *Contribution à l'étude du traitement des troubles de la ménopause naturelle par l'opothérapie ovarienne*. Thèse (Paris: Jouve & Boyer, 1899); Édouard Lévy, *Les*

nineteenth century, increasing numbers of women were also attracted from Russia, Romania, and Bulgaria to study medicine at the universities of Paris and Montpellier, following the official acceptance of women into graduate pathways of the medical faculties; and this in turn encouraged more French women, like Darcanne-Mouroux, to apply to train as doctors as well.[135] However, Darcanne-Mouroux's most memorable work was not her medical thesis but her semi-autobiographical fictional writing of the 1920s published under the pseudonym Marthe Bertheaume, as we consider in the next chapter, which, unique among the women discussed in this book, crossed squarely between the worlds of medical and literary evocations of women's ageing.

Another Paris candidate, Madeleine Tessier, focused on the onset of menopause in her 1911 thesis, rehearsing a similar historical story to that found in the many nineteenth-century theses produced at the Paris faculty, which blamed the pathological view of menopause on ancient and early modern medicine, referring to the description of uterine diseases in Hippocrates, Galen, Rhazes, Forestus, and Ambroise Paré, none of whom actually discussed the final cessation of menses much at all.[136] Tessier was supervised by the pioneering surgeon-doctor Samuel Pozzi, who, along with Félix Jayle, pioneered the combined use of hysterectomy, oophorectomy, and ovarian-opotherapy in women of various ages during the 1890s (discussed in our final chapter). Tessier emphasised that the majority of women suffered no diseases in the natural transition to menstrual cessation, proposing that the view of it as a time of cancer and gynaecological disorders had formed in modern medicine from the observation of a small minority of clinically diagnosed individuals.[137] Her thesis drew from Pozzi's case examples at the Broca hospital, including a group of 170 women who were at the hospital for other reasons, unrelated to gynaecological disorders, and so could be taken to be more representative of the general population than the cohorts on which much previous generalisation about menopause gynaecology had been based.

Nonetheless, Tessier appears not to have considered that if these women were in hospital due to other diseases, their menopause might still not be representative of healthy individuals. Jayle's subset of eighty-nine patients on which her thesis most focused were also in fact specifically referred to him for opotherapy

Bouffées de chaleur de la ménopause opératoire (Paris: Georges Carré & C. Naud, 1900); Jean Pignod, *Des troubles oculaires de la femme non diathésiques coïncidant avec les troubles de la menstruation et la ménopause.* Thèse (Lyon: Imprimerie Paul Legendre, 1900); Georges Siracoff, *Brachialgie de la ménopause.* Thèse (Lausanne: Imprimerie G. Varney-Burnier, 1902); René Bailleau, *Des tachycardies de la ménopause.* Thèse (Paris: L. Boyer, 1901); Louis Drevet, *Effets thérapeutiques du corps jaune de l'ovaire, en particulier dans l'hypofonction de la glande ovarienne, la ménopause naturelle, la ménopause post-opératoire.* Thèse (Paris: G. Steinheil, 1907); Adolphe Charreire, *Myomes et ménopause, atrophie, dégénérescences malignes, indications.* Thèse (Montpellier: G. Firmin, Montane & Sicardi, 1907); Maurice Godart, *Ménopause précoce et obésité.* Thèse (Paris: Steinheil, 1908).

135 Fontaine, *Les Étudiantes en médecine à la faculté de Montpellier*, 60–61.

136 Madeleine Tessier, *Établissement de la ménopause.* Thèse (Paris: Ollier-Henry, 1911), 12–14.

137 Ibid., 12.

treatment, suggesting they were actually from the cohort she had already identified as a specific, minority subset of women who were most impacted by menopausal symptoms.[138] Indeed she listed the percentages of each of the following symptoms from which they reported suffering (most likely via a specific checklist to which they were asked to respond positively or negatively): hot flushes (73%), nervous disorder or headaches (36.7%), poor sleep (36.7%), neuromuscular asthenia (28.5%), changes in character (26.6%), weaker memory (34.6%), obesity (24.4%), gastrointestinal problems (12.2%), hearing loss (23.7%), and vision problems (64.1%).[139] Of those women who permitted a genital examination, they found 36.9 per cent normal, 36.9 per cent with sclerosis of the vulva, 9.23 per cent with redness, 12.3 per cent with mild *colpocèle* (scarring from previous birth trauma), and 4.6 per cent with eczema.[140]

It was also around this time that the unusual medical family Gaboriau began studying, publishing, and clinically practising. Both parents Hélina (1869–1952) and Auguste were pharmacist-doctors, graduating from the Paris faculty within one year of each of other in 1897–1898,[141] and proud parents of a doctor daughter, Isabelle, who graduated from the same faculty in 1919, with both mother and daughter making contributions to the medical understanding of gynaecology and women's ageing.[142] In her history of medicine thesis of 1898, Hélina had critiqued the insistence often made in modern medicine of rupture with folk traditions and the 'abjection' with which those called 'empirics' were 'unjustly condemned'.[143] She said that the nineteenth-century revival of Hippocrates had produced little of value to modern medicine and that Galen's influence was positively retrograde, with the only 'refuge' of 'enlightenment' in the premodern sciences being the Arab world.[144] Needless to say, this was a very unconventional narrative about the medical past relative to the celebratory and self-proclaimed 'Hippocratic' accounts that prevailed in French writing on women's health throughout the nineteenth century, as we saw in Chapter 6.

Although it was not part of her initial medical interest, Hélina turned later in her career towards women's health, following a similar pattern observed of women doctors in both France and Switzerland, as Begert, Demirbas, and Fauvel have suggested, because it was much harder for them to make a successful career as general clinicians, whereas they were viewed as appropriate for the medical care of women's diseases.[145] This may have been so for Hélina Gaboriau, or

[138] Ibid., 54–55. [139] Ibid., 58–66. [140] Ibid., 66.

[141] Auguste Clément Marie Gaboriau, *Du surmenage intellectuel et de son traitement préventif par l'emploi simultané du phosphure de zinc et de l'arséniate de strychnine*. Thèse (Paris: Jouve, 1897); Hélina Gaboriau, *Essai sur la genèse et l'évolution de la thérapeutique* (Paris: A. Maloine, 1898).

[142] Isabelle Gaboriau, *Contribution à l'étude des métrorragies dites essentielles de la ménopause*. Thèse (Paris: Jouve, 1919); Hélina Gaboriau, *Les Trois Âges de la femme: Puberté, maternité, ménopause* (Paris: Larousse, 1923).

[143] Gaboriau, *Essai sur la genèse et l'évolution de la thérapeutique*, 7.

[144] Ibid., 12–14. [145] Begert, Demirbas, & Fauvel, 'Terre promise ou terre interdite?', 78.

perhaps it was because she was inspired by her daughter's emerging specialisation in gynaecology, that she chose to publish a 1923 manual on *Les Trois Âges de la femme* (The Three Ages of Women)—now reducing women's lifespan only to puberty, maternity, and menopause. This work proposed a number of quite radical challenges to conventional medical ideas about women's physiology, showing detailed diagrams of the female genitalia with clitoris,[146] and another diagram of 'normal' (lean) torso proportions in women to indicate how unnatural was the shape produced by the wearing of corsets.[147] But the final chapter on menopause referred to Pierre Roussel in the view that 'once the wish of nature is fulfilled', there was a sudden neglect of all sexual motivation, as well as a loss of beauty, vigour, and seductive charm,[148] though Gaboriau did also note Roussel's observation that this process was gradual, not immediate upon the end of menstruation.[149] Her account of the mechanisms of the cessation of menses was aligned to the new model of ovarian depletion reflected in other works of gynaecology since the 1890s, with the uterus now seen as far less significant.[150] She too referred to the age of menopause as beginning at 40, but said that in Paris it was later than in the provinces, most commonly occurring around 50–52 years, even if none of the various theories attempting to explain such differences had managed to prove anything.[151] Charmingly, she began her section on 'the symptoms of menopause' with the matter-of-fact statement quoted at the start of this chapter: 'The principle symptom of menopause is the cessation of the menstrual flux.'[152] Nonetheless, she thereafter listed among the possible effects of the cessation of menstruation every single negative symptom that had ever been evoked by doctors of menopause throughout the entire nineteenth century,[153] including 'psychical troubles', especially 'religious madness', which she said was one of the worst forms and very widespread.[154] There was also a substantial hygienic advice section which included vaginal douches of hot, aromatic plant decoctions, moderate conjugal relations, moderate exercise daily, hot baths, and everything culinary in moderation, with restriction of dairy and eggs if tending towards fatness (*embonpoint*).[155]

Her daughter Isabelle had a somewhat more specialised and nuanced approach in her 1919 thesis, focusing on the role of uterine haemorrhages in menopause and proposing that these were not necessarily pathological.[156] She specified the term menopause to refer to the time between regular menstruation and its definitive cessation, a 'period of perturbation' that could occur anytime between the

146 Gaboriau, *Les Trois Âges de la femme*, 38–46. 147 Ibid., 19.

148 Ibid., 178–218. 149 Ibid., 179.

150 Ibid., 180. Dr Charles Barbaud & Dr A. Rouillard, *Histoire clinico-thermale de la femme aux trois grandes périodes de sa vie: Puberté, union sexuelle, ménopause. Troubles et accidents de la ménopause (âge critique de la femme), traitement thermal aux eaux de Luxeuil* (Paris: Jouvet, 1895).

151 Gaboriau, *Les Trois Âges de la femme*, 181.

152 Ibid., 183. 153 Ibid., 184–189. 154 Ibid., 188. 155 Ibid., 188–192.

156 Gaboriau, *Contribution à l'étude des métrorragies dites essentielles*, 11.

ages of 40 and 50.[157] She listed numerous causes of haemorrhages, including due to fibroids, polyps, ovarian cysts, and cancers, as well as unrelated diseases such as syphilis and pathologies of the lungs, veins, or digestive tract.[158] Nonetheless, she proposed that menopause haemorrhages were so common and sometimes without lesions or other symptoms, as to suggest they were not, per se, pathological—though only speculum examination could confirm this. She cited various statistical accounts from English and American gynaecology clinical records, while astutely noting that no systematic attempt had in fact been made to account for their statistical prevalence in the general population.[159] Gaboriau-the-younger too had a substantial section of hygienic advice, borrowing explicitly from the 1911 gynaecology treatise of the Paris professors Jean-Louis Faure and Armand Siredy, with one important exception: she did not repeat their recommendation for the use of ovarian opotherapy pharmacy of the kind that was now for sale in Paris to all menopausal women who could afford it.[160] Other novel therapies were promoted by women doctors in the 1920s for menopause too: the Paris candidate Georgette Perrin wrote about the therapeutic effect of thermal baths for the treatment of hypertension in menopause, drawing on patient records from a clinic in Royat in the Auvergne-Rhône-Alos region.[161] German women too now were studying medicine, with a focus on ageing, such as the 1925 Göttigen student Else Scherer who wrote her dissertation on blood pressure during the climacteric (here referring to men's midlife) and during women's menopause.[162] Another Swiss francophone woman doctor, Marie Florin, wrote her 1929 Geneva thesis on the use of radioactive *curiethérapie* in the treatment of menopausal uterine pathologies—this was similar to the 'rejuvenation' treatment of irradiation applied to the ovaries used by the German-American endocrinologist Harry S. Benjamin, and which was described by the American writer Gertude Atherton in her 1923 novel *Black Oxen* (about an older women who has this treatment), which was made into a movie.[163] But these therapies appeared to have little uptake in the French context, enamoured as it was becoming instead with the new exogenous hormone discoveries (discussed in the next chapter).

[157] Ibid., 9. [158] Ibid., 12. [159] Ibid., 29–32.

[160] Ibid., 47–51; Jean-Louis Faure & Armand Siredy, *Traité de gynécologie médico-chirurgicale* (Paris: Octave Doin et fils, 1911), 234.

[161] Georgette Perrin, *L'Hypertension de la ménopause, son traitement à Royat.* Thèse (Paris: Jouve, 1926).

[162] Else Scherer, *Über das Verhalten des Blutdruckes im Klimakterium und der Menopause.* Dissertation (Göttingen: Fritz Scherer, 1925).

[163] Marie Florin, *La Curiethérapie dans le traitement des métropathies hémorragiques de la ménopause.* Thèse (Geneva: Benno Schwabe, 1929); Susan Squier, 'The Traffic Between Technologies of Reproduction and Age-Extension', in Kathleen Woodwood, ed., *Figuring Age, Women, Bodies, Generations* (Bloomington & Indianapolis: Indiana University Press, 1999), 86–99; Chandak Sengoopta, *The Most Secret Quintessence of Life: Sex, Gonads and Hormones, 1850–1950* (Chicago: University of Chicago Press, 2006), 90–94.

By the turn of the twentieth century there were also an increasing number of works, from outside France, part hygiene, part proto-feminism, referring to women's ageing in novel ways for French readers: Maria Maiocchi Plattis (1864–1917), writing under the pseudonym Jolanda, was an Italian journalist whose works were frequently translated into French, such as the book published in 1910, *Talisman de jeunesse* (Talisman of Youth), which was a sort of advice manual about the types of femininity and women's roles in the changing times of industrial modernity.[164] Jolanda was probably around 46 years old when this work appeared in France, with a preface by the Baronesse d'Orchamps, who was probably the one who translated it from Italian. Like some of the other idiosyncratic women discussed in this chapter, Jolanda has attracted some recent attention among gender historians, but which has mostly focused on the more superficial aspects of these writers in their advice about clothes and beauty.[165] But this was not all that Jolanda was talking about. She acknowledged that, although women generally aspired to remain youthful and beautiful, it was not the fresh-faced youth with vacuous smiles who inspired great works of literature and philosophy, citing the example of the Ferrarese noblewoman Eleonora d'Este (1515–1575), the muse of Tacitus, who she said was 'ugly, sickly and aged'.[166] And she blamed men's disdain for women's character, from Diogenes to Lombroso, for the limited prospects they had in modern society.[167] Jolanda reiterated the old medical hygienic idea that peasant lifeways provided a model for city women in finding ageing less sombre. But she offered no hygienic advice modelled on peasants' bodily lifeways in the manner of the medical writers, instead implying it was their psychological attitude that caused them to complain less about the ills of ageing.[168]

A 1901 book by the American doctor, suffragist, and prohibitionist Emma F. Angell Drake (1849–1934) entitled *What a Woman of Forty-Five Ought to Know* was also translated into French by a Geneva press in 1908, providing francophone readers with the first feminist account of the medical concept of menopause, a concept which by this time, had become a marginal topic in US medicine.[169] While Drake's account specifically rejected the idea that women entered a 'critical' time or climacteric in the late forties, the French translation

[164] Jolanda (Maria Plattis), *Talismans de jeunesse (les raffinements de la femme): conseils et règles de la vie féminine contemporaine, mondanité, éducation, maternité, hygiène* (Paris: A. Méricant, *c.*1910).

[165] Also discussed by Stewart, *For Health and Beauty*, 13; Louise Foxcroft, *Hot Flushes, Cold Science: A History of the Modern Menopause* (London: Granta Books, 2011), no page numbers; and Valerie Steele, *Paris Fashion: A Cultural History* (Oxford: Oxford University Press, 1988), 296.

[166] Jolanda, *Talismans de jeunesse*, 33. [167] Ibid., 14. [168] Ibid., 65.

[169] Emma Angell Drake, *What a Woman of Forty-Five Ought to Know* (Philadelphia: Vir Publishing, 1901); Emma Angell Drake, *Ce que toute femme de 45 ans devrait savoir (l'âge critique)* (Geneva: J. H. Jeheber, 1908). Chad Pearsall, 'Biography of Emma F. Angell Drake, 1849–1934', in National Woman Suffrage Association, *Biographical Database of NAWSA Suffragists, 1890–1920.* <https://documents.alexanderstreet.com/d/1009656460>.

assimilated the work, in its title, to *l'âge critique*.[170] Drake pondered how the lifespan could be divided into phases, proposing the same three as had Madame Gensse just two years earlier, but proposed that the final phase should be divided again to give a 'meridian period' that she described as 'a great table-land, where all sort and kinds of opportunities lie in waiting, and where women may roam at will, recognising and seizing upon the things they could find time heretofore to look upon at a distance'.[171] Thus was born the notion of the positive 'midlife'—menopause as a unique post-reproductive, existential opportunity for professional women, which, as Susanne Schmidt has shown, became an important part of American feminist theories of ageing in the second half of the twentieth century.[172]

Two significant chapters of Drake's book were devoted to the questions of 'auto-suggestion' and 'self-induced diseases'—referring to the power of the mind both to cure disease and to cause it.[173] Here she proposed that women around 45 years old needed particularly to avoid the expectation of their cessation of menses as a time of suffering, which she acknowledged was difficult given the vast medical description of it as such. By Drake's account, the medical concept of menopause had acquired a significant and very problematic nocebo power—the negative form of placebo, or what Drake herself called 'auto-suggestion'—that women should avoid as much as possible. A woman must apply 'all her good sense and willpower to the issue in order to tide her safely over this period, with health and strength assured'.[174] Drake herself refused to describe any menopause 'symptoms' or their hygienic management, instead proposing a broad prescription of existential reorientation to stay healthy and happy through the change, by enjoying more time to oneself, withdrawing from domestic duties, cultivating friendship, regular exercise, as well as both general temperance and dietary caution (no pies and cakes).[175] It is not clear how many women in France read the 1908 translation of Drake's book (which, apart from the addition of the 'critical age' subtitle, was otherwise very close to the original). But as we will see in the next chapter, French women writers and doctors too around this time were now beginning to realise their own accounts of how the cessation of menses could herald new forms of personal agency.

[170] Drake, *What a Woman of Forty-Five Ought to Know*, 29. [171] Ibid., 43.
[172] Susanne Schmidt, *Midlife Crisis: The Feminist Origins of a Chauvinist Cliché* (Chicago: University of Chicago Press, 2020), 49–59.
[173] Drake, *What a Woman of Forty-Five Ought to Know*, 129–171.
[174] Ibid., 167. [175] Ibid., 97.

9

Women Writers' Fictional, Autobiographical, and Epistolary Responses to Medical Discourses About Women's Ageing, 1900–1930

> 'En effet, mon cher ami, c'est une vanité sotte, puérile et pénible, de lutter contre le temps qui nous fane et nous désagrège, mais c'est vous, les hommes, qui nous obligez à nous défendre contre les ans qui nous attaquent. C'est vous qui nous y forcez, par le dédain que vous avez de nos automnes.... Faut-il renoncer, au lendemain de la trentaine, à la sentimentalité exquise de l'existence? Mais c'est l'âge où nous avons le plus et le mieux conscience des bontés de la vie.'
>
> ('Indeed, my dear friend, it is a foolish, puerile and painful vanity to struggle against the time that wilts and disaggregates us; but it is you men who oblige us to defend ourselves against the years that attack us. It is you who force us into it, by the disdain that you have for our autumn.... Must one renounce the exquisite sentimentality of existence after one's thirties? But it is also the age when we are the most and the best aware of the bounties of life.')
>
> Yvette Guilbert, *Les Demi-vieilles*, 1902.[1]

This chapter considers how other kinds of women writers, who were not medical researchers, doctors, or midwives, responded to medical discourses about their ageing during the period of particular French fascination with women's reproductive ageing in the late nineteenth century and up to 1930. Diverging from the medical works primarily discussed in the book, we turn now to literary, autobiographical, and epistolary works which engaged with French medical concepts of women's ageing. We will focus on some highly unusual individuals on whom there is little existing scholarship, as well as on several more iconic or canonical figures who have been widely discussed in relation to ageing, but not specifically to medical discourses of menopause.

[1] Yvette Guilbert, *Les Demi-vieilles* (Paris: Félix Juven, 1902), 286–287.

The French Invention of Menopause and the Medicalisation of Women's Ageing: A History. Alison M. Downham Moore, Oxford University Press. © Alison M. Downham Moore 2022. DOI: 10.1093/oso/9780192842916.003.0010

These women's responses were highly varied. They are a non-homogeneous group, not only in terms of educational backgrounds, professional opportunities, and styles of writing, but also in relation to their individual experiences and expectations of ageing. One thing they all had in common, however, is that, each in different ways, they responded to the increasingly cohering and publicly circulating negative medical discourse of women's final cessation of menses: as the end of being truly a woman, as the end of being desirable to men, as the beginning of decrepitude, as a time of sexual renunciation, of necessary morbidity, of withdrawal from the world and from the pleasures of city life, or of nervous crisis and depression. All were educated and literate women who seemed well aware of what medical men were saying about their ageing. In having powerful intellectual ambitions and complex forms of existential meaning in their lives, they also all had their own unique ways of challenging or transcending the view of women as useless and irrelevant on account of no longer menstruating, which medicine claimed to be challenging but actually continually elaborated and reproduced. It is not possible to know much about how non-literate, non-writing women experienced the final cessation of menses or ageing, aside from the occasional accounts of them in doctors' case examples discussed throughout this book. This chapter thus does not claim to represent anything like the full spectrum of French women's responses to the concept of menopause in this period, but to ponder the thoughts of some particularly thoughtful women who took the trouble to unpack the complex emotional, philosophical, cultural, and physiological implications of the expanding French medicalisation of women's ageing.

This chapter compares four women writers who were all born and raised in the nineteenth century and who wrote about ageing in fictional, epistolary, or autobiographical ways through the peak period of French medical discourses of the critical age, the *âge de retour*, and menopause. They are Yvette Guilbert (1865–1944), the Comtesse de Tramar (pseudonym of Marie-Fanny de Lamarque de Lagarrigue, 1843–1911), Anne Darcanne-Mouroux (pseudonym of Marthe Bertheaume, 1878–1963), and Colette (Sidonie-Gabrielle Colette, 1873–1954). In doing so we will consider what impact medical discourses appeared to have on their own reported experiences of, and reflections about, feminine ageing. As a field of inquiry, women's writing on ageing and menopause could easily have filled a whole book of its own by including discussion of the later works of Simone de Beauvoir (1908–1986), whose four books *Le Deuxième Sexe* (1949), *La Force de l'âge* (1963), *Une mort très douce* (1964), and *La Vieillesse* (1970) have attracted the most scholarly attention of any of the women writers to address women's ageing;[2] or the writer Violette Leduc (1907–1972), who, like Colette, viewed her

[2] Simone de Beauvoir, *Le Deuxième Sexe*, 2 vols (Paris: Gallimard, 1949); Simone de Beauvoir, *La Force de l'âge* (Paris: Gallimard, 1963); Simone de Beauvoir, *Une mort très douce* (Paris: Gallimard, 1964); Simone de Beauvoir, *La Vieillesse* (Paris: Gallimard, 1970); Diana Holmes, 'Colette, Beauvoir

own ageing relatively positively (or at least, no more negatively than she viewed the rest of her life!).[3] And indeed, Oliver Davis's 2006 monograph *Age Rage and Going Gently* carefully considers both Beauvoir's and Leduc's imaginaries of ageing.[4] We might also consider more recent and diverse francophone writers such as the Algerian novelist Maïssa Bey (b. 1950), the Mauritian novelist Ananda Devi (b. 1957), and the French novelist Michèle Sarde (b. 1939), whose ideas about menopause are discussed by Maria Kathryn Tomlinson in a broader study of the female fertility cycle in contemporary francophone fiction.[5] Nonetheless, all of these worthy figures fall outside the temporal scope of the current book, with its focus on the long eighteenth and nineteenth centuries, and were significantly exposed to more global and twentieth-century public and medical concepts, rather than the nineteenth-century French discourses that dominated up until the 1920s but less so thereafter. There are earlier possible examples too, such as Madame de Lambert (Anne-Thérèse de Marguenat de Courcelles, 1647–1733) who wrote a short epistolary essay in 1736 on old age,[6] and the Marquise du Deffand (Marie de Vichy-Chamrond, 1696–1780), who was known for her long platonic relationship and correspondence with the much younger British writer Horace Walpole between 1742 and 1777.[7] But these women had absolutely nothing to say about medical concepts of women's ageing or the end of fertility and menstruation, as these were topics that held negligible currency in France before the 1780s. This chapter thus focuses on women who were themselves children of the nineteenth century, born long enough after the invention of menopause to have been exposed to the increasingly public circulation of discourses medicalising women's ageing after the 1850s.

and the Change of Life', *French Studies*, 53/4 (1999): Penelope Deutscher, 'Beauvoir's Old Age', in Claudia Card, ed., *Cambridge Companion to Beauvoir* (Cambridge: Cambridge University Press, 2003), 286–304; Oliver Davis, *Age Rage and Going Gently: Stories of the Senescent Subject in Twentieth-Century French Writing* (Amsterdam/New York: Rodopi, 2006), 113–138; Sylvie Chaperon, 'Simone de Beauvoir, la promesse faite aux femmes', *L'Humanité* (9 January 2008): 1–4. <https://www.humanite.fr/node/384540> (viewed 11 May 2020): 430–443; Anne Strasser, 'Simone de Beauvoir, du *Deuxième Sexe* à *La Vieillesse*: quand l'intime gagne le politique', *Itinéraires*, 2 (2012): 93–103; Armelle Brad-Chopard, 'Le Vieillissement au féminin et au masculin chez Simone de Beauvoir', *Recherches féministes*, 26/2 (2013): 37–50; Silvia Stoller, ed., *Simone de Beauvoir's Philosophy of Age: Gender, Ethics, Time* (Berlin: De Gruyter, 2014); Stephen Katz, 'Simon de Beauvoir's *The Coming of Age*: The Humanities and Gerontology's Diagram of Science', *Age, Culture, Humanities: An Interdisciplinary Journal*, 3 (2016): 1–10.

3 Violette Leduc, *La Bâtarde* (Paris: Gallimard, 1964), 462.

4 Davis, *Age Rage and Going Gently.*

5 Maïssa Bey, *Hizya* (Paris: Aube, 2015); Ananda Devi, *Indian Tango* (Paris: Gallimard, 2007); Michèle Sarde, *Françoise et la cinquantaine* (Paris: Seuil, 2003); Maria Kathryn Tomlinson, *From Menstruation to Menopause: The Female Fertility Cycle in Contemporary Women's Writing in French* (Liverpool: Liverpool University Press, 2021).

6 Madame de Lambert (Anne-Thérèse de Marguenat de Courcelles), *De l'amitié, suivi de Traité de la vieillesse* [1736] (Paris: Payot, 2018).

7 Madame du Deffand (Marie de Vichy-Chamrond), *D'Éros à Agape, où les correspondances de Mme du Deffand avec Horace Walpole*, ed. Olivier Deshayes (Paris: L'Harmattan, 2011).

It may seem jarring to move in this chapter towards the consideration of autobiographical, fictional, and epistolary representations of women's ageing, which differ significantly from the medical sources thus far considered in this book, and which would be worthy of a whole book in themselves. Our aim here is to consider these works in relation to the medical concept of menopause, identifying the extent to which medical discourses formed part of scholarly women's imaginaries. The final decade of the nineteenth century saw new forms of women's writing, both autobiographical and fictional, in which themes relating to bourgeois life that were not previously part of women's contributions to literature were broached. One of these was the question of women's transition to post-reproductive existence. Menstruation was patently not so broached, and none of the writers discussed here addressed the matter in such explicit terms. For the generation of elite French women born in the second half of the nineteenth century, reaching midlife between 1880 and 1930, the medical suggestion that they could expect to experience a 'critical age' around the ages of 45–50 years, when their ageing would suddenly begin—something that at the same time they should not worry about, because that too would make them sick—was now widely disseminated. Popular hygiene manuals and guides to women's health or their critical age published between 1860 and 1901, like those we considered in the previous chapter, as well other medical professionals who now sought to write in the genre of medical *vulgarisation*, were all part of the cultural landscape in which bourgeois and aristocratic women were raised (and some of the working classes too, as literacy had begun to increase), telling them what it meant to live beyond the cessation of menses.[8] What, then, did these new kinds of women writers make of this discourse?

[8] Amélie Wion-Pigalle, *Le Conseiller secret des femmes, ou Conseils sur les moyens de se préserver des maladies qui atteignent spécialement les femmes* (Paris: Chez l'auteur, 1861); Théophile-Charles-Emmanuel Édouard Auber, *Hygiène des femmes nerveuses, ou Conseils aux femmes pour les époques critiques de leur vie* (Paris: Germer Baillière, 1841); Émile Bertin, *De la ménopause considérée principalement au point de vue de l'hygiène* (Montpellier: C. Coulet/Paris: Adrien Delahaye, 1866); Mme Delestrée, *Le Conseiller secret des femmes, ou Conseils sur les moyens de se préserver des maladies qui atteignent spécialement les femmes*, 7th ed. (Paris: Chez l'auteur, 1875); Alex Mayer, *Conseils aux femmes sur l'âge de retour: Médecine et hygiène* (Paris: J. B. Baillière et fils, 1875); Anon., *Les Âges critiques de la femme: Puberté—Ménopause. Guides des mères de famille, des maîtresses de pension et des directrices d'établissements religieux* (Paris: V. Goupy et Jourdan, 1878); Alexis Clerc, *Hygiène et médecine des deux sexes; suivies d'un Dictionnaire d'hygiène et de médecine*, 2 vols (Paris: Jules Rouff et cie, 1885); Marcellin Camboulives, *L'Homme et la femme à tous les âges de la vie: Étude hygiénique, médicale, physiologique, sociale et morale* (Paris: E. Flammarion, 1890); Ernest Monin, *L'Hygiène des riches* (Paris: A. Silvestre, 1891); Hayès, *Hygiène de l'âge critique* (Paris: Librairie des publications modernes, 1891)Dr; Marie de Thilo, *L'Hygiène de la femme* (Paris: Fishbacher, 1891); Anon., *Accidents du retour d'âge et maladies du système véneux; varices et ulcères variqueux; hémorroïdes, varicocèle; phlébites, œdèmes chroniques; congestions; hémorrages, etc.; Leur traitement par l'Élixir de Virginie* (Paris: Moride, 1894); Mme A. Gensse, *Les Quatre Âges de la femme au point de vue physiologique, cinquième édition* (Corbeil: E. Crété, 1899); André Castan, *Hygiène de l'âge de retour* (Paris: J. B. Baillière et Fils, 1901).

Yvette Guilbert, *Les Demi-vieilles*, 1902

One of the most curious writers to consider in relation to medical discourses of menopause is the late nineteenth-century Parisian actress, singer, writer, and producer Yvette Guilbert (b. Emma Laure Esther Guilbert, 1865–1944). Guilbert (Image 9.1), in many respects, embodied the very archetype of the decadent, modern, urban bourgeois woman that so many doctors warned women against, on the threat of suffering a miserable litany of menopausal symptoms in their critical age. Guilbert is most known for her performances at the Moulin Rouge and Le Chat Noir in Paris at the *fin de siècle* (when Toulouse-Lautrec painted a watercolour portrait of her); but her career in *café-concert* and music theatre spanned nearly fifty years throughout the late 1880s (Image 9.2) until the mid-1930s, and she was made *Chevalier de la légion d'honneur*, a high state honour, in 1932.[9] Nonetheless, as Geraldine Power has shown, and like many

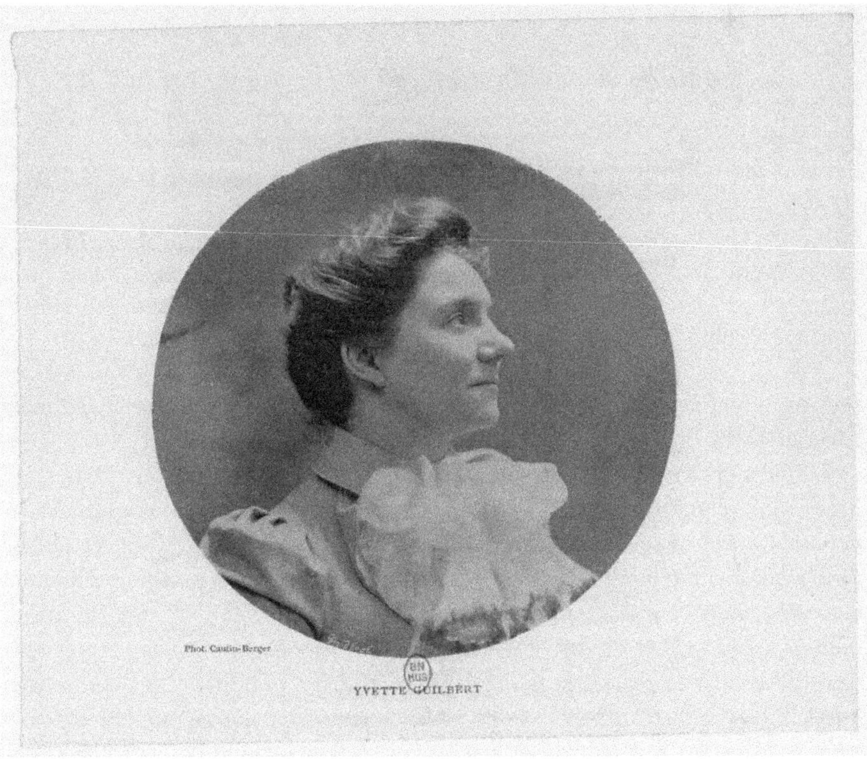

Image 9.1 Cautin-Berger photograph of Yvette Guilbert, 1900. Courtesy of the Bibliothèque Nationale de France.

[9] Geraldine Power, 'Yvette Guilbert: A Career of Public Applause and Personal Disappointment', *Context*, 27 & 28 (2004): 31–41.

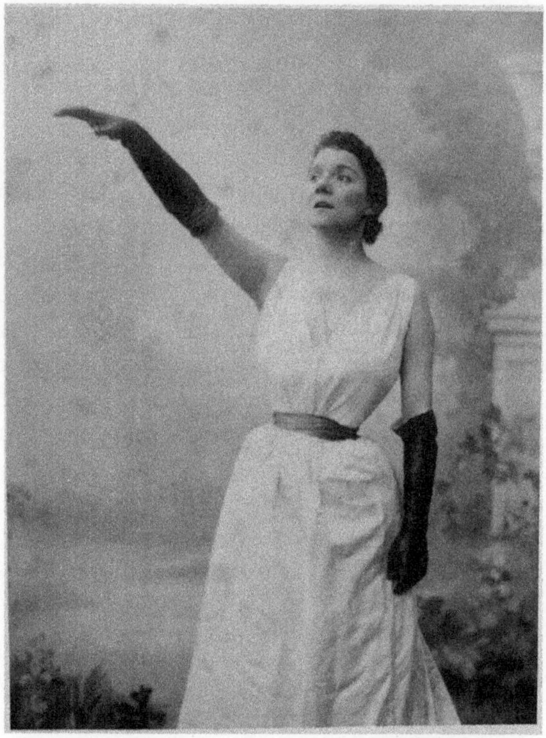

Image 9.2 Unidentified artist, Yvette Guilbert, *c.*1895. Photograph on paper Image: 12.7 × 9.3 cm (5 × 3 11/16 in.) Sheet: 16 × 12.5 cm (6 5/16 × 4 15/16 in.). Collection Zimmerli Art Museum at Rutgers University, Gift of Herbert D. and Ruth Schimmel 1990.0122. Photo Peter Jacobs.

successful women theatre professionals in this time, Guilbert experienced many frustrations throughout her career and ultimately died in poverty.[10]

Guilbert spoke of no symptoms or diseases in women in their forties and fifties, nor of menstruation or its stoppage, either in her autobiographical or fictional works. She did, however, have much to say about women's ageing, particularly with reference to the public pressure on actresses to stay youthful and beautiful, and to the lack of respect many men had for older women. Her fusion of ideas about women's creative agency and professionalism in ageing represented a powerful counter-discourse to the medical tendency of bifurcating older women into either modern, urban, worldly decadence—which was thought to cause women to suffer in menopause on account of their wounded vanity and over-stimulated nerves—or the contrasting image, repeatedly painted in medical

[10] Ibid., 31.

works on women's health, of the model selfless, peasant grandmother role, proposed as the only possible compensation for women's drastic loss of femininity, meaning, and purpose after the end of their fertility (as we considered in Chapters 4 and 5). Guilbert's 1902 book *Les Demi-vieilles* (The Half-old Women) portrayed a very different kind of path for a woman in her mid- and late forties, one buzzing with erotic and romantic possibilities—but above all one where older women could ambitiously pursue creative work in the theatre as a higher purpose, making meaningful, unique, and ground-breaking contributions to culture.

Les Demi-vieilles was published when Guilbert, aged 37, was already a household name in Paris, and was known in theatre scenes throughout Europe and even in New York. It was not her first book, as she had already published several successful autobiographical works about her busy, successful theatre career.[11] She said that, unlike her previous books, it was not an autobiography—and indeed, its central character, who is aged between 43 and 45 years in the temporal range of the narrative, is 6–8 years older than Guilbert was when she wrote it. She explained that the story and its characters were all a pastiche of details from the lives of two friends of hers who were older theatre women, with parts of her own experience included.[12] The book alluded to the relaxed sexual morals of the theatre world, to serial monogamy, non-monogamy, homosexuality, women choosing to remain childless, and romantic bonds outside marriage. It portrayed women who made no attempt to avoid the powerful chagrins and passions that doctors warned would destroy women's nerves, and even give them cancer, in their forties.[13]

Les Demi-vieilles tells the story of a successful theatre actress and singer named Esther Renot (Esther was one of Guilbert's middle names). At the start of the book she is 43 years old and at the peak of her successful career thus far, but already worrying that she may be perceived as too old for the glamorous roles for which she is known by an adoring public. Her hair is dyed with henna to cover the greys.[14] She feels as if she is suffocating from the tight corset she uses to look more hourglass-shaped, and choking from the pearls she wears high around her neck to hide her ageing skin. Nonetheless, she reaffirms her commitment to glamour, which is both a burden and a weapon in her fight to maintain her status as a star. But she also wonders when she will be permitted 'to grow old at her

[11] Yvette Guilbert, *Comment on devient une étoile* (Paris, 1893); Yvette Guilbert, *La Vedette*, 7th ed. (Paris: H. Simonis Empis, 1902). This was a work which had previously been self-published many years earlier—in her preface, Guilbert refers to being 25 when she wrote it (in around 1890).

[12] Guilbert, *Les Demi-vieilles*, 'Préface', unpaginated.

[13] The cancer claim is found in Louis Chandelux, *L'Âge critique de la femme (ménopause)*. Thèse (Paris: Irgnoux, 1850), 27; Laurent Martin, *Les Dangers de l'amour, de la luxure et du libertinage pour l'homme, pour la femme, pendant la jeunesse, pendant l'âge mûr, pendant la vieillesse* (Paris: Lebigre-Duquesne Frères, 1865), 380–381.

[14] Guilbert, *Les Demi-vieilles*, 6.

leisure'. After all, she has an adult son from a previous marriage, and is soon to become a grandmother.[15] But the decadent authorial voice proposes that her very appeal to the theatre world is precisely 'that slimness that age transforms into a sort of misplaced skinniness', and which is a 'caricature of grace', making her both 'lamentable and desirable' in her impassioned struggle to remain relevant and pursue further glory: 'Pauvre lutteuse! Pauvre délicieuse demi-vieille de la Rampe! ('Poor fighter! Poor delicious half-old woman of the stage!')'[16] Other older women, too, are scrutinised and appraised. A socialite woman she encounters at a soirée is 'resplendent', with firm skin and powdered hair, and seems 'well preserved' for her 53 years. Esther attributes this to her remaining healthy and happy, which gives her 'a youthful air' ('un air jeunet').[17] Another woman, whose age is not specified but who has a 35-year-old son (and so is probably at least in her fifties), is estimated to weigh 120 kilograms—which, Esther notes, does not stop her from being someone who 'wants to matter'.[18]

Already here there is a clear divergence from the simplistically negative view of women's ageing proposed in medical writing throughout the nineteenth century. The character of Esther perhaps fits the negative medical image of glamorous bourgeois women for whom ageing is a 'hell', as Pierre Roussel first proposed, since it is a loss of youthful beauty and the power it gives women to command the hearts of men.[19] And yet the authorial voice of ambivalent desire and pity for Esther presents her appeal as a unique aesthetic that only an older woman can provide. This is in tune with the romantic and decadent appreciation of decay as part of the full spectrum of earthly life epitomised by Charles Baudelaire's 1857 poetry collection *Les Fleurs du mal* (the flowers of evil).[20] Indeed, at several points, Guilbert cites Baudelaire's poems 'Le Serpent qui danse' and 'Réversibilité'.[21] Guilbert's perspective was far from the medical tendency in works on menopause to bifurcate older women into either the frumpish and virtuous or the vain and immoral, and to represent them either as without any sexual desire or as mad because they still had it, as we saw in the previous chapter. Guilbert's libidinous older women are neither mad nor immoral, and there is never any suggestion that they suffer in ageing because of their sexual activity—on the contrary, the most vibrant are those who are still taking lovers. Instead of the medical-moral view of older coquettish women as pathetic in their pursuit of youthful appearance and behaviour, this pursuit is instead reframed as a deliberate strategy to resist the pull of death—Esther and her friends are forever only 'half-old' because they refuse to renounce their youthful spirit.[22]

[15] Ibid., 2–3. [16] Ibid., 4. [17] Ibid., 11. [18] Ibid., 12.
[19] Pierre Roussel, *Système physique et moral de la femme* (Paris: Chez Vincent, 1775), 85.
[20] Charles Baudelaire, *Les Fleurs du mal* (Paris: Poulet-Malassis & de Broise, 1857).
[21] Ibid., 121, 233. [22] Ibid., 290–291.

All the older women described in *Les Demi-vieilles* are unlike the images of women in medical works on menopause, which systematically portrayed urban elite modern women as ageing poorly and suffering a precipitous demise after the cessation of menses because of both their wounded vanity and their unhealthy lifestyles. The 'well-preserved' 53-year-old socialite in Guilbert's book is surely precisely such a *bourgeoise* from the medical men's perspectives, but here she is represented as triumphing over her ageing through youthfulness of spirit. This was a view of ageing that doctors never appeared to have considered, though the suggestion that she also cared for her health was closer to the hygienic view of ageing prescriptions found in most medical works. The Marquise de Lapic (*la pique* = the pike, someone who makes cutting remarks) is 50 years old with a lover who is ten years younger. Her youthfulness is attributed to her being in love.[23] Nonetheless, she judges Esther's sensuality as a sort of desperation: 'ce désir perpétuel, jamais assouvi, cette chair toujours prête à vouloir du plaisir' ('this perpetual desire, never satisfied, this flesh always ready to want pleasure').[24] But even this character's perspective is not exactly the same as that of doctors who judged libidinous older women mad or immoral; instead she seems to detect in Esther a terror of ageing that is driving her to pursue pleasure at all costs, and thus to choose lovers who will hurt her. And indeed, at the climax of the narrative, Esther's boyfriend turns out to be just such a hurtful choice, something Esther herself predicted when she first met him. The 120 kg woman is depicted as purposeful and powerful—also not an image of fat women that doctors ever evoked, instead always focusing on their propensity for disease and troublesome symptoms in menopause. 'La mère Roset' is a woman of 80 years who has a jolly gait and walks without a cane, while her daughter Adèle is 60 and is dying painfully of a breast cancer that has gnawed away at her for years.[25] The older women characters in Guilbert's book are anything but homogeneous, but they also seem designed to push against many of the medical clichés. A peasant woman—the most idealised model of ageing in almost all of the medical works on women's health from the mid-eighteenth century onwards—is represented here instead as haggard and used-up at the age of 32, seeming vastly older than her years on account of her many pregnancies, back-breaking labour, and the contempt with which her husband treats her.[26]

Les Demi-vieilles centres on Esther's love affair with a successful playwright, Maurice Roval, who is eight years younger than her. Maurice woos Esther to become both his lover and his muse in the writing of his new play on the theme of 'la femme de quarante ans' ('the woman of forty years'), in which he wants Esther

[23] Ibid., 124. [24] Ibid., 127. [25] Ibid., 112. [26] Ibid., 143.

to star, since she fits the part of a mature women who has remained 'coquettish'.[27] The provisional title of Roval's play references the earlier comic play by Faciolle *La Femme de quarante ans, ou Les Femmes à vapeurs* (The Woman of Forty Years, or The Women with Vapours) which was performed at the Palais-Royal in 1805.[28] The title of Guilbert's novel, too, references another well-known novel about women by Marcel Prévost, *Les Demi-vierges* (The Half-virgins) of 1894, which focused on the ravages of Parisian life and the effect of modern education on girls who were both sexually mature and under pressure to attract a husband but expected to remain virgins in the meantime.[29] *Les Demi-vieilles*, on the other hand, focuses on older women who were still sexually attractive and motivated, but were widely, according to nineteenth-century medicine, expected to renounce all sexual and romantic pursuits. In the preface of the book Guilbert said it was a work of 'natural history' written for women who were 'sensitive, impressionable, pained, amorous and tender ones',[30] referencing both the Roussel-inspired concept of women as the more sensitive and emotional sex, as well as the whole nineteenth-century genre of natural histories of the sexes, and especially of women.[31] This was the idea underpinning the 'naturalism' of Émile Zola too. However, Guilbert's was a book written not only about older women, but also for them. The character Esther agrees to the muse-affair with Roval only so that they can create a great work of theatre together, but she worries about his 'youthful male bestiality, idealising, despite himself, her already-russet autumn' ('son automne déjà roussi').[32] Her friends worry for her that Roval is merely using here as a 'lapin d'essais' (a rabbit for medical testing—or a 'guinea pig' as we say in English).[33] Indeed, Roval proves to be a manipulative and cruel person who had judged Esther all along for her efforts to disguise her age. He writes a role for her in his play which shows her 'magnificent soul and heart', but also her 'puerilities', her 'painful defences', her 'tenacious struggle against time', her 'exasperated will toward youth at all times', her 'hidden motherhood', and her gestures of a 'faded lover/woman in love' ('une amoureuse fanée').

[27] Ibid., 28.

[28] C. A. Faciolle, *La Femme de quarante ans, ou Les Femmes à vapeurs: Comédie en un acte et en prose, représentée pour la première fois, à Paris, sur le théâtre des Variétés, au Palais-Royal* (Paris: Delauney, 1805).

[29] Marcel Prévost, *Les Demi-vierges* (Paris: Alphonse Lemerre, 1894).

[30] Guilbert, *Les Demi-vieilles*, 'Préface', unpaginated.

[31] Georges-Louis Leclerc de Buffon, *Histoire naturelle de l'homme et de la femme: d'après nos plus grands naturalistes*, 2nd ed. [1786] (Paris: Armand-Aubrée, 1834); Gabriel Jouard, *Essai sur quelques points de l'histoire naturelle médicale de la femme, considérés sous les rapports physique, anatomique, physiologique, avec des applications à la pathologie.* Thèse (Paris: S. A. Huguelet, 1803); Jacques Louis Moreau (de la Sarthe), *Histoire naturelle de la femme, suivie d'un traité d'hygiène appliqué à son régime physiques et moral aux différentes époques de la vie*, 3 vols (Paris: Duprat, 1803); Auguste Debay, *Histoire naturelle de l'homme et de la femme* (Paris: E. Dentu, 1862). See Sean Quinlin, *Morbid Undercurrents: Medical Subcultures in Postrevolutionary France* (Ithaca, NY: Cornell University Press, 2021), 68–94.

[32] Guilbert, *Les Demi-vieilles*, 76.

[33] Ibid., 151.

Esther's letter in reply to him many years after their breakup acknowledges his perspective on women like her, but asks why it should be otherwise, and proposes that it is men like him (and perhaps like Roussel), rather than age itself, that have made getting older such a hell for them:

> Indeed, my dear friend, it is a foolish, puerile and painful vanity to struggle against time as it wilts and disaggregates us, but it is you men who oblige us to defend ourselves against the years that attack us. It is you, by the disdain in which you hold our autumn.[34]

She appears to directly challenge the entire corpus of medical advice for menopausal women about avoiding all forms of urban stimulus, powerful emotions, and love affairs:

> Must one renounce the exquisite sentimentality of existence after one's thirties? But it is also the age when we are most and best aware of the bounties of life. Our flourishing delivers to us new understandings of happiness; are we then reproachable for doing all we can to tenderly prolong it?[35]

In addition to answering back to many of the nineteenth-century medical forms of contempt, Guilbert also provides numerous portraits of alternative lives of older women, and indeed of other realities of nineteenth-century bourgeois norms relative to those described in medical sources. Esther knows a perfectly dull bourgeois family who, becoming worried about their son being too long a virgin (implying that he may be homosexual), slip him some money to fund his first 'débauche' with a prostitute, which they see as a matter of 'hygiène'.[36] At a soirée in the home of a Paris socialite, an intriguing conversation occurs on the subject of women's gynaecological matters and ageing between several of the women and two rather inelegantly named doctors: a surgeon Dr Lecoupeur (*le coupeur* = the cutter), and a medical professor Lafrousse (*la frousse* = the terror), as well as another medically trained writer named Wladimir Meridione (his name suggesting he may be both East-European and Mediterranean). The group speculates on what ages women and what preserves them. Professor Lafrousse thinks it is just a matter of remaining thin. One of the young women present, Élodie, who is a performer of both Turkish belly-dance and a Spanish 'dance of the hips', thinks having babies will age her and expresses the desire never to have any. Esther speculates that this is why Élodie has befriended Dr Lecoupeur, who is infatuated with her, since she wants to have the operation 'to cut out all one wants'—implying the new practices of hysterectomy or oophorectomy for which

[34] Ibid., 286. [35] Ibid., 287. [36] Ibid., 105.

gynaecologists had become enthusiastic in the 1890s. But one of the older women present, Countess Malpocet (*mal posé* = badly placed), says this operation 'fades one's traits and causes poor health', referring to the growing body of medical evidence, since the last years of the nineteenth century, of the iatrogenic effects of such surgeries, particularly prior to menopause.[37] The writer Meridione thinks if women stop wanting to have babies it will only lead to 'debauchery', but he is put in his place by the hostess, herself an older woman who has mothered four children and says motherhood is indeed exhausting and that having any more than two consigns a woman to 'servitude'.[38]

Medicine is also satirised elsewhere in the book, at one point relative to older women specifically: the writer Wladimir complains of doctors who prey upon women in their 'retour d'âge'. Doctors are depicted deliberately cultivating profitable patients by stimulating their health anxieties. He knows one clinician who makes 55,000 francs a year, with a large part of that owing to a single rich patient who pays 50 francs per daily visit just to be reassured that he is not about to die. The biggest sources of income for doctors, he says, are 'les gogos de pharmacie'—people who absolutely want to take chemical remedies, on whom doctors can experiment with new pharmaceutical products.[39] Here Guilbert added to a growing naturalist tradition within French (and German) literature of engaging with modern biomedicine, such as in the work of Émile Zola and Thomas Mann, or in the more scathing critique of doctors' coldness and predatory drives in the royalist writer Léon Daudet's 1894 novel *Les Morticoles*.[40] But Guilbert's satirical observations were not fantastical like Daudet's, and speak far more directly to the question of women's ageing as a specific target of medicalisation in the nineteenth century.

Comtesse de Tramar (Marie-Fanny de Lamarque de Lagarrigue), *L'Amour obligatoire*, 1900

Several of the themes raised by Guilbert are also a feature of the 1900 work *L'Amour obligatoire* (Obligatory Love), published in three editions up to 1913, by the writer known as the Comtesse de Tramar, a pseudonym of the aristocrat

[37] Félix Jayle, 'Opothérapie ovarienne dans la ménopause artificielle post-opératoire et la ménopause naturelle', *Revue de gynécologie et chirurgie abdominale*, 2 (1898): 239–272; Marcel Molk, *Kritik der vaginalen und abdominalen totalen Hysterectomie in Fällen von Fybromyomen*. Dissertation (Strasbourg: J. Singer, 1901).

[38] Guilbert, *Les Demi-vieilles*, 22–23.

[39] Ibid., 261–262.

[40] Larry Duffy & Catherine Emerson, eds, *La Nature dévoilée: French Literary Responses to Science* (Hull: Hull University Press, 2000); Mary Donaldson-Evans, *Medical Examinations: Dissecting the Doctor in French Narrative Prose, 1857–1894* (Lincoln, Nebr.: University of Nebraska Press, 2000); Dietrich von Engelhardt, 'Krankheit und Heilung bei Thomas Mann', *Praxis*, 95/1 (2006): 13–21; Léon Daudet, *Les Morticoles* (Paris: Bibliothèque Charpentier, 1894).

Marie-Fanny de Lamarque de Lagarrigue, Baronne d'Ysarn de Capdeville and Marquise de Villefort (1843–1911).[41] But this was a very different kind of work from Guilbert's. Tramar's other works mostly engaged with the ideal of *galanterie* in epistolary writing in which the life experience of virtuous aristocrats served as moral advice on how to live well, particularly in relation to amorous matters and the condition of women.[42] As Alain Viala has shown, *galanterie* was always a highly malleable concept.[43] *L'Amour obligatoire: Les Étapes de la vie d'une femme, la carrière de l'homme* (The Stages of the Life of a Woman, the Career of Man), like Tramar's 1911 work *Que veut la femme? Être jolie, être aimée et dominer* (What does a Woman Want? To be Pretty, to be Loved and to Dominate), extended the concept of epistolary writing into new domains of erotic evocation, misanthropy, and pathological description.[44] Both *Que veut la femme?* and *L'Amour obligatoire* stretched the bounds of what might be expected from an epistolary work, considering a variety of ways women might accommodate ageing, ranging from a transcendent, ecstatic religiosity to a form of sadistic libertinage. There was still a tone of moral instruction, but it was set mostly by providing evocative portraits of how *not* to live, rather than of how to live well. Unlike all the medical, hygienic works and popular health manuals, which focused on the reproductive phases of women's conventional lives, or else divided the lifespan into septenaries, Tramar divided women's lifespan according simply to decades, with the 'âge du déclin' ('the age of decline') from 40 to 49 years,[45] the age of 'l'abdication' from 50 to 59 years,[46] 'la première vieillesse' ('the first old age') from 60 to 69,[47] and the second and final old age from 70 until death.[48] But she also included a separate chapter on the 'époque critique', which mentioned nothing to do with age or the cessation of menstruation and instead focused on the general question of dealing with life disappointments, and on hypochondria.[49]

Tramar emphatically insisted that women began to age in widely variable ways: 'There are women who are absolutely finished at forty', whereas others 'who forgo the roses of spring' could aspire to remain beautiful into old age; and it was only after the age of 40 that women could appreciate the value of love.[50] She then illustrated a mode of being for women in this decade which is reminiscent of some of the psychiatric works discussed in the previous chapter about

[41] Comtesse de Tramar (Marie-Fanny de Lamarque de Lagarrigue), *L'Amour obligatoire: Les Étapes de la vie d'une femme, la carrière de l'homme* [1900], 3rd ed. (Paris: Librairie Universelle, 1913). See Marie-Claire Grassi, 'L'Art épistolaire français (XVIIIe et XIXe siècles)', in Alain Montadon, ed., *Pour une histoire des traités de savoir-faire en Europe* (Clermont-Ferrand: Association des publications de la Faculté des Lettres et Sciences humaines de Clermont-Ferrand, 1994), 301–331.

[42] Comtesse de Tramar (Marie-Fanny de Lamarque de Lagarrigue), *Que veut la femme? Être jolie, être aimée et dominer* (Paris: Malet, 1911).

[43] Comtesse de Tramar (Marie-Fanny de Lamarque de Lagarrigue), *Règles du savoir-vivre dans la société moderne* (Paris: Havard, 1905).

[44] Alain Viala, *La Galanterie, une mythologie française* (Paris: Seuil, 2019).

[45] Tramar, *L'Amour obligatoire*, 411–422. [46] Ibid., 423–438.

[47] Ibid., 440–445. [48] Ibid., 446–447. [49] Ibid., 281–282. [50] Ibid., 411, 440.

menopausal 'erotomania'. It is certainly possible that Tramar had read such works, but since she referenced no other works of literature or scholarship, it is difficult to know what had inspired her. In this version of feminine ageing, the woman,

> ... throws herself headlong into the melee, happening by chance on the prey that lands within her reach. She makes herself an educator of adolescents. She vitiates and fades everything she touches, happy still to find love again; experiencing no shame for her criminal practices. Traversing the full spectrum of vicious and vitiating vice. Giving herself over to incest, covered in the muck of ignorant ingenuous love, which receives from her the first lesson in a repulsive and tiresome venery.[51]

Women who were thus inclined had only one way of avoiding such perverse behaviour: to take instead a path of mystical transcendence and sexual renunciation, which provided a 'voluptuous joy' in which one's soul 'glides among the higher spheres and cannot descend'. It made one susceptible to 'disincarnating oneself' ('se désincarner') in a continual flight ('envolement') that was 'full of charm'. Nonetheless, she also characterised this mode of being in a similar way to mid-century alienist/psychiatric scholars who pathologised older women's religiosity, such as Étienne Esquirol and Pierre Berthier, further suggesting that psychiatric texts may have been among Tramar's readings.[52] Such women, said Tramar, found 'an attraction bordering on eroticism' in Catholic confession, turning it into a form of vice in itself. It was 'a dangerous monomania', and priests were 'often the victims of these maniacs'.[53] But while psychiatric works provided a clear moral order within which such 'pathologies' were to be understood, Tramar's account was riddled with ambiguity. She described the religious-mania pathway both as a charming source of joy and transcendence and as a solution to the 'repulsive' perversion of paedophilic incestuous desire in older women, and yet also as its own kind of pathology.

Another kind of early-ageing woman was 'she who fights'. Here the author evokes a model similar to Yvette Guilbert's character Esther, describing those who 'do not accept the brutalities of time, who want to fight against it, hoping to vanquish and turn it backwards' ('le faire rétrograder'). She appeared to consider this a legitimate option: 'One can always try, it is not forbidden to mount a fine defence.'[54] During one's fifties, this would become harder though, she warned, as women would 'suffer incommensurably from the progression toward the death of

[51] Ibid., 412.

[52] Étienne D. Esquirol, *Des maladies mentales considérées sous les rapports médical, hygiénique et médico-légal*, 2 vols (Paris: J. B. Baillière, 1838), vol. 1, 503; Pierre Berthier, *Médecine mentale* [1857], 2nd ed. (Paris: V. Masson, 1860), 61.

[53] Tramar, *L'Amour obligatoire*, 414.

[54] Ibid., 420–421.

one's being', losing every day 'a parcel of the elements' of one's previous capacities for seduction. She who sought to remain coquettish in this decade would 'fall into the abysmal depths of love', relying only on the 'fiction of sentiment' provided by the 'parasitic milieux' of the deity who would accept her servitude, 'the alms of love paid to this unsatisfied woman who tumbles into the fetid mire' ('l'aumône de l'amour faite à cette inassouvie qui dégringolera dans la fange fétide'). Such women were 'thirsty for love and lust, their flesh is consumed and burns like a parched old bundle of sticks.... Love is indispensable to them like opium to those in the dens of the Levant.'[55] Such a struggle could not persist beyond the fifties, since this was the 'autumn of life, the march toward the tomb, the sunset that brings down the shadows of the night that follows. Nature dies without revolt.'[56]

Nonetheless there was still 'the old coquettish one' who was 'the wound of humanity' who fancied her appeal as like 'a flower of love, late to close among the ruins', but was really an 'audacious libertine, Cupid, the desperate adventurer ('l'aventurière aux abois')'.[57] Evoking both Gothic fiction and the aesthetic of the Grand Guignol theatre in Paris of the late 1890s[58]—or perhaps thinking of performers like Yvette Guilbert and Sarah Bernhardt—she said such a woman was sometimes also a 'dominatrix, vain, ambitious, an extortionist. By love, by threats, by betrayal, she succeeds in her goal, paving her path with corpses', she was a 'vampire drinking human blood down to the last drop'.[59] But 'after the revolts, the struggles, the despair, there comes a calm'. Eventually even this figure of defiance would have to renounce 'the feverish anxiety, the unrealizable expectations... the chimeric hopes, the malignant dreams', and 'understand that everything is finished', at which point there would be a 'return of wisdom'.[60] Thereafter and for the remainder of her life, a woman could experience peace, happy memories of her youth, and enjoy being a grandmother, albeit always accompanied by a sense of doom about approaching death.[61] Those who had always taken care of their health (she offered no specific prescriptions here) could expect to remain 'captivating and seductive' even in their sixties, until a time when a 'sudden crack appears', one's 'being dislocates', 'the mask falls' and the entire 'academy bends' ('l'académie s'infléchit').[62] There is also a short chapter at the end of this book which focused on men's ageing, but here Tramar seemed far less interested in differentiating such a wide and eccentric spectrum of possibilities—men simply became lonely and sad once their careers ended, only finding solace in religious piety.[63] The abject language and unusual portraits of women's ageing in *L'Amour obligatoire* clearly distinguish it both from the tone of nineteenth-century medical writing on the critical age and from the fictional style of Tramar's contemporary

[55] Ibid., 424–425. [56] Ibid., 430. [57] Ibid., 430–431.
[58] Agnès Pierron, *Les Nuits blanches du Grand-Guignol* (Paris: Seuil, 2002).
[59] Tramar, *L'Amour obligatoire*, 432. [60] Ibid., 438. [61] Ibid., 446–447.
[62] Ibid., 440. [63] Ibid., 573–575.

Yvette Guilbert. But it was not entirely dissimilar to some forms of psychiatric and popular medical writing on menopause, which appeared to relish the details of older women's sexual variations.[64]

While Tramar appeared to condemn as 'repulsive' and 'desperate' the modes of women's ageing that either preyed sexually on young people, pestered priests for confession in the pursuit of sexual arousal, or held on too long to a 'coquettish' demeanour, she also provided no clearly preferable pathway for handling the effects of ageing. Just not worrying about it, for instance, was not one of the possibilities she discussed; and while she promoted the idea of women in their seventies finding peaceful joy as grandmothers, she did not appear to imagine the possibility of any kind of contented mode for women prior to this time, after the age of 40. The title of her book, *L'Amour obligatoire*, suggested that in every decade, love was women's refuge; but then she also used the word *amour* in different ways, variously to refer to piety (love of God), to conjugal bonds, to cosmetic glamour, or to eroticism—even of a perverse kind—and she clearly indicated a way in which the pious kind of 'love' too was in reality a form of perverse 'monomania'. So it is not entirely clear what kind of 'love' Tramar thought obligatory for ageing women. Perhaps indeed her general misanthropic point was that there was no way to be either content or admirable in midlife, since it was an inherently uncomfortable time in between youthful splendour and ageing demise.

Marthe Bertheaume (Anne Darcanne-Mouroux), *L'Âge mystique*, 1928

Anne Darcanne-Mouroux was altogether a different kind of writer from both the Comtesse de Tramar and Yvette Guilbert. Born thirteen years after Guilbert and thirty-five years after Tramar, she had made her debut in the scholarship of menopause with her 1904 Paris medical thesis, defended when she was 26 years old, as we considered in the previous chapter; but around the age of 50, following her separation from her husband (the psychiatrist Gustave Darcanne), she began writing autobiographical-fictional works looking at women's ageing, such as *Oublie ce que tu sais* (Forget What You Know, 1928) and *L'Âge mystique* (The Mystical Age, 1930) under the pseudonym Marthe Bertheaume. The use of a pseudonym may have been, as Thomas Bauer suggests, designed to protect her clinical reputation, which her novels might be seen to compromise; or it may have been to protect those in Darcanne-Mouroux's own life, given that her fictional characters tended to be based on them. This includes her estranged husband, himself a well-known clinical psychiatrist who Darcanne-Mouroux refused to

[64] Henri Guimbail, *De la folie à la ménopause*. Thèse (Paris: A. Delahaye, 1884); Hayès, *Hygiène de l'age critique*.

divorce on account of her Catholic morals.[65] She had also become a suffragist and hygiene activist after the First World War, remaining ever a devout Catholic, but also very much a modern woman, working as a Paris clinical gynaecologist while campaigning both for women's rights and for the improvement of the public health of the French population through sporting organisations.[66]

Bertheaume's (Darcanne-Mouroux's) 1928 novel *Oublie ce que tu sais* featured as its central character Dr Chantal, a woman who, arriving at a 'certain age', is not feeling as vibrant as before, though she also does not believe herself ill.[67] It tells the story of her struggle to find social solace as a Catholic woman in the largely atheistic circles of interwar feminism, and seems to be quite closely modelled on Darcanne-Mouroux's own life as a doctor, a suffragist, a pious Catholic, and a mother. But the 1930 novel *L'Âge mystique*, while still somewhat autobiographical, seems to be considerably more fictional and focuses far more specifically on the existential questions of women's end of fertility. It tells the story of Bérengère Audierne, who is a 'conférencière et suffragiste' (speaker and suffragist—just as Darcanne-Mouroux was, although in this novel the central character is not a doctor). Bérengère's daughter Odette is a 'bold and very modern young woman' ('une jeune femme hardie et bien moderne'), married and pregnant.[68] Bérengère will thus soon be a grandmother. This produces the despondent sense that her youth has suddenly ended; but she resists these thoughts, since she feels too vital and still worthy of love to accept the identity of an old woman. She still has a magnificent neck, a firm face, and not a single white hair—she is only 43, after all. Her estranged husband died in a train accident some years earlier, and she wonders if she might soon meet someone else. She does not feel entitled to her sadness about growing older, and feels guilty that she is not simply happy for her daughter.[69]

After the birth of her grandchild, Bérengère feels rejected by her daughter, whose entire attention is now focused on the new baby. When the baby becomes ill, a doctor is called, who (bizarrely) is a psychiatrist, Daniel Xambaud.[70] When, later, Bérengère goes to see this man on the pretext of talking about the baby's recovery, she ends up disclosing to him all her own struggles of late. These include unexplained crying, an inexplicable loss of motivation, hypersensitivity ('les nerfs sont à fleur de peau'), a capricious appetite, sleeping badly, waking in the night

[65] Marthe Bertheaume (Anne Darcanne-Mouroux), *Oublie ce que tu sais* (Paris: Éditions de la vraie France, 1928); Marthe Bertheaume (Anne Darcanne-Mouroux), *L'Âge mystique* (Paris: Éditions de la vraie France, 1930); Thomas Bauer, *La Sportive dans la littérature française des Années folles* (Lille: Presses Universitaires de Septentrion, 2011), 64.

[66] Annabelle Caprais, *La Place et le rôle des femmes dans la gouvernance des fédérations sportives françaises*. Thèse, Education, Université de Bordeaux (2020). HAL Archives ouvertes, Id: tel-03114344. <https://hal.archives-ouvertes.fr/tel-03114344v2>, 212.

[67] Marthe Bertheaume (Anne Darcanne-Mouroux), *Oublie ce que tu sais*, 131; Bauer, *La Sportive dans la littérature française*, 62–63.

[68] Bertheaume (Anne Darcanne-Mouroux), *L'Âge mystique*, 9.

[69] Ibid., 14–16. [70] Ibid., 24.

with violent palpitations that make her think she is going to die, feelings of suffocation in her throat, jumping at the slightest noise, and finding it intolerable to be alone whereas she has always previously liked it.[71] The doctor tells her that while pharmacological remedies may be able to alleviate her symptoms, the only cure is for her to remarry.[72] Thus begins a flirtatious courtship between Bérengère and Dr Xambaud which occupies much of the first half of the book and appears to go on for about two years, in which time Xambaud continues to try to convince Bérengère that what she needs is neither medication nor philosophical wisdom, but simply his own erotic affection and romantic attachment. Finally, he proposes to her in a letter, and she ambiguously only half-refuses.[73]

Bérengère then takes a holiday alone in Italy and becomes fascinated by the attractive nuns she meets staying at a convent, one of whom causes Bérengère to shiver on account of the 'svelte and young' body that she can imagine under the nun's long black gown.[74] She confides in an older nun, Sister Saint-Ignace, about her recent mysterious symptoms, and the nun confirms to her that many women around the same age (now 45) suffer such illnesses, wishing her a rapid recovery of her 'air de jeunesse'.[75] Bérengère and Sister Saint-Ignace engage in a long dialogue about the nature of love and of Catholic piety, in which Bérengère speculates that religious devotion is really 'earthly affection' channelled into a higher purpose. Sister Saint-Ignace acknowledges that 'one can only go to God with the aid of the sentiments of our poor human nature', and that one cannot love God with reason alone: 'it is with the heart that one must seek him, since he has given us one'.[76] Bérengère, still determined to find the erotic in divine worship, refers to the 'great joy' of 'l'ivresse mystique' ('mystical intoxication/euphoria'); but the austere nun will have none of this, and discourages Bérengère from her own aspirations to monasticism, telling her she is probably too old and independent for the necessary obedience.[77] Nonetheless, Bérengère experiences a new serenity and feelings of transcendence while staying at the convent; and when she returns to Paris, it is with the conviction that she does not need to marry Daniel, telling him 'you see how I have aged, I am not the same person that you loved'.[78] Ever the materialist psychiatrist, Daniel recoils in horror at her renewed religious mysticism, which he sees (as Bérengère had predicted) as a form of mental pathology.[79] Great works of literature, too, had suggested that women's religiosity in the critical age was precipitated by the loss of their minds, as in the Goncourt brothers' *Madame Gervaisais*, whose unusual intellectual talents evaporate in a religious fervour caused by the 'revolution of her moral temperament, a sort of returning to her nature' once she reaches 'the age when she redescends in life'.[80] But Bérengère

[71] Ibid., 32. [72] Ibid., 38. [73] Ibid., 88, 119.
[74] Ibid., 105–106. [75] Ibid., 107. [76] Ibid., 180.
[77] Ibid., 188. [78] Ibid., 204. [79] Ibid., 206–207.
[80] Edmond de Goncourt & Jules de Goncourt, *Madame Gervaisais* (Paris: A. Lacroix, Verhoeckhoven & Cie, 1869), 205–206.

does not care about such judgements of her piety, and the novel ends with her confiding in a close woman friend and experiencing a renewed sense of peace and happiness.

L'Âge mystique attempts to elaborate a pathway for mature, independent Catholic women facing the sense of their reproductive ageing as a moment of nervous and emotional crisis, the answer to which is an intensified mystical piety, without shame relative to the growing atheistic norms both of modern medicine and of feminism—two worlds Darcanne-Mouroux inhabited. The book appears clearly to engage with many of the negative discourses about women's 'critical age' elaborated in medicine of the long nineteenth century, and which were still active in the first three decades of the twentieth century: ideas of women's reproductive changes resulting in a sudden rather than gradual ageing, and entailing nervous symptoms, personal crisis, changes in sexual relations, and increased religious fervour. There is no mention of menstruation or its cessation, still hardly an acceptable topic of fictional writing in this period, in contrast to more recent women's fiction in French.[81] But the description of Bérengère's symptoms and the remarks about these being common in women 'around her age' make it clear that what is being discussed is the very same 'crisis' described in works on menopause and on women's *âge de retour*. Darcanne-Mouroux, herself a doctor who in her youth had written her own Paris thesis on the topic of 'early menopause', appeared thus to absorb and replicate, more than any of the other women writers discussed here, the masculine account of women's sudden entrance into old age with the loss of fertility.[82] But in other respects, the novel challenged many of the ideas found in that medical corpus, proposing a revision of the meaning of religious piety for older women, and showing the psychiatric perspective to have its own biased agendas.

The flirtation with the psychiatrist Daniel Xambaud, in effect, plays out one of the recurrent debates among nineteenth-century doctors and psychiatrists about the value or danger of menopausal sexual relations—Daniel speaks for the liberal (or perhaps libertine) view that conjugal union can help alleviate menopause symptoms, and that midlife remarriage is thus a healthy option for older women. Bérengère engages with the Catholic expectation of menopause as the 'death of sex', which in her account women can try to resist, but only by becoming ridiculous and by bending to the will of others, and especially the men who desire them. The more truly independent path, which brings peace and contentment as a cure for the nervous perturbation of the critical age, Bérengère suggests, is the path of devotion to God and of friendship with other women. As in Guilbert's novel, bonds with other women friends appear crucial to the central character's

[81] Tomlinson, *From Menstruation to Menopause*.

[82] Anne Darcanne-Mouroux, *Contribution à l'étude clinique de la ménopause précoce*. Thèse (Paris: H. Jouve, 1904).

capacity to transcend masculine judgements of her approach to ageing. The nineteenth-century psychiatric view that women's madness in menopause is often expressed as religious fervour is represented too in the judgements of the character of Daniel who (like Darcanne-Mouroux's actual estranged husband) is a psychiatrist.[83] But this perspective is itself shown to be partisan, representing men's desire for older women to remain erotically available to them, rather than devoted to God, as well as evincing medicine's failure to appreciate how soothing prayer and religious contemplation may be for the nervousness of older Catholic women. Bérengère does not entirely accept the loss of sexuality which so many of the menopause doctors asserted was necessary during menopause, since she appears to experience her mysticism erotically; but she certainly rejects the idea that she must re-couple with a man and seek to resume the conjugal life which she enjoyed in her youth. Her description of mystical erotic experience is also considerably more positive than that of the Comtesse de Tramar—there is no mania or perversion here. Notably too, though pharmaceutical treatments for menopause are alluded to in Bérengère's first conversation with Dr Xambaud, these are represented as having only partial remedial powers, and are summarily dismissed as inadequate for the larger existential questions the character appears to face.

Colette, *La Naissance du jour*, 1928

Another book, published like Bertheaume's in 1928, and presenting an equally unusual French woman's account of her ageing, is nonetheless considerably more known in literary and feminist scholarship: *La Naissance du jour*, by Colette (Sidonie-Gabrielle Colette, 1873–1954). Colette (Image 9.3) was primarily a writer, and a very successful one, with a skilled refinement and a literary drive vastly greater than any of the writers discussed thus far, who were all considerably more amateur in their writing pursuits—Guilbert as an actress and singer; Bertheaume as a doctor and activist; Tramar as an aristocrat who dabbled in the epistolary genre. Numerous scholars have pondered Colette's unique take on women's ageing. There would thus be little point in rehearsing here plot lines and characters that have already been widely discussed elsewhere.[84] However, what

[83] Esquirol, *Des Maladies mentales*, vol. 1, 503; Michel-Victor Barbier, *De l'influence de la menstruation sur les maladies mentales*. Thèse (Paris: Rignoux, 1848), 14; Berthier, *Médecine mentale*, 61; Guimbail, *De la folie à la ménopause*, 27, 29, 49–50, 69–70.

[84] Carla Carlino, 'Écrire la catastrophe du vieillir: Le Cas de Colette', in A. Soncini Fratti, ed., *Horizons de recherche/Research Horizons* (Bologna: Emil, 2014), 173–182; Francine Dugast-Portes, 'Colette: Écrire le vieillir', in Alain Montandon, ed., *Écrire le vieillir* (Clermont-Ferrand: Presses Universitaires Blaise Pascal, 2005), 159–170; Claude Benoit, 'L'Art de "bien vieillir" chez deux grandes femmes de lettres: George Sand et Colette', *Gérontologie et société*, 28/114 (2005): 167–193; Bethany Ladimer, *Colette, Beauvoir and Duras: Age and Women Writers* (Gainsville, Fla: University of Florida

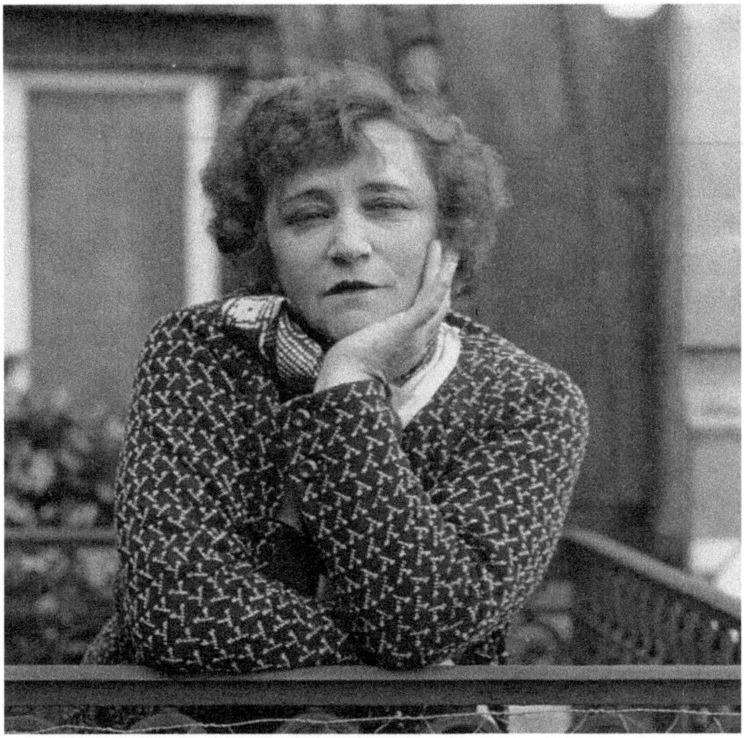

Image 9.3 Colette photographed aged 59 (photographer unknown), 1932. Courtesy of the Bibliothèque Nationale de France.

does remain to be explored of Colette's work is the consideration of how it may have been influenced by the prevalent, now more than 100-year-old French medical discourse about menopause and women's ageing that persisted throughout the early twentieth century, into the period of Colette's forties and fifties—a focus not hitherto brought to her work. To be clear, Colette was not nearly as interested in medicine as Bertheaume, who was also a doctor, or even Guilbert, who criticised and satirised doctors like other writers of the *fin de siècle*, and she most certainly did not replicate/pervert any psychiatric ideas about older women's sexuality in the manner of the Comtesse de Tramar. But she did appear, gently, to connect her own experiences of ageing to medical concepts of menopause symptomology, though only to look through them to find her own unique strategies for embracing the plenitude of being in midlife, what she referred to as 'le chic suprême du savoir-décliner' ('the supreme chic of knowing how to decline').[85]

Press, 1999); Diana Holmes, 'Colette, Beauvoir and the Change of Life', *French Studies*, 53/4 (1999): 430–443; Lois W. Banner, *In Full Flower: Aging Women, Power, and Sexuality* (New York: Vintage Books, 1993), 267–272.

[85] Colette, *La Naissance du jour* [1928] (Paris: Flammarion, 1984), 166.

As Francine Dugast-Portes, Carla Carlino, and Claude Benoit have described, there are reflections on ageing throughout Colette's oeuvre, even in some of her earliest published works.[86] Colette was indeed intensely conscious of ageing throughout her own adult lifespan (even undergoing the supposedly anti-ageing medical procedure of injections of young people's blood when she was 51), and in her fictional writing she developed both a unique fascination with older bodies and a complex spectrum of images of ageing that ranged from catastrophising to sublime.[87] Several of her works depicted sexual relationships between older women and young men.[88] *La Naissance du jour*, published when Colette was 55 years old, depicts the infatuation of 35-year-old Vial with the 50-year-old central character, who is broadly Colette herself, in a work of autobiographical fiction filled with rapturous evocations of the sensuality of ageing bodies.

La Naissance du jour, by its title, and by much of its content, referred to women's time of life post-fertility as the dawning of a new sense of self, a time of increased self-definition, of becoming more exhilarated by the natural world and freer to choose how and who to be. Colette's very use of the term 'climatérique' to describe the age of 50 indicated an important rejection of the dominant French medical discourse of women's ageing, which almost always referred to it as heralded by the cessation of menses, entailing sudden losses of charm, beauty, and vitality, and requiring elaborate hygienic regimes to manage. The terms 'critical age', 'âge de retour', and menopause were used in almost all such medical works. The term 'climacteric', on the other hand, was very rarely used in French medicine, though it was more common in the scant works on women's cessation of menses in English, Irish, and American medicine of the nineteenth century, and the Austrian doctor Enoch Kisch had used its German form (*klimakterische Alter*) in his book of 1874;[89] it was, as we saw in Chapter 1, also the term (in its Latin form) invoked by Friedrich Hoffmann in 1704 to describe the septenary years in the life cycle (though without reference to the final cessation of menses).[90] Indeed, the 'climacteric' conveyed the early modern Ptolemaic astrological concept of the lifespan divided into septenary years at the cusp of each of which the organism was thought to renew itself—making the forty-ninth year especially salient, since

[86] Dugast-Portes, 'Colette: Écrire le vieillir', 160; Carlino, 'Écrire la catastrophe du vieillir', 176–177; Benoit, 'L'Art de "bien vieillir" chez deux grandes femmes de lettres', 182–193.

[87] Benoit, 'L'Art de "bien vieillir"', 175.

[88] Dugast-Portes, 'Colette: Écrire le vieillir', 160–166; Davis, *Age Rage and Going Gently*, xxxi.

[89] H. Halford, 'On the Climacteric Disease', *Medical Transactions*, 4 (1813): 316–328; Henri Kennedy, 'Observations on Climacteric Disease', *Dublin Journal* of *Medical Science*, 25/74 (1844): 245; Enoch Heinrich Kisch, *Das klimaterische Alter der Frauen in physiologischer und pathologischer Beziehung* (Erlangen: Ferdinand Enke, 1874).

[90] Friedrich Hoffmann, *De Annorum climactericorum rationali & medica explicatione. Opera omnia physico, tomus quintus* (Geneva: Fratres de Tournes, 1704); Stolberg, Michael, 'Von den "Stufenjahren" zur "Menopause"': Das Klimakterium im Wandel der Zeit', *Würzburger Medizinhistorische Mitteilungen*, 24 (2005): 41–50.

it was the seventh septenary and hence more astrologically powerful.[91] Something of this idea was also present in the Montpellier vitalist accounts of 'critical times', referring to a positive revolution of the entire economy of an organism, in the movement from one phase of life into another.[92] Nineteenth-century doctors too conveyed something of this when they referred to menopause as a kind of second puberty, with a small minority of scholars sometimes even proposing that it thus rejuvenated women.[93] Colette's climacteric was precisely such a time, and she likened her discovery of a new mode of being to rebirth,[94] to acquiring a 'new skin',[95] and to the autumn harvest.[96] She presented the loss of her maternal capacity as heralding a life phase of liberation to become whoever she now wanted to be, without the overbearing expectation of the one thing women have often been told is the singular meaning of their lives.[97]

This book, like many of Colette's other works, contains portraits of others' ageing too. She observed the resilience of a 72-year-old Provençal woman who walked four kilometres every day to take her mixed collection of farm produce to the port market.[98] But this was no idealised abstract vision of peasant virtue; rather it was Colette enjoying the beauty of older people around her, and enjoying their appreciation of the beauty of life itself, in describing the elderly woman appreciatively caressing 'un des lys des rivages qui s'élancent de la terre, grandissent si vite qu'on n'ose pas les regarder, épanouissent leur corolla et leur parfum maléfique de fruit mûr blesse, puis retournent au néant...' ('one of those sea-shore lilies that shoot out of the earth, grow so fast that one dare not look at them, spread forth their corollas and their maleficent odour of bruised ripe fruit, and then return to nothingness').[99] The Provençal woman's own ageing is thus situated within a luxurious reverie of the cycle of life in which, in our fruition and emergence, we are already half-decayed in our ripeness, after which there is annihilation. In this respect Colette was much closer to Baudelaire than to medical views of ageing and death. Colette's writing is filled with descriptions of transcendence, ecstatic bliss in enjoyment of the natural world, the land, the sea, plants, and animals, and the sensation of merging herself with the earth and its bounty, which permit her to embrace her aliveness as an older woman

[91] Colette, *La Naissance du jour*, 48; Max Engammare, *Soixante-trois: La Peur de la grande année climactérique à la Renaissance* (Geneva: Droz, 2013); Daniel Schäfer, *Old Age and Disease in Early Modern Medicine*, trans. Patrick Baker (London: Routledge, 2015).

[92] Théophile de Bordeu, *Recherches sur le pouls par rapport aux crises* (Paris: De Bure l'aîné, 1756); J. B. D. Létu, *Essai sur la doctrine des crises et des jours critiques dans les maladies aiguës*. Thèse (Montpellier: Jean Martel aîné, 1816); Nicolas-Marie Grévin, *Essai sur les crises*. Thèse (Montpellier: Jean Martel, 1825).

[93] Joseph-Marie-Joachim Vigarous, *Cours élémentaire de maladies des femmes, ou Essai sur une nouvelle méthode pour étudier et pour classer les maladies de ce sexe*, 2 vols (Paris: Deterville, 1801), vol. 1, 47; Joseph-Lazare-Jacques Coural, *Considérations générales sur les phénomènes physiologique et pathologique de la femme aux divers âges de la vie*. Thèse (Montpellier: Jean Martel, 1822), 36.

[94] Colette, *La Naissance du jour*, 134. [95] Ibid., 133. [96] Ibid., 49.

[97] Ibid., 53, 35. [98] Ibid., 68. [99] Ibid., 69.

wholeheartedly. Every place where a woman has felt love, or where she has been healed from love, becomes a native land to her. Thus, she says, 'ce rivage bleu de sel, pavoisé de tomates et de poivrons, est deux fois mien' ('this salt-blue shore, bedecked with tomatoes and peppers, is twice mine').[100]

Other passages in *La Naissance du jour* suggest that Colette was very aware of the possibility of viewing her midlife experience according to the medical perspective of menopause symptomatology. But no sooner does she evoke tropes of medical pathology than she brushes them aside in favour of ecstasy. She experiences insomnia every night—one of the recurrent symptoms cited by doctors writing on the 'critical age'. But rather than seeing this as something to be remedied, she relishes the unusual experience of the night, its sounds and odours, of being awake for the dawn light, imagining her Parisian friends with their nocturnal social world who never get to have that pleasure.[101] Indeed, the book's title references this moment in the transition from night to the break of day, not only as a metaphor of her newfound agency but also in reference to the disturbed sleep pattern that fortuitously permits her to enjoy the nocturnal countryside and the appearance of the very first light. After a confrontation with Vial in which she explains to him why she will not be his lover, she processes complex regrets, longing, satisfaction, and sweetness, but also sleeps very little. She experiences this sleep loss as a new super-power, declaring 'I need little sleep; naps, for the last few weeks, have been all I need. When the desire for sleep returns, I will sleep vehemently and voluptuously.' She has but to wait for her previous rhythm to return—that is the lesson of 'la grande élégance des mœurs' ('the great elegance of habits'), 'le chic suprême du savoir-décliner' ('supreme chic of knowing how to decline'), which she learnt from her own ageing mother.[102] She wonders if she began ageing at 40, imagining herself as an 'ageing woman in love' ('amoureuse vieillissante') who, might become pale with 'noble consumption' so as to leave her place to a rosy young rival; her generosity is a 'sort of neurosis', but should the young lover refuse it, she threatens that she will perish from 'plethora'.[103] But she spares only a fleeting moment for such thoughts, in contrast to her extensive rhapsodic revelling in the natural and provincial world and her own place in it as an ageing woman:

> ... cette fraicheur de poudre d'eau, ce doux leurre, cet esprit de province, cette innocence enfin, n'est-ce pas l'appel charmant de la fin de la vie? Que tout est devenu simple ...[104]
>
> (... that misty freshness, that sweet lure, that spirit of the provinces, that innocence, is it not the charming call of the end of life? How simple everything has become ...)

She is now in a time of life where there is nothing left to do but enrich her spirit.[105]

[100] Ibid., 29. [101] Ibid., 36–38. [102] Ibid., 166.
[103] Ibid., 50–51. [104] Ibid., 25. [105] Ibid., 53.

Like Guilbert, Colette saw herself as more of an 'old girl' than an ageing woman.[106] Nonetheless, much of *La Naissance du jour* is about her renunciation of romantic attachment, not dissimilar to that of Bertheaume, though without the latter's Catholicism: 'il me semble qu'entre l'homme et moi, une longue récréation commence' ('it seems to me that, between men and me, a long time of recreation is beginning').[107] She finds men to be good companions but plans to take leave of them ('courteously').[108] She has lived all her life since the age of 16 in the pursuit of love and enmeshed in romantic bonds, having been told that to do otherwise would be 'the worst affront' ('la pire outrecuidance').[109] But she now feels liberated from this and is ready to embark on something she has never done before: living her life without being bonded to a love partner.[110] It is a 'climacteric commandment', she says; she no longer wishes automatically to couple with anyone. She describes precisely how she is becoming 'a woman who is escaping from the age of still being a woman', she is now a 'compère' of a man (the masculine counterpart to the friendly/positive *commère*), she celebrates her thick neck like a man's and her bodily strength from which grace is progressively disappearing, as signs of an authority that shows men can no longer cause her to despair. The *récréation* is not a pause but a shift to a situation of shared leisure. Lying awake in the predawn hours, she revels in the sounds of fighting felines in the street around her house, and fantasises about marrying a very large cat.[111]

Like Bertheaume, what she renounces in her sexual relations, she finds elsewhere in ecstatic rhapsody. But this is even less like the medical image of older women's 'death of sex' than Bertheaume's, in that she does not appear to be announcing a permanent abandonment of love affairs, but a new agential approach to them in a genuine relinquishment of the psychological attachment she has hitherto felt compelled to romance. She is not avoiding sex in the view that it would be bad for her health, as medical texts often claimed about women in menopause, rather she is embracing a 'tremendous' achievement. She has not lost her sexual desire, but nor is she denying herself anything.[112] The final word of the novel is 'oasis'.[113] Lois Banner seems to read this aspect of *La Naissance du jour* simply as sexual renunciation and as Colette's acceptance of her descent into old age, pointing to a similar theme of the older women characters in Colette's other novels.[114] But there are reasons to doubt this interpretation. Notably, Colette did have a relationship during and after the writing of *La Naissance du jour*—with a man sixteen years younger than her.[115] In the book, she refers to her aversion for the mundane and dependent properties of relationships in general, from which she seeks respite: 'n'importe quel amour, si on se fie à lui, tend à s'organiser à la manière d'un tube digestif' ('any love, if one relies on it, tends to

[106] Ibid., 35. [107] Ibid., 34. [108] Ibid., 39. [109] Ibid., 71.
[110] Ibid., 133. [111] Ibid., 48, 65. [112] Ibid., 134. [113] Ibid., 167.
[114] Banner, *In Full Flower*, 271. [115] Dugast-Portes, 'Colette: Écrire le vieillir', 160.

become organised like a digestive tube').[116] The suffering of hurt lovers, adultery, abandonment are less 'venerable' than growing older and dying, which she feels will be upon her soon anyway. But they are forms of suffering with much the same stench, and she plugs her nose at the approach of them all.[117] Her need to break from this pattern of automatic relations in order to claim her new, older selfhood is a clear theme throughout *Naissance du jour.*

The autobiographical novels of Marthe Bertheaume and Colette, both written in 1928, were already finding their own forms of transcendence of the catastrophising medical discourses about menopause that were elaborated throughout the nineteenth century and as late as the interwar period. They were both thus able to carve their own paths to midlife self-realisation, undeterred by the medical view of their time of life as miserable, humiliating, desperate, or morbid. Nonetheless, Bertheaume was clearly more conscious of the medical concept of menopause symptomatology than the Comtesse de Tramar, Guilbert, or Colette, on account of her medical training and practice. Throughout the first decades of the twentieth century, a different set of discourses was becoming established globally: the idea of menopause as a state of universal hormone depletion that could be remedied simply with the emergent endocrine pharmaceuticals. French medicine was rapidly eclipsed in that medical industrialism, even as it was largely responsible for inspiring it (as we consider in the next chapter). In France, too, with the substantial diminution of the folk healers and charlatans who had so stimulated nineteenth-century doctors' drives to carve out new patient markets among urban elites, there was now less impetus to medicalise the daily lives of older women. The concept of hygiene moved away from the nineteenth-century model of preventive health for ageing women in relation to diet, sleep, beverages, sexual activity, and exercise. Women writers of the 1920s were thus already less exposed to this kind of advice about their ageing. But we should be wary of generalising that French women generally no longer bore a burden from the nocebo effect, or 'auto-suggestion', of nineteenth-century ideas about their ageing, as the American doctor Emma Drake had described it.[118] Colette and Bertheaume were both clearly idiosyncratic individuals with their own considerable psychological resources for metabolising and transcending prevalent views of older women's nature. In this chapter we have not considered the later examples of Violette Leduc and Simone de Beauvoir, who fall outside our temporal scope, whose respective writings on ageing have attracted far more scholarly interest than all the women discussed here (except for Colette). Both of these extraordinary writers, born in the twentieth century and reaching their forties after the Second World War, might have been expected to be less burdened by the

[116] Colette, *La Naissance du jour*, 49. [117] Ibid., 36–37.

[118] Emma Angell Drake, *What a Woman of Forty-Five Ought to Know* (Philadelphia: Vir Publishing, 1901), 161–171.

nineteenth-century French medicalisation of menopause, and indeed Leduc appeared, like Colette, to find her own ways of relishing the pleasures of post-fertility life.[119] Beauvoir, on the other hand, clearly dreaded growing older, even from quite a young age, and experienced it as a humiliation, only much later in life finding a greater curiosity about her own ageing, as well as a passion for the defence of older people from the prevailing negative social valuation of them.[120] Just as nineteenth-century doctors were not united on the meaning of menopause and women's ageing, so too women themselves have responded to it in different ways.

[119] Leduc, *La Bâtarde.*

[120] Beauvoir, *Le Deuxième sexe*, vol. 2, 456–462; Beauvoir, *La Vieillesse.* As Oliver Davis has shown, the earlier and more negative view has been a disproportionate focus of most scholarship on Beauvoir's view of ageing: Davis, *Age, Rage and Going Gently*, 1–30.

10
Fibroids, Hysterectomy, and the Opotherapy-Surgical Technology Nexus

While general French medical theses describing women's critical age and its hygiene became less common in the final three decades of the nineteenth century, this was not the end of the French invention of menopause. Two new disciplines took it on as important pedagogic and clinical focus after this time: psychiatry, as we considered in Chapter 7, and gynaecological surgery, which expanded massively from the 1870s until the 1920s. In the second half of the nineteenth century, the French dominion over the topic of menopause had begun gradually to diminish, even as those writing about it were floridly generating new topics in relation to novel concepts such as erotomania and degeneration. German, English, Italian, and American writers had begun occasionally to discuss women's final cessation of menses, though never with the level of fascination that French medicine continued to show towards it. But the new rise of gynaecological surgery in the second half of the nineteenth century produced an important surge of international research and intercultural communication between medical scholars with an interest in women's ageing reproductive organs. Women in their forties were now seen by some surgeons in many countries, especially in France and England, as important targets for the experimental surgical removal of the uterus and ovaries. In French medicine, these organs had long been seen as monstrous and troublesome throughout women's lifespan, from puberty to pregnancy, in menstruation, lactation, and menopause, causing nervous and mental illnesses as well as cancers and other gynaecological pathologies. In young women they were deemed necessary for conception, particularly in the intensifying pronatalist culture of the late nineteenth century and increasing anxieties about negative population growth, with the resulting major focus in women's medicine on questions of fertility.[1] In older women, on the other hand, the uterus and ovaries were often described by doctors as shrivelled and useless at best, often perverting, cancerous, or degenerate at worst.

[1] Henri Leridon, 'Théories de la fécondité: Des démographes sous influence?' *Population*, 70/2 (2015): 331–373; Andrea A. Rusnock, *Vital Accounts: Quantifying Health and Population in Eighteenth-Century England and France* (Cambridge: Cambridge University Press, 2002), 179–209; Patrice Bordelais, *Le Nouvel Âge de la vieillesse* (Paris: Éditions Odile Jacob, 1993), 117–131; Karen Offen, 'Depopulation, Nationalism and Feminism in Fin-de-Siècle France', *American Historical Review*, 89/3 (1984): 648–676.

The French Invention of Menopause and the Medicalisation of Women's Ageing: A History. Alison M. Downham Moore, Oxford University Press. © Alison M. Downham Moore 2022. DOI: 10.1093/oso/9780192842916.003.0011

In French gynaecology from the 1870s, benign uterine fibroid tumours (leiomyomas) became the most common condition for which women were prescribed the new but still very dangerous surgeries of hysterectomy and oophorectomy, often in their thirties and forties, well before the natural cessation of menses with ageing. But by the turn of the twentieth century, several influential French surgeons had begun to insist that these common tumours were a specific pathology of menopause itself, even as a vast statistical dataset suggested exactly the opposite—that they stopped growing or even disappeared with the end of menstruation and fertility. Hysterectomy with oophorectomy was the solution proposed for fibroids and several other benign (non-cancerous) growths and disorders. But this surgery performed on a woman before the age of menopause, if she survived it, artificially created a state similar to natural menopause, only far more abruptly and with long-term consequences for ageing morbidity. This was no longer just about the medical invention of a novel concept of menopause or a critical age, as had been the case thus far throughout the nineteenth century. There was now a surgically created population of women whose medical treatments actually put them into menopause, in the nineteenth-century sense of this concept: the definitive cessation of menstruation, the end of fertility, and the loss of systemic activity of the uterus and ovaries, but also uncomfortable physical and nervous symptoms, fat gain, memory problems, and loss of vitality. French medicine, by the 1890s, was also beginning to see menopause in relation to the loss of the ovaries' internal secretions, which were understood to be both health-preserving and prosexual,[2] thus opening the possibility of their novel pharmacological replacement in women who had their organs surgically excised. It was a whole new level of disease-mongering: no longer simply contenting itself with the reconstruction of concepts about women's ageing that made them targets for medical surveillance, hygiene, and psychiatric incarceration, instead it introduced a far more aggressive, novel iatrogenesis of premature ageing morbidity in women who would not otherwise have suffered it. Clearly, none of these early surgical innovators had access to any of the vast data available to patients and clinicians in the twenty-first century indicating long-term increased risks for ageing women's morbidity following premenopausal hysterectomy and oophorectomy for benign conditions.[3] But their

[2] Chandak Sengoopta, *The Most Secret Quintessence of Life: Sex, Glands and Hormones, 1850–1950* (Chicago: University of Chicago Press, 2006), 33–49.

[3] To cite just a portion of recent research referring to increased risks of thyroid and brain cancer, cardiovascular disease, mental health conditions, dyslipidaemia, hypertension, urinary incontinence, dementia, osteoporosis, and general ageing multi-morbidity: Sabbir T. Rahman et al., 'Risk of Thyroid Cancer Following Hysterectomy', *Cancer Epidemiology*, 72 (2021): 1–8. Article 101931; Martha Hickey & Gita D. Mishra, 'Timing and Type of Menopause and Risk of Cardiovascular Disease', *Menopause: The Journal of the North American Menopause Society*, 28/5 (2021): 477–479; Shannon K. Laughlin-Tommaso et al., 'Long-Term Risk of De Novo Mental Health Conditions after Hysterectomy with Ovarian Conservation: A Cohort Study', *Menopause: The Journal of the North American Menopause Society*, 27/1 (2020): 33–42; Marios K. Georgakis et al., 'Surgical Menopause in Association with Cognitive Function and Risk of Dementia: A Systematic Review and Meta-analysis', *Psychoneuroendocrinology*

own concepts about the decline of the uterus and ovaries heralding a sudden 'death of sex' and the advent of old-age illness should have been sufficient to cause doctors to pause over the ethics of inducing early menopause artificially in women who had no life-threatening diseases. Indeed, many doctors did pause over it, particularly in France and Germany, and hysterectomy and oophorectomy remained controversial treatments until the early twentieth century, not least because of how risky they remained. In 1883, in the ninety-three published case observations of hysterectomy in the international medical literature, mortality was as high as 67 per cent, and it still remained around 14 per cent in 1941 despite massive improvements in surgical technique, aseptic procedure, antibiotics, anaesthetics, and patient aftercare.[4]

But another development in French and German medicine in the 1890s, alongside the improved survival rates for hysterectomy between 1870 and 1900, helped to soften some of the opposition to the increasingly widespread radical gynaecological surgeries for benign conditions. This was the commercialisation of ovarian hormonal opotherapy products, 'ovarian juice' (*le suc ovarien*) as it was called in the 1890s, which over the following fifty years became the source of multi-billion-dollar profits for global pharmaceutical conglomerates.[5] It was only in 1924 that the French biochemist Robert Courrier (1895–1986) isolated the specific ovarian hormone which he named 'folliculine', later known as oestrogen, which became the backbone of the global pharmaceutical enterprise of menopause hormone

106 (2019): 9–19; Pei-Chen Li et al., 'Risk of Hyperlipidemia in Women with Hysterectomy: A Retrospective Cohort Study in Taiwan', *Nature Scientific Reports*, 8 (2018): 1–9. Article 12956; D.-C. Ding et al., 'Risk of Hypertension after Hysterectomy: A Population-Based Study', *BJOG: International Journal of Obstetrics & Gynaecology* (2018): 1–8; Shannon K. Laughlin-Tommaso et al., 'Cardiovascular and Metabolic Morbidity after Hysterectomy with Ovarian Conservation: A Cohort Study', *Menopause: Journal of the North American Menopause Society*, 25/5 (2017): 483–492; Walter A. Rocca et al., 'Accelerated Accumulation of Multimorbidity after Bilateral Oophorectomy: A Population-Based Cohort Study', *Mayo Clinic Proceedings*, 91/11 (2016): 1577–1589; Daniel Altman, Li Yin, and Henrik Falconer, 'Long-Term Cancer Risk after Hysterectomy on Benign Indications: Population-Based Cohort Study', *International Journal of Cancer*, 138 (2016): 2631–2638; Riley Bove et al., 'Age at Surgical Menopause Influences Cognitive Decline and Alzheimer Pathology in Older Women', *Neurology*, 82 (2014): 222–229; Catharina Forsgren and Daniel Altman, 'Long-Term Effects of Hysterectomy: A Focus on the Aging Patient', *Aging Health*, 9/2 (2013): 179–187; Erik Ingelsson et al., 'Hysterectomy and Risk of Cardiovascular Disease: A Population-Based Cohort Study', *European Heart Journal*, 32 (2011): 745–750; T. K. T. Phung et al., 'Hysterectomy, Oophorectomy and Risk of Dementia: A Nationwide Historical Cohort Study', *Dementia and Geriatric Cognitive Disorders*, 30/1 (2010): 43–50; Jeannette S. Brown et al., 'Hysterectomy and Urinary Incontinence: A Systematic Review', *The Lancet*, 356/9229 (2000): 535–539.

[4] Ornella Moscucci, *The Science of Woman: Gynaecology and Gender in England, 1800–1929* (Cambridge: Cambridge University Press, 1993), 67, 82.

[5] André Marchand, *Opothérapie: Émergence et développement d'une technique thérapeutique (France, 1889–1940)*. Thèse (Paris: Conservatoire national des arts et métiers, 2015); Elizabeth Siegel Watkins, *The Estrogen Elixir: A History of Hormone Replacement Therapy in America* (Baltimore: Johns Hopkins University Press, 2009); Celia Roberts, *Messengers of Sex: Hormones, Biomedicine and Feminism* (Cambridge: Cambridge University Press, 2007); Ilana Löwy and Jean-Paul Gaudillière, 'Médicalisation de la ménopause, mouvements pour la santé des femmes et controverses sur les thérapies hormonales', *Nouvelles Questions féministes*, 25/2 (2006): 48–65.

replacement therapy in the twentieth century.[6] But the precedents of this practice had unfolded in France of the 1890s, in response, in turn, to the innovation of surgical hysterectomy and oophorectomy from the 1870s onwards. It was in the context of developing ovarian opotherapy in the 1890s that the iatrogenic side effects of surgeries to remove women's reproductive organs became an object of scientific study, thanks to the pioneering work of several Paris gynaecologists working under Samuel Pozzi (1846–1918), particularly Félix Jayle (1866–1945).[7] Almost immediately, these therapies were extrapolated to the small number of women whose menses had naturally ceased with ageing and who complained of debilitating symptoms of hot flushes, night sweats, headaches, joint pain, memory problems, and sleep disturbance. Menopause was thus radically reconfigured in French medicine in the final decade of the nineteenth century in response to an emerging interrelated endocrine-surgical nexus of treatments; and the surgical menopause created artificially in premenopausal women and then 'remedied' by ovarian opotherapy became the template for the treatment of older women as well.

The Emergence of Gynaecological Surgery and Artificial Menopause

It might be assumed that the practice of hysterectomising all women presenting with uterine tumours of any kind was a product of the emergence of gynaecological surgery in the context predating the histological distinctions later made between cancerous and non-cancerous cell types. But this was patently not so. From early in the nineteenth century, uterine fibroids were widely observed to be a distinct type of non-cancerous tumour that could certainly grow and replicate its own cells,[8] but that could not metastasise to neighbouring tissues or invade the lymphatic system to produce distal metastasis, as malignant cancers of the breast had been observed to do. French microbiologists had debated the nature of cancer cells throughout the 1840s, following the Paris histopathologist Herman Lerbert's experiments showing unique cell types present in the uterine tumours that had been clinically identified as malignant.[9] Uterine fibroid tumours lacked these cancerous cell types and had a unique fibrous tissue structure all of their

[6] Robert Courrier, *La Physiologie de l'ovaire* (Alençon, Imprimerie alençonnaise, 1948).

[7] Samuel Pozzi & Félix Jayle, *Traité de gynécologie clinique et opératoire* [1890], 4th ed., 2 vols (Paris: Masson et Cie, 1905–1907), vol. 2, 779; Félix Jayle, *Opothérapie ovarienne dans la ménopause artificielle post-opératoire et la ménopause naturelle* (Paris: Masson, 1898).

[8] Jean Buisson, *Contribution à l'étude des fibromes après la ménopause*. Thèse (Paris: Jouve, 1927).

[9] Ann La Berge, 'Dichotomy or Integration? Medical Microscopy and the Paris Clinical Tradition', in Caroline Hannaway & Ann Le Berge, eds, *Constructing Paris Medicine* (Amsterdam: Rodopi, 1998), 275–312 [298–300]; Ornella Moscucci, *The Science of Woman: Gynaecology and Gender in England, 1800–1929* (London: Palgrave, 2016), 53–54.

own.[10] This was not something that could be used for diagnosis, since it required the tumour to be extracted first. But that the vast majority of fibroids had a recognisable, non-malignant histological presentation—with the clinical features of slow-growing benign masses producing only local pressure and haemorrhage symptoms—was widely understood well before hysterectomy or oophorectomy were commonly performed in France. Uterine cancer, on the other hand, was viewed as having 'clearly accusable symptoms' which were not easily confused with those of benign fibroid tumours.[11] The practice of hysterectomising women in their thirties and forties for benign conditions, which became common in France from the mid-1870s, did not emerge as a result of any ambiguity about what constituted cancerous tumours and what did not. Gynaecologists certainly recognised that a tiny percentage of apparently benign uterine tumours would turn out to be malignant on histological analysis, just as they do today.[12] But this was not the justification offered by the first surgeons and gynaecologists who performed this radical and dangerous surgery. Rather, their rationales focused on the symptoms of which the patients complained (especially constipation and haemorrhagic bleeding), on the purported uselessness of the uterus and ovaries once a woman approached menopause (even within ten to fifteen years), on the general greater prevalence of cancer later in women's old age, and on the technical difficulties of selectively removing just the tumour itself (myomectomy) while conserving the uterus and ovaries.

Gynaecology in the broadest sense was an ancient field and was distinguished throughout the history of medicine, with the Latin word becoming increasingly common from the early seventeenth century and the French word appearing in the 1830s. Up to this time, the term referred broadly to the diseases of women including, but not limited to, those relating to their reproductive organs.[13] While numerous nineteenth-century French doctors had addressed questions of gynaecological pathology, including the age-related cessation of menses (which, as we have seen, was viewed as 'not a disease' but was treated like one anyway), before the 1880s few doctors considered themselves solely experts in the care of women's reproductive organs. French obstetrics had emerged as a discipline of its own since the seventeenth century, becoming fully medically professionalised by the beginning of the nineteenth century.[14] Given that many matters relating to pregnancy, fertility, menstruation, and childbirth were already covered by obstetrics,

[10] Georges Pouchet, *Précis d'histologie humaine d'après les travaux de l'école française* (Paris: Masson, 1864), 100; Jean Casimir Félix Guyon, *Des tumeurs fibreuses de l'utérus* (Paris: Adrien Delahaye, 1860), 21–22.

[11] F. L. Pichot, *Étude clinique sur le cancer du corps et de la cavité de l'utérus* (Paris: Henri Rey, 1876), 18.

[12] Jonas Abeille, *Des corps fibreux de l'utérus* (Paris: E. Thunot, 1868), 7.

[13] Helen King, *Midwifery, Obstetrics and the Rise of Gynaecology* (London: Routledge, 2007).

[14] Nathalie Sage Pranchère, *L'École des sages-femmes: Naissance d'un corps professionnel (1786–1917)* (Tours: Presses Universitaires, 2017).

gynaecology only made sense as a distinct discipline if there were substantial women's health conditions it pertained to treat that went clearly beyond this. Menopause, like hysteria and nymphomania, was just such a condition. The growing association of uterine and ovarian pathologies with it, both benign though sometimes symptomatic conditions such as uterine fibroids, ovarian cysts, and uterine prolapse, and deadly forms of cancer, suggested an important patient cohort of women in their forties and fifties, who thus attracted the attention of this new and expanding surgical discipline.

Late nineteenth-century gynaecological monographs, textbooks, theses, and articles in medical journals had a notably different tone from much of the medical writing on menopause up to this time. Devoting far less space to characterising women's general 'nature' with reference to ideas about their nervousness and sensibility inspired by Pierre Roussel, they instead focused far more on technical description and surgical skills, showing more nuance in the denomination of specific pathologies and greater cognisance of changing, global research trends. The growth of gynaecological surgery in the second half of the nineteenth century was an international and intercultural movement, and major French gynaecologists were far more aware of clinical practices and research trends in other countries—especially the work of surgeons and gynaecologists in Germany, Austria, England, Scotland, Italy, and the United States—than were general menopause medical and hygiene writers.[15] Consequently, they appear far more medically serious than the often lyrical, speculative, and repetitious French medical writing on menopause or women's critical age from 1799 to 1880. There was (mostly) no longer any talk of supposedly Hippocratic aphorisms, nor insistent correctives of supposed past medical errors of the kind that characterised nineteenth-century French menopause doctors' historical stories about their own revolutionary historical importance.

Numerous doctoral dissertations and books on surgical techniques of hysterectomy and oophorectomy were written between 1842 and 1900, not only by French but also by German, American, Irish, Scottish, Italian, Spanish, and English doctors.[16] Such surgeries, conducted before the advent of aseptic

[15] Surgeons' travel writings summarising gynaecological practices in other countries were common: e.g. Dr Poullet, *La Gynécologie à l'étranger* (Lyon: Riotor, 1879); A. Brissay, *Fragments de chirurgie et de gynécologie opératoire contemporaines* (Paris: O. Doin, 1887).

[16] Eugène Kœberlé, *Documents pour servir à l'histoire de l'extirpation des tumeurs fibreuses de la matrice par la méthode sus-pubienne* (Paris: J. B. Baillière et fils, 1864); Horatio Robinson Storer, *Successful Removal of the Uterus and Both Ovaries* (Boston: David Clapp & Son, 1866); Stanislas Caternault, *Essai sur la gastrotomie dans les cas de tumeurs fibreuses péri-utérines; précédé des 8 premières observations relatives aux 8 premières ablations de la matrice pratiquées par E. Kœberlé* (Paris: J. B. Baillière et fils/London: Hippolyte Baillière, 1866); Jules Émile Péan and Léopold Urdy, *Hystérotomie: De l'ablation partielle ou totale de l'utérus, etc.* (Paris: Adrien Delahaye, 1873); Alfred Hegar, 'Zur Ovariotomie, die intraperitoneale Versorgung des Stiels der Ovarientumoren; Schicksale und Effecte versenkter Ligaturen, abgeschnürter Gewebsstücke, Brandschorfe, vollständig getrennte Massen oder zurückgelassener Flüssigkeiten in der Bauchhöhle', *Gynäkologie*, 36, *Klinische Vorträge*,

technique or antibiotics, were almost always deadly; but doctors began taking new risks with them in French, English, and German medicine after the 1840s, approaching them as experimental surgeries that could help to develop general abdominal laparotomic technique.[17] While many such surgeries were initially without success in terms of patient survival, in the 1860s reports began accumulating of successful operations, at least with short-term post-operative survival—long-term follow-up was rare. Fibroid tumours that dangled into the vagina from pedicles attached to the inner surface of the uterus could more easily be removed by dilating the cervix and incising the tumour from its pedicle, without the need for hysterectomy or indeed for any excision of the organs. Other pedunculated tumours on the outer surface of the uterus could also be removed without hysterectomy, although this required the far more dangerous laparotomy (sometimes also called either *gastrotonomie* or *gastrotomie*)—abdominal incision. But both of these kinds of fibroids together accounted for less than half of the very common benign tumours that many women developed in their thirties and which continued to grow into their forties. While a few surgeons focused on removing just the tumour, while conserving the uterus and ovaries in the surgery known as myomectomy,[18] most did not even try to do this, opting instead for complete excision of the offending organs themselves—both the uterus and ovaries. For modern medicine, abdominal hysterectomy and oophorectomy were undoubtedly the most exciting surgeries in terms of general abdominal technical advancement given that women's reproductive organs were among the few abdominal organs (unlike the stomach, kidneys, heart, lungs, liver, spleen, or most of the bowel) that could be surgically removed without fatally impacting the patient's individual physiological function—assuming they survived the surgery. Given too how powerful were the prevalent negative nineteenth-century medical views of the uterus as a morbid organ that deranged women's overall physiology throughout the lifespan and as atrophying suddenly with the final cessation of menses, it is perhaps unsurprising that it was targeted for removal in women defined as approaching menopause and deemed no longer capable of, or appropriate for, conception.

109 (1877): 811–830; A. P. Gavilan, *De l'hystérectomie vaginale dans les cas de fibromes utérins* (Paris: Berthier, 1888); J. C. Irish, *Treatment of Uterine Fibro-Myomata by Abdominal Hysterectomy* (Boston: Damrell & Upham, 1890); Sébastien Le Moinet, *Hystérectomie abdominale totale et hystérectomie abdomino-vaginale pour fibromes de l'utérus* (Paris: G. Steinheil, 1894); Albert Ramon, *Hystérectomie abdomino-vaginale: Méthode Péan dans les cas de gros fibromes utérins* (Paris: G. Steinheil, 1893); Jules-Henri Pigeonnat, *Gros fibromes utérins (Hystérectomie abdominale, méthode-péritonéale)* (Paris: Henri Jouve, 1896); Paul George Caboche, *Hystérectomie abdominale totale (procédé de Doyen); Manuel opératoire et résultats* (Paris: G. Steinheil, 1897).

[17] Moscucci, *The Science of Woman*, 170.

[18] Oscar Larcher, *Contributions à l'histoire des polypes fibreux intra-utérins à apparitions intermittentes* (Paris: Asselin, 1867); Louis Dartigues, *Chirurgie conservatrice de l'utérus et des annexes dans le traitement des fibromes* (Paris: Maloine, 1901).

The conceptual ground was laid in medical writing on the diseases of women even well before the practice of hysterectomising women around menopause became common. In 1858 the work of the renowned Würzburg professor of obstetrics/gynaecology Friedrich Wilhelm Scanzoni von Lichtenfels (1821–1891) on the diseases of women's sexual organs, published the previous year,[19] was translated from German to French. It conveyed something of the views about women's ageing and cancer prevalence which were significant in German medicine of the early nineteenth century but with which French scholars, even those writing about menopause, had hitherto only rarely engaged.[20] Scanzoni referred repeatedly throughout his *Practical Treatise on the Diseases of Women's Sexual Organs* to the idea that although certain kinds of women's diseases became rarer after the final cessation of menses due to the diminished influence of the uterus, other pathologies became more common in older women. Those approaching the final cessation but still menstruating irregularly were at particularly high risk of troublesome fibroid tumours, polyps, and cysts, as well as haemorrhagic complaints and dangerous cancers of the breast, uterus, or ovary.[21] He said that the perturbation of menstrual function with the approach of menopause caused an 'excess of nutrition' that fed the growth of cancer cells, resulting in breast cancer being more common in women between the ages of 40 and 50 years than at any other age.[22] Pathologies emerging during the critical age before the menses ended should be watched very closely, Scanzoni advised, since they had a tendency to progress rapidly at this time of life.[23] Surgeries entailing extirpation of the uterus and ovaries, which Scanzoni said were the best chance medicine had of curing dangerous cancers, were discussed throughout the book; but he acknowledged that most of the surgeries of this kind of the uterus which had been attempted were for cancers that were already well developed, and that there were as yet few cases in which the patient had survived the surgery. Fibroid tumours occurring during the critical age, he noted, were not dangerous even though they sometimes entailed troublesome symptoms, which generally diminished, along with the volume of the tumour, following menopause. He considered surgeries to remove such tumours to be the best cure in the case of symptomatic fibroids, saying this was an approach with which 'everyone agrees'; though he did not appear to consider it either desirable or necessary to remove the uterus or ovaries along with the tumour. He asserted that fibroids did not generally recur after being extirpated—possibly because he had mostly treated women close to menopause, when recurrence was uncommon.[24]

[19] Friedrich Wilhelm Scanzoni (von Lichtenfels), *Lehrbuch der Krankheiten der weiblichen Sexualorgane* (Vienna: Wilhelm Braumüller, 1857).

[20] Friedrich Wilhelm Scanzoni (von Lichtenfels), *Traité pratique des maladies des organes sexuels de la femme*, trans. M. Dor & A. Socin (Paris: J. B. Baillière et fils, 1858), 72, 144, 215, 252.

[21] Ibid., 168, 543. [22] Ibid., 543. [23] Ibid., 272. [24] Ibid., 215.

The Strasbourg professor of medicine Eugène Kœberlé (1828–1915) was the first French surgeon to publish on his attempts at abdominal hysterectomy for the treatment of benign uterine fibroids. He proposed that this was the best method for removing large tumours of this kind, since attempting to extract just the tumour itself required it to be morcellated, which was too dangerous, causing massive haemorrhage.[25] There was no point trying to treat cancerous tumours with this surgery, he noted, since cancer was impossible to cure.[26] He claimed instead that hysterectomy was needed for benign fibroid tumours that were not easily separable from the uterus, whatever their size.[27] But Kœberlé viewed these growths as most common in women in their thirties, and made no mention of them having any relationship to menopause.[28] While he initiated the dangerous French experiment on women that was the nineteenth-century practice of hysterectomy, he was not the one to target older women in relation to menopause as his non-consensual experimental subjects—he extended that honour instead to younger women.

However, from early in the development of the practice of gynaecological surgical removal of the uterus and or ovaries, the question of menopausal women as a group likely to require such surgeries was raised. The 1866 *Practical Treatise of Disease of the Uterus, Ovaries and Fallopian Tubes* by the Montpellier professor of medicine and clinical surgery Amédée Courty addressed the question of whether gynaecological diseases could be expected to improve or become exacerbated by menopause. He said that some uterine diseases could persist for many years after menopause without causing any pain or 'provoking any sympathetic troubles' (e.g. hysteria), remaining in a sort of latent state,[29] but he also said that menopause brought new risks of disease:

> The *âge de retour* certainly helps make some [uterine diseases] disappear via the cessation of periodic ovulation as well as the menstrual flux…But it does not always make the usual flux cease; far from it, it can sometimes increase in intensity, no longer having any regulator…Moreover, this *âge de retour* often itself produces a predisposition toward diathetic afflictions, and consequently, if it suppresses one danger, it brings another.[30]

Courty identified non-cancerous masses growing on the uterus and ovaries as particularly common in women approaching menopause. While most fibroid tumours and ovarian cysts were clearly 'benign', he said, if they grew to a large volume, distending the abdomen or continuing to grow indefinitely, it was

[25] Kœberlé, *Documents pour servir à l'histoire de l'extirpation*, 11. [26] Ibid., 3.
[27] Ibid., 9. [28] Ibid., 4.
[29] Amédée Courty, *Traité pratique des maladies de l'utérus, des ovaires et des trompes* [1866] (Paris: P. Asselin, 1872), 309.
[30] Ibid., 176–177.

impossible for it not to have a profound impact on the patient's general health. He identified three specific ways in which such formations 'altered the constitution' of the patient: 'by its mechanical interference with the movements of the organs' and their 'performance of their functions'; by the 'irritation or sympathetic troubles' it provoked in some organs; and by its consumption of nutrients, which deprived the woman's other tissues of nourishment. He emphasised that this was particularly a concern in young women whose tumours had grown rapidly, but he also joined in the physiognomic speculations about gynaecological disease that had been suggested by English surgeons enthusiastic to perform oophorectomy on women in their forties in this same period.[31] Here the idea was that women whose uterus or ovaries were diseased would develop certain facial characteristics of premature ageing: the face became wrinkled, the lips thinner, the nose pointier, the eye sockets deeper, and the eyes themselves more protruding. These were 'the traits of premature old age', juxtaposed with eyes that still shone like those of a younger person. These were the signs 'that bear witness to a vitality suffocated by the development of a parasite', the tumour. Courty here even reproduced a drawing of a 42-year-old woman with the 'facies ovarien'—someone with a gynaecological tumour as indicated by her supposedly haggard face—produced by Thomas Spencer Wells in his 1865 book on *Diseases of the Ovaries*, of which a short summary appeared in French translation in 1867, with a full French translation following in 1883.[32] Courty's qualifications about younger women being the group of greater concern thus appear less resounding, as he referred to the notion that the signs of facial premature ageing in women in their forties might be taken as indicators of gynaecological pathologies in need of surgery. Nonetheless, Courty remained conservative in his recommendations of surgeries such as hysterectomy and oophorectomy, considering the substantial mortality risk they entailed still in the France of the 1860s and early 1870s (around 60%—slightly lower than the European average),[33] remarking of the many attempted surgeries of this kind where the patient had not recovered: 'it is not possible to encourage surgeons to follow this path until the causes of death following the operation, being better known, can be more effectively avoided or fought', or until cases where success was more probable became better identified.[34]

[31] Ibid., 1069.

[32] Ibid., 1070; Thomas Spencer Wells, *Diseases of the Ovaries* (London: John Churchill, 1865), 288; Thomas Spencer Wells, *Du traitement des kystes et des tumeurs ovariques* (Paris: Leclerc, 1867); Thomas Spencer Wells, *Des tumeurs de l'ovaire et de l'utérus, leur diagnostic et leur traitement* (Paris: G. Masson, 1883).

[33] Courty, *Traité pratique des maladies de l'utérus, des ovaires et des trompes*, 298–299, 443.

[34] Ibid., 1121. Percentage figure is calculated from the total reported deaths within the total reported cases in Jules Péan & Léopold Urdy, *Hystérotomie: De l'ablation partielle ou totale de l'utérus par la gastrotomie: Étude sur les tumeurs qui peuvent nécessiter cette opération* (Paris: Adrien Delahaye, 1873).

Jules Péan's Dangerous Experimental Surgeries and Their Rationales

Other doctors citing both Courty and Spencer Wells were even less cautious than they. The renowned Paris surgeon Jules Péan (1830–1898) was one who urged doctors to show 'sang-froid' and determination towards the experimental practice of laparotomic hysterectomy—removal of the uterus and ovaries via abdominal incision (which he called *hystérotomie*), despite the high mortality risk it entailed.[35] Péan performed surgeries for public viewing at the Hôpital Saint-Louis in Paris, which is how Toulouse-Lautrec's 1891 painting of him in the act came into existence (Image 10.1).[36] The medical satirist Léon Daudet, in his memoires of 1914, wrote of Péan 'effortlessly removing half a dozen uteruses and a few pairs of ovaries' in a single session, describing him as a 'tragic prestidigitator' and the results as a 'scientific massacre'.[37] Péan's 1873 book on this new gynaecological surgery written with his intern, the Montpellier-trained surgeon Léopold Urdy, proposed to provide an account of all the situations in which partial or full hysterectomy, with removal of both ovaries as well, was 'necessary'. He appeared to view the advancement of the practice of removing women's reproductive organs as 'the glory of contemporary surgery', with a 'brilliant future', remarking that it 'should definitively be classed among the great surgical operations'.[38] He said that the 'law of surgical progress' dictated that, since oophorectomies by laparotomy (abdominal incision) were already being performed (particularly in England), hysterectomy by laparotomy now had to be advanced as well.[39] Numerous surgeons in various national contexts had removed uteri in recent years without initially intending to, having operated for a different reason, but Péan took pride in what he claimed was the fact that it was a Frenchman, Kœberlé, who performed thefirst intentional and successful hysterectomy in 1863.[40] In fact Kœberlé himself acknowledged the Manchester surgeon A. M. Heath in 1843 as the first.[41] In one of his case examples, Péan mentions first being keen to perform the surgery himself to impress a distinguished professor who was observing him.[42] Like Courty, he too cited the *facies ovarium* idea—that uterine and ovarian pathologies marked women's faces with premature ageing and bulging eyes (Image 10.2).[43] Perhaps it was for this reason that he so commonly performed the surgery on women in their forties who, as *demi-vieilles* (half-old-women, as Yvette Guilbert called them) fitted that visual portrait better than either younger or much older women. He extended the idea further too, adding that women with malignant

[35] Ibid., 14.

[36] Jeffrey K. Aronson & Manoj Ramachandran, 'The Diagnosis of Art: Dr. Péan's Operation', *Journal of the Royal Society of Medicine* (2008): 423–424.

[37] Léon Daudet, *Devant la douleur* (Paris: Nouvelle librairie nationale, 1914), 65–66.

[38] Péan & Urdy, *Hystérotomie*, v–vi. [39] Ibid., 2. [40] Ibid., 8.

[41] Kœberlé, *Documents pour servir à l'histoire de l'extirpation*, 9.

[42] Péan & Urdy, *Hystérotomie*, 63. [43] Ibid., 105.

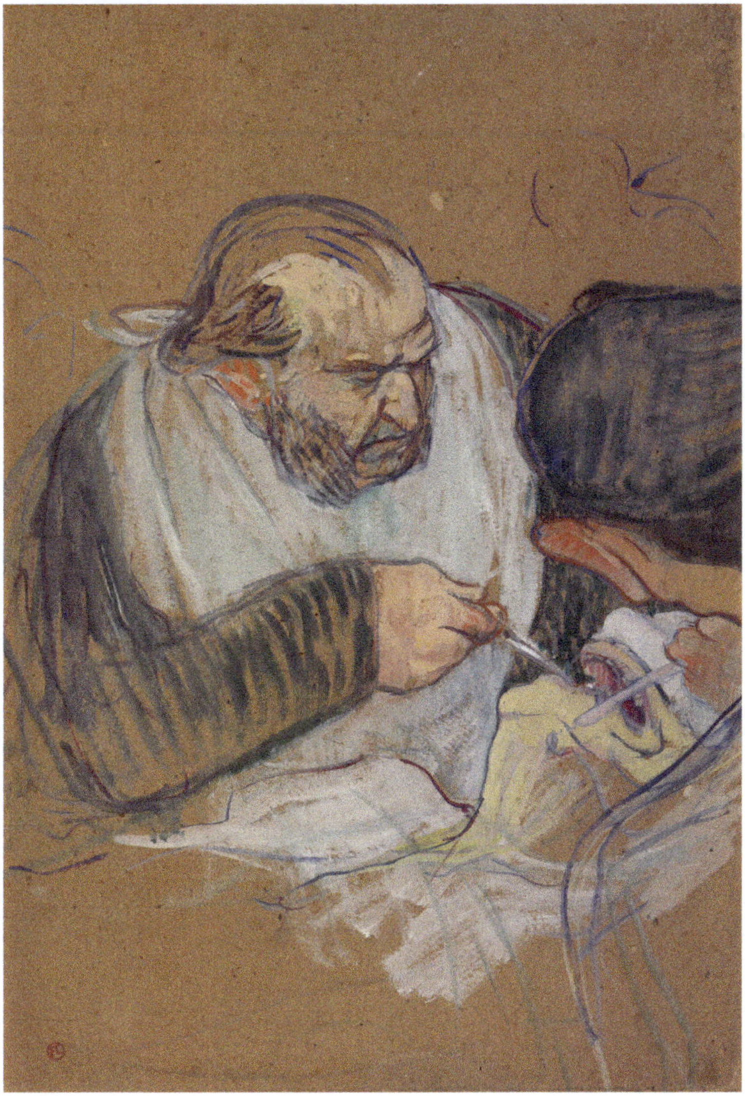

Image 10.1 Henri Toulouse-Lautrec, *Une opération par le Docteur Péan à l'Hôpital International*, *c.*1891. Courtesy of Wikimedia, Creative Commons Attribution-ShareAlike 4.0 International.

uterine cancers had a different look again to those with the *facies ovarium*. These women instead were pale, jaundiced, underweight, and exhausted.[44]

Péan, like Courty and other surgeon-gynaecologists, insisted that he only performed hysterectomy when a woman's life was already threatened by an existing

[44] Ibid., 113.

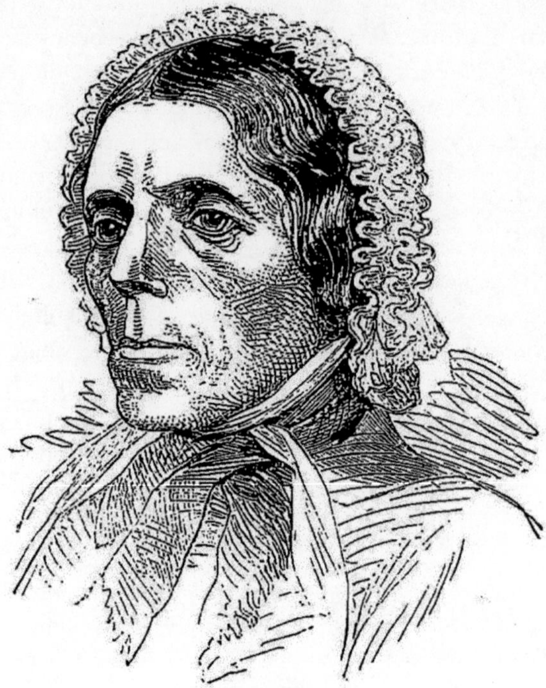

Fig. 263 (*).

Image 10.2 Thomas Spencer Wells, drawing of a 42-year-old woman with the '*facies ovarium*'. Reproduced in Courty, *Traité pratique des maladies de l'utérus et ses annexes*, 1872, Fig. 286. With permission from the Bibliothèque Nationale de France.

gynaecological pathology. In practice, however, this was difficult because most gynaecological conditions were not cancer and nor were they lethal. Deaths from gynaecological cancer constituted less than half of the 2.2 per cent general women's cancer mortality in English statistics, whereas benign fibroid tumours had been observed in between 25 and 40 per cent of all women by the time they reached menopause.[45] All those practising the surgery appeared to agree on the ethical parameter of only performing dangerous surgeries if a woman's pathologies already threatened her life, but this sat in tension with the availability of patients on whom they could practice the surgery, and with surgeons' enthusiasm and ambition for performing it. Their need to practice it more often was not only a product of careerist ambition, since the surgeon with greater skill in performing the surgery was also assumed to be able to lower the mortality rate and cure more women of their diseases. It was a complex ethical conundrum, mixing some

[45] David Berry Hart & Alexander Hugh Freeland Barbour, *Manual of Gynecology* [1882], 2nd ed. (Edinburgh: W. & A. K. Johnston, 1883), 436; Amédée Dechambre, ed., *Dictionnaire encyclopédique des sciences médicales*, Series 5, vol. 2 (Paris: G. Masson & P. Asselin, 1886), 81.

amount of genuine concern for helping patients with a lot of professional pride and ambition, all in the face of no available knowledge of any long-term effects of the surgeries they were performing. By way of justification for his own enthusiasm for hysterectomy, Péan noted that the uterus did not 'represent an indispensable function for the conservation of the individual', and that its absence was 'perfectly compatible with life'. This was particularly relevant for older women because 'once the sexual life of women is terminated after menopause' and the uterus no longer has any role, 'it becomes useless and even dangerous through the numerous afflictions of which it can be the seat'.[46]

From the many discussions about mortality rates of different surgeries in the writings of Péan and other scholars, it was clearly the single most significant number from the point of view of gaining prestige as a gynaecological surgeon—surely a good marker that was also in the interest of women's health? The only issue was that it was widely recognised that those women suffering from the most active and dangerous cancers were also the least likely to survive abdominal surgery, making them a potential liability for surgeons wishing to present a better percentage of successful surgeries in their publications. So while all the surgeons agreed in principle that hysterectomy was only to be used in cases where women's lives were already at risk, women presenting with signs of advanced malignancy represented only a small minority of Péan's and other surgeons' case observations.[47] As Péan himself noted, such clearly malignant growths were uncommon compared to the far more ubiquitous benign uterine fibroids and ovarian cysts.[48] Péan said that of the seventeen cases of advanced uterine cancer that another French surgeon Philippe Boyer had attempted to treat, only three of the patients had survived the operation, and even those did not live for more than a year or so after their surgery, and it was for this reason that Péan himself tried to avoid operating on such patients.[49] Péan also said that he refused to operate on women older than about 55 for a similar reason, because if the patient was of a 'too-advanced age', she would be in 'a considerable state of weakness'.[50] He, on the other hand, was able to boast seven successful surgeries out of the nine he had recently performed—only a 22.2 per cent mortality rate, much lower than any other surgeon had yet reported, although he acknowledged it could just be due to a lucky streak.[51] His success was perhaps surprising indeed given that infections causing fever were already understood to be one of the major causes of death in surgery, and Péan was an opponent of the microbial theory of Louis Pasteur, rejecting the emerging antiseptic surgical methods about which other doctors such as the

[46] Péan & Urdy, *Hystérotomie*, 12. [47] Moscucci, *The Science of Woman*, 67.
[48] Péan & Urdy, *Hystérotomie*, 80.
[49] Ibid., 32. Philippe Boyer, *Traité des maladies chirurgicales* [1818], 7 vols, 5th ed. (Paris: Labé, 1846), vol. 5, 942–958.
[50] Péan & Léopold, *Hystérotomie*, 51. [51] Ibid., 24.

Scottish surgeon Joseph Lister (1827–1912) had already written, and about which his French compatriots Ulysse Trélat (1828–1890) and the young Samuel Pozzi (1846–1918) were at this same time becoming enthusiastic.[52] Péan's trick instead may have been his careful patient selection.

With so many of the patients who most needed gynaecological surgeries, as well as all women over age 55, excluded from his surgical list, how indeed could Péan find enough women to hysterectomise successfully? He evoked a portrait of a hypothetical woman approaching menopause, perhaps summing up his ideal target for hysterectomy: one suffering fatigue, a feeling of heaviness in the abdomen, constipation, some loss of appetite, perhaps a little nausea. Such a woman, he noted, would not be easily convinced that she needed to let a doctor examine her genital organs. But he emphasised that catching uterine disease in the very early stages implied the best chance of a cure. Such a woman generally only became concerned once a mass in her belly started to grow while she continued to menstruate (indicating it could not be a pregnancy).[53] Péan's eighteen cited cases where the age was recorded, which included nine of his own and nine cases of the other surgeons who had hitherto recorded such surgeries for tumour removal, comprised ten women (55.5%) in the age range of 40–53 years, and eight (45.5%) women in their thirties. But several of the younger women, such as a Mlle Chaux, aged 38, who died from her surgery, presented with more worrying symptoms suggestive of possible malignancy, such as a rapidly growing mass in their abdomen, recent sudden weight loss, and substantial ascites (fluid in the abdominal cavity).[54] The success rate in such surgical patients was widely recognised to be lower than in women with large, slow-growing abdominal masses and haemorrhagic bleeding or regular heavy, painful periods—who tended more often to be women in their forties or early fifties.[55] Women viewed as approaching the 'critical age' or menopause were to some extent then targeted for the dangerous experimental surgery that was hysterectomy in this period, but an almost equivalent number of women in their thirties were also subjected to it. However, there was an important difference in the kinds of growths for which the older women were prescribed this radical surgery.

Women in their forties and fifties were clearly more likely to be prescribed hysterectomy with oophorectomy for conditions that were widely recognised as

[52] Joseph Lister, 'Observations on Ligature of Arteries on the Antiseptic System', *The Lancet*, 3 April (1869): 451–455; Joseph Lister, 'The Antiseptic Method of Dressing Open Wounds', *Medical Record*, 11 (1876): 695–696; Lindsay Fitzharris, *The Butchering Art: Joseph Lister's Quest to Transform the Grisly World of Victorian Medicine* (London: Penguin, 2018), 227–228; Samuel Pozzi, *Quelques observations à propos du pansement de Lister appliqué aux plaies d'amputation et d'ablation de tumeurs* (Paris: la Veuve A. Delahaye, 1876); Caroline de Costa & Francesca Miller, *The Diva and Doctor God: Letters from Sarah Bernhardt to Doctor Samuel Pozzi* (Bloomington: Xlibris, 2010), 99–101.

[53] Péan & Léopold, *Hystérotomie*, 103.

[54] Ibid., 73–78.

[55] Ibid., 32; Kœberlé, *Documents pour servir à l'histoire de l'extirpation*, 15; Louis Bourlet, *Étude sur la métrite interne chronique après la ménopause*. Thèse (Paris: A. Parent, 1879).

benign (meaning non-lethal), as the clinical medicine of this time defined slow-growing uterine and ovarian tumours, cysts, and polyps. This choice drew on the justification provided by Péan of older women's uteri and ovaries as now 'useless' and a potential liability for future hypothetical rare lethal diseases. Numerous doctors had described fibroids (which were frequently diagnosed by palpation), as not particularly dangerous, and only sometimes even symptomatic, noting that they were widely reported in autopsies of women who had died of tuberculosis and other unrelated diseases, without ever having caused suspicion of their presence—something Péan himself acknowledged.[56] He also acknowledged a widely agreed medical fact about fibroids (both then and now) that they were rarely found in women older than 55, and had often been observed to atrophy and even disappear completely after the final cessation of menses.[57] Selecting such patients for abdominal hysterectomy made little sense if they were close to menopause as predicted by their age; it might be expected that gynaecologists would advise such women simply to wait it out, rather than risk a 60 per cent likelihood of dying in surgery for the treatment of a benign growth, something Péan himself acknowledged to be a sensible conclusion.[58] Indeed he cited one such case of a woman who had already ceased menstruating, whom he persuaded not to have surgery and whose fibroid disappeared some time afterwards.[59] And yet in all his other case observations of hysterectomy for fibroid treatment in women in their forties, he did not mention any such conversations, appearing instead rather enthusiastic to offer them a surgical solution: hysterectomy.

Péan described conversations in which he recommended abdominal surgery to women in their forties with likely benign tumours who had not previously considered it, as well as conversations with women who came to the hospital with the preformed intention to have some sort of surgery to remove their tumour.[60] Did he inform these women of the danger that awaited them in submitting to such a surgery and of how experimental it still was? Péan, choosing his words carefully here, said of one such patient, 'I concealed from her neither the difficulties nor the dangers', and that he only proceeded with the surgery after obtaining her *husband's* consent.[61] But it is not clear what, if anything, Péan told the patient herself about the specific surgery he planned to give her, either its permanent sterilising

[56] Péan & Léopold, *Hystérotomie*, 47; Marie Anne Victoire Boivin & A. Dugès, *Traité pratique des maladies de l'utérus et de ses annexes, accompagné d'un atlas de 41 planches in-fol. gravées et coloriées, représentant les principales altérations morbides des organes génitaux de la femme*, 2 vols (Paris: J. B. Baillière, 1833), vol. 1, 327; Kœberlé, *Documents pour servir à l'histoire de l'extirpation*, 4–6.

[57] Péan & Urdy, *Hystérotomie*, 33–35; Kœberlé, *Documents pour servir à l'histoire de l'extirpation*, 4–6; Abeille, *Des corps fibreux de l'utérus*, 4; Charles Henry F. Routh, *On Some Points Connected with the Pathology, Diagnosis and Treatment of Fibrous Tumours of the Womb: Lettsomian Lectures on Midwifery and Diseases of Women* (London: T. Richards, 1864), 38; Mara Ulin et al., 'Uterine Fibroids in Menopause and Perimenopause', *Menopause*, 27/2 (2020): 238–242.

[58] Péan & Léopold, *Hystérotomie*, 36. [59] Ibid., 36. [60] Ibid., 53, 179.

[61] Ibid., 53–54.

effect or its extreme danger. Some patients clearly understood that surgeons could remove their unsightly and uncomfortable tumours, but there is no indication that they were aware that their uteri and ovaries would also be removed, or that they were advised that their tumour was most likely not going to kill them, whereas they were more likely to die from the procedure than to recover from it. Such clear communication would perhaps be surprising for nineteenth-century surgeons, given the low esteem in which so many doctors held women's intelligence, which they viewed as naturally inferior to men's and similar to that of a child; and given that the concept of informed consent was not clearly part of French doctors' ethical training, having cohered in biomedicine only in the second half of the twentieth century (though antecedents have been found throughout medical history).[62] Certainly, Péan appeared to have a sense that he owed women some amount of information before risking their lives to reduce their symptoms, while advancing surgical knowledge and his own career.

On the other hand, according to Péan's and others' own explicit ethical frame, selecting older women with benign conditions for this surgery clearly contradicted the stated criteria of only practising dangerous abdominal hysterectomy in patients whose lives were already threatened by their existing gynaecological pathologies. Péan's solution to that problem was to exaggerate the risks and symptoms of uterine fibroids—against the grain of a widespread medical consensus which affirmed their benignity—and to speak of them together with malignant tumours in relation to his proposed therapeutic surgical solution. He said that any kind of tumour could cause debilitating enough symptoms to justify the dangerous experimental use of abdominal hysterectomy.[63] Because fibroids sometimes produced appetite suppression, constipation, or diarrhoea, they therefore potentially could be, eventually, a cause of death, implying that the surgery was necessary to save women from starvation.[64] He said that although most uterine tumours and ovarian cysts were not cancerous, representing an 'inconvenience rather than a disease', they could also cause haemorrhages so severe as to threaten women's lives, and pain so intense as to prevent women from sleeping, and compression of the digestive organs so extreme as to result in malnutrition.[65] He claimed that most of his case examples were of this kind, and he saw it as a 'cruel alternative' from which he had to choose in either letting the women 'suffer and succumb' to their benign tumours/cysts, or risk the operation which he assumed to be as dangerous as the existing reports suggested (around 60%

[62] Alexander Morgan Capron, 'Where Did Informed Consent for Research Come From?' *The Journal of Law, Medicine & Ethics*, 46/1 (2018): 12–29; P. Dalla-Vorgia et al., 'Is Consent in Medicine a Concept Only of Modern Times?', *Journal of Medical Ethics*, 27/1 (2001): 59–61. Doi:10.1136/jme.27.1.59.

[63] Péan & Léopold, *Hystérotomie*, 228. [64] Ibid., 40. [65] Ibid., 47.

mortality).[66] However, the case observations he provided in this very publication tell a somewhat different story of patient presentation.

Undoubtedly some of his patients had indeed grappled with painful and heavy bleeding for many years, such that they may possibly have chosen a life-threatening treatment that offered some hope of a cure, though it does not appear that Péan ever explained to them exactly how high this risk of death from surgery was. Mme Cornau, aged 42 (Observation IV) who survived her oophorectomy surgery, had complained of haemorrhages that made it difficult for her to 'practice her occupation as a concierge'; she was clearly anaemic, and Péan said that she had begged him to operate on her (without explicit mention of what the surgery would be).[67] Nonetheless, after her surgery, Péan said she still suffered similar symptoms every menstrual period, albeit with less blood loss.[68] Mlle Virginie Gauthier, aged 45 (Observation VII) was also fortunate to be one who survived the abdominal hysterectomy with oophorectomy that Péan gave her in 1870 as a cure for her apparently asymptomatic uterine fibroid which had slowly grown to a considerable size. Péan described her appearance as 'debilitated', with a hunched posture and rickets, and said that she had a weak pulse, but he referred to no gynaecological symptoms, pain, or digestive symptoms associated with her benign tumour.[69] Mlle Thérèse Lefèvre, aged 41 (Observation VI), had developed metritis along with the slow growth of an abdominal mass, but suffered no gastrointestinal symptoms or bloating, no weight loss or decline in strength, only a certain breathlessness when climbing stairs, and her complexion was described as 'yellow'. She too survived her hysterectomy with oophorectomy surgery.[70] Mme Baldé, aged 38 (Observation IX), was less fortunate, having suffered painful periods that had become heavier in recent years, with a rapidly growing tumour; she died shortly after her surgery, in a fever.[71] Péan also described a patient of Demarquay reported in the *Union médicale* of 1868, Mlle M., aged 43 (Observation XVIII), whose large, slow-growing uterine tumour (initially thought to be an ovarian cyst) had been accompanied by just one symptom—heavy painful periods, with mildly painful haemorrhages at other times. She too died in a fever the night after her surgery.[72] Notably, often the removed ovaries were observed to be entirely healthy.[73] Péan said this was done because, if the uterus was already being removed, the ovaries 'are no longer of any use', their presence being merely a cause of 'periodic congestion', and it was easier to cut it all out at once rather than detach the uterus from its appendages.[74]

Later Péan found a new idea for defending his practice of using the most dangerous surgical procedure known to medicine in the treatment of benign growths

[66] Ibid., 48. [67] Ibid., 66–73. [68] Ibid., 72. [69] Ibid., 135–142.
[70] Ibid., 124–135. [71] Ibid., 153–156. [72] Ibid., 178–183. [73] Ibid., 58, 73.
[74] Ibid., 217.

in women in their forties. In an 1893 article in the *Annales de gynécologie et d'obstétrique* entitled 'On the supposed benignity of uterine fibroids', he argued against the grain of most medical scholarship about these tumours, which considered them most commonly to atrophy after menopause.[75] He pointed to his own surgical record as proof that this could not be true, since of his 250 patients given hysterectomies for fibroid, 100 were in their forties, 70 in their thirties, 30 in their twenties, and 10 between the ages of 50 and 70.[76] His data actually conformed very well to the majority view that fibroids were a tumour of the fertile years and much less troubling to women after the cessation of menses; but he appears to have thought that their apparent prevalence among his patients of women in their forties presenting with symptomatic or large fibroids meant that the tumours must have something to do with menopause. It was a legacy of the past century of medical ideas about menopause as a critical age, which, despite referring to the final cessation of menses, actually focused far more on the hygienic management of women well before it. 'Menopause is thus in fact a critical age and not a beneficial age, as certain surgeons have pretended in order to disguise their impotence instead of admitting it,' Péan said, evoking the masculine prowess of the surgeon who was not afraid to penetrate with his scalpel.[77] Léon Daudet's memoir cited earlier said that Péan's displays of surgical prowess were much admired by silly women (*les femmes sottes*) who saw in 'crazed butchery…a spectacle of strength'.[78] As Bertrand Gibert has shown, surgeons performing hysterectomies and oophorectomies were widely satirised and characterised both by novelists and by the popular presses of the *fin de siècle*, which often implied that it was the desire of decadent women to acquire permanent contraception that provided the clientele for such clinicians.[79] But surgeons' own patient observations give no indication of this.

Péan also related his account of the danger fibroids posed to ongoing psychiatric theories of menopausal madness, here suggesting that it was these common uterine tumours which in fact caused the nervous complications associated with the genital influences on women's minds, resulting in hysteria, hypochondria, suicide attempts, sleepwalking, and precocious senility, as well as morphine addiction and alcoholism.[80] But he did not elaborate on this, perhaps aware that in French psychiatry of the 1890s hysteria was viewed as a nervous disease and was mostly no longer ascribed to the influence of the uterus. He seems rather to have grasped at every possible justification as to why women with non-lethal conditions should be exposed to such high risks of death in surgery. After twenty

[75] Jules Péan, 'De la prétendue bénignité des fibromes utérins', *Annales de gynécologie et d'obstétrique*, 39/1 (1893): 460–466.

[76] Ibid., 461. [77] Ibid., 462. [78] Daudet, *Devant la douleur*, 67.

[79] Bertrand Gibert, 'Des avatars littéraires: Le Cas du Docteur Pozzi', *Poétique* 2/190 (2021): 171–202.

[80] Péan, 'De la prétendue bénignité des fibromes utérins', 463.

years of practising abdominal hysterectomies, Péan's mortality rate in 1893 still sat at 15 per cent (30 deaths out of 200 surgeries), though he claimed (as in his 1873 work) that it was better in his most recent series.[81] Perhaps just another lucky streak? In 1895 he explained his turn away from abdominal hysterectomy to the vaginal entry form which was less lethal, exaggerating the risks of fibroids even more, claiming that it was necessary to remove even small tumours of this kind with hysterectomy to rescue 'these poor miserable sick women whose life is constantly menaced and poisoned by all sorts of ills' from succumbing to death before their tumours had grown large.[82]

Relative to surgical norms of his day, Péan was clearly viewed as something of a reckless cowboy. In 1872, as he and Urdy were preparing their 1873 manuscript on hysterectomy for publication, the Paris Académie de Médecine formally condemned the practice, following an oral report on the surgeries of Péan and Kœberlé presented to them by the eminent senior surgeon Jean Nicolas Demarquay (1814–1875).[83] Hysterectomy and oophorectomy remained vehemently opposed by many physicians and surgeons, who often pointed to the many lethal failures of both vaginal hysterectomy and especially abdominal laparotomy relative to the non-lethal gynaecological conditions they mostly pertained to treat,[84] as well as posing moral objections to the sterilising effect of the surgeries, particularly when used on women young enough to conceive. This was also probably why Péan focused so much on women in their forties, whom he viewed as already approaching menopause—after all, who would object to these women being made sterile? Even Péan's contemporaries who were themselves enthusiasts of rapid gynaecological surgical advancement were nonetheless critical of his experiments with hysterectomy, which they viewed as showing an excess of surgical aggression.[85] Major gynaecologists, such as Auguste Nonat in his 1,100-page *Practical Treatise of the Diseases of the Uterus, its Appendages, and the External Genital Organs* (1874), reiterated the common medical consensus that fibroids were primarily a tumour of the reproductive lifespan, diminishing or even disappearing after menopause.[86]

The young Paris graduate Samuel Pozzi in 1875 had accused Péan of exaggerating the danger of haemorrhagic bleeding caused by fibroids to justify his experimental hysterectomy technique on women with benign conditions, even as he credited

[81] Ibid., 465.

[82] Jules Péan, 'Les Fibromes utérins', *Annales de gynécologie et d'obstétrique*, 44/1 (1895): 345–350.

[83] Auguste Nonat, *Traité pratique des maladies de l'utérus, de ses annexes, et des organes génitaux externes* (Paris: Adrien Delahaye, 1874), 1021; M. Tillaux, 'Communications: De l'hystérectomie au traitement des tumeurs fibreuses utérines', *Bulletin de l'Académie de Médecine*, 8 (1879), 1035–1048.

[84] Alphonse-Alexandre Boinet, *De la gastrotomie dans les cas de tumeurs fibreuses utérines interstitielles, péri-utérines et dans les tumeurs dites fibro-cystiques* (Paris: G. Masson, 1873).

[85] L. Prévost Coyteux, 'On Hysterectomy', *American Gynaecological and Obstetrical Journal* (1897): 1–16.

[86] Nonat, *Traité pratique des maladies de l'utérus*, 613, 845.

Péan with being the most accomplished French surgeon to date with the technique of abdominal hysterectomy.[87] He expressed horror too at the rashness of Kœberlé's extirpations of the ovaries and uterus, with their attendant 75 per cent mortality.[88] Pozzi was one who kept in mind the proportional danger of a surgery relative to the danger of the disease it was supposed to treat, which led him to reserve high-risk surgeries (as were both hysterectomy and myomectomy) only for the specific cases that required it, preferring the surgically less dangerous oophorectomy as a treatment for most symptomatic fibroids.[89] The rationale for that choice was clear: it put women in 'artificial menopause', which resulted in the atrophy of their fibroids and a reduction of haemorrhagic bleeding.[90] But Pozzi was also one of the few surgeons in France who practised the often technically more complex myomectomy favoured by several German gynaecologists, and he provided detailed instructions with precise drawings in his 1890 *Treatise of Gynaecology*, showing how to perform this fertility-conserving surgery which he reserved for young women with benign fibroids.[91] 'It would be useless to undertake a laborious enucleation, instead of an efficient hysterectomy, if a woman were close to menopause or had already passed it', he affirmed.[92] So while older women should not be used as experimental guinea pigs for a dangerous surgery they did not necessarily require (as in Péan's approach), it was legitimate to hysterectomise them if they sought any kind of surgical removal of their fibroids, since myomectomy was a similarly risky procedure. Pozzi also corrected Péan's false nationalist historical attribution of the first deliberate hysterectomy to Kœberlé in 1863, arguing that it was in fact to several English surgeons twenty years earlier that the honour belonged.[93] This kind of corrective recognition of international surgical innovations remained an important feature of Pozzi's interventions into the historical description of gynaecology's recent intercultural emergence, a perspective which he took pains to impress upon medical students at the University of Paris.[94]

Péan clearly had many eminent opponents, which was reflected in his long struggle to acquire the official recognition of the Académie de Médecine (finally accorded in 1887) and to obtain a university post (he never did). It seems likely that his cavalier approach to dangerous and unnecessary surgeries was the primary reason. Even in the 1890s, the renowned Paris-trained southern gynaecologist

[87] Samuel Pozzi, *De la valeur de l'hystérotomie dans le traitement des tumeurs fibreuses de l'utérus*. Thèse (Paris: G. Masson, 1875), 15, 40.

[88] Ibid., 38–39.

[89] Paul Robert Charrier, *Revue critique du Traité de Gynécologie du Docteur Pozzi* (Paris: Asselin & Houzeau, 1890), 7.

[90] Samuel Pozzi & Félix Jayle, *Traité de gynécologie clinique et opératoire* [1890], 4th ed., 2 vols (Paris: Masson et Cie, 1905–1907), vol. 1, 313, 325, 379.

[91] Ibid., 385, 389–424. [92] Ibid., 424. [93] Ibid., 425.

[94] Samuel Pozzi, *Progrès et évolution de la gynécologie contemporaine, extrait de la leçon d'ouverture d'un cours libre de gynécologie fait à la Faculté de médecine de Paris* (Paris: P. Dupont, 1887); Pozzi & Jayle, *Traité de gynécologie*, vol. 1, 424–435.

Jacques Amédée Doléris, who had founded the *Archives d'obstétrique et de gynécologie*, later becoming a Radical Party deputy for the Basses-Pyrénées and who was an expert on both uterine fibroids and on medical education for gynaecologists, opposed the generalisation of hysterectomy to patients with benign conditions. In an 1892 article partly entitled 'Too many useless mutilations', Doléris complained that surgeons were removing healthy reproductive organs from women's bodies, often without a clear diagnosis of their pathology.[95] The popularity of organ removal surgeries for benign conditions such as fibroids reflected an entirely non-therapeutic motive, Doléris said. It was purely for surgeons to gain experience in the technique of hysterectomy and oophorectomy, since surgery was, after all, a trade (*un métier*) in which 'skill is only acquired with practice'. He remarked of their choice of patients that 'subjects are needed to lend themselves to these surgical exercises, and lacking legitimate indications, one is obliged to content oneself with what one finds'. The surgeons who did this found 'no lack of justifications' for doing so, he said.[96] Notably though, Doléris seemed more concerned about women young enough to reproduce being subjected to these surgeries, rather than women around menopause, remarking that 'it is certainly not the moment for doctors to aid depopulation in any way by resorting in all instances to castration'.[97]

From the late 1880s to the 1920s, the chorus of objections to hysterectomy for fibroid treatment became substantial indeed. Numerous French, German, American, and English gynaecologists condemned the new rash enthusiasm for the removal of women's ageing reproductive organs, developing alternative surgical or non-surgical treatments for common conditions, such as fibroids and dysmenorrhea, that were now already being widely treated with hysterectomy or oophorectomy.[98] Some of the new women gynaecologists were among them—Isabelle Gaboriau, whom we met in the Chapter 8, wrote her 1919 Paris thesis on uterine haemorrhages in menopause transition, arguing that these were not even generally pathological or in need of surgery.[99] The surgeon Alfred Boiffin had noted in his 1893 book about fibroids that there had been 'a new evolution of minds' in international gynaecology in relation to them which 'manifested in the

[95] Jacques Amédée Doléris, 'Trop de mutilations inutiles…pas assez de gynécologie conservatrice', *Nouvelles Archives d'obstétrique et de gynécologie*, 6 (1892):378–384.

[96] Ibid., 383. [97] Ibid., 381.

[98] Georges Apostoli, *Sur une nouvelle application de l'électricité après les accouchements: communication faite à l'Académie de médecine de Paris* (Paris: H. Lauwereyns, 1881); Georges Apostoli, *Sur un nouveau traitement de la métrite chronique et en particulier de l'endométrie par la galvano-caustique chimique intra-utérine* (Paris: O. Doin, 1887); Franklin H. Martin, *Lectures on the Treatment of Fibroid Tumours of the Uterus: Medical, Electrical and Surgical* (Chicago: W. T. Keener, 1897); Paul Morély, *Essai sur l'ouverture des collections annexielles par la voie vaginale* (Paris: G. Steinheil, 1899); Marcel Molk, *Kritik der vaginalen und abdominalen totalen Hysterektomie in Fällen von Fybromyomen.* Dissertation (Strasbourg: J. Singer, 1901); Marius Bonier, *De la myomectomie abdominale dans le traitement des fibromes utérins* (Lyon: Imprimerie Schneider, 1904).

[99] Isabelle Gaboriau, *Contribution à l'étude des métrorragies dites essentielles de la ménopause.* Thèse (Paris: Jouve, 1919).

very marked tendency to directly attack the tumour and to demand a radical cure as treatment', eschewing palliative care via 'castration' (hysterectomy, oophorectomy, or both) in favour of the specific removal of the offending growth while preserving reproductive function where possible.[100] By the 1890s such surgeries were now somewhat less dangerous—thanks largely to the aseptic turn in European surgery, and despite his reservations, Boiffin noted that some surgeons still considered hysterectomy to be 'a veritable method of choice' for many gynaecological pathologies, particularly for women close to menopause for whom the sterilisation effect was less consequential.[101] But other gynaecologists were considerably more resistant to the practice. Roland Pichevin was one who criticised the 'abuses of castration' in Paris medicine in an 1890 book published by the reputable press Steinheil. He claimed that many of the conditions that oophorectomy and hysterectomy were designed to treat, such as inflammation of the fallopian tubes and ovarian cysts, actually healed themselves over time, and that surgeons' insistence that gynaecological disorders had already rendered such women sterile were completely false—he cited a case of one of his own patients who had been prescribed such a surgery and who had refused it, becoming pregnant afterwards.[102] A major 1900 French gynaecology by the physiologist Albert Robin (1847–1928) and the gynaecologist Paul Dalché (1858–*c.*1930), which was published in multiple editions up to 1922 and used in medical pedagogy at the Paris Faculty throughout this time, sniped repeatedly throughout its 500 pages about the overuse of hysterectomy to treat benign conditions. The authors deemed such surgeries worthless in all but a few cases on the grounds that three-quarters of gynaecological diseases were 'fausses utérines'—disturbances of menstrual function actually deriving from systemic physiological disorders, such as diabetes, undernutrition, digestive disorders, or infectious diseases. They did not actually originate from the uterus, the authors explained, and therefore could not be cured by its removal.[103] The hysterectomy/oophorectomy naysayers and all the many developers of novel myomectomy, cauterisation, electrical, intra-uterine device and chemical therapies were, in a sense, the first wave of the 'minimally invasive' surgery movement which has grown again in Europe, Asia, and North America since the 1990s.[104] Its first iteration represented an important constraining influence on the rapidly expanding international field of ambitious gynaecological surgeons focused on hysterectomy and oophorectomy. Here, France still had

[100] Alfred Boiffin, *Tumeurs fibreuses de l'utérus* (Paris: Rueff et cie., 1893), 146–148.

[101] Ibid., 146.

[102] Roland Pichevin, *Les Abus de la castration chez la femme* (Paris: G. Steinheil, 1890), 43.

[103] Paul Dalché & Albert Robin, *Gynécologie médicale: Traitement des maladies des femmes* (Paris: J. Rueff, 1900), 23, 104, 124, 468, 471.

[104] Sally Frampton & Roger L. Kneebone, 'John Wickham's New Surgery: "Minimally Invasive Therapy", Innovation, and Approaches to Medical Practice in Twentieth-Century Britain', *Social History of Medicine*, 30/3 (2017): 544–566. Doi:10.1093/shm/hkw074; Botros Rizk et al., eds, *Advances in Minimally Invasive Gynecologic Reproductive Surgery* (Boca Raton, Fla/London: CRC Press, 2021).

one last major role to play, in wedding endocrine ovarian treatments to the iatrogenesis of surgical menopause.

The Internationalism and Caution of Samuel Pozzi

The Paris gynaecologist Samuel Pozzi (Image 10.3), who treated the famous French actress Sarah Bernhardt (1844–1923) for her massive benign ovarian cyst in 1898 (he was initially her lover in the 1860s and remained her lifelong friend), was another leading figure in controversial French experiments with hysterectomy and oophorectomy in the 1880s and 1890s. He was known for implementing the new antiseptic surgery procedures of the English surgeon Joseph Lister (whom he visited), with resulting dramatic improvements in patient survival. Pozzi was clinical professor of gynaecology at the University of Paris, a member of the Académie de Médecine, and in 1898 an elected senator of the Dordogne, of which

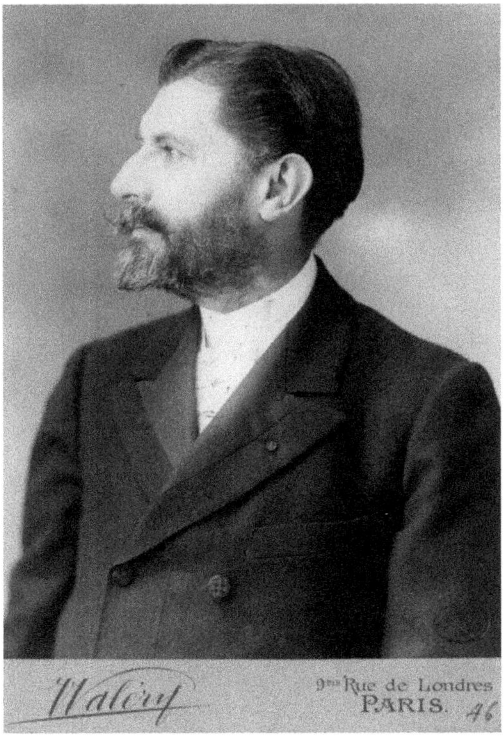

Image 10.3 Walery (Stanisław Julian Ignacy Ostroróg), photograph of Samuel Pozzi, *c.*1900. Image ref.: CIPH0046. Courtesy of the Bibliothèque Nationale de France.

he was a native (Bergerac). Like Sarah Bernhardt, he was an ardent Dreyfusard.[105] He was a prolific scholar, and authored with his intern Félix Jayle the 1890 two-volume textbook of gynaecological surgery that was reprinted in four French editions up to 1907, translated into English (1892 and 1899), German (1892), Italian (1895), Russian (1897), Polish (1907), and widely used in both French and international medical pedagogy until around 1930.[106] He, more than any other French surgeon, was responsible for the massive leap in the development of abdominal surgery technique using aseptic protocols, which increased patient survival in laparotomy and other major gynaecological procedures by 300 per cent (Image 10.4). In a tragic irony, he himself died from abdominal injury when a mentally ill ex-patient shot him multiple times in his Paris clinical rooms in 1918. His assistant and co-author Félix Jayle was one of the surgeons who tried to save his life in the emergency operation in which the multiple intestinal perforations of the bullets were masterfully repaired, but Pozzi nonetheless died due to massive internal haemorrhaging.[107]

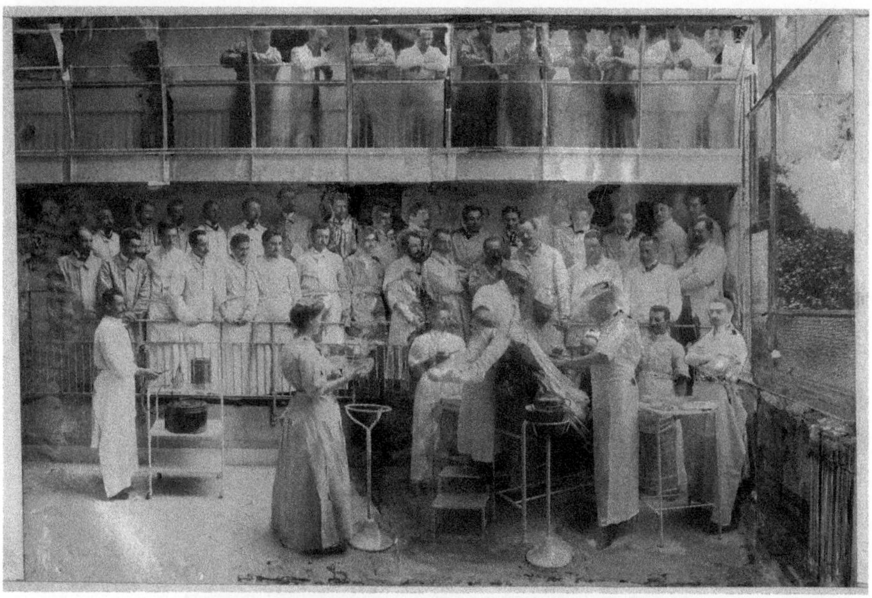

Image 10.4 Samuel Pozzi photographed performing laparotomy surgery in teaching theatre, *c.*1890s. Image ref.: CIPD0004. Courtesy of the Bibliothèque Interuniversitaire de Santé.

[105] Claude Vanderpooten, *Samuel Pozzi, chirurgien et ami des femmes* (Paris: Éditions In Fine, 1992); De Costa & Miller, *The Diva and Doctor God*, 106.

[106] Samuel Pozzi & Félix Jayle, *Traité de gynécologie clinique et opératoire* [1890], 4th ed., 2 vols (Paris: Masson et Cie, 1905–1907).

[107] De Costa & Miller, *The Diva and Doctor God*, 244–247.

Pozzi was certainly not alone in the surgical revolution that he led. He travelled globally throughout his successful career as a general surgeon, specialist gynaecologist, and medical professor at the Paris faculty, visiting the most accomplished centres of surgical excellence in England, the USA, and South America to exchange knowledge of novel procedures and emerging science.[108] Without the enormous improvements in surgical practices that occurred during this period, the ensuing story of the surgical-endocrine nexus treatment for older women would never have unfolded. These were the early beginnings of the global development of new twentieth-century ways of medicalising menopause with hysterectomy and hormone replacement therapy, which French doctors, like Pozzi and his students, initiated, though they were not to remain for long at its helm.

Pozzi's entrance into Paris medicine in the 1870s formed part of a significant shift towards more rigorous medical ethics in women's health, more sophisticated surgical technique, and more international collaboration and knowledge exchange in relation to global gynaecology. He completed two theses as qualifications for his surgical career, the first for his *licence* in 1873 on the infectious fistulas that formed in some patients after abdominal surgeries, and the second for his Paris faculty professorial *agrégation* in 1875 on the value of hysterectomy in the treatment of uterine fibroids.[109] Pozzi, unlike Péan, was deeply afraid of the often-deadly surgery that was late nineteenth-century laparotomic hysterectomy, and he found Péan's and others' claims to surgical triumph to be utterly appalling when the general mortality rate for even the much less dangerous oophorectomy still sat at 34 per cent.[110] Fibroid tumours alone were not a sufficient cause for conducting hysterectomy, he said, while admitting that some of his own and others' attempts to remove just the tumour sometimes became hysterectomies due to surgical complications.[111] He said that fibroids often grew in a triphasic pattern, beginning as asymptomatic in their initial phase of genesis, becoming potentially symptomatic in the second phase, followed by a diminution of volume and symptomatology in the phase after menopause. But at the end of the second phase, he said, there was often a 'last ascending oscillation in the development of the tumour', in the years approaching menopause.[112] He cited a case example of this, a patient of Paul Broca's treated at the Pitié hospital around 1850: a woman, aged 50 at the time, who had several large fibroids that had undergone a growth surge around the approach of her final menstruation. Some time later these tumours spontaneously diminished, and she never suffered any symptoms, either when they were large or after they shrank. She had been followed up and was now

[108] Ibid., 98–99, 105.

[109] Samuel Pozzi, *Étude sur les fistules de l'espace pelvi-rectal supérieur, ou fistules pelvi-rectales supérieures*. Thèse (Paris: G. Masson, 1873); Samuel Pozzi, *De la valeur de l'hystérotomie dans le traitement des tumeurs fibreuses de l'utérus*. Thèse (Paris: G. Masson, 1875).

[110] Pozzi, *De la valeur de l'hystérotomie*, 40–43.

[111] Ibid., 29, 49.

[112] Ibid., 19.

(in 1875) 75 years old, active, healthy, living independently, and still doing her own housework.[113] Pozzi certainly always treated some fibroids with hysterectomy, particularly in older women, if he deemed them too risky to remove selectively due to greater blood loss, or the longer surgical time required—both factors that increased the risk of death. But over his career he appears to have increasingly favoured alternative treatments - both myomectomy and oophorectomy, or even partial ovarian ablation, wherever possible.[114] Haemorrhagic bleeding, though alarming, he said, was never lethal, and should not be taken as justification for risking women's lives in hysterectomy, which he said was a common error of other surgeons, particularly Péan.[115] Fibroids could affect intestinal and bladder function too, Pozzi acknowledged, but he did not consider this cause for surgery either, unless there was very serious bowel obstruction which put women at risk of peritonitis.[116]

Pozzi and Jayle also affirmed the ages from 40 to 50 years as the peak time of susceptibility to uterine cancer, which they observed to be the most common form of cancer in women, followed by breast cancer, drawing on the English statistics of J. Y. Simpson from 1847 to 1861.[117] They followed the English gynaecologists David Berry Hart and Alexander Hugh Freeland Barbour in the view that women were more than twice as prone to cancer as men up to the age of 50, on account of the 'sexual organs' being particularly susceptible to it during the reproductive years, based on Simpson's data which recorded 87,348 fatal carcinomas of which 61,715 were among women, accounting for 2.2 per cent of all female deaths.[118] As Ornella Moscucci notes, this gendered belief about cancer, which had been argued by the Irish physician Walter Hayle Walshe in 1846, persisted in medicine from the mid-nineteenth century until the 1920s, when new Swiss and Norwegian statistical data indicated that cancer prevalence was actually similar both in men and women, while in the 1930s prostate cancer prevalence in men was found in Britain to be 365 per cent higher than had previously been realised.[119] Nonetheless, public health campaigns both in England and France continued to focus on women's cancers far more than men's up until the 1950s, including the recommendation of prophylactic hysterectomy and oophorectomy, based on the old conceptual layer of medical ideas about women's greater morbidity (despite their longer life expectancy) due to the supposedly morbid nature of their reproductive organs.[120]

[113] Ibid., 19.

[114] Samuel Pozzi, *Relevé statistique des opérations pratiquées dans le service de gynécologie de l'hôpital Broca* (Paris: Masson, 1899), 11–23.

[115] Pozzi, *De la valeur de l'hystérotomie*, 14.

[116] Ibid., 14.

[117] Pozzi & Jayle, *Traité de gynécologie*, vol. 1, 515.

[118] Ibid., 515–516; Berry Hart & Freeland Barbour, *Manual of Gynecology*, 436.

[119] Walter Hayle Walshe, *The Nature and Treatment of Cancer* (London: Taylor & Walton, 1846), 152–153; Moscucci, *The Science of Woman*, 8–9, 36–37; see also Ilana Löwy, *Preventive Strikes: Women, Precancer, and Prophylactic Surgery* (Baltimore: Johns Hopkins University Press, 2010), 10–13.

[120] Moscucci, *The Science of Woman*, 2–3.

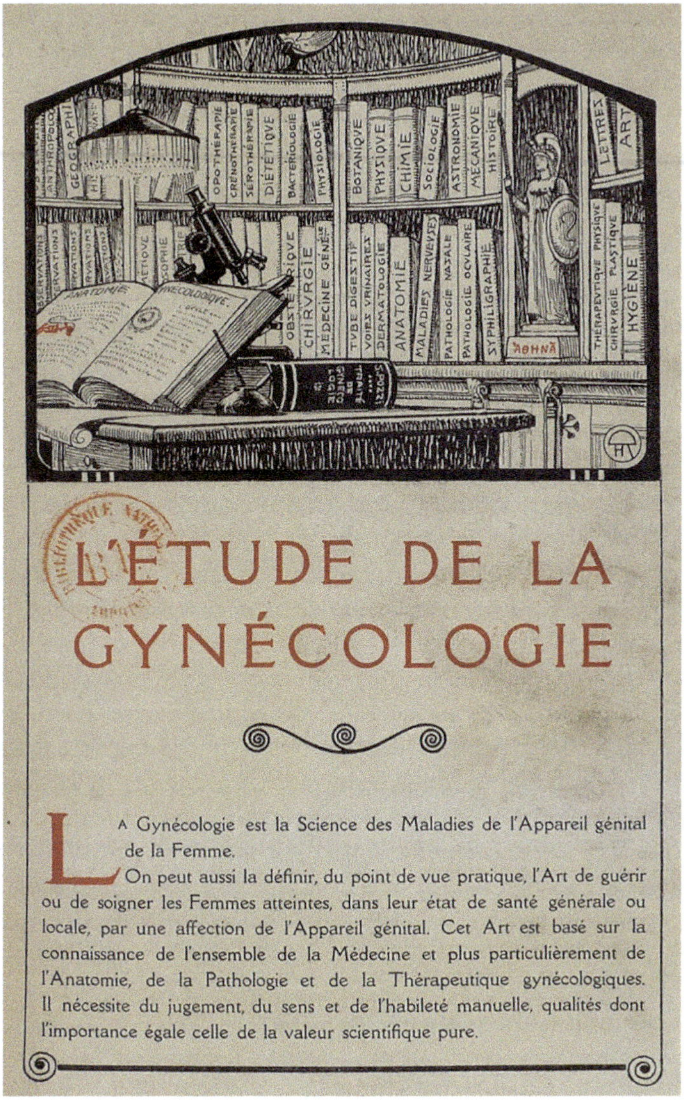
L'ÉTUDE DE LA GYNÉCOLOGIE

La Gynécologie est la Science des Maladies de l'Appareil génital de la Femme.

On peut aussi la définir, du point de vue pratique, l'Art de guérir ou de soigner les Femmes atteintes, dans leur état de santé générale ou locale, par une affection de l'Appareil génital. Cet Art est basé sur la connaissance de l'ensemble de la Médecine et plus particulièrement de l'Anatomie, de la Pathologie et de la Thérapeutique gynécologiques. Il nécessite du jugement, du sens et de l'habileté manuelle, qualités dont l'importance égale celle de la valeur scientifique pure.

Image 10.5 Félix Jayle Frontispiece of textbook, *Gynécologie*, 1918. Courtesy of the Bibliothèque Nationale de France.

In Pozzi's 1899 statistical account of all the operations he had performed and overseen in the women's diseases wing of the Broca hospital between 1890 and 1899, it is clear that he was favouring surgeries of the ovary (either unilateral or bilateral oophorectomy, or partial resection of the ovary) over extirpation of the uterus in the treatment of uterine fibroids, ovarian cysts, and inflammations of the fallopian tubes. He was able to show 100 per cent survival of his patients using these methods, followed up for one year after surgery. He also documented recurrences in patients whose ovaries had been extirpated due to malignant tumours—clearly indicating the need for adjunct therapies in the case of these dangerous cancers that almost always killed women.[121] Nonetheless, the cancer-focused prophylactic removal of healthy women's sexual organs, described in the excellent studies of both Moscucci and Löwy, does not appear to have been the only driver of hysterectomy and oophorectomy in women approaching menopause in France between 1890 and 1920.[122] As we have seen, however, these organs' propensity to develop cancer with ageing was indirectly evoked by surgeons as part of their complex web of justifications for extirpating the organs of women in their forties rather than simply removing the benign tumours that grew on them, as some, like Pozzi, were prepared to do for younger women.

In his early work, Pozzi considered myomectomy with conservation of the uterus and ovaries to be the best treatment for uterine fibroids, but worried about the practice of morcellating them, which caused much greater blood loss, though he noted the advantage of the technique for reducing incision size, which was another important factor in patient survival at this time.[123] Conserving the uterus was something worth considering, he said: 'one can always hope... that the patient will escape the incidents that menace her and will be able to attain menopause'. The conservative approach, he noted, would invariably leave some women to die in their forties or fifties from the rare cancerous forms of these common tumours, but this would still be a much smaller number than those dying from hysterectomy, given the 64 per cent mortality risk he identified for it in the 1870s.[124] There was rarely any long-term follow-up of those patients who had survived the procedure either, he noted.[125] On the other hand, if a tumour had rapidly grown in a woman who was already past menopause, causing haemorrhages long after the final cessation of the menses, he considered hysterectomy with oophorectomy to be absolutely 'authorised', given that such a presentation very likely indicated an aggressive malignant cancer.[126]

Pozzi, even early in his career, pointed to the high number of deaths from post-surgical fever indicative of 'septicaemia' as the figure most likely to be easily improvable through the application of aseptic methods, for which he later became a major advocate, transforming Paris surgical practices dramatically.[127] In his 1899 *Relevé statistique* he displayed his own and other surgeons' successes and failures over time transparently and in great detail. He thereby showed the difference in patient survival made by the massive upgrading of surgical equipment,

[121] Pozzi, *Relevé statistique*, 6.

[122] It did become a more common practice, however, towards the end of the 1920s, e.g. Jean-Eugène Proust, *Influence de la ménopause sur le cancer du sein et castration ovarienne thérapeutique par les rayons X*. Thèse (Bordeaux: Impr. de l'Académie et des Facultés, 1929).

[123] Pozzi, *De la valeur de l'hystérotomie*, 30. [124] Ibid., 49. [125] Ibid., 21.

[126] Ibid., 50. [127] Ibid., 44–46.

accommodation, and procedure that he led at the Broca hospital in the last decade of the nineteenth century, with much improved outcomes in the patient datasets from the final three years of the century.[128] But Pozzi is primarily of interest to us here because he helped to train some of the most important figures in French medical research on the effects of hysterectomy, oophorectomy, and the use of ovarian opotherapy in both surgical and in natural menopause: Félix Jayle, Paul Charrier, Maurice Lissac, and others. He was thus a crucial vector for the entanglement of surgical and endocrinological technologies around the treatment of menopause and of older women, which heralded the end of French dominance over the topic by sparking a whole new era of global pharmaceutical commercial interest in women's ageing. Notably too, Pozzi's concern about the excessive mortality entailed in hysterectomy when used for benign tumours (except for the most technically simple ones) meant that he often turned instead to the less risky oophorectomy, which had always entailed roughly half the mortality of hysterectomy, and which he was able to perfect to a reliably survivable standard (100%) in the treatment of benign conditions by the end of his time at the Broca hospital.[129]

This surgery, too, even though it preserved the uterus, mimicked many of the effects of menopause, which was precisely Pozzi and Jayle's rationale for performing it, since fibroids were known to shrink after natural menopause:

> Clinical medicine has long understood that the cessation of the sexual life of woman quite often brings a remarkable sedation of the incidents caused by fibroid bodies . . . Hence came the idea to hasten the appearance of this favourable period by provoking an *artificial menopause* through ablation of the ovaries.[130]

Notably, the idea of treating fibroids with surgical 'castration' (oophorectomy) to produce a 'premature menopause' was precisely the thesis topic of the Bordeaux doctoral candidate Jean-Albert Pascal in 1887.[131] Pozzi and Jayle did not perhaps invent the idea, but they certainly helped to disseminate it widely, contributing to the iatrogenic creation of a new population of women placed surgically in menopause. They were also the first group of clinicians to observe and document the symptoms suffered by many of the women thus treated, but not before their approach of inducing artificial menopause was followed by countless other surgeons.[132] To their credit, these two gynaecologists accurately recognised that this

[128] Pozzi, *Relevé statistique*, 3. [129] Ibid., 21–23.

[130] Pozzi & Jayle, *Traité de gynécologie*, vol. 1, 379, emphasis in original.

[131] Jean-Albert Pascal, *La Ménopause prématurée par la castration ovarienne: Contribution à l'étude du traitement des fibromes utérins*. Thèse (Bordeaux: Veuve Cadoret, 1887).

[132] Sébastien Le Moniet, *Hystérectomie abdominale totale et hystérectomie abdomino-vaginale pour fibromes de l'utérus* (Paris: G. Steinheil, 1894); Edgar Garceau, *Vaginal Hysterectomy as Done in France*

was a matter requiring its own research investigation—a task which Félix Jayle initiated at the Broca hospital, as we consider in the final section of this chapter.[133]

In 1897, a Paris doctoral thesis written by Émile Canu (who said he had previously been a primary school teacher in the Saint-Denis quarter of Paris for ten years before studying medicine) heavily criticised the widespread use in France of oophorectomy and hysterectomy on nationalist pro-natal grounds, claiming that the nation's negative population growth of the late nineteenth century was a direct consequence of the fad for castration surgeries in gynaecology since the 1870s; but he also emphasised the widespread practices of lack of patient information or consent in such surgeries.[134] Much of the thesis was a series of case observations based on a survey that Canu had posted (along with a stamped, self-addressed envelope) to women who had received such surgeries in the Paris hospital system between 1892 and1896. It appears he had access to their addresses via a Dr Bec (no doubt Édouard Le Bec (1851–1941)) who performed the surgeries, as well as through several individuals who assisted him in the Office of General Statistics at the Ministry of Commerce.[135] But he also said that he had used his neighbourhood contacts as a schoolteacher to speak personally with women who had had such surgeries.[136] The survey, like all checklist questionnaires, suffered from being highly suggestive to the patients of symptoms they could expect to have as a result of their surgery, and so should not be straightforwardly taken as indicative of patient experience. Canu was primarily concerned about women of childbearing age being deprived of their conceptive capacities, rather than about women close to menopause, although he also published the responses he received from older women. Clearly he was a fan of the non-surgical, electrical treatment for fibroids that was in vogue at this time as an alternative to hysterectomy/oophorectomy, pioneered by the Paris gynaecologist Georges Apostoli (1847–1900).[137]

But several things are noteworthy about the cases of the women who responded to Canu's inquiries, both in answering the checklist questions but also, in some cases, providing credible narrative accounts of their treatment. Many of the forty-two women whose cases Canu described said that they had not been told what the surgery was that they would be given until after they had received it,[138] several

(New York: William Wood & Co, 1895); Constantin Angelesco, *Hystérectomie abdominale totale pour tumeurs fibreuses de l'utérus* (Paris: Georges Carré, 1897).

[133] Félix Jayle, *Opothérapie ovarienne dans la ménopause artificielle post-opératoire et la ménopause naturelle* (Paris: Masson, 1898).

[134] Étienne Canu, *Résultats thérapeutiques de la castration chez la femme: Conséquences sociales et abus de cette opération* (Paris: Ollier-Henry, 1897), 126–133.

[135] Ibid., 7. [136] Ibid., 14.

[137] Ibid., 121, 153; Apostoli, *Sur un nouveau traitement de la métrite chronique*; Dr Delétang, *Du traitement des fibromes utérins par la méthode d'Apostoli* (Paris: O. Doin, 1889).

[138] Canu, *Résultats thérapeutiques de la castration chez la femme*, 28 (Observation 6), 33 (Observation 8), 35 (Observation 9), 39 (Observation 10), 41 (Observation 12), 45 (Observation 14), 48 (Observation 15), 52 (Observation 17), 65 (Observation 23), 76 (Observation 29), 83 (Observation 33), 94 (Observation 39).

said that only their husband's consent had been obtained but not theirs,[139] while a substantial number said they had indeed been told.[140] Canu clearly wanted to portray the surgeons as reckless and irresponsible, but the claim that they were often not informing their patients that their reproductive organs would be removed, with both a sterilising effect and with potential consequences for their subsequent health, is consistent with the obfuscation of patient consent found in the writing of gynaecological surgeons themselves, particularly Péan. However, many of the cases referred to surgeries received at the Broca hospital during the 1890s, when Samuel Pozzi oversaw the gynaecology wing there and when Félix Jayle was working there too. One woman, 'C', aged 30, who had not been told that her surgery would sterilise her, said that she was delighted when she found out, since she did not want to have any more children (Observation 5).[141] But others were not so lucky. One of those, 'G', a woman of 51 years (Observation 20), who was not told what her surgery would be, also expressed reluctance to blame her surgeon, not wishing to bring disrepute to him, despite suffering severe new symptoms since her hysterectomy with oophorectomy and regretting having had the surgery.[142] Another woman, 'Mme. R', aged 40, who named the surgeon who had hysterectomised her in 1892 as a Dr Terrillon at the Salpêtrière hospital, said she was told that she would die unless she had 'the operation' but was not informed of what the operation would consist, even after asking. She said that she had become completely debilitated since the surgery, suffering a wide variety of symptoms: sleeping only three hours a night, memory loss, irascibility, prematurely reaching 'old age'; she had become so 'useless' that she and her husband had been forced to abandon their family business.[143] 'Madame R', aged 52 (Observation 27), who was ovariectomised by a renowned surgeon at the Broca hospital (whom Canu indicated simply as 'X'), said that she was not told what her surgery was until afterwards when she asked what the word 'ovariotomie' meant, after seeing it written on her patient card.[144] Another woman aged 52 from Fribourg in Switzerland, 'Mme. X', was diagnosed with a fibroid in 1892, though she had no symptoms relating to it. She was told she needed a surgery to remove it but was not informed what surgery she would be given; she guessed that they had removed her uterus. Before the surgery her only symptom was heavy menstruation and some mild hot flushes, but three days after the surgery she suffered a 'congestion of the brain', and had since experienced daily headaches, palpitations, and a massive loss of strength and memory function, 'conjugal relations are impossible', and her 'general state [was] worse than before'. She said that she had paid 3,500 francs for the operation (equivalent to just over one kilogram of gold, and more than many

[139] Ibid., 17 (Observation 1), 18 (Observation 2), 25 (Observation 5).
[140] Ibid., 40 (Observation 11), 50 (Observation 16), 55 (Observation 18), 70 (Observation 26), 77 (Observation 30).
[141] Ibid., 25. [142] Ibid., 58. [143] Ibid., 69–70. [144] Ibid., 74.

doctors earned in a month), and afterwards also required 600 francs per month for ongoing medical treatments that she did not need before the surgery.[145] Her operation took place in the rue de Ranelagh, in the 16th arrondissement, a rich area.

The French medical controversy around the practice of hysterectomising and ovariectomising menopausal women did not end here. In the first decade of the twentieth century, doctoral theses now picked up the debate about the effect of menopause on uterine fibroids and the necessity or abuse of hysterectomy and oophorectomy. The first, by the Montpellier candidate Adolphe Charreire in 1907, provided a balanced account of the opposing arguments, concluding that 'since they can decrease in size on the approach of age 50, myomas are not per se an indication for [surgical] intervention'.[146] But he also considered the new histological analyses of tumour tissues which appeared to show that both the rare cancerous form of fibroid and the common benign form shared more similar cellular features than had previously been identified microscopically.[147] Much of his thesis focused on the question of whether an existing benign tumour could transform into a sarcoma as a result of menopause, which Charreire admitted was possible in a small number of cases. While it was clear that menopause brought atrophy of fibroids, it could also rarely, in some cases, see alteration of the tumour into a malignant form characterised by a sudden increase in its rate of growth.[148] He noted a wide variability in surgeons' reports about the ubiquity of such cancerous fibroids,[149] which no doubt reflected the speculative nature of much diagnosis, and the important divide between ethical and careful surgeons versus those who overemphasised the dangerousness of fibroids generally in order to justify their removal with high-risk hysterectomy in all women in their forties. Charreire declared himself opposed to such recklessness: 'the womb, though not an indispensable organ, should be conserved as long as possible, in the absence, of course, of any harmful changes, even in women who have 'passed the age of making it operate'.[150] He discussed several of the alternative treatments for fibroids and the symptoms that they caused, such as curettage of the uterus, ligature of the uterine arteries, electrical treatments, and the use of oophorectomy, the less dangerous surgery favoured both by the German gynaecologist Alfred Hegar and by Samuel Pozzi.[151] But notably he made no mention of the other alternative surgery

[145] Ibid., 171–173; Rodney Edvinsson, *Historical Currency Converter* (test version 1.0). Historicalstatistics.org: <https://www.historicalstatistics.org/Currencyconverter.html|> (viewed 30 November 2021). Highly successful doctors' salaries in mid-nineteenth-century France ranged from 4,000 to 7,000 francs per month, but were more often as low as 2,000 francs. See Matthew Ramsey, *Professional and Popular Medicine in France, 1779–1830* (Cambridge: Cambridge University Press, 1988), 113.

[146] Adolphe Charreire, *Myomes et ménopause, atrophie, dégénérescences malignes, indications*. Thèse (Montpellier: G. Firmin, Montane & Sicardi, 1907), 45.

[147] Ibid., 18. [148] Ibid., 12–15. [149] Ibid., 19–26. [150] Ibid., 47–48.

[151] Ibid., 46–47.

available in this time, myomectomy (removal of just the tumour and no organs), which remained so rare as to be very often ignored in French gynaecological works (apart from Pozzi's).

The Lyon surgical candidate Émile Guillaume, on the other hand, was one who took sides with the Péan current of surgical hubris, restating the importance of hysterectomy in the treatment of benign conditions such as fibroids, despite the many deaths this continued to cause, and denigrating the lower-risk use of oophorectomy or partial ovarian ablation, such as Pozzi practised, to cure women of their menstrual disorders by inducing surgical menopause.[152] Guillaume's thesis centred on hysterectomy for any woman over the age of 40 presenting with a uterine fibroid (*myome utérin*), extending Péan's argument that these tumours' benignity had been much exaggerated. His thesis too was specifically about the relationship between menopause and fibroid growths: he strongly challenged the common medical understanding that such tumours stopped growing and even tended to shrink, along with the atrophy of the uterus itself, after the final cessation of menses. He said that on the contrary, fibroids were a disease of menopause itself, and occurred in 40 per cent of women by the age of 50 years.[153] While menopause often brought relief from the haemorrhagic bleeding that fibroids sometimes caused, many women assumed they were cured thereafter, whereas their tumours had merely entered a new phase, continuing 'to evolve insidiously' to reappear 'at a more advanced age' as malignant cancers.[154] Guillaume argued that fibroids of all kinds in fact had the potential to become malignant, and that it was 'false to affirm that [they] always regress around menopause'.[155] It was a peculiar kind of malignancy, he suggested, which did not metastasise and instead remained local. He would not go so far as the Brussels surgeon Jacobs, who in 1906 had claimed that fibroids *always* became malignant in menopause, but he insisted nonetheless that menopause indeed had a dangerous impact on their evolution, and that deadly forms were more common than most gynaecologists realised.[156]

Hysterectomy was the treatment of choice to cure fibroids, which Guillaume claimed was now 'accepted everywhere'.[157] He was particularly keen on what he called 'the American procedure' of 'subtotal hysterectomy' practised by the Lyon surgeon Henri-Alphonse Albertin (1860–1939), referring to removal of both the uterus and ovaries via abdominal laparotomy, severing the uterus above the

[152] Émile Guillaume, *Le Myome utérin à la ménopause* (Lyon: J. Prudhomme, 1910), 14.

[153] Ibid., 9.

[154] Ibid., 34. The topic also of another Paris thesis around this same time: François Frédéric Cocheret, *De la valeur des métrorragies après la ménopause comme signe de cancer de l'utérus et comme indication de l'hystérectomie totale abdominale*. Thèse (Paris: H. Jouve, 1909).

[155] Guillaume, *Le Myome utérin à la ménopause*, 17–18.

[156] Ibid., 21; C. Jacobs, 'Fibrome utérin: Quelques observations cliniques tirées de 633 opérations abdominales', *Bulletin de la Société Belge de Gynécologie et Obstétrique*, 8 (1905–1906): 73–79.

[157] Guillaume, *Le Myome utérin à la ménopause*, 12.

cervix (while the term 'total hysterectomy' referred to incision below and including the cervix, which was most often done via a vaginal route).[158] Vaginal hysterectomy was less common, though highly regarded by gynaecologists, he said, with those still performing it doing so as an expression of their 'personality'.[159] Common pharmacological remedies prescribed for fibroids such as potassium iodide, calcium chloride, cannabis tincture, hydrastis, and ergot were all useless.[160] And while electrical treatments could bring temporary relief of pain and haemorrhages, they could not cure fibroids, and sometimes even made then gangrenous. The proponents of such treatments, he said, had campaigned on the idea that they offered an alternative to the drastic cure of surgery, chanting 'No more oophorectomies', but their results did not live up to their promise.[161] He said the alternative surgery of myomectomy (removal of just the fibroid, leaving all the organs in place) had been definitively discredited. Its principal advantage was that it preserved fertility, he said, but most women did not conceive after the surgery anyway, and many simply grew new fibroids in the place of those that had been removed. The operation was also more prone to complications.[162] He said that women often came asking for a myomectomy but were instead given hysterectomy, citing a case of this happening to a patient treated by Alphonse Albertin when he was practising in Paris—again confirming Canu's account that the question of women's consent for such surgeries was often ignored.[163]

While Guillaume acknowledged that many of the most symptomatic cases of fibroids were found in patients who had suffered from them since early in their thirties, nonetheless he said that 'at the approach of menopause, the genital organs of woman are the seat of an intense congestion', resulting in exacerbation of any existing gynaecological pathologies.[164] The main symptoms he described were heavy menstruation with intermittent haemorrhages resulting in anaemia, as well as intestinal and bladder problems caused by pressure from the growing tumour. Most of the women who sought surgery, he said, were those suffering virtually constant haemorrhaging. He acknowledged that haemorrhagic bleeding had never actually killed anyone, but insisted that it could do so potentially because the low blood volume it created in women might cause venous thrombosis and cardiac problems in menopause. He claimed that Albertin had followed 'several' women who 'had obstinately refused the intervention' (hysterectomy) and they all succumbed to fatal venous or cardiac diseases around the time of menopause.[165] Any uterine pathology could cause heart troubles, he said, via sympathy of the uterus with the hypogastric plexus, pointing to Pozzi's observations of palpitations as a frequent symptom of gynaecological lesions.[166] By way of example he cited the case of a 40-year-old woman described by the Paris surgeon Violet at a meeting of the Société des Sciences Médicales in 1905. She was diagnosed with a

[158] Ibid., 12. [159] Ibid., 40. [160] Ibid., 36. [161] Ibid., 37. [162] Ibid., 39.
[163] Ibid., 41. [164] Ibid., 22. [165] Ibid., 24–25. [166] Ibid., 31.

painful fibroid which caused her belly to swell and led to more frequent urination, but these symptoms 'in the eyes of the patient were not very worrisome'. Then the fibroid grew and when a surgeon examined her heart, he found it beating 'frantically' ('affolé')—rapidly and irregularly, with intermittent palpitations. After calming down, he explained, she 'resigned herself' to the surgery that she had previously refused. 'This observation shows us evidently just how far one can push surgical audacity,' Guillaume said, though it was regrettable that so many sufferers waited so long for menopause to cure their fibroids instead of entrusting themselves to a surgeon.[167]

While Guillaume acknowledged that the average age of the final cessation of menses in French women in this time was generally agreed to be 48 (ranging from 46 to 52), he appears to have forgotten this throughout his study, referring also in his thesis to 'the age of menopause (40–50 years)'.[168] His slippage from the average age based on the range of 46–52 years to a whole decade beginning six years younger than this had important implications for the kinds of gynaecological conditions that could now be ascribed to 'menopause', helping to justify the expansion of hysterectomy in a context where it remained a controversial procedure. Guillaume even said that none of his own patients in the age range of 40–50 years had yet reached menopause (in the sense of having ceased menstruating), nor indeed had several aged between 50 and 55 years; nonetheless, his argument about the close relationship between 'menopause' and fibroids focused on the group aged 40–50, who he said were the most afflicted.[169] This was only made to make sense by construing the moment of menopause as lasting an entire decade or more, defined by the very gynaecological symptoms that were being blamed on it, rather than by the final cessation of menses itself. Medical scholarship on fibroid tumours of the uterus had flourished in multiple European scientific contexts in the last decades of the nineteenth century. They were widely understood to be a kind of benign growth that closely followed women's reproductive lifespan, never appearing before the age of 20, frequently emerging during pregnancy, and rarely seen after the age of 50.[170] So if surgeons wanted to make the case that fibroids were a disease of menopause that required surgical treatment with hysterectomy—justifying the sterilisation effect as of no consequence to women

[167] Ibid., 32. [168] Ibid., 73. [169] Ibid., 33.

[170] Léon Brachet, *Myôme utérin délogé par le travail de l'accouchement et opéré avec succès* (Paris: J. B. Baillière et fils, 1870); William Netzel, *Opération césarienne rendue nécessaire par un myome incarcéré dans le petit bassin*, trans. H. Cazin (Paris: V. A. Delahaye, 1876); Adrien Phelippeaux, *Histoire clinique d'un fibrome utérin du poids de 150 grammes, opération et guérison: Considérations sur quelques faits de gynécologie. Discussion. Commentaires* (Paris: V. Adrien Delahaye, 1878); H. Chassigny, *Régression de myome utérin* (Lyon: Association typographique, 1883); Joseph Fabricius, *Über Myome und Fibrome des Uterus und deren Einfluss auf die Umgebung* (Vienna/Leipzig: W. Braumüller, 1895); Franklin H. Martin, *Lectures on the Treatment of Fibroid Tumours*; C. J. Bond, 'On the Results of 50 Cases of Abdominal Hysterectomy for Fibroid Disease of the Uterus: With Remarks on the After-History of the Patients and on the Artificial Menopause', *The Lancet*, 161/4142 (1903): 162–167.

in their forties, since they were no longer fertile anyway—then some serious revision of the definition of menopause was needed. Even older women might have been made a target in this way too, except that it was harder to find patients suffering symptomatic fibroids who were older than their early fifties, and the surgical survival rate declined in a linear fashion with age. No doubt some women in their forties, particularly those with severe symptoms, were keen to have their tumours surgically removed once knowledge of this possibility became known. But given that most French surgeons only offered hysterectomy with oophorectomy as a surgical solution, elaborate justification was required for the view of the uterus and ovaries as inherently pathological in women in their forties, underpinning the practice of their wholesale removal.

Péan too in 1893 had criticised the 'supposed benignity of uterine fibroids' and the 'illusory role of menopause' in shrinking them, and Guillaume leaned heavily on his account, pointing to his surgical statistics of 100 hysterectomies conducted on women in their forties, compared to 70 such surgeries done on women in their thirties, 30 on women in their twenties, and only 10 on women over the age of 60.[171] Guillaume discussed Péan's data alongside datasets from several other surgeons which also privileged women in their forties for hysterectomy. Notably, the one decade missing from most of their statistics was the group aged 50–60 years which—assuming a cessation of menses at an average age of 48—would be the relevant group for observing whether or not fibroid atrophy had occurred following the end of menstruation. Only one dataset, that of the British surgeon Francis William Nicol Haultain (1861–1921), included a group aged specifically between 50 and 60 years—eight cases, compared to the 80 Haultain had treated who were in their forties, and only one of the eight women in their fifties had even in fact ceased menstruating.[172] In fact, out of all of the many hundreds of hysterectomies performed by the four surgeons Guillaume cited, only this one patient had actually reached her final menstruation.[173] These numbers were hardly compelling as evidence of the role of the final cessation of menses in causing or exacerbating fibroids, but Guillaume seemed to think they were. Perhaps he justified this both by assuming that fibroid shrinkage, were it real, should occur abruptly sometime in the ten or so years *before* the final cessation of menses, and also by defining 'menopause' in this remarkably vague way with reference to an entire decade or more. In fact, the most obvious connection between menopause and fibroids appearing at this moment in medical history was that women with these tumours were now vulnerable to being put into surgical menopause as a result of their treatments—a far more abrupt and symptomatic transition to post-fertile life than any woman ageing without surgery. Guillaume finished his thesis with the

[171] Guillaume, *Le Myome utérin à la ménopause*, 50.
[172] Ibid., 51. [173] Ibid., 51.

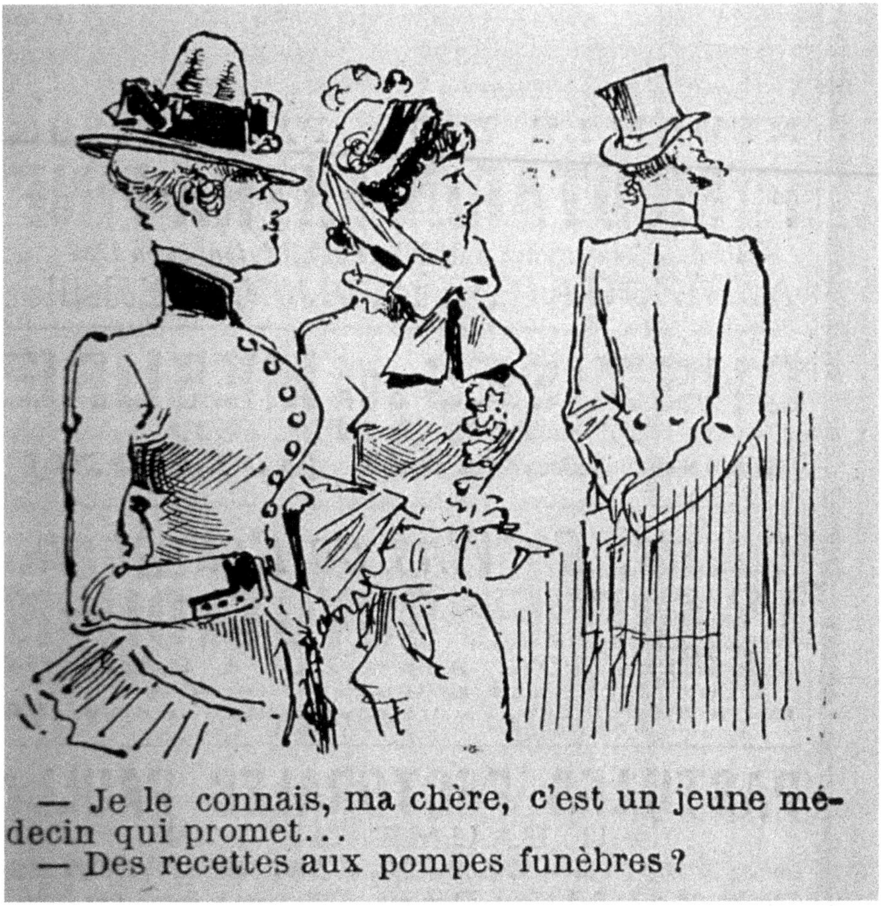
— Je le connais, ma chère, c'est un jeune médecin qui promet...
— Des recettes aux pompes funèbres ?

Image 10.6 Renard, two women commenting on a young ambitious doctor, *c.*1890. The dialogue reads with one women beginning, 'I know him, darling. He is a young doctor who promises...', and the other interrupts, '... revenues to funeral directors?'. Courtesy of the Bibliothèque Nationale de France.

suggestion that it might even be better to remove all of women's reproductive organs *before* their forties, at the first signs of even small fibroids,[174] thus increasing the number of women who could be surgically targeted and expanding the population of post-menopausal women to include an even larger number of those placed surgically into a similar state. It was a remarkable new definition indeed of the medicalisation of menopause.

By the 1890s, there were many gynaecologists treating older women with benign conditions such as fibroids and ovarian cysts using hysterectomy with

[174] Ibid., 74.

oophorectomy, in the view that these organs were by now useless in any case and that there was little point in removing only the tumour, which was a more technical operation to be reserved for young women only. One such doctor was Émile Baudron, who had been an intern in the Paris hospital system under the surgeon Paul Segond (1851–1912). Baudron described two cases of women, one with large uterine fibroids and another with ovarian cysts, both with bleeding and pain, who had recently ceased menstruating and whom he treated using Péan's method of vaginal hysterectomy with double oophorectomy, most likely prescribing this as the only available treatment. He described their recovery from these recent surgeries as 'marvellous', but admitted that had not seen them since and so could not know anything of their long-term well-being.[175] But he said the vaginal and abdominal hysterectomy were both so much less dangerous than before that surgeons like Paul Segond, Samule Pozzi, Ulysse Trélat, Auguste Nélaton, and Paul Reclus were all commonly prescribing them for a wide variety of gynaecological disorders in older women 'now that the technique is well established'.[176] The question of the long-term after-effects of radical gynaecological surgeries was yet to change the course of medical mechanistic concepts of menopause.

Ovarian Opotherapy in the Treatment of Surgical and Natural Menopause

Félix Léon Jayle, Samuel Pozzi's intern, was a Paris gynaecological researcher who made his debut in the 1890s, documenting the physiological effects of the 'castration' of women—the marked iatrogenic symptoms his and Pozzi's patients reported following the surgical removal of their uterus and ovaries, or the ovaries alone.[177] The surgical gynaecologist Baudron included some discussion in his 1894 work on vaginal hysterectomy of his case observations from the long-term follow-up of patients whose uteri and ovaries had been removed one to three years earlier; many mentioned weight gain, hot flushes, nervousness, and other symptoms—which Baudron minimised in his account of their cases as successfully curing their gynaecological disorders.[178] Jayle, it seems, with Pozzi's encouragement, sought to account more seriously for the after-effects of these surgeries, and to experiment with pharmacological remedies to counteract them. Jayle had defended his specialist thesis on peritoneal septicaemia at the Paris faculty in

[175] Émile Baudron, *De l'hystérectomie vaginale appliquée au traitement des annexes de l'utérus (Opération de Péan): Étude basée sur les 200 premières observations du Docteur Paul Segond* (Paris: Société d'Éditions Scientifiques, 1894), 177, 369.

[176] Ibid., 13.

[177] Félix Léon Jayle, *Opothérapie ovarienne dans la ménopause artificielle post-opératoire et la ménopause naturelle* (Paris: Masson, 1898).

[178] Baudron, *Hystérectomie vaginale appliquée au traitement des annexes de l'utérus*, 88–99.

1895, though he had been working already as hospital intern for several years before this and had already co-authored a book on breast cancer in 1894 with the Paris medical professor Charles Monod.[179] He worked at the Broca hospital in Paris from at least 1894, and he was the editor of the *Revue de gynécologie et de chirurgie abdominale* (Review of Gynaecology and Abdominal Surgery) from 1896. His specialist work after graduation focused on a pharmacological therapy intended to counteract the side effects of the 'castration' of women (oophorectomy) using the new ovarian opotherapy products derived from sheep organs, such as the product sold by the German Merck chemical company, called Ovariin (or Ovarine in France), which was available in Germany by 1895.[180] Jayle first began publishing his clinical findings on this topic in 1896 just as another Paris doctoral candidate supervised by Louis Landouzy (1845–1917) was writing on exactly the same theme—Maurice Lissac (1870–*c.*1940).[181] It was Landouzy who had created the word 'opothérapie' to refer to all of the many glandular animal tissues which were now being used as medicaments.[182]

These scholars writing about ovarian replacement for surgical and natural menopause were no longer a French exception, as medical specialists of menopause up to this time had mostly been. Several German, Austrian, and Swiss gynaecologists were also simultaneously experimenting with similar ovarian pharmacy products for surgical menopause patients in the new opotherapy craze that had emerged at this time for a wide range of diseases, using a wide variety of animal organs and glands as medicaments, particularly following the success of animal thyroid extracts in the treatment of deficiencies of that gland in humans.[183] The use of gonadal extract was, however, an idea that French medical scholars had recently revived, following the self-injections of the French-American physiologist Charles-Édouard Brown-Séquard (1817–1894) of guinea pig testicle extract in 1889, which immediately inspired the French doctor Gaston Variot (1855–1930) to experiment with testes extracts as rejuvenation medications in a

[179] Félix Léon Jayle, *Septicémie péritonéale aiguë post-opératoire*. Thèse (Paris: Carré, 1895); Charles Monod & Félix Jayle, *Cancer du sein* (Paris: Rueff & Cie, 1894).

[180] Jayle, *Opothérapie ovarienne dans la ménopause*; Richard Mond, 'Kurze Mittheilungen über die Behandlung der Beschwerden bei natürlicher oder durch operation veranlasster Amenorrhee mit Eierstocksconserven (Ovariin Merck)', *Münchener medizinische Wochenschrift*, 14 (1896): 314–316.

[181] Félix Léon Jayle, 'Résultats éloignés de la castration chez la femme', *Bulletin de l'Académie de Médecine* (1896): 196–197; Félix Léon Jayle, 'Opothérapie ovarienne contre les troubles consécutifs à la castration chez la femme', *Presse médicale* (1896): 221–222; Maurice Lissac, *Traitement des troubles consécutifs à la castration chez la femme: Opothérapie ovarienne*. Thèse (Paris: Georges Carré, 1896).

[182] Louis Landouzy, *Les Sérothérapies: Leçons de thérapeutique et matière médicale* (Paris: Georges Carré et C. Naud, 1898), 12. See Marchand, *Opothérapie*, 365, 532.

[183] Mond, 'Kurze Mittheilungen über die Behandlung'; F. Mainzer, 'Vorschlag zur Behandlung der Ausfallserscheinungen nach Castration', *Deutsche medizinische Wochenschrift*, 22/12 (1896): 188; Rudolph Chrobak, 'Über Einverleibung von Eierstockgewebe', *Centralblatt für Gynäkologie*, 20 (1896): 521–524; Maurice Muret, *De l'organothérapie par l'ovaire? Communication faite à la reunion de la Société vaudoise de médecine à Lavey le 18 juin 1896* (Lausanne: Georg, 1896); W. Latzko & J. Schnitzler, 'Ein Beitrag zur Organotherapie bei Osteomalacie', *Deutsche medizinische Wochenschrift*, 23/37 (1897): 587–592.

group of elderly men.[184] But in the same series of discussions of this controversial and well-known experiment, Brown-Séquard had also mentioned the possibility of a similar experiment using ovarian extracts in women, proposing that the same rejuvenation effect of testicular juice injected into elderly men could be expected of ovarian juice injected into elderly women, though animal experiments would be required before this could be tested on human subjects.[185] In his 1898 Bordeaux thesis published as a book on ovarian opotherapy, Louis Bestion de Camboulas claimed that Brown-Séquard had in fact proceeded with human experiments of ovarian juice the same year as he experimented with the testes extract in men, injecting forty-six elderly women with it in 1889, though notably Brown-Séquard does not appear to have published on any such experiment.[186] A Marseille doctor certainly did though, publishing a short pamphlet on his experiment of ovarian injections in three elderly women in 1889. The results were underwhelming, since he was not targeting the specific population most starkly deprived of their own ovarian secretions: women whose ovaries had been surgically removed in midlife.[187] The first doctor to do so was probably the Lausanne gynaecologist Maurice Muret, who began experimenting with ovarian extracts from around 1893, only publishing his findings in 1896, his patients being young women with amenorrhea, ovariectomised young women, and women in natural menopause; he indicated that the extracts were effective in reducing symptoms in both of the latter two groups, and in resuming the menses of the amenorrhea patients.[188] By 1897 the practice was unfolding in at least seven different major European clinics, including Jayle's and Pozzi's.

Lissac had worked closely with Jayle, who had encouraged him to undertake the thesis topic. Most of the case observations discussed in this thesis were Jayle's patients, while several were patients of the Kiel surgeon Richard Mond, and several were Émile Baudron's.[189] Lissac said that all surgeons involved in the use of

[184] Charles-Édouard Brown-Séquard, 'Note on the Effects Produced on Man by Subcutaneous Injections of Liquid Obtained from the Testicles of Animals', *The Lancet*, 2 (1889): 105–107; Gaston Variot, 'Trois expériences sur l'action physiologique du suc testiculaire injecté sous la peau, suivant la méthode de M. Brown-Séquard', *Comptes rendus des séances de la Société de Biologie et de ses filiales*, 41 (1889): 451–454; Charles-Édouard Brown-Séquard, 'Remarques à l'occasion du travail de M. Variot, sur les injections de liquide testiculaire chez l'homme', *Comptes rendus des séances de la Société de Biologie et de ses filiales*, 41 (1889): 454–455.

[185] Charles-Édouard Brown-Séquard, 'Seconde note sur les effets produits chez l'homme par des injections sous-cutanées d'un liquide retiré des testicules frais de cobaye et de chien', *Comptes rendus des séances de la Société de Biologie et de ses filiales*, 41 (1889): 420–422.

[186] Louis-Alexandre-Philippe Bestion de Camboulas, *Le Suc ovarien, effets physiologiques et thérapeutiques: Organothérapie ovarienne* (Paris: J. B. Baillière et fils, 1898), 14.

[187] Louis André Félix Villeneuve, *Quelques faits pour servir à l'histoire des injections sous-cutanées de suc de tissu testiculaire et ovarien par la méthode Brown-Séquard: Observations recueillies par MM. Vaudey et Lachaud* (Marseille: Barlatier & Barthelet, 1889).

[188] Muret, *De l'organothérapie par l'ovaire.*

[189] Lissac, *Traitement des troubles consécutifs à la castration*, 6; 53–56; 58–59.

castration surgeries in women had been singularly focused on the question of mortality from the surgery itself, ignoring the other important matter of how the patients fared after recovering from the surgery. The reason for this, he said, was that the women themselves were so fixated on getting rid of the most terrible symptoms for which they sought a life-threatening surgical solution that they 'neglected to speak with their surgeon' about all the other minor symptoms from which they had suffered and which they expected the surgery to cure, only reporting these after the surgery.[190] He said that his thesis would withhold all judgement about the cause of the many problems he would describe or their relation to the surgeries the women had received, reminding the reader that both age and individual constitution could account for some of the reported symptoms of women following surgical 'castration'.[191] The operations that caused 'castration' were a 'wonderful surgical achievement...which are of great service in many cases', and he did not wish to imply that there was any reason not to use them.[192] Nonetheless, he affirmed the view that 'one must never think of ablation of the ovaries without ensuring that it is manifestly not possible to undertake a more conservative surgery', adding that 'this sage precept has sometimes been forgotten' both in France and in Germany.[193]

Lissac claimed there was much disagreement about the matter of side effects of oophorectomy among surgeons, with some, such as Alben Martin, finding all his castrated patients reporting post-surgical symptoms such as hot flushes, dyspepsia, psychological problems, changes in character, memory loss, and hypochondria, while others such as Baudron claimed that only a small minority of patients had such problems (around 12%, in Baudron's case).[194] Lissac acknowledged too that French gynaecologists were not alone in investigating the treatment of side effects of oophorectomy with ovarian opotherapy. But he said that Richard Mond's data from the University of Kiel was of limited value, since the German surgeons were in the practice of performing only partial ablations of the ovary and administering Ovarine several years after the surgery.[195] French psychiatry had also not entertained the view espoused by the American surgeon William Goldwell that all mad women should be ovariectomised, Lissac said, pointing to Charcot's rejection of this practice and the widespread observation that hysterectomy and oophorectomy in fact exacerbated mental illness.[196]

Lissac's thesis focused on a description of the function of the ovaries, noting the recent recognition that these were the organs that regulated menstruation, and were a kind of 'lymphatic gland' which secreted a special, though unknown,

[190] Ibid., 7. [191] Ibid., 8. [192] Ibid., 15.
[193] Ibid., 15–16. [194] Ibid., 8.
[195] Ibid., 17. See Mond, 'Kurze Mittheilungen über die Behandlung'.
[196] Lissac, *Traitement des troubles consécutifs à la castration chez la femme*, 16.

'chemical product' that had systemic effects in women's bodies.[197] This product clearly also regulated women's 'femininity', since many surgeons had noticed their castrated patients developing gravelly voices, hairs on their chins, and exaggerated skeletal growth.[198] These were the same changes that occurred in women after menopause, he said, indicating that the ovaries, whether absent or deficient, produced a substance that made women feminine and protected them from various symptoms.[199] This was the birth of the definition of menopause as a state of hormone deficiency based on the comparison with women who had been hysterectomised and ovariectomised. Lissac admitted (remarkably!) that he and a male friend had once eaten minced ovary, and said that the following night the friend experienced a most uncharacteristic terrible nightmare, while Lissac's own sleep was disturbed all night by a 'nervous irritation'; from which Lissac speculated that ovarian secretions may be a nervous toxin to men.[200] He also gave a detailed description of the main symptoms following oophorectomy, classing headaches, insomnia, and facial paralysis, as well as changes of character, melancholy, and suicidal thoughts among the signs of 'neurasthenia', and considering the memory problems reported by many women to be a sign of madness.[201] He classed digestive problems, constipation, facial acne, and obesity as 'Nutritional Disturbances', and said that sexual effects were highly varied, with many women reporting no change, around half reporting a complete abolition of all desire, and a small number reporting intensified desire.[202] He claimed that many of these symptoms fell under the category of 'plethora' and were often treated with blood-letting or leeches.[203] Old conceptual layers, it seems, take a long time to die.

Félix Jayle, on the other hand, had taken his inspiration in 1895 for the treatment of surgically induced menopause from the recent successful uses shown for thyroid opotherapy: his idea was to 'supplement' the absent secretions of the missing ovary with an opotherapy ovarian replacement.[204] In addition to accounting for all the various experiments of 1896 being conducted in other countries with ovarian opotherapy, Jayle undertook his own series of studies between 1895 and 1898 under the supervision of Samuel Pozzi at the Broca hospital. This entailed following the treated patients for several months or even years after their oophorectomies, which he said was designed to avoid the most common errors made in medicine in the treatment of uterine-ovarian diseases, where long-term follow-up was generally entirely absent.[205] He documented in great detail the symptoms reported by the hysterectomy and oophorectomy patients at the hospital, it seems, using an open-ended interview method in which he asked them if they had noticed anything new following their surgery, rather than simply giving

[197] Ibid., 19–20. [198] Ibid., 21–22. [199] Ibid., 22. [200] Ibid., 29.
[201] Ibid., 11–13. [202] Ibid., 14–15. [203] Ibid., 24–25.
[204] Reported by Lissac, ibid., 25–26.
[205] Ibid., 244; Félix Léon Jayle, 'Effets physiologiques de la castration chez la femme', *Revue de gynécologie et de chirurgie abdominale*, 3, May–June (1897): 403–436.

them a pre-written checklist survey, as became the standard in menopause research thereafter (with its attendant problems of suggestion).[206] The results of his and others' research were quite clear, Jayle said. The ovarian extracts had few side effects reported by patients who were treated with them and were particularly effective in the reduction of the vaso-motor symptoms caused by surgical castration in pre-menopausal women—hot flushes.[207] 'Nervous phenomena' were not affected by the medicament, however, and Jayle never saw any improvement in the patients he treated with ovarian opotherapy for 'neurasthenia' triggered by castration. He said he had also tried giving the extracts to several 'elderly women' with no success, matching the German researchers Latzko and Schnitzler's negative result from an attempt to reverse osteoporosis in elderly women using Ovariin.[208] In one of his initial 1896 papers he had concluded that his own patient data showing marked novel symptoms in 'castrated' women -not all of which were remediable through ovarian medicaments—indicated a need to reconsider the widespread practice of oophorectomy. 'There is cause to ask whether it would not be useful, anytime it is materially possible, to respect the ovary in the course of operations practiced on the utero-ovarian apparatus.'[209]

Jayle's twenty-nine case observations of ovarian medicaments given to women suffering surgical menopause symptoms, reported in his 1898 book, are noteworthy in several other respects. He recommended not telling the patients what the medication was that they were being given, in order to avoid them reacting with repugnance.[210] This was not unusual given that other surgeons reported not even telling their patients with fibroids that their reproductive organs would be removed in the surgery to excise their tumours. Many women were in their early to mid-twenties and were now being prescribed oophorectomy for a wide variety of benign conditions (dysmenorrhea, painful periods, white discharge, non-cancerous tumours, cysts, and inflammations). Their post-surgical symptoms (hot flushes, night sweats, headaches, insomnia, nightmares, mood changes, pelvic pain, leg neuralgia, vision problems, facial neuralgia, impaired memory, migraines, weight gain, and acne) seem to have been quite severe; although Jayle reported several of them to be 'satisfied with' the surgery they had received, suggesting that, for some at least, its immediate post-surgical side effects were not as debilitating as the conditions that it was meant to cure.[211] It is also clear that for most of those who suffered extreme symptoms, the remedial effect of the ovarian treatment Jayle gave them only worked for as long as they kept taking it, indicating that the

[206] See Mwenza T. Blell, 'Menopausal Symptoms Among British Pakistani Women: A Critique of the Standard Checklist Approach', *Menopause*, 22/1 (2015): 79–87.
[207] Jayle, *Opothérapie ovarienne dans la ménopause artificielle*, 244.
[208] Ibid., 245; Latzko & Schnitzler, 'Ein Beitrag zur Organotherapie bei Osteomalacie'.
[209] Jayle, 'Opothérapie ovarienne contre les troubles consécutifs à la castration', 222.
[210] Jayle, *Opothérapie ovarienne dans la ménopause artificielle*, 244.
[211] Ibid., 243 (Observation I), 253 (Observation VI), 254 (Observation VII), 259 (Observation XIV), 261 (Observation XVII).

surgery had created a lifelong need for medication that they did not previously have—surely a true example of iatrogenesis.[212] While numerous patients complained that they felt dreadful whenever they stopped taking the Ovarine, not all of them could afford the continual expense.[213] The surgery or the medication, or the combination of them both, seems to have caused several of the patients to become considerably overweight.[214] Some patients clearly considered the side effects excessive and insufficiently remedied by the ovarian medication, and one woman, 'G' (Observation VIII), aged 39 years, given hysterectomy with oophorectomy for fibroids, told Jayle she would never have consented to the surgery had she known how many new problems it would cause her.[215]

Jayle also described 'frequently' giving ovarian medicaments to women in their late forties and early fifties who had not undergone surgeries but who nonetheless suffered hot flushes and other menopause symptoms. He noted that the other doctors to date who had reported similar findings, Muret, Mond, and Jacobs, had merely summarised their patient outcomes without specific case observations, and had failed to 'control for time', by which he seems to have meant that theirs were short-term treatments without any follow-up months or years later.[216] Jayle provided only three case observations, saying these were representative of the three kinds of responses he had seen among the larger cohort, with little variation: either Ovarine worked initially in reducing their symptoms but then stopped working; or it improved things somewhat continuously; or else it was completely successful. But Jayle said that however well the medication worked in reducing hot flushes in these women (which was variable), few of them considered it worth the bother and expense to keep taking Ovarine continuously as it appeared was necessary to maintain its effect.[217] This is perhaps unsurprising given that each of these case examples described patients who were clearly dealing with several different illnesses not obviously related to their menstrual status. 'P' (Observation XX), who was 52 years old and a day labourer (*journalière*), had suffered hot flushes, pelvic pain, and haemorrhagic bleeding since the cessation of her menses, as well as suicidal thoughts which had previously led her to be interned for a month in the Sainte-Anne asylum. Jayle gave her Ovarine for one month and her hot flushes ceased altogether, but then returned even as she increased the dosage of Ovarine. She gained weight and began experiencing nightmares.[218]

'F' (Observation XXI), who was 49 and had given birth seven times, with two miscarriages, had recently ceased menstruating and begun experiencing pelvic pain, loss of appetite, constipation, bad digestion, frequent urination, nervousness,

[212] Ibid., 245 (Observation I), 247 (Observations III and IV), 247 (Observation V), 253 (Observation VII), 255 (Observation IX), 260 (Observation XIV), 263 (Observation XIX).
[213] Ibid., 260–262 (Observation XVII).
[214] Ibid., 246 (Observation II), 257 (Observation XII), 259 (Observation XIV).
[215] Ibid., 255. See also 263 (Observation XIX). [216] Ibid., 263. [217] Ibid., 263–264.
[218] Ibid., 264–265.

fevers, and most recently hot flushes, neuro-muscular asthenia, melancholy, insomnia, and nightmares. On gynaecological examination, she was diagnosed with inflammation of the left ovary and Fallopian tube, but she refused the operation (presumably oophorectomy) that was prescribed to her. Jayle gave her a series of 'artificial serum injections' (a filtered proprietary ovarian product designed for injection), one per day; on the fourth day she began to experience relief of her symptoms, which increased up to the thirteenth day of injections, after which he switched her to the injections of whole-ovary liquid. Jayle said the two kinds of injections had identical effects, only the ovarian liquid injections were more painful to receive (because they contained more organic matter, they would have provoked localised inflammation around the injection site). Her hot flushes were improved, but her pain increased and her strength diminished. This patient also received massages and laudanum rubs, which she found particularly soothing.[219]

'Mme. K' (Observation XXII), aged 47, had never had children, and was treated by a Dr Bonneau in Mantes, who reported her case to Jayle.[220] She was still menstruating, albeit irregularly, and suffering hot flushes and night sweats around the time of her menses, along with unexplained crying, grumpiness, excessive salivation, mysterious pains in her hands with very brittle nails, palpitations, insomnia, trembling, and suicidal thoughts. She had been gaining considerable weight over the past five or six years, was suspected of a thyroid disorder, and was found to have a highly irregular heartbeat.[221] Bonneau prescribed hydrotherapy treatments as well as ovarian injections, and after the fourth session of these, she appeared to him much improved; after one month of treatment her hot flushes, night sweats, and sleep were considerably improved. Bonneau tapered her off the ovarian injections and ceased them entirely once she appeared to have few remaining symptoms. Sometime later the symptoms returned but the patient was reluctant to undergo further injections, so Bonneau gave her two weeks of Ovarine pills instead. Two years later she was followed up and reported suffering no more hot flushes or sweats.[222] She later returned to the hospital for treatment of a heart condition, but Bonneau considered this unrelated to her menopause.[223]

Notably, neither Jayle nor Lissac related their ovarian research to the testicular extract experiments of Brown-Séquard that had occurred just seven years earlier, except with reference to 'la méthode Brown-Séquard et d'Arsonval'—a specific mode of glandular extraction to produce an injectable liquid that was named after both Brown-Séquard and the physician-inventor Jacques Arsène d'Arsonval (1851–1940).[224] This relative dissociation from the testicular-extract experiments no doubt reflected a desire to avoid the reputation of early gonadal-glandular

[219] Ibid., 265–267. [220] Ibid., 267. [221] Ibid., 267–269.
[222] Ibid., 270. [223] Ibid., 270–271.
[224] Jayle, *Opothérapie ovarienne dans la ménopause artificielle*, 243.

therapy as a source of embarrassment to French academic institutions on account of the view that testes extracts were nothing more than both an elaborate placebo and a form of aphrodisiac.[225] Single-remedy medicaments claiming to fix numerous conditions all at once were strongly associated in Paris medicine with empirics and charlatans. This was part of the reason for the disrepute into which Brown-Séquard's testicular opotherapy had fallen.[226] It was thus important for Jayle and others promoting ovarian extracts to be both circumscribed in their claims to efficacy and specific in the ailments they pertained to treat with them. Another doctoral candidate, Manuel S. Gomès in 1898, who also worked with Pozzi and Jayle at the Broca hospital, and who also wrote his thesis on the ovarian organotherapy treatment they were trialling, referred to the problem of the 'sceptical reception' received by Brown-Séquard in Paris medicine and biology to his hypothesis of the gonadal organs, including the ovary, as secretory glands.[227]

Gomès also reported several of the most recent case observations of Samuel Pozzi prescribing Ovarine to women in natural menopause suffering hot flushes, headaches, and other symptoms. One woman aged 54 years (Observation 1) who was still being treated by Pozzi as Gomès's thesis went to press, said she was 'in paradise' since she had started the ovarian therapy, though Gomès said it was too soon to say how long she would need to take it.[228] The second observation was a woman aged 47 years who had been suffering hot flushes, headaches, pelvic pains, weight gain, and 'nervous crises' since her menses had ceased. Pozzi's notes, as conveyed by Gomès, succinctly summed up the new approach to medicating women's final cessation of menses: 'Diagnosis: Menopause troubles. Treatment: Ovarine'. She was seen again after 100 days of Ovarine treatment and reported fewer hot flushes and had lost some weight.[229] An 1899 book summarising the current state of medical knowledge of ovarian opotherapy by the Toulouse doctor Prosper Mossé affirmed the new approach as well: 'The troubles of the menopause relate not only to a perturbation of the circulatory equilibrium caused by the cessation of the catamenial haemorrhagic flux; they seem to result from the deficiency of a secretion', which could (at least sometimes) be compensated by Ovarine.[230] Another 1899 publication by the Bordeaux chemist A. Flourens,

[225] Merriley Borell, 'Brown-Séquard's Organotherapy and its Appearance in America at the End of the Nineteenth Century', *Bulletin of the History of Medicine*, 50 (1976): 309–320; Merriley Borell, 'Organotherapy and the Emergence of Reproductive Endocrinology', *Journal of the History of Biology*, 18 (1985): 1–30; John Hoberman, *Testosterone Dreams: Rejuvenation, Aphrodisia, Doping* (Berkeley: University of California Press, 2005), 2; Sengoopta, *The Most Secret Quintessence of Life*, 36–40; Celia Roberts, *Messengers of Sex: Hormones, Biomedicine and Feminism* (Cambridge: Cambridge University Press, 2007), 114.

[226] As explicitly noted in Marcellin Bertholet, *Notice sur la vie et les travaux de M. Brown-Séquard* (Paris: Institut de France, 1898), 256.

[227] Manuel S. Gomès, *De l'opothérapie ovarienne, contribution à l'étude physiologique et thérapeutique de l'ovarine*. Thèse (Paris: Georges Carré & C. Naud, 1898), 8–9.

[228] Ibid., 22–23. [229] Ibid., 25.

[230] Prosper Mossé, *État actuel de l'opothérapie ovarienne: Étude expérimentale et clinique* (Paris: J. B. Baillière et fils, 1899), 62.

whose laboratory manufactured ovarian pills containing ten centigrams of fresh sheep ovary, also promoted their use in treating 'troubles of the menopause', for which the standard dose was two pills per day.[231]

The new Broca researcher-clinicians working with ovarian opotherapy appeared wary of the attempts by some psychiatrists to enlist both oophorectomy and ovarian extracts in the treatment of mental pathologies in women attributed to the influence of their genital organs. This mid-nineteenth-century concept was held in relative contempt by the leading figures of neurology and psychiatry, such as both Jean-Martin Charcot and the Paris faculty professor Charles Souleyre, but persisted as a fringe theory entertained by number of doctors at the *fin de siècle*, especially the Bordeaux psychiatrist Emmanuel Régis whom we met in Chapter 7. He published papers throughout the 1890s on the idea of ovarian pathologies as the cause of women's madness, including one which reported a partially positive outcome of injecting ovarian juice into a single patient whose mental illness was attributed to her oophorectomy.[232] The Montpellier surgeon Dr Henri Castagné was also a rare proponent in France of the practice that was widespread in North American psychiatry at the time, of hysterectomising and ovariectomising women diagnosed with hysteria, inducing artificial menopause on the basis of the belief that it was a time when hysteria naturally reduced or resolved.[233] Nonetheless, even Castagné concluded that it was much too dangerous an operation to be used as a common treatment for mental pathologies, and should be reserved only for those patients in whom all other therapies had failed and who also had gynaecological pathologies worthy of surgery in themselves.[234] Souleyre published his major work in 1898 on the 'genito-pathologies' of neurasthenic women, in which he affirmed the more widespread view that surgical castration aggravated female mental pathologies, surveying a wide range of psychiatric and surgical views on the matter and citing only one French author, Auguste Lutaud, who regarded the surgery as an 'ultimate resource'.[235] Nonetheless, it was hard to deny that ovarian opotherapy might be of value to women whose novel nervous pathologies had followed their surgical castration. Souleyre thus considered ovarian juice as just one of many possible pharmacological remedies with promise in the treatment of women's nervous and mental diseases, but he said that the evidence for it was still insufficient and unclear on account of the role of

[231] A. Flourens, *De l'opothérapie* (Bordeaux: G. Gounouilhou, 1899), 8.

[232] Émmanuel Régis, 'Cas de folie consécutive à une ovaro-salpingectomie', *Journal de médecine de Bordeaux*, 37/10 September (1893), 413–417.

[233] Henri Castagné, *De l'ablation des annexes de l'utérus dans l'hystérie* (Montpellier: Charles Boehm, 1891). See Wendy Mitchinson, *The Nature of Their Bodies: Women and Their Doctors in Victorian Canada* (Toronto: University of Toronto Press, 1991).

[234] Castagné, *De l'ablation des annexes de l'utérus dans l'hystérie*, 77.

[235] Charles Souleyre, *Neurasthénie et génitopathies féminines, étude des formes utérines secondaires de la névrose* (Paris: Bailliere, 1898), 190–192.

'auto-suggestion' that may explain the effects of the ovarian injections used in most of the small clinical experiments to date.[236]

Brown-Séquard was revived in other major 1898 publications in France on questions relating to ovarian opotherapy and menopause, most notably of the book by Bestion de Camboulas, published by the eminent Paris medical press J. B. Baillière et fils, which summarised the significance of the various European experiments on this theme, relating both to natural and to surgical menopause (and which was immediately—and rather negatively—reviewed in the *British Medical Journal*).[237] The similarity of the symptoms experienced by the two groups clearly indicated that the mechanism of menopause was a natural process of ovarian decline, Bestion said, explicitly connecting this new theory to the discovery of Brown-Séquard and the French physiologist's hypothesis of 1889 that the ovary was another secretory gland which deposited into the bloodstream its very own special substance.[238] Jayle too had insisted on the nature of the ovary as a secretory gland comparable to the thyroid.[239] Bestion de Camboulas mentioned four other commercial ovarian products in addition to Ovarine that were already in circulation in French pharmacy by 1898: Ovaraden, Oophorine, Ovigénine, and Ovairine.[240] It was clearly already a thriving and expanding commercial enterprise before the century's end. Bestion even revived the 'Propter uterum' aphorism here too, now relating it to the new evidence of the importance of the ovarian secretions for women's femininity, vitality, sanity, and ageing well-being.[241] Most of his book, however, focused on Bestion's own animal experiments, injecting supraphysiological amounts of ovarian extract into crows and rabbits of both sexes, with mostly disastrous consequences for the poor beasts, which was the focus of the *British Medical Journal*'s contempt for the book.[242] But he also provided an inventory of several of the Aquitaine clinicians now prescribing ovarian juice to menopausal women and who had transmitted their private case notes to him, including the Bordeaux university professors Anozan and Boursier, Dr Monod of the Maison protéstante de Bordeaux, Dr Courtin, and Dr Rogée in Saint-Jean-d'Angély, just north of Bordeaux.[243]

The use of ovarian opotherapy was also most certainly becoming more common even before 1898 in other parts of France in the treatment of women who had not been hysterectomised. But this was not yet based on the idea of ovarian deficiency, which only became the central rationale of ovarian and hormone replacement after Jayle's work at the Broca hospital, and the similar experiments of

[236] Ibid., 200.

[237] Bestion de Camboulas, *Le Suc ovarien*; Anon., 'Le Suc ovarien, effets physiologiques et thérapeutiques (The Physiological and Therapeutic Effects of Ovarian Juice) by L. Bestion de Camboulas', *British Medical Journal*, 2/1958 (1898): 87–88.

[238] Bestion de Camboulas, *Le Suc ovarien*, 23.

[239] Jayle, *Opothérapie ovarienne dans la ménopause artificielle*, 239.

[240] Bestion de Camboulas, *Le Suc ovarien*, 27. [241] Ibid., 21. [242] Ibid., 35–64.

[243] Ibid., 67–111.

German, Swiss, and Belgian doctors. For instance, in his 1896 book of *Consultations on the Diseases of Women*, the Mâcon medical gynaecologist Auguste Joseph Lutaud (1847–1925), mentioned by Souleyre as an enthusiast of surgical castration, prescribed ovarian products for acute (but not chronic) metritis.[244] Lutaud, who published several major works on women's gynaecological health and edited the *Paris Journal of Medicine* (among several journals), was, like Péan, an ardent opponent of Pasteur's theory of bacteria as the cause of disease, as well as a moral campaigner against prostitution, which he considered would be made redundant by the legalisation of divorce without cause.[245] He said that haemorrhagic bleeding was almost always a sign of serious uterine pathology, so that opotherapy medications for this condition were at best an adjunct therapy. The exception was in women around the time of menopause, for whom haemorrhages were often 'essential', in which case these were amenable to a purely pharmaceutical treatment with ovarian opotherapy. Medicating menopause with ovarian extract was thus assimilated into his gynaecology practice simply as one of the many 'relative particularities' to take into account in the judgement of clinical diagnoses and therapeutic determinations.[246] Lutaud did, however, also make special mention of older women among his patients in the section of his *Consultations* on nymphomania, for which the treatments ranged from the pharmacological (strontium, bitter orange, potassium bromide, camphor, Indian hemp, etc.) to the moral (behavioural change, recommendation of marriage) to the surgical (especially clitoridectomy, which he said was a very effective cure).[247] Uteruses and ovaries, it seems, were not the only organs being cut out of older women in the medical view of their genital organs as monstrous, diseased, or useless.

Hysterectomies were by this time widely prescribed to older women too, not only for fibroids but also for uterine prolapse. This condition was not uncommon among older working-class mothers who had endured numerous long and difficult labours during their childbearing years, though these were already becoming less common due to the increasing use of Caesarean section in obstetrics from the end of the nineteenth century—which were also sometimes combined with hysterectomy and oophorectomy.[248] The Nancy gynaecological surgeon Gaston Lanique described nine such cases of women with uterine prolapse in his

[244] Auguste Joseph Lutaud, *Consultations sur les maladies des femmes* (Paris: Rueff, 1895), 81.
[245] Auguste Joseph Lutaud, *Études sur la rage et la méthode Pasteur* [1887], 2nd ed. (Paris: Journal de médecine de Paris, 1891).
[246] Lutaud, *Consultations sur les maladies des femmes*, 176. [247] Ibid., 99.
[248] Charles Maygrier, *Étude sur l'opération de Porro: Opération césarienne suivie de l'amputation de l'utérus et des ovaires* (Paris: A. Delahaye et L. Lecrosnier, 1880); V. Duchamp, *De l'amputation par le vagin de l'utérus artificiellement inversé comme complément de l'opération césarienne* (Saint-Étienne: J. Pichon, 1886); Julien Potocki, *De l'opération césarienne, et, en particulier, de l'opération césarienne avec double suture de l'utérus, par la méthode de Saenger* (Paris: G. Steinheil, 1886); Émile Blanc, *De l'opération césarienne, méthodes opératoires et indications* (Paris: Lecrosnier et Babé, 1890).

case observations in an 1894 book about vaginal hysterectomy.[249] He clearly distinguished the validity of the surgery based on the age of the patient: after menopause, the womb 'is no longer a useful organ', whereas for younger women it was 'still good for fecundation'.[250] He claimed that almost all doctors were now in favour of removing the uterus and ovaries of all older women at any sign of gynaecological disorder, saying that 'practically everyone agreed on the completely innocuous character of the operation'. Nonetheless, Lanique also noted the continuation of a marked medical opposition to the practice by several physiologists and gynaecologists who he said viewed it as a 'pis-aller thérapeutique' ('crappy therapeutic solution').[251]

By 1900 numerous studies, both Jayle's and others', had indicated that many women whose uterus and/or ovaries had been removed were complaining of post-surgical symptoms that were sometimes very serious. The acknowledgement by Jayle and other surgeons that removal of women's reproductive organs was not without serious negative effects disturbed the view of them as dispensable defended by most other pro-hysterectomy voices. The new opotherapy pharmaceuticals provided a partial solution to the problem in the form of ovarian supplementation—the precursor of oestrogenic hormone replacement therapies marketed by pharmaceutical companies after 1939.[252] But ovarian products were not a rejuvenation elixir, and could not offset all the iatrogenic effects of surgical castration, even if they clearly were a partially effective remedy for menopausal hot flushes, particularly those provoked by the abrupt loss of ovarian function due to the ovaries' removal during the fertile years of a woman's lifespan. Importantly though, while ovarian therapies were initially developed for women of menstruating ages who had undergone hysterectomy and oophorectomy, they were then very quickly extrapolated to all post-menopausal women, who were now theorised to be 'ovarian deficient' according to a presumed (though never defined) endocrine norm of young (non-hysterectomised/ovariectomised) women. From this moment onwards, the surgical removal of uteruses and ovaries knew no bounds in French, German, and American gynaecology. A 1960 American gynaecological society narrative about the history of the discipline acknowledged that the 'sudden burst of endocrines' in the early twentieth century was responsible for the massive increase in gynaecological surgeries thereafter.[253] Hysterectomy/oophorectomy and pharmaceutical ovarian replacement thus represented a mutually reinforcing medico-technological complex, an entanglement of two forms of treatment that

[249] Gaston Lanique, *De l'hystérectomie vaginale totale appliquée au traitement du prolapsus utérin complet* (Nancy: Imprimerie Coopérative de l'Est, 1894), 32, 41, 48, 63, 74–78, 85–86.

[250] Ibid., 86. [251] Ibid., 85–86.

[252] Borell, 'Organotherapy and the Emergence of Reproductive Endocrinology'; Sengoopta, *The Most Secret Quintessence of Life*, 154–194.

[253] Theodore Cianfrani, *A Short History of Obstetrics and Gynecology* (Springfield Ill.: Charles C. Thomas, 1960), xi.

would be rapidly globalised in the second half of the twentieth century. This chapter does not proceed beyond the first decade of the twentieth century, since from this moment onwards the elaboration of menopause as an object of medicalisation was no longer a specifically French phenomenon. Their work was done in putting into place an elaborate accumulation of conceptual layers relating to women's ageing and the inherent morbidity of their reproductive organs.

Conclusion

While French doctors did not stop entirely writing about menopause and women's ageing after the 1920s, they were, after this time, neither an exception or at the forefront of international medical research on such questions. Moreover, the number of specialist works had trickled down to just a handful published from 1920 to 1945, even including re-editions of earlier works.[1] Therefore, a natural closure is suggested following the final set of ideas French medicine had contributed at the *fin de siècle* (along with a few in other European cultures), about hysterectomy for women in their forties, with ovarian replacement proposed as the answer to its side effects, and which was then generalised to women in natural menopause. This development became a massive global enterprise in the twentieth century because of the uptake of sex-steroid hormones by pharmaceutical companies proposing to offer the solution to all the complaints of ageing women thereafter. Gynaecological surgery development was also led by North American clinicians as much as European ones after the 1910s, and proliferated exponentially throughout the global south between 1960 and 2020.[2] There is excellent research already available on the wider topic of menopausal hormone replacement in the twentieth century, especially Elizabeth Siegal Watkins's book about the American history of oestrogen, and Chandak Sengoopta's book about the intercultural European scientific development of sex-steroid hormones, with its focus on the interwar period.[3] The French researchers who were part of the global story of twentieth-century menopause medicine did not lead or dominate the development of sex-steroid hormone replacement in the way they had dominated nineteenth-century menopause medicine.

Menopause has now acquired the status of a medical given in global research and clinical practice but its origins lay firmly in the unique preoccupations of French medicine of the long nineteenth century—accommodating new

[1] Arthur Leclercq, *L'Âge critique, goutte, affections paragoutteuses, obésité* [1911], 2nd ed. (Paris: Octave Doin, 1922); Jean Pierre Charles Callen, *De la rareté des fibromes purs de l'utérus après la ménopause.* Thèse (Bordeaux: V. Cambette, 1924); Victor Pauchet, *L'Automne de la vie; l'homme et la femme à l'âge critique*, préface de M. Brieux de l'Académie Française (Paris: Editions J. Oliven, 1932); Claude Béclere, *Les Hémorragies utérines avant et après la ménopause* (Paris: Masson, 1936).

[2] Alison Downham Moore, Fouzieyha Towghi, Holly Ashford, Tinashe Dune, & Rashmi Pithavadian, 'The Global Proliferation of Radical Gynaecological Surgeries: A History of the Present', *History & Anthropology*, 32/4 (2021): 1–25.

[3] Elizabeth Siegel Watkins, *The Estrogen Elixir: A History of Hormone Replacement Therapy in America* (Baltimore: Johns Hopkins University Press, 2009); Chandak Sengoopta, *The Most Secret Quintessence of Life: Sex, Glands and Hormones, 1850–1950* (Chicago: University of Chicago Press, 2006).

The French Invention of Menopause and the Medicalisation of Women's Ageing: A History. Alison M. Downham Moore, Oxford University Press. © Alison M. Downham Moore 2022. DOI: 10.1093/oso/9780192842916.003.0012

physiological and statistical models, instantiating emerging specialist fields, asserting its legitimacy over competing health practitioners, championing medicine's status as revolutionary while also claiming ancient inheritance, and developing professional identities, intuitional rivalries, and competitive patient markets that, while part of many European cultures of this time, were particularly acute in the French context after the political events of the revolutionary period. Menopause was an exemplary topic for numerous medical agendas, not least helping to justify a gender order in which older women were more than ever patients and less than ever health practitioners themselves. French medical thought of the nineteenth century told fanciful stories about how it had derived the concept of menopause symptomatology from ancient scholars, transmitted via early modern luminaries of gynaecology. This book has shown how these stories about the medical past came to be constructed in the legitimation of doctors' insistences that older women required both elaborate regimes of self-care and regular medical surveillance, both in approaching and following their final cessation of menses. Menopause was broadly part of a particular fixation of French medical culture of the long nineteenth century with the peculiar 'nature' and vital force of women, defined as utterly distinct from that of men, and as determined by their reproductive organs, which were thought to influence women's entire physiology and psychology. At the same time, menopause was frequently defined as the masculine period of a woman's lifespan, since the decline of the uterus or ovaries meant that the very thing that defined her as feminine was lost. Through this perspective, menopause came to be seen as a deficiency condition, necessarily in need of medical, hygienic, and self-disciplined attention, an assumption that continues today to underpin both biomedical and many alternative health approaches to treating or managing it.

Menopause was a particularly important ground through which doctors and medical scholars accommodated the unique pressure on medical culture in the aftermath of the French Revolution and the dissolution of university faculties and societies. Unlike any other cultures of this time, French medicine underwent a radical rewriting of narratives about its own historical importance, towards an account that simultaneously emphasised both rupture and continuity. In the post-revolutionary need for new curriculum and methods, and for a competitive edge in the unregulated market following the collapse of state regulation, scholars such as Philippe Pinel, Pierre-Jean-Georges Cabanis, Joseph-Marie-Joachim Vigarous, and their students, were keener than ever to align themselves to an idea of Hippocratic physiological medicine and to insist on the superiority of their systemic nosological approach relative to the work of empirics, charlatans, and folk healers. The first doctoral theses on women's final cessation of menses between 1799 and 1840 were filled with statements of commitment to physiological and vitalist principles (especially the idea of uterine sympathy), Hippocratic or pseudo-Hippocratic aphorisms, hygienic advice, denigration of charlatans and *commères*, and self-proclamations of modern scientific corrective to traditional myths.

Nonetheless, older currents of thought clearly contributed to the assemblage of the concept of menopause, some derived from Ptolemaic astrology in its early modern revival, which highlighted the forty-ninth year as a major 'climacteric'; while scholars of the eighteenth century's own particular feminine pathology—the vapours—had elaborated much of the therapeutic prescription later transferred to women in menopause to follow the lifeways of the peasantry. Vitalist philosophy of medicine espoused at both the universities of Halle and Montpellier throughout the eighteenth century clearly provided much of the conceptual ground for the new (since 1775) particularly French genre of 'natural histories of women', and for the later elaboration of menopause, both of which characterised the female life essence as peculiarly determined by the uterus. This was an organ, it was thought, that influenced their entire 'animal economy' through sympathy with the other parts of the body, making them the nervous sex, and binding women's vitality tightly to their phase of conceptive capacity. The vitalist preoccupation with distinguishing patients on the basis of sex, age, temperament, profession, and character also importantly permitted the focus on older women to become imaginable as a specialist topic, while the unique Montpellier concept of crisis as a productive, transitory state informed many of the early attempts to define menopause as a critical life stage, even as it was, on the surface, apparently reduced to the mere fact of no longer menstruating. Encyclopedist attempts to redefine the life cycle importantly contributed to the emerging view of the cessation of menses as heralding the beginning of women's ageing, even as they considered sex differences rather minimally.

Menopause was also part of the difficulty that nineteenth-century French masculine medicine had in accommodating the demographic indication of women's superior resilience to death in almost every age band, and particularly in the older ages. It was thus an important topic for the bifurcation of morbidity from mortality, permitting a wider embrace of disciplines concerned not only with pathology and longevity but also with good health, such as the nineteenth-century field of *hygiène*, which justified itself partly with reference to the older-age patient cohorts, and particularly women.[4] Both were categories of people thought more receptive to, and more in need of, hygienic intervention. Effectively a form of preventive medicine, hygiene—in that older sense of the word—was largely lost after the nineteenth century, becoming the domain of new forms of popular and alternative healthcare instead, while medical hygiene turned its attention primarily to

[4] Rudolf Gerhard, 'Santé publique et éducation: Notions d'hygiène sociale au XVIIIe et au XIXe siècle. Étienne Tourtelle (1756–1800), Jules Levy (1805–1872), Jules Rochard (1819–1896)', *Histoire des sciences médicales*, 17/A1 (1982): 146–150; Franck Thénard-Duvivier, ed., *Hygiène, santé et protection sociale de la fin du XVIIIe siècle à nos jours* (Paris: Ellipses, 2012).

public sanitation, epidemics, and eugenics. Indeed, many of the preoccupations that brought menopause into being are no longer general principles of twenty-first-century biomedicine. And yet, the underlying and still present assumptions of women as the sicker sex in ageing, as needing special regimes around the final cessation of menses, as best served by the removal of their uterus and/or ovaries, as deficient once their conceptive capacity ends, or as prone to mental illness in menopause, all have important nineteenth-century origins.

The competitive environment that French clinicians faced, especially during the revolutionary period when their privileges were dissolved, but also throughout the nineteenth century as the medical faculties turned out graduates at a faster rate than the market for their services grew, meant that new patient groups among the largest sections of affluent society may have been accurately apprehended as an important source of potential revenue. While it is not clear that any doctors were deliberately disease-mongering to drum up work for themselves, it is also hard to ignore the potential benefit they might derive from convincing women that their normal ageing (from as young as 40 years) required medical attention. At the same time, elite women in this new era of heightened industrialisation and urbanisation clearly were facing important changes in their bodily lifeways, having fewer children, becoming more sedentary, spending more time indoors, or out in the city at night, and consuming more processed foods and alcoholic beverages than in earlier eras. Many menopause doctors showed heightened awareness of these important impacts of industrialisation on French society and urged women to move more, sleep enough (but not too much), avoid alcohol, and eat fresh food. Numerous medical writers identified menopause symptoms as a disease of civilisation, leaning on comparisons between urban elite lifeways and the healthy ageing of peasant women. Of all the nineteenth-century ideas about women's ageing relative to the growing health data accumulation throughout the twentieth and twenty-first centuries, the view that regular exercise improves menopause symptoms and long-term health outcomes for women post-menopause is the one that has proven most resilient.[5]

[5] F. B. Hu, M. J. Stampfer, & G. A. Colditz et al., 'Physical Activity and Risk of Stroke in Women', *Journal of the American Medical Association*, 283/22 (2000): 2961–7. E. J. Aiello, Y. Yutaka, S. S. Tworoger, et al., 'Effect of a Yearlong, Moderate-Intensity Exercise Intervention on the Occurrence and Severity of Menopause Symptoms in Postmenopausal Women', *Menopause*, 11 (2004): 283–288; Kristina L. Kendall & Ciaran M. Fairman, 'Women and Exercise in Aging', *Journal of Sport and Health Science*, 3/3 (2014): 170–178; Virginia Overdorf, Betty Kollia, Katherine Makarec, & Cassandra Alleva Szeles, 'The Relationship Between Physical Activity and Depressive Symptoms in Healthy Older Women', *Gerontology and Geriatric Medicine*, 1/4 (2016): 1–8. Doi: 10.1177/2333721415626859; Saori I. Braun, Youngdeok Kim, Amy E. Jetton, et al., 'Sedentary Behavior, Physical Activity, and Bone Health in Postmenopausal Women', *Journal of Aging and Physical Activity*, 25/2 (2017): 173–181; Helena Hörder, Lena Johansson, & Xin Guo, 'Midlife Cardiovascular Fitness and Dementia: A 44-year Longitudinal Population Study in Women', *Neurology*, 90/15 (2018): e1298-e1305; Juliana S. Oliveira, Marina B. Pinheiro, Nicola Fairhall, et al., 'Evidence on Physical Activity and the Prevention of Frailty and Sarcopenia Among Older People: A Systematic Review to Inform the World Health Organization Physical Activity Guidelines', *Journal of Physical Activity and Health*, 17/12 (2020): 1247–1258;

Nineteenth-century doctors both in France and elsewhere also worried about older women's nerves and sexuality in ways that were clearly important both in the gendered insistence of women's inferiority to men, and for the psychiatric dogma which defined menopause as a time of psychopathology and perversion, with reference to ageing as a form of degeneration. Some doctors objected to the attempt to pin hysteria on menopausal women, generating an important counter-discourse to the view espoused by scholars like Alexandre Brierre de Boismont and Noël Guéneau de Mussy. However, an entire century of previous French vapours writing had helped to justify the focus on women's nervous and mental pathologies at all times of uterine change. The marked degeneration current in *fin-de-siècle* psychiatry was also common in German, Austrian, and Italian psychiatry, where older women were sometimes held in suspicion with resort to similar rationales. In France, psychiatric writers identified a particular form of mental illness they ascribed to menopausal women, referring to sexual desire after the cessation of menses as inherently perverse. Some sexually active older women may thus have been viewed as automatically mentally ill. Notably though, French psychiatrists largely rejected the view that women's mental illness could be cured with hysterectomy or oophorectomy which was practised in several English and North American contexts,[6] and on the contrary, worried about the potential of such surgeries to perturb women's nervous systems and brains.

While many of these preoccupations spoke to markedly nineteenth-century values, the story told in this book has important legacies for current medical practice. Hysterectomy, whose French origins we considered in the final chapter, is the most common surgery among French women today, with 85 per cent of these performed for benign conditions and most of them on women between the ages of 45 and 50 years.[7] While the surgical mortality today for such procedures is low and the techniques incomparably improved relative to the danger hysterectomy posed to French women of the late nineteenth century, the rationales underpinning the practice have changed little: the ageing uterus is still viewed as both redundant and disease-prone, with 'fertility-conserving' procedures

Marianne Huebner, David Meltzer, Wenjuan Ma, & Holly Arrow, 'The Masters Athlete in Olympic Weightlifting: Training, Lifestyle, Health Challenges, and Gender Differences', *PLoS One*, 15/12 (2020): Article e0243652; Mikel Izquierdo, R. A. Merchant, J. E. Morley, et al., 'International Exercise Recommendations in Older Adults (ICFSR): Expert Consensus Guidelines', *The Journal of Nutrition, Health and Aging*, 25 (2021): 824–853.

[6] Wendy Mitchinson, *The Nature of their Bodies: Women and Their Doctors in Victorian Canada* (Toronto: University of Toronto Press, 1991), 77–98; Regina Morantz-Sanchez, *Conduct Unbecoming a Woman: Medicine on Trial in Turn-of-the-Century Brooklyn* (New York: Oxford University Press, 1999), 104–127; Sally Frampton, *Belly-Rippers, Surgical Innovation and the Ovariotomy Controversy* (London: Palgrave, 2018), 130–150.

[7] Audrey Chevron et al., 'Hystérectomie: Évolution des pratiques entre 2009 et 2019 en France', *Gynécologie obstétrique fertilité & sénologie*, 49 (2021): 816–822; Ilana Löwy and George Weisz, 'French Hormones: Progestins and Therapeutic Variance in France', *Social Science and Medicine*, 60 (2005): 2609–2622.

provided to younger women often advised against for women close to menopause. There is little recent data on the percentage of French women using menopausal HRT, though it has been observed to have enjoyed high esteem among them relative to populations in other countries, used by up to 52 per cent of women between the ages of 50 and 69 years, but to have declined following the publication of two large UK and US studies of the early 2000s which indicated increased cancer and cardiovascular disease risks with the use of combined oestrogen-progesterone therapy with Equine oestrogen in overweight women up to 60 years of age.[8] The largest pharmaceutical supplier of HRT in France, Besins Healthcare Ltd, was founded in Paris 1885, but was not one of the early innovators of ovarian opotherapy. There is more that clearly could be said in this book about the twentieth-century French medical researchers whose work was important in the development of sex-steroid hormone discovery: Robert Courrier's research between the 1920 and 1940s on the physiology of the ovary; on the approach to ageing hygiene of the interwar Amiens surgeon Victor Pauchet (1869–1936);[9] on the uptake, in French psychoanalysis and hygiene, of the work of the Spanish endocrinologist Gregorio Marañon (1887–1960), who wrote about the sexes in ageing, extending the idea that was common in nineteenth-century menopause medicine that ageing reduced differences between the sexes, making all older people intersexual.[10]

The rehearsal of nineteenth-century hygienic and moral advice about the 'âge de retour' was also even sometimes revived by French writers after the Second World War, such as in Michel Ducet's 1964 *The Climacteric Age of Man and Woman: The Turn of Age and Sexual Crisis.*[11] Notably though, none of these thinkers considered menopausal or ageing women to require special attention; in part because they were just as interested in men's or in young women's physiology and psychology, and in part because they rejected the idea which had so fascinated many nineteenth-century doctors—that men and women represented practically different species and that—*especially* in ageing—they followed utterly distinct paths. The interwar period saw many expressions of what the historian Thomas Laqueur called 'the one-sex model' of homologous views of men and women, but this was precisely at the time in which Laqueur claimed the 'two-sex model' was most triumphant—an objection that other medical historians have

[8] Angèle Gayet-Ageron et al., 'Estimated Numbers of Postmenopausal Women Treated by Hormone Therapy in France', *Maturitas*, 52/2–3 (2005): 269–305; Virginie Ringa, Noëlle Varnoux, Stéphanie Paiult, & Gérard Bréart, 'Hormone Therapy Use Among Postmenopausal French Women Before the Publication of the Women's Health Initiative Study: Duration of Use and Factors Associated with Discontinuation', *Reproductive Endocrinology*, 83/6 (2005): 1771–1779.

[9] Pauchet, *L'Automne de la vie.*

[10] Gregorio Marañon, *L'Âge critique (étude pathogénique et clinique)*, trans. J. Sanjuro D'Arella (Paris: Librarie Félix Alcan, 1934).

[11] Michel Ducet, *L'Âge climatérique de l'homme et de la femme, retour d'âge et crise sexuelle* (Soissons: Aubenas, 1964).

made about Laqueur's take on the interwar period too.[12] Both Victor Pauchet and the later Michel Ducet even revived the early modern idea of the unisex 'climacteric' crisis around the 49th and 63rd years which referenced ancient Ptolemaic astrology and which was so rarely cited in nineteenth-century menopause medicine. Might conceptual layers in the history of medicine be as cyclical as young women's menses? Might some of those cycles, like the menses of women as they start to diminish, come around at a slower pace than others, and eventually come to rest?

The five-year process of writing this book was a continual exercise in abstention from beliefs about how women themselves should or should not regard, treat, medicate, or live their time of life around or after the final cessation of menses. But a certain hope has underpinned this inquiry that its historical unpacking of the conceptual layers that are compressed within modern medical menopause might help to demystify and thus neutralise its nocebo powers to inflect women's experience of their ageing as deficiency or as disaster. As Dominique Dirlewanger notes in his 2018 study of diversity and health in older French and Swiss populations, ageing is a multi-coloured phenomenon, therefore no singular sets of recommendations can possibly serve it.[13] Cécile Charlap's recent sociological work examining French menopause through a lens of African-French cultural diversity is also a powerful call to revise the set of concepts that were inherited from a French medical past that pre-dated the large waves of immigration that have transformed the contemporary spectrum of French women's expectations and needs in ageing.[14] People over 50 years of age in 2021 number around 40 per cent of the population of France, as they do in most affluent countries, and French women have a life expectancy of around 85 years, with more humans living to older ages than ever before in human history.[15] Many of the medical models of treating older bodies as degenerated exceptions to the youthful ideal were developed in a historical period when movement in this direction had already begun transforming European demographic rations but had not yet become so stark as it is today. The most insightful French medical clinicians of the nineteenth century often recognised the wide diversity of ways women aged and of their individual medical needs in later life, though this approach was more pronounced in Montpellier vitalism than it was in the Parisian hygienic discourses that became dominant in the nineteenth century. There was also a marked trend towards

[12] Howard Chiang, 'Epistemic Gender, Sex Beyond the Flesh: Science, Medicine, and the Two-Sex Model in Modern America', *eSharp*, 9 (2007): 1–34 [6–16].

[13] Dominique Dirlewanger, *Les Couleurs de la vieillesse: Histoire culturelle des représentations de la vieillesse en Suisse et en France (1940–1990)* (Neuchâtel: Alphil-Presses universitaires suisses, 2018).

[14] Cécile Charlap, *La Fabrique de la ménopause.* Thèse de sociologie (Strasbourg: Université de Strasbourg, 2015); Cécile Charlap, *La Fabrique de la ménopause* (Paris: CNRS, 2019).

[15] <https://fr.statista.com/statistiques/472349/repartition-population-groupe-dage-france/>; Dirlewanger, *Les Couleurs de la vieillesse*, 39–67.

population-based, rather than precision, personalised medicine, emerging from the end of the nineteenth century and with important legacies into the present—such as in the still-prevalent gynaecological recommendation to women in their forties to undergo hysterectomy for benign tumours and as a prophylactic measure again uterine cancers that affect only 3 per cent of the population of people with uteruses, and despite ever mounting evidence of increased risks for multiple forms of ageing morbidity resulting from such surgeries.[16] Can the medical concept of women's ageing as something which must be universally—and in just one way—medically treated, like Colette, release its attachment to the past and awaken to a new break of day?

[16] Elizabeth A. Stewart, Stacey A. Missmer, & Walter A. Rocca, 'Moving Beyond Reflexive and Gynecologic Prophylactic Surgery', *Mayo Clinic Proceedings*, 96/2 (2021): 291–294.

Bibliography

Primary Sources

Abeille, Jonas, *Des Corps fibreux de l'utérus* (Paris: E. Thunot, 1868).

Actualités médicales, 'La Première doctoresse française: Conversations avec Mme Madeleine Brès, docteur en médecine', *La Chronique Médicale: Revue bi-mensuelle de médecine scientifique, littéraire et anecdotique*, 2/7 (1 April 1895): 190–196.

Alaize, Pierre, *Le Rôle de la fonction interne de l'ovaire et les essais d'opothérapie ovarienne en pathologie nerveuse et mentale* (Montpellier: Imprimerie générale du Midi, 1906).

Alibert, Jean Louis, *Nouveaux Elémens de thérapeutique et de matière médicale, suivis d'un nouvel essai sur l'art de formuler*, 3 vols (Paris: Crapart, Caillet et Ravier, 1804).

Alibert, Jean Louis, 'Eloge historique de Pierre Roussel', in Pierre Roussel, *Système physique et moral de la femme, ou Tableau philosophique de la constitution, de l'état organique du tempérament, des mœurs et des fonctions propres au sexe*, 3rd ed. [1775] (Paris: Crapart, Caillet et Ravier, 1803).

André, Mathieu, *Quelques Propositions sur l'hygiène en général*. Thèse (Montpellier: Publisher not identified, 1807).

Angelesco, Constantin, *Hystérectomie abdominale totale pour tumeurs fibreuses de l'utérus* (Paris: Georges Carré, 1897).

Anglade, Jean Baptiste, *Considérations sur les effets que peut produire la cessation des règles*. Thèse (Montpellier: Jean Martel, 1812).

Anon., *Accidents du retour d'âge et maladies du système véneux; varices et ulcères variqueux; hémorroïdes, varicocèle; phlébites, œdèmes chroniques; congestions; hémorrhages, etc.; Leur Traitement par l'Elixir de Virginie* (Paris: Moride, 1894).

Anon., *Les Âges critiques de la femme: Puberté—ménopause. Guides des mères de famille, des maîtresses de pension et des directrices d'établissements religieux* (Paris: V. Goupy et Jourdan, 1878).

Anon., *Annuaire statistique du département de la Vienne pour 1833* (Poitiers: Saurin Frères, 1833).

Anon., *Aristotle's Masterpiece, or the Secrets of Generations Display'd in all the Parts thereof* [1684] (London: no publisher, 1704).

Anon., *Bibliothèque du médecin-praticien, ou résumé général de tous les ouvrages de clinique médicale et chirurgicale, de toutes les monographes, de tous les mémoires de médecine et de chirurgie pratiques, anciens et modernes, publie en France et à l'étranger*, 15 vols (Paris: Bureau de la Gazette des Hôpitaux, 1842–1851).

Anon., *Cinquantième anniversaire du mariage de M. et Mme Charié-Marsaines: Souvenir du 29 avril 1889* (Paris: E. Plon Nourrit, 1889).

Anon., *Consultation de plusieurs médecins célébrés de l'Université de Montpellier sur des maladies aigues et chroniques*, 9 vols (Paris: Durand & Pissot fils, 1748–1750).

Anon., *Dictionnaire universel françois et latin, contenant la signification et la définition tant des mots de l'une et l'autre langue, avec leurs différents usages, que des termes propres de chaque estat et de chaque profession; la description de toutes les choses naturelles et artificielles; l'explication de tout ce que renferment les sciences et les arts; Avec des remarques d'érudition et de critique*, 3 vols (Paris: Estienne Ganeau, 1704).

Anon., *Dr. Chamberlain's Midwife's Practice. Or, a Guide for Women in that High Concern of Conception, Breeding, and Nursing Children* (London: J. Clowes, 1665).

Anon., *Encyclopédie méthodique*, 17 vols (Paris: Pancoucke, 1792).

Anon., *Encyclopédie, ou Dictionnaire raisonné des sciences, des arts et des métiers*, vol. 17 (Paris: Samuel Faulche, 1765).

Anon., 'Hygiène physiologique de la femme', *Revue encyclopédique ou analyse raisonnée des productions les plus remarquables dans les sciences, les arts industriels, la littérature et les beaux-arts* (Paris: Bureau central de la revue encyclopédique, 1825), 468–469.

Anon., 'Literarische Nachrichten: 1. Französische Literatur', *Allegemeine Literatur-Zeitung*, 125 (29 August 1798): 1033–1046.

Anon,, 'Mlle de Thilo, Docteur-Médecin spécialiste', *L'Impartial* (Thursday, 18 February 1892): 6.

Anon., *Nouveau Dictionnaire de l'Academie Françoise, dedié au roy*. 2 vols, vol. 2: M–Z (Paris: Coiganrd, 1718).

Anon, 'Variétés', *Journal de médecine, chirurgie, pharmacie*, 26 (1813): 422–429.

Apostoli, Georges, *Sur une nouvelle application de l'électricité après les accouchements: communication faite à l'Académie de médecine de Paris* (Paris: H. Lauwereyns, 1881).

Apostoli, Georges, *Sur un nouveau traitement de la métrite chronique et en particulier de l'endométrie par la galvano-caustique chimique intra-utérine* (Paris: O. Doin, 1887).

Arago, François, 'Notices bibliographies: Poisson', in *Œuvres complètes de François Arago*, 16 vols (Paris: Gide et J. Baudry, 1854), vol. 2, 593–698.

Armand, P., *Considérations sur l'âge critique des femmes, et sur les moyens de prévenir les maladies qui peuvent survenir à cette période de la vie*. Thèse (Paris: Didot Jeune, 1820).

Assegond, Albert, *De la femme, considérée à l'âge critique: Changements physiologiques qui s'opèrent dans on etat physiques et moral, et de l'application des règles de l'hygiène à cette principale époque de la vie*. Thèse (Paris: Didot Jeune, 1821).

Astruc, Jean, *Tractatus de motus fermentativi causa, novam et mechanicam hypothesim continens* (Montpellier: H. Pech, 1702).

Astruc, Jean, *Traité de maladies des femmes*, 6 vols (Paris: P. Guillaume Cavelier, 1761–1765).

Auber, Théophile-Charles-Emmanuel-Édouard, *Hygiène des femmes nerveuses ou Conseils aux femmes pour les époques critiques de leur vie* (Paris: Germer Baillière, 1864).

Aulagnier, Alexis-François, *Nouveau Recueil d'observations et de consultations sur les maladies des femmes, et spécialement sur celles qui se déclarent vers l'âge critique* (Paris: l'auteur, 1821).

Aulagnier, Alexis-François, *Considérations sur l'âge critique qui amène la suppression absolue du flux périodique* (Paris: Gabon, 1824).

Auvard, Alfred, *Traité pratique de gynécologie*, 2nd ed. (Paris: Octave Doin, 1894).

Bachot, Gaspard, *Erreurs populaires touchant la médecine et régime de santé* (Lyon: Barthelemy Vincent, 1626).

Baglivi, Giorgio, *De praxi medica ad priscam observandi rationem revocanda: Libri duo. Accedunt dissertationes novae* (Leiden: Fredericum Haringium, 1700).

Bailleau, René, *Des tachycardies de la ménopause*. Thèse (Paris: L. Boyer, 1901).

Ball, Benjamin, *Des embolies pulmonaires*. Thèse (Paris: Rignoux, 1862).

Ball, Benjamin, *La Folie érotique* (Paris: J. B. Baillière, 1888).

Ball, Benjamin, *Leçons sur les maladies mentales*, 2nd ed. (Paris: Asselin & Houzeau, 1890).

Balzac, Honoré de, *Physiologie de l'amour* (Paris: Chapentier, 1828).

Barbaud, Dr Charles & Dr A. Rouillard, *Histoire clinico-thermale de la femme aux trois grandes périodes de sa vie: Puberté, union sexuelle, ménopause. Troubles et accidents de la*

ménopause (âge critique de la femme), traitement thermal aux eaux de Luxeuil (Paris: Jouvet, 1895).
Barbey d'Aurevilly, Jules, *Premier Memorandum: 1836–1828* (Paris: Alphonse Lemerre, 1900).
Barbier, Michel-Victor, *De l'influence de la menstruation sur les maladies mentales*. Thèse (Paris: Rignoux, 1848).
Bardout, Claude-Martial, *Considérations générales sur la cessation du flux menstruel, et sur les précautions à prendre pour en prévenir les accidens ou les maladies*. Thèse (Paris: Didot Jeune, 1816).
Barié, Ernest, *Étude sur la ménopause* (Paris: V. Adrien Delahaye, 1877).
Baron, Joseph Stéphane, *De la ménopause (âge critique)*. Thèse (Paris: Rignoux, 1851).
Barthez, Paul-Joseph, *Nouveaux Eléments de la science de l'homme* (Montpellier: J. Martel aîné, 1778).
Barthez, Paul-Joseph, *Consultations de médecine*, ouvrage posthumé, 2 vols, ed. J. Lordat (Paris: Michaud et Frères, 1810).
Baudelaire, Charles, *Les Fleurs du mal* (Paris: Poulet-Malassis & de Broise, 1857).
Baudron, Émile, *Hystérectomie vaginale appliquée au traitement des annexes de l'utérus (Opération de Péan): Étude basée sur les 200 premières observations du Docteur Paul Segond* (Paris: Société d'Éditions Scientifiques, 1894).
Bayard, Henri-Louis, *Essai médico-légal sur l'utéromanie-nymphomanie*. Thèse (Paris: Didot Jeune, 1836).
Beauchène, Edme-Pierre Chauvot de, *De l'influence des affections de l'âme dans les maladies nerveuses des femmes, avec le traitement qui convient à ces maladies* [1781], 2nd ed. (Montpellier & Paris: Méquignon, 1783).
Beauvoir, Simone de, *Le Deuxième Sexe*, 2 vols (Paris: Gallimard, 1949).
Beauvoir, Simone de, *La Force de l'âge* (Paris: Gallimard, 1963).
Beauvoir, Simone de, *Une mort très douce* (Paris: Gallimard, 1964).
Beauvoir, Simone de, *La Vieillesse* (Paris: Gallimard, 1970).
Béclard, Pierre A., *Essai sur les maladies auxquelles les femmes sont le plus fréquemment exposées à l'époque de la cessation des menstrues*. Thèse (Paris: Pancoucke, 1802).
Béclere, Claude, *Les Hémorragies utérines avant et après la ménopause* (Paris: Masson, 1936).
Becquerel, Louis Alfred, *Traité élémentaire d'hygiène privée et publique* (Paris: Labé, 1851).
Becquerel, Louis Alfred, *Traité clinique des maladies de l'utérus et de ses annexes*, 2 vols (Paris: G. Baillière, 1859).
Bell, B. W., *The Sex-Complex: A Study of the Relationship of the Internal Secretions to the Female Characteristics and Functions in Health and Disease* (New York: William Wood & Co., 1916).
Belliol, Jean-Alexis, *Maladies des femmes, traité des maladies utérines*, 4th ed. (Paris: E. Dentu, 1858).
Bennet, James Henry, *Traité pratique de l'inflammation de l'utérus, de son col et de ses annexes, et des rapports de cette inflammation avec les autres affections utérine*, 4th ed. Trans. Michel Peter (Paris: P. Asselin, 1864).
Benoiston de Châteauneuf, Louis-François, *Recherches sur les consommations de tout genre de la ville de Paris en 1817, comparées à ce qu'elles étaient en 1789* (Paris: chez l'auteur, 1820).
Benoiston de Châteauneuf, Louis-François, *Mémoire sur la mortalité des femmes de l'âge de quarante à cinquante ans, lu à l'Académie des sciences, dans la séance du 13 mai 1818* (Paris: Martinet, 1822).
Benoiston de Châteauneuf, Louis-François, *Extraits des recherches statistiques sur la ville de Paris et le département de la Seine* (Paris: Bureau du Bulletin, 1824).
Benoiston de Châteauneuf, Louis-François, 'Note lue à l'Académie royale des sciences dans sa séance du 30 janvier 1826, sur les changemens qu'ont subies les lois de la mortalité en Europe, depuis un demisiècle (1775–1825)', *Le Moniteur*, 6 February 1826, 1–10.

Berger, Émile, *Les Troubles oculaires d'origine génitale chez la femme* (Paris: Félix Alcan, 1905).

Bertheaume, Marthe (Anne Darcanne-Mouroux), *L'Âge mystique* (Paris: Éditions de la vraie France, 1930).

Bertheaume, Marthe (Anne Darcanne-Mouroux), *Oublie ce tu sais* (Paris: Éditions de la vraie France, 1928).

Berthier, Pierre, *Médecine mentale* [1857], 2nd ed. (Paris: V. Masson, 1860).

Berthier, Pierre, *Des névroses menstruelles, ou La Menstruation dans ses rapports avec les maladies nerveuses et mentales* (Paris: Delahaye, 1874).

Bertholet, Marcellin, *Notice sur la vie et les travaux de M. Brown-Séquard* (Paris: Institut de France, 1898).

Bertin, Émile, *De la ménopause considérée principalement au point de vue de l'hygiène* (Montpellier: C. Coulet/Paris: Adrien Delahaye, 1866).

Bertrand, Pierre-Jean-Baptiste, *Dissertation sur l'aménorrhée définitive ou âge critique des femmes sur les accidents auxquels elles sont exposées à cette époque, et sur les moyens thérapeutiques, hygiéniques et prophylactiques les plus appropriés à leur situation.* Thèse (Paris: Didot le Jeune, 1824).

Bestion de Camboulas, Louis Alexandre Philippe, *Le Suc ovarien, effets physiologiques et thérapeutiques, organothérapies ovarienne* (Paris: J.-B. Baillière et fils, 1898).

Bey, Maïssa, *Hizya* (Paris: Aube, 2015).

Bienaymé, Gustave, 'Le Coût de la vie à Paris à diverses époques', *Journal de la Société Statistique de Paris*, 37 (1896): 375–390 [379].

Binet, Louis, Louis Berthet, Louis Papin, and Nicolas-Edmé Restif de la Bretonne, *Illustrations de Les Contemporaines ou Aventures des plus jolies femmes de l'âge présent* (Paris: No publisher identified, 1780–1782).

Blanc, Émile, *De l'opération césarienne, méthodes opératoires et indications* (Paris: Lecrosnier et Babé, 1890).

Bland-Sutton, J., 'An Address on the Perils and Complications of Fibroids after the Menopause', *The Lancet*, 161/4162 (1903): 1571–1572. Doi: 10.1016/S0140-6736(01)73078-4.

Boerhaave, Herman, *Boerhaave's Medical Correspondence Containing the Various Symptoms of Chronical Distempers, the Professor's Opinion, Method of Cure and Remedies, to which is added Boerhaave's practice in the hospital at Leyden, with his manner of instructing his pupils in the cure of diseases* (London: John Nourse, 1745).

Boerhaave, Herman, *Aphorismes de Monsieur Herman Boerhaave sur la connaissance et la cure des maladies* (Paris: Huart, Briasson & Durand, 1745).

Boiffin, Alfred, *Tumeurs fibreuses de l'utérus* (Paris: Rueff et Cie, 1893).

Boissier de Sauvages, François de, *Nosologie méthodique, dans laquelle les maladies sont rangées par classes, suivant le système de Sydenham, & l'ordre des botanistes*, 10 vols (Paris: Hérissant le fils, 1771).

Boivin, Marie Anne Victoire, *Mémorial de l'art des accouchements, suivi des Aphorismes de Mauriceau* (Paris: Méquignon père, 1812).

Boivin, Marie Anne Victoire, *Mémoire sur les hémorragies internes de l'utérus, qui a obtenu le prix d'émulation au concours ouvert (en 1818) par la Société de médecine de Paris, par Mme veuve Boivin, suivi des Aphorismes d'Andrew Blake sur les hémorragies utérines* (Paris: Gabon, 1819).

Boivin, Marie Anne Victoire Gillain, *Dell'Arte di assistere ai parti opera classica della signora Boivin*, trans. Domenico Meli (Milan: Giovanni Silvestri, 1822).

Boivin, Marie-Anne-Victoire, *Handbuch der Geburtshülfe, nach den Grundsätzen der Entbindungs-Anstalt zu Paris, und denen der berühmtesten in- und ausländischen Geburtshelfer: Mit 106 lithographirten Abbildungen, welche die Behandlung aller Arten der Entbindung zeigen, 6 synoptischen Tabellen, das Ergebniß von 24,214 Fällen darbietend, und einem Anhange: die Aphorismen von Mauriceau und Orazio Valota enthaltend*, trans. Robert Ferdiand, ed. Dietrich Wilhelm Heinrich Busch (Marburg: Johann Christian Krieger, 1829).

Boivin, Marie Anne Victoire & A. Dugès, *Traité pratique des maladies de l'utérus et de ses annexes, accompagné d'un atlas de 41 planches in-fol. gravées et coloriées, représentant les principales altérations morbides des organes génitaux de la femme*, 2 vols (Paris: J.-B. Baillière, 1833).

Boivin, Marie & A. Dugès, *A Practical Treatise on the Diseases of the Uterus and its Appendages; translated from the French of Mme. Veuve Boivin, Sage-femme Surveillante en Chef de la Maison de Santé, etc. and A. Dugès, Professeur a la Faculté de Médecine de Montpellier, etc. With Copious Notes, by G. O. Heming, F.L.S. Consulting Accoucheur to the St. Pancras Infirmary, etc* (London: Sherwood, Gilbert & Piper, 1834).

Bomare, Jacques C. Valmont de, *Dictionnaire raisonné universel d'histoire naturelle, avec L'Histoire des trois règnes, et le détail des usages de leurs productions dans la médicine, dans l'économie domestiques & champêtre, et dans les arts & métiers*, vol. 7 (Lyon: Bruyset, 1791).

Bompard, Alexis, *Cours théorique et pratique sur les maladies des femmes* (Paris: Rouvier, 1834).

Bond, C. J. 'On the Results of 50 Cases of Abdominal Hysterectomy for Fibroid Disease of the Uterus: With Remarks on the After-History of the Patients and on the Artificial Menopause', *The Lancet*, 161/4142 (1903): 162–167. Doi 10.1016/S0140-6736(00)50285-2

Bonafous, J. B. H., *Considérations physiologiques et générales sur les diverses époques de la vie de la femme*. Thèse (Paris: Didot Jeune, 1817).

Bond, C. J., 'On the Results of 50 Cases of Abdominal Hysterectomy for Fibroid Disease of the Uterus: With Remarks on the After-History of the Patients and on the Artificial Menopause', *The Lancet*, 161/4142 (1903): 162–167.

Boinet, Alphone-Alexandre, *De la gastrotomie dans les cas de tumeurs fibreuses utérines interstitielles, péri-utérines et dans les tumeurs dites fibro-cystiques* (Paris: G. Masson, 1873).

Bonier, Marius, *De la myomectomie abdominale dans le traitement des fibromes utérins* (Lyon: Imprimerie Schneider, 1904).

Bontemps, Dr F., *De l'hygiène des âges extrêmes et de la nécessité des services d'enfants dans les hôpitaux, conférence aux femmes de France* (Saumur: L. Picard, 1892).

Bordeu, Théophile de, *Recherches sur le pouls par rapport aux crises* (Paris: De Bure l'aîné, 1756).

Bordeu, Théophile de, *Recherches sur le pouls par rapport aux crises* [1756], new ed., 3 vols (Paris: Didot Jeune, 1779).

Bordeu, Théophile, 'Recherches anatomiques sur la position des glandes, et sur leur action, in idem', *Œuvres complètes*, vol. 1 [1752] (Paris: Caille et Ravier, 1818).

Bordeu, Théophile, *Œuvres complètes de Bordeu, précédées d'une notice sur sa vie et sur ses ouvrages*, ed. M. le Chevalier, 2 vols (Paris: Caille et Ravier, 1818).

Börner, Ernst, *Die Wecheseljahre der Frau* (Stuttgart: Ferdinand Enke, 1886).

Börner, Ernst, *The Menopause*, trans. H. Egbert (New York: William Wood, 1887).

Bossu, Antonin, *Anthropologie, ou Étude des organes, fonctions et maladies de l'homme et de la femme, comprenant l'anatomie, la physiologie, l'hygiène, la pathologie et la thérapeutique*, 2 vols (Paris: Comon, 1846).

Bouchardat, Apollinaire, *Traité d'hygiène publique et privée basée sur l'étiologie* [1881], 3rd ed. (Paris: Félix Alcan, 1887).

Bouchut, Eugène, *Du nervosisme aigu et chronique et des maladies nerveuses* (Paris: J. B. Baillière et fils, 1877).

Boude, Jean-Antoine, *Quelques Propositions sur l'hygiène des vieillards et des gens faibles*. Thèse (Montpellier: Jean Martel aîné, 1813).

Bouffier, Prosper & Madame Bouffier, *Maladies des femmes: Métrite chronique* (Paris: J. B. Baillière, 1862).

Boulenger, J.-B.-M.-N.-D., *Essai sur la doctrine des crises*. Thèse (Paris: Didot le Jeune, 1831).

Bourlet, Louis, *Étude sur la métrite interne chronique après la ménopause*. Thèse (Paris: A. Parent, 1879).

Boussi, Raoul, *Étude sur les troubles nerveux Réflexes observés dans les maladies utérines* (Paris: V. Adrien Delahaye, 1880).

Boyer, Philippe, *Traité des maladies chirurgicales* [1818], 7 vols, 5th ed. (Paris: Labé, 1846).

Boyveau-Laffecteur, Pierre, *Essai sur les maladies physiques et morales des femmes* (Paris: Chez l'auteur, 1789).

Brachet, Jean-Louis, *Traité de l'hystérie* (Paris: Baillière, 1847).

Brachet, Léon. *Myôme utérin délogé par le travail de l'accouchement et opéré avec succès* (Paris: J. B. Baillière et fils, 1870).

Brame, Caroline, *Le journal intime de Caroline B.* [*c.*1865], ed. Georges Ribeill & Michelle Perrot (Paris: Montalba, 1985).

Brantôme, Pierre de Bourdeille seigneur de, *Vies des dames galantes* [*c.*1666] (Paris: Victor Bunel, 1880).

Brierre de Boismont, Alexandre F., *De la menstruation, considérée dans ses rapports physiologiques et pathologiques* (Paris: Germer Baillière, 1842).

Brierre de Boismont, Alexandre F., 'Recherches bibliographiques et cliniques sur la folie puerpérale, précédées d'un aperçu sur les rapports de la menstruation et de l'aliénation mentale', *Annales médico-psychologiques* (1851): 574–610.

Brillat-Savarin, Jean Anthelme, *Physiologie du goût, avec une notice sur l'auteur par Émile de Labédollière* (Paris: G. Barba, 1851).

Briquet, Pierre, *Traité clinique et thérapeutique de l'hystérie* (Paris: J. B. Baillère et Fils, 1859).

Brissay, A., *Fragments de chirurgie et de gynécologie opératoire contemporaines* (Paris: O. Doin, 1887).

Broussais, Casimir Anne Marie, *De la Statistique appliquée à la pathologie et à la thérapeutique* (Paris: J.-B. Baillière, 1840).

Broussais, François-Joseph-Victor, *Histoire des phlegmasies ou inflammations chroniques, fondée sur de nouvelles observations de clinique et d'anatomie pathologique: Ouvrage présentant un tableau raisonné des variétés et des combinaisons diverses de ces maladies, avec leurs différentes méthodes de traitement*, 2 vols (Paris: Gabon, 1808).

Broussais, François-Joseph-Victor, *De l'irritation et de la folie: Ouvrage dans lequel les rapports du physique et du moral sont établis sur les bases de la médecine physiologique* (Paris/Brussels: Mlle Delauney/Librairie Médicale Française, 1828).

Broussais, François-Joseph-Victor, *Cours de pathologies et thérapeutique générales*, 2 vols (Paris: J. B. Baillière, 1834).

Brown-Séquard, Charles-Édouard, 'Note on the Effects Produced on Man by Subcutaneous Injections of Liquid Obtained from the Testicles of Animals', *The Lancet*, 2 (1889): 105–107.

Brown-Séquard, Charles-Édouard, 'Remarques à l'occasion du travail de M. Variot, sur les injections de liquide testiculaire chez l'homme', *Comptes rendus des séances de la Société de Biologie et de ses filiales*, 41 (1889): 454–455.

Brown-Séquard, Charles-Édouard, 'Seconde Note sur les effets produits chez l'homme par des injections sous-cutanées d'un liquide retiré des testicules frais de cobaye et de chien', *Comptes rendus des séances de la Société de Biologie et de ses filiales*, 41 (1889): 420–422.

Broye, Nicolas, *Considérations sur la cessation des règles.* Thèse (Montpellier: Jean Martel Aîné, 1813).
Bruant, Paul, *De la mélancolie survenant à la ménopause.* Thèse (Paris: Henri Jouve, 1888).
Brühl, Julius, *Über die psychischen Störungen des Klimakteriums.* Dissertation (Würzburg: A. Memminger, 1887).
Brunet, Alexis, *Contribution à l'étude des métrorragies d'origine ovarienne: Parallèle entre la radiothérapie et la curiethérapie dans les métrorragies de la ménopause.* Thèse (Montpellier: Emmanuel Montane, 1927).
Buchan, Alex P., *Observations on Indigestion in which is satisfactorily shewn the efficacy of Ipecacuan, believing this, as well as its connected train of complaints peculiar to the decline of life*, translated from the French memoir of Mr Daubenton, 1st ed. (London: J. Callow, 1807).
Buffon, Georges-Louis Leclerc Comte de & Louis-Jean-Marie Daubenton, *Histoire naturelle générale et particulière*, 15 vols (The Hague: Pierre de Hondt, 1750), vol. 3.
Buffon, Georges-Louis Leclerc de, *Histoire naturelle de l'homme et de la femme: D'après nos plus grands naturalistes*, 2nd ed. [1786] (Paris: Armand-Aubrée, 1834).
Buisson, Jean, *Contribution à l'étude des fibromes après la ménopause.* Thèse (Paris: Jouve, 1927.
Cabanis, Pierre-Jean-Georges, *Coup d'œil sur les révolutions et sur la réforme de la médecine* (Paris: Crapart, Caille & Ravier, 1804).
Cabanis, Pierre-Jean-Georges, *Rapports du physique et du moral de l'homme*, 2 vols (Paris: Crapelet, 1805).
Cabanis, Pierre-Jean-Georges, *Œuvres complètes de Cabanis*, 5 vols (Paris: Bossanges Frères/Firmin Didot, 1823–1825).
Caboche, Paul George, *Hystérectomie abdominale totale (procédé de doyen): Manuel opératoire et résultats* (Paris: G. Steinheil, 1897).
Callen, Jean Pierre Charles, *De la rareté des fibromes purs de l'utérus après la ménopause.* Thèse (Bordeaux: V. Cambette, 1924).
Camboulives, Marcellin, *L'Homme et la femme à tous les âges de la vie: Etude hygiénique, médicale, physiologique, sociale et morale* (Paris: E. Flammarion, 1890).
Canstatt, K. F., *Die Krankenheiten des höheren Alters und ihre Heilung*, 2 vols (Erlangen: Ferdinand Enke, 1839).
Canu, Étienne, *Résultats thérapeutiques de la castration chez la femme: Conséquences sociales et abus de cette opération* (Paris: Ollier-Henry, 1897).
Capuron, Joseph, *Traité des maladies des femmes, depuis la puberté jusqu'à l'âge critique inclusivement.* Thèse (Paris: Croullebois, 1812).
Carnot, Hector, *Mouvement de la population féminine de 1813 à 1855, dans la ville de Paris et mortalité comparée de la jeunesse de 15 à 25 ans dans cet intervalle* (Paris: Moquet, 1857).
Carriat, René, *Une complication des fibromes utérins après la ménopause (leur gangrène et leur nécrobiose).* Thèse (Bordeaux: Victor Cambett, 1923).
Castagné, Henri, *De l'ablation des annexes de l'utérus dans l'hystérie* (Montpellier: Charles Boehm, 1891).
Castan, (Dr) André, *Hygiène de l'âge de retour* (Paris: J. B. Baillière et Fils, 1901).
Caternault, Stanislas, *Essai sur la gastrotomie dans les cas de tumeurs fibreuses péri-utérines; précédé des 8 premières observations relatives aux 8 premières ablations de la matrice pratiquées par E. Koeberlé* (Paris: J.-B. Baillière et fils/Londres: Hippolyte Baillière, 1866).
Chahinian, Yervant-Vahram, *Contribution à l'étude de la neurasthénie liée aux trois grandes étapes génitales de la femme, puberté, union sexuelle, ménopause, considérée plus spécialement dans ses rapports avec l'éducation.* Thèse (Bordeaux: J. Pechade, 1899).

Chaix (Laboratoire), *Manuel de l'opothérapie: Revue des médications thyroïdienne, ovarienne, testiculaire ou orchitique, thymique* (Paris: Chaix Dépositaires, 1910).

Chamberlain, Geoffrey, *From Witchcraft to Wisdom: A History of Obstetrics & Gynaecology in the British Isles* (London: Royal College of Obstetrics and Gynaecologists Press, 2007).

Chambon de Montaux, Nicolas, *Des maladies des femmes*, 2 vols (Paris: Rue et Hôtel Serpente, 1784).

Chambon de Montaux, Nicolas, *Des maladies des filles*, 2 vols (Paris: Rue et Hôtel Serpente, 1785).

Chambon de Montaux, Nicholas, *Les Maladies de la grossesse* (Paris: Rue et Hôtel Serpente, 1785).

Chambon de Montaux, Nicholas, *Maladies chroniques à la cessation des règles* (Paris: Dugour et Durand, 1798).

Chomel, Auguste François, *Éléments de pathologie générale* [1817], 2nd ed. (Paris: Crochard, 1824).

Chandelux, Louis, *L'Âge critique de la femme (ménopause)*. Thèse (Paris: Irgnoux, 1850).

Chapiro, Aron, *La Physiologie de l'ovaire dans ses rapports avec le traitement des troubles de la ménopause*. Thèse (Lausanne: Imprimerie de l'Université, 1912).

Charcot, Jean-Marie, *Leçons du mardi à la Salpêtrière. Policlinique 1888–1889*. Notes de cours de M. M. Blin (Paris: Bureaux du Progrès médicale/E. Lecrosnier & Babé, 1889).

Charcot, Jean-Marie, *Leçons sur l'hystérie virile*, introd. M. Ouerd (Paris: Le Sycamore, 1984).

Charreire, Adolphe, *Myomes et ménopause, atrophie, dégénérescences malignes, indications*. Thèse (Montpellier: G. Firmin, Montane & Sicardi, 1907).

Charrier, Paul Robert, *Revue critique du Traité de gynécologie du Docteur Pozzi* (Paris: Asselin & Houzeau, 1890).

Charrier, Paul Robert, *De la castration tubo-ovarienne comme traitement radical des salpingites chroniques non suppurées, des métrorrhagies causées par les fibromes et de la dysménorrhée ovarienne, d'après les documents et observations recueillis dans le service du Dr Pozzi* (Paris: Topographie A. Davie, 1892).

Chaslon, Maurice, *Essai sur la menstruation* (Paris: Didot Jeune, 1803).

Chassigny, H., *Régression de myome utérin* (Lyon: Association typographique, 1883).

Chastelain, Jean, *Traité des convulsions et des mouvemens convulsifs, qu'on appelle à présent vapeurs* (Paris: J. Annison, 1691).

Chatelain, J.-Victor, *Essai sur la menstruation*. Thèse (Paris: Didot Jeune, 1827).

Chazal, S. G., *De l'hygiène des femmes à l'époque de la cessation des menstrues*. Thèse (Paris: Didot Jeune, 1826).

Chéneaux, Marie-Gustave Léopold, *De la menstruation et de la ménopause, au point de vue de la physiologie et de l'hygiène*. Thèse (Paris: Rignoux, 1859).

Chéreau, Achille, *Mémoires pour servir à l'étude des maladies des ovaires; Première Mémoire* (Paris: Fortin & Masson, 1844).

Chéreau, Georges, *Notions d'hygiène, suivies d'un bref raccourci des origines et de l'histoire des Français* (Caen: Maurice Toutain, 1921).

Chouffe, Jean-Baptiste-P., *Des accidents et des maladies qui surviennent à la cessation de la menstruation*. Thèse (Paris: Croullebois & Gabon, 1802).

Chrobak, Rudolph, 'Über Einverleibung von Eierstockgewebe', *Centralblatt für Gynäkologie*, 20 (1896): 521–524.

Cianfrani, Theodore, *A Short History of Obstetrics and Gynecology* (Springfield, Ill.: Charles C. Thomas, 1960).

Clair, Antoine, *Essai sur les vapeurs en général, et sur l'hystérie en particulier* (Montpellier: Jean Martel aîné, 1814).

Clément, Étienne, *Cardiopathie de la ménopause* (Paris: G. Masson, 1884).

Clerc, Alexis, *Hygiène et médecine des deux sexes; suivies d'un Dictionnaire d'hygiène et de Médecine*, 2 vols (Paris: Jules Rouff et Cie, 1885).

Cocheret, François Frédéric, *De la valeur des métrorragies après la ménopause comme signe de cancer de l'utérus et comme indication de l'hystérectomie totale abdominale*. Thèse (Paris: H. Jouve, 1909).

Cohnstein, 'Zur Physiologie der Menopause', *Archiv für Pathologische Anatomie und Physiologie und für Klinische Medicin*, 61/1 (1874): 100–109.

Colette (Sidonie-Gabrielle), *La Naissance du jour* (Paris: Flammarion, 1993).

Collinet, Marc, *Des modifications des organes génitaux de la femme à l'époque de la ménopause*. Thèse (Paris: Librairie Ollier-Henry, 1887).

Colombat de l'Isère, Marc, *L'Hystérotomie ou l'amputation du col de la matrice dans les affections cancéreuses, suivant un nouveau procédé, avec la description de l'hystérotome et de plusieurs autres instrumens nouveaux présentés à la faculté de médecine de Paris* (Paris: Mansut Fils, 1828).

Colombat de l'Isère, Marc, *Traité des maladies des femmes et de l'hygiène spéciale de leur sexe*, 2 vols (Paris: Librairie médicale de Labé, 1838–1843).

Colombat de l'Isère, Marc, *A Treatise on the Diseases of Women and Special Hygiene of Females*, trans. Charles D. Meigs (Philadelphia : Lean & Blanchard, 1850).

Combemale, Pierre & Henri Demacon, *La Sécretion interne de l'ovaire et l'entretien de l'activité intellectuelle* (Lille: Imprimerie centrale, 1927).

Combres, Jean-Louis-Victor, *Dissertation sur la médecine conservatrice, ou l'hygiène*. Thèse (Montpellier: Jean Martel, 1813).

Corbichon, Jean, *Le Grand Propriétaire de toutes choses, Isidore de Seville* (Paris: Jean Longis, 1556).

Corvisart, Jean-Nicholas, *Essai sur les maladies et les lésions organiques du cœur et des gros vaisseaux* (Paris: Imprimerie Migneret, 1806).

Coste, Jean-Paul-Édouard-Boniface, *Considérations générales sur la menstruation*. Thèse (Montpellier: Boehm, 1837).

Coste, Jean-Paul-Édouard-Boniface, *Histoire générale et particulière du développement des corps organises, publiée sous les auspices du Ministre de l'instruction publique* (Paris: Victor Masson, 1847).

Coural, Joseph-Lazare-Jacques, *Considérations générales sur les phénomènes physiologique et pathologique de la femme aux divers âges de la vie*. Thèse (Montpellier: Jean Martel, 1822).

Courrier, Robert, *La Physiologie de l'ovaire* (Alençon : Imprimerie alençonnaise, 1948).

Courty, Amédée, *Traité pratique des maladies de l'utérus, des ovaires et des trompes* [1866] (Paris: P. Asselin, 1872).

Cros, F., *Du rhumatisme coïncidant avec l'âge critique et de son traitement par les eaux de Lamalou-l'Ancien* (Nice: V.-E. Gauthier, 1884).

Crosilhes, Hippolyte Pierre, *Hygiène et maladies des femmes* (Paris: Moquet, 1850).

Currier, Andrew Fay, *The Menopause* (New York: D. Appleton & Co.: 1897).

Dagassan, Daniel, *Dissertation sur l'hystérie, vulgairement connue sous le nom de vapeurs* (Montpellier: Jean Martel aîné, 1819).

Dagonet, Henri, *Traité élémentaire et pratique des maladies mentales, suivi de considérations pratiques sur l'administration des asiles d'aliénés* (Paris: J. B. Baillière et fils, 1862).

Daignan, Guillaume, *Tableau des variétés de la vie humaine* (Paris: Chez l'auteur, 1786).

Dalché, Paul, *Troubles gastriques de la ménopause et leur traitement* (Paris: G. Maurin, 1900).

Dalché, Paul, *Gynécologie médicale; opothérapie; puberté; glandes endocrines* (Paris: Vigot, 1915).

Dalché, Paul & Albert Robin, *Gynécologie médicale: Traitement des maladies des femmes* (Paris: J. Rueff, 1900).

Daléas, Pierre, *Accidents tardifs de la castration ovarienne et ménopause physiologique.* Thèse (Toulouse: Impr. Du Centre, 1922).

Dallemagne, Jules, *Dégénérés et déséquilibrés* (Brussels: H. Lamertin, 1895).

Dalsace, Jean, *Castration ovarienne et troubles du métabolisme minéral: A propos d'ostéopathies douloureuses succédant à la ménopause artificielle. Travail du service du professeur agrégé Lévy-Solal.* Thèse (Paris: Louis Arnette, 1926).

Dalsace, Jean, *De certaines algies de la ménopause, essai pathogénique et thérapeutique* (Paris: Masson, 1927).

Darcanne-Mouroux, Anne (Marthe Bertheaume), *Contribution à l'étude clinique de la ménopause précoce.* Thèse (Paris: H. Jouve, 1904).

Dartigues, Louis, *Chirurgie conservatrice de l'utérus et des annexes dans le traitement des fibromes* (Paris: Maloine, 1901).

Daubenton, Louis-Jean-Marie, *Histoire naturelle des animaux*, vol. 1 of the *Encyclopédie méthodique*, ed. Denis Diderot & Jean le Rond D'Alembert (Paris: Panckoucke, 1782).

Daubenton, Louis-Jean-Marie, *Mémoire sur les indigestions qui commence à être plus fréquents, pour la plupart des hommes, à l'âge de quarante ou quarante-cinq ans* (Paris: Pierres, Debure, Didot, Goué & Née de la Rochelle, 1784).

Daudet, Léon, *Le Stupide dix-neuvième siècle: Exposé des insanités meurtrières qui se sont abattues sur la France depuis 130 ans, 1789–1919* (Paris: Nouvelle Librairie Nationale, 1922).

Daudet, Léon, *Les Morticoles* (Paris: Bibliothèque Charpentier, 1894).

Daudet, Léon, *Devant la douleur* (Paris: Nouvelle librairie nationale, 1914).

Debay, Auguste, *Histoire naturelle de l'homme et de la femme* (Paris: E. Dentu, 1862).

Debourge, Jean Baptiste, *L'Hygiène de la vieillesse et les conseils pour la longévité, causeries du dimanche* (Montdidier: Mérot, 1869).

Dechambre, Amédée, ed., *Dictionnaire encyclopédique des sciences médicales*, 27 vols in 5 series (Paris: G. Masson & P. Asselin, 1874–1889).

Deffand, Madame du (Marie de Vichy-Chamrond), *D'Éros à Agape, où les correspondances de Mme du Deffand avec Horace Walpole*, ed. Olivier Deshayes (Paris: L'Harmattan, 2011).

Dejerine, Jules, *L'Hérédité dans les maladies du système nerveux* (Paris: Asselin et Houzeau, 1886).

Delagénière, Henri, *Supériorité de la laparotomie sur l'hystérectomie vaginale dans les cas de suppurations pelviennes* (Paris: F. Alcan, 1893).

Delestrée, Mme, *Le Conseiller secret des femmes, ou Conseils sur les moyens de se préserver des maladies qui atteignent spécialement les femmes* [1861 Wion Pigalé], 7th ed. (Paris: Chez l'auteur, 1875).

Delétang, Dr, *Du traitement des fibromes utérins par la méthode d'Apostoli* (Paris: O. Doin, 1889).

Demangeon, Jean-Baptiste, *Anthropogénèse ou génération de l'homme, avec des vues de comparaison sur les reproductions des trois règnes de la nature, et des recherches sur la conservation des espèces et des races* (Paris: Rouen Frères, 1829).

Deparcieux, Antoine, *Essai sur les probabilités de la durée de la vie humaine, d'où l'on déduit la manière de déterminer les rentes viagères, tant simples qu'en Tontines* (Paris: Frères Guerin, 1746).

Deslandes, Pierre-Joseph, *An Morborum, cessante mensium fluxu, therapeia, quae difficillema, rationali medicina duce, felicior?* (Paris: Quillau, 1786).

Desmarres, 'Clinique ophtalmologique: Amaurose cérébrale double, due à la suppression de l'époque menstruelle. Guérison. Par M. le Docteur Xavier Galezowski', *Gazette des Hôpitaux* (1864): 138.

Desruelles, H. M. J. '*De la ménopause ou l'âge critique des femmes*, par Ch. P.L. De Gardanne, D.M.P; seconde édition, Paris, 1821. In-8° de 447 pages', in J.-B. Regnault, *Journal universel des sciences médicales*, 25 (Paris: Baudouin Frères, 1822), 170–186.

Devay, Francis, *Traité spécial d'hygiène des familles: particulièrement dans ses rapports avec le mariage au physique et au moral et les maladies héréditaires* (Paris: Labé, 1858).

Devergie, Alphonse, *Médecine légale, théorique et pratique, avec le texte et l'interprétation des lois relatives à la médecine légale*, 2 vols (Brussels: H. Dumont, 1837).

Devers, Jacques, *Essai sur la cessation des règles*. Thèse (Paris: Didot le Jeune, 1822).

Devi, Ananda, *Indian Tango* (Paris: Gallimard, 2007).

Dewees, William M. Potts, *Treatise on the Disease of Females* (Philadelphia: H. C. Carey & I. Lea, 1826).

Dezeimeris, Jean-Eugène, *Dictionnaire historique de la médecine ancienne et moderne*, 3 vols (Paris: Béchet Jeune, 1837).

D'Hooghe, 'De l'influence des maladies zygomatiques sur la grossesse, la parturition et ses suites', *Annales de la Société de Médecine d'Anvers*, 36 (1874): 70–86.

Diderot, Denis, ed., *Encyclopédie, ou Dictionnaire raisonné des sciences, des arts et des métiers par une société de gens de lettres*, 17 vols (Neuchâtel: Faulche, 1765).

Dionis, Pierre, *Cours d'opérations de chirurgie démontrées au Jardin royal* (Paris: Laurent d'Houry, 1714).

Dionis, Pierre, *Traité général des accouchements, qui instruit de tout ce qu'il faut faire pour être habile accoucheur* (Paris: C.-M. d'Houry, 1718).

Dioscorides of Anazarbus, Petanius, *De materia medica*, trans. Lily Y. Beck (Hildesheim: Georg Olms Verlag, 2017).

Dirlewanger, Dominique, *Les Couleurs de la vieillesse: Histoire culturelle des représentations de la vieillesse en Suisse et en France (1940–1990)* (Neuchâtel: Alphil-Presses universitaires suisses, 2018).

Docé, Lucien-Hector, *Dissertation sur la cessation des menstrues vulgairement appelée âge critique, et sur les moyens hygiéniques que réclame la santé de la femme à cette époque*. Thèse (Paris: Didot Jeune, 1831).

Doisy, Edward A. & J. O. Ralls, 'The Extraction of Some Properties of an Ovarian Hormone', *Journal of Biological Chemistry*, 61 (1924): 711–727.

Domont, Antoine Joseph, *Dissertation sur la menstruation*. Thèse (Paris: Didot Jeune, 1807).

Dostoyevsky, Fyodor, *Buried Alive, or, Ten Years Penal Servitude in Siberia*, trans. Marie von Thilo (London: Longmans, Green, and Co., 1881).

Drake, Emma Angell, *What a Woman of Forty-Five Ought to Know* (Philadelphia: Vir Publishing, 1901).

Drake, Emma Angell, *Ce que toute femme de 45 ans devrait savoir (l'âge critique)* (Geneva: J. H. Jeheber, 1908).

Drevet, Louis, *Effets thérapeutiques du corps jaune de l'ovaire, en particulier dans l'hypofonction de la glande ovarienne, la ménopause naturelle, la ménopause post-opératoire*. Thèse (Paris: G. Steinheil, 1907).

Dubois d'Amiens, F., *Histoire philosophique de l'hypochondrie et de l'hystérie* (Paris: Deville Cavellin, 1833).

Dubreuilh, Charles, *Quelques Considérations sur le développement de la sensibilité aux diverses époques de la vie de la femme* (Bordeaux: Crugy, 1859).

Ducet, Michel, *L'Âge climatérique de l'homme et de la femme, retour d'âge et crise sexuelle* (Soissons: Aubenas, 1964).

Duchamp, V., *De l'amputation par le vagin de l'utérus artificiellement inversé comme complément de l'opération césarienne* (Saint-Étienne: J. Pichon, 1886).

Ducuing, Joseph, *Les Indications du traitement des fibromes utérins en dehors de la grossesse*. Thèse (Bordeaux: Imprimerie de l'Université, 1935).

Ducuing, Joseph, *Le Fibro-myome utérin: Statistiques, critiques et commentaires sur une série personnelle de 1.300 cas dont 547 inédits: Fibromatose expérimentale, physiologie de l'ovaire irradié* (Paris: Masson, 1946).

Dumas, Charles Louis, *Questiones medicinae duodecim* (Montpellier: J.-F. Tournel, 1790).

Dumas, Charles-Louis, *Principes de physiologie, ou Introduction à la science expérimentale, philosophique et médicale de l'homme vivant*, 2 vols (Paris: Crapelet, 1800).

Dumoulin, *Nouveau Traité du rhumatisme et des vapeurs* [1703], 2nd ed. (Paris: d'Houry, 1710).

Duncan, Daniel, *Seconde et troisième partie de la chimie naturelle, ou l'Explication chimique et mécanique de l'évacuation particulière aux femmes et de la génération* (Paris: L. d'Houry, 1687).

Duplessis, E., *De l'Âge critique et des soins hygiéniques que réclament les femmes à cette époque*. Thèse (Paris: Didot Le Jeune, 1828).

Duprat, Frank, *La Puberté tardive dans ses rapports avec la fonction menstruelle, la fécondité et la précocité de la ménopause*. Thèse (Paris: Vigot Frères, 1911).

Dupuy, Henri-Paul-Marie, *Métrite hémorrhagique de la ménopause et de la vieillesse*. Thèse (Bordeaux: Imprimerie du Midi, 1897).

Durieux, Etienne-Paul-Jean, *La Fonction ovarienne et les troubles de la ménopause dans leurs rapports avec la radiothérapie des fibro-myomes utérins*. Thèse (Paris: Louis Arnette, 1920).

Dussault, *Essai sur les hémorrhagies actives du système muqueux considérées comme crises dans les maladies aiguës*. Thèse (Paris: Didot Jeune, 1818).

Edvinsson, Rodney, *Historical Currency Converter* (test version 1.0). <Historicalstatistics.org>: <https://www.historicalstatistics.org/Currencyconverter.html> (viewed 30 November 2021).

Esquirol, Étienne D., *Des maladies mentales considérées sous les rapports médical, hygiénique et médico-légal*, 2 vols (Paris: J. B. Baillière, 1838).

Fabricius, Joseph, *Über Myome und Fibrome des Uterus und deren Einfluss auf die Umgebung* (Vienna/Leipzig: W. Braumüller, 1895).

Faciolle, C. A., *La Femme de quarante ans, ou Les Femmes à vapeurs: Comédie en un acte et en prose, représentée pour la première fois, à Paris, sur le théâtre des Variétés, au Palais-Royal* (Paris: Delauney, 1805).

Farbe, François, *Bibliothèque du médecin-praticien, ou résumé général de tous les ouvrages de clinique médicale et chirurgicale*. Tome II: *Maladies des Femmes, maladies de l'appareil urinaire* (Paris: Libraire le Boucher, 1844).

Faure, Jean-Louis & Armand Siredy, *Traité de gynécologie médico-chirurgicale* (Paris: Octave Doin et fils, 1911).

Féré, Charles, *La Famille névropathique: Théorie tératologique de l'hérédité et de la prédisposition morbides et de la dégénérescence*, 2nd ed. (Paris: F. Alcan, 1898).

Féré, Charles, *L'Instinct sexuel: Évolution et dissolution* (Paris: Félix Alcan, 1899).

Ferenczi, Sandor, 'Die psychiatrische Schule von Bordeaux über die Psychoanalyse', in Sandor Ferenczi, *Bausteine zur Psychoanalyse*, 4 vols (Bern: Hans Huber, 1939), vol. 4, 12–24.

Fiessinger, Dr Ch., 'L'Inaptitude médicale des femmes', *La Médecine moderne: Journal de thérapeutique, de médecine, de chirurgie, d'accouchements et de pharmacologie*, 11/11 (7 February 1900), 81.

Fitzgerald, Gérard, *Tractatus pathologicus de affectibus feminarum praeternaturalibus* (Paris: J. Neaulme, 1754).

Fitzgerald, Gérard, *Traité des maladies des femmes* (Paris: Duchesne, 1758).

Florin, Marie, *La Curiethérapie dans le traitement des métropathies hémorragiques de la ménopause*. Thèse (Genève: Benno Schwabe, 1929).

Flourens, A. *De l'opothérapie* (Bordeaux: G. Gounouilhou, 1899).

Fodéré, François-Emmanuel, *Traité de médecine légale et d'hygiène publique ou de police de santé* (Paris: Mane, 1813).

Forbes, John, Alexander Tweedie, & John Conolly, *Cyclopedia of Practical Medicine, comprising treatises on the nature and treatment of disease, materia medica and therapeutics, medical jurisprudence, etc, etc.*, 4 vols (London: Sherwood, Gilbert & Piper, 1833).

Force, Victor, *Du rhumatisme à la ménopause*. Thèse (Paris: A. Parent, 1877).

Fothergill, John, 'On the Management Proper at the Cessation of the Menses', *Medical Observations and Inquiries*, 5 (London: Cadell, 1776): 160–186.

Fothergill, John, *Conseils pour les femmes de quarante-cinq à cinquante ans, ou conduite à tenir lors de la cessation des règles* [1778] (Paris: Briand, 1778).

Fothergill, John, *Conseils aux femmes sur les moyens de prévenir ou d'arrêter les suites facheuses de leur temps critique*, trans. Charles François Simon Giraudy (Paris: Crochard, 1805).

Fougerolles, François de, *De senum affectibus prœcavendis, nonnullisque curandis enarratio* (Lyon: J. de Gabiano et L. Durand, 1610).

Fouquet, Marie, *Recueil des remèdes faciles et domestiques*, 5th ed. (Dijon: Jean Ressayre, 1704).

François, Simon, *Essai sur les crises*. Thèse (Paris: Didot Jeune, 1831).

Froment, N., *Dissertation sur la métrite chronique*. Thèse (Paris: Didot Jeune, 1828).

Furetière, Antoine, 'Climacterique', *Le Dictionnaire universel* [1690] 3rd ed., 3 vols, vol. 1 (Rotterdam: Leers, 1708).

Gaboriau, Auguste Clément Marie, *Du surmenage intellectuel et de son traitement préventif par l'emploi simultané du phosphure de zinc et de l'arséniate de strychnine*. Thèse (Paris: Jouve, 1897).

Gaboriau, Hélina, *Essai sur la genèse et l'évolution de la thérapeutique* (Paris: A. Maloine, 1898).

Gaboriau, Hélina, *Les Trois Ages de la femme: Puberté, maternité, ménopause* (Paris: Larousse, 1923).

Gaboriau, Isabelle, *Contribution à l'étude des métrorragies dites essentielles de la ménopause*. Thèse (Paris: Jouve, 1919).

Gagnebé, Joseph, *Exposition de quelques maladies qui attaquent les femmes à la cessation des règles*. Thèse (Montpellier: Imprimerie de Tournel, 1801).

Gallais, Jean-Pierre, *Mœurs et caractères du dix-neuvième siècle*, 2 vols (Paris: Belin-leprieur, 1817).

Gallard, Théophile, *Mesures à prendre pour diminuer le mortalité parmi les femmes en couche*, discours prononcé à la Société médicale des hôpitaux, dans la séance du 11 février 1870 (Paris: J. B. Baillière, 1870).

Gallard, Théophile, *Pathologie des ovaires: Leçons cliniques sur la menstruation et ses troubles* (Paris: Baillère, 1885).

Garat, *Influence de la ménopause sur le développement de l'aliénation mentale*. Thèse (Paris: G. Steinheil, 1898).

Garceau, Edgar, *Vaginal Hysterectomy as Done in France* (New York: William Wood & Co., 1895).

Gardanne, Charles-Pierre-Louis de, *Dissertation sur les avis à donner aux femmes qui entrent dans l'âge critique*. Thèse (Paris: Didot Jeune, 1812).

Gardanne, Charles-Pierre-Louis de, *Avis aux femmes qui entrent dans l'âge critique* (Paris: Gabon, 1816).

Gardanne, Charles-Pierre-Louis de, *De la ménopause ou de l'âge critique des femmes* (Paris: Méquignon-Marvis, 1821).

Gerdessus, Alexandre-Jacques-Bernard, *La Ménopause et son rôle en psychiatrie* (Toulouse: Dirion, 1910).

Gardien, Claude Martin, *Traité d'accouchemens et des maladies des filles, des femmes et des enfans*, 4 vols (Paris: Crochard, 1807).

Garnier, Joseph-François, *Considérations sur l'âge critique, et sur l'hygiène des femmes à cette époque*. Thèse (Paris: Didot Jeune, 1820).

Gaudin, Jean, *Contribution à l'étude du traitement actuel des troubles produits par la ménopause opératoire*. Thèse (Bordeaux: Y. Cadoret, 1930).

Gaume, Jean-Clément-Jules, *Contribution à l'étude de l'action du bain carbo-gazeux naturel sur les troubles de la ménopause*. Thèse (Nancy: C. Thomas, 1930).

Gavilan, A. P., *De l'hystérectomie vaginale dans les cas de fibromes utérins* (Paris: Berthier, 1888).

Gellius, Aulus, *Les Nuits attaques*, trans. Mm. E. de Chaumont, Félix Flambart, & E. Buisson (Paris: C. L. F. Pancoucke, 1846).

Gendrin, Augustin Nicolas, *Traité philosophique de médecine pratique*, 3 vols (Paris: G. Baillière, 1839).

Gendrin, Augustin Nicolas, *De l'influence des âges sur les maladies* (Paris: Baillère, 1840).

Genest, Dr Louis, *Comment prévenir et guérir les maladies du retour d'âge: Hygiène préventive; les soins spéciaux; les meilleurs remèdes* (Paris: M. Drouin, *c.*1920).

Gensse, Mme A., *La Femme et la génération* (Paris: J.-B. Baillière et fils, 1894).

Gensse, Mme A., *Les Quatre Ages de la femme au point de vue physiologique, cinquième édition* (Corbeil: E. Crété, 1899).

Gensse, Mme A., ed., *La Beauté par l'hygiène: Journal de la famille: Médecine, littérature, sciences, arts*, 15 Janvier (1900), mensuel, 28cm.

Gentilhomme, Ernest-Jules-Henri, *Hystérectomie abdominale: Technique, critique, résultats* (Paris: Georges Carré, 1894).

Georget, Étienne-Jean, *De la folie, considérations sur cette maladie, suivies de recherches cadavériques* (Paris: Crevot, 1820).

Georget, Étienne-Jean, *De la physiologie du système nerveux et spécialement du cerveau, recherches sur les maladies nerveuses en général et en particulier sur le siège, la nature et le traitement de l'hystérie, de l'hypochondrie, de l'épilepsie et de l'asthme convulsif*, 2 vols (Paris: J.-B. Baillière, 1821).

Georget, Étienne-Jean, *De la folie ou aliénation mentale* (Paris: Rignoux, 1823).

Gérard, Bernard-Eugène, *De l'âge critique chez la femme, et des maladies qui l'accompagnent*. Thèse (Paris: Rignoux, 1849).

Giehm, Gerhard, *Überwindung der Wechseljahre bei Mann und Frau (keine Wechseljahre mehr)* (Hanover: Wilkens, 1952).

Gilibert, Jean-Emanuel, *L'Anarchie médicinale, ou, La Médecine considérée comme nuisible à la société*, 3 vols (Neuchatel: No publisher stated, 1772).

Giraud, Jean-Claude, *Essai sur la ménespausie ou cessation des menstrues*. Thèse (Montpellier: Jean Martel, 1824).

Giraudy, Charles-François-Simon, *Conseils aux femmes sur les moyens de prévenir ou d'arrêter les suites fâcheuses de leur temps critique par le Docteur Fothergill de Londres, traduit de l'anglais* (Paris: Crochard, 1805).

Glisson, Francis, *Tractatus de natura substantiae energetica, seu de vita naturae* (London: Flesher, 1672).

Glinel, P. N., *Sur l'âge critique des femmes*. Thèse (Paris: Didot Jeune, 1818).

Godart, Maurice, *Ménopause précoce et obésité*. Thèse (Paris: Steinheil, 1908).

Gomès, M. S., *De l'opothérapie ovarienne, contribution à l'étude physiologique et thérapeutique de l'ovarine*. Thèse (Paris: Georges Carré & C. Naud,1898).

Goncourt, Edmond de & Jules de Goncourt, *Madame Gervaisais* (Paris: A. Lacroix, Verhoeckhoven & Cie, 1869).

Goubelly, Claude André, *Connoissances nécessaires sur la grossesse, sur les maladies laiteuses et sur la cessation des règles; ouvrage utile au sexe, et aux gens de l'art*, 2 vols (Paris: Chez l'auteur, 1785).

Goulin, Jean and Anselme L. B. Bréchillet Jourdain, *Le Médecin des dames, ou l'art de les conserver en santé* (Paris: Vincent, 1771).

Graaf, Reinier de, *A New Treatise Concerning the Generative Organs of Women* [1668], trans. H. D. Jocelyn and B. P. Setchell, *Journal of Reproduction and Fertility*, 17 (1972): 1–222.

Gravis, J.-P., *Dissertation sur la cessation des menstrues, et sur les conseils à donner aux femmes pour les préserver des accidents ou maladies dont elles sont menacées à cette époque*. Thèse (Paris: Didot Jeune, 1813).

Grévin, Nicolas-Marie, *Essai sur les crises*. Thèse (Montpellier: Jean Martel, 1825).

Grisolle, Augustin, *Traité de pathologie interne* [1844], 8th ed., 2 vols (Paris V. Masson et fils, 1862).

Gubian, Louis, *Considérations générales sur l'état physiologique de la femme parvenue à l'âge critique, et sur les moyens hygiéniques qui lui conviennent*. Thèse (Paris: Didot Jeune, 1816).

Guéneau de Mussy, Noël, 'Remèdes secrètes' (Séance du 11 Novembre 1847, Académie royale de médecine), *Archives générales de médecine*, 18 (Paris: Béchet jeune, 1928), 581–585.

Guéneau de Mussy, Noël, 'L'Érotisme de la ménopause', *Gazette hebdomadaire de médecine et de chirurgie*, 37 (13 October 1871): 591–595.

Guilbert, J. N., *Des purgatifs à la cessation des menstrues*. Thèse (Paris: Imprimerie de la Bibliothèque Médicale, 1803).

Guilbert, Yvette, *Comment on devient une étoile* (Paris, 1893).

Guilbert, Yvette, *La Vedette*, 7th ed. (Paris: H. Simonis Empis, 1902).

Guilbert, Yvette, *Les Demi-vieilles* (Paris: Félix Juven, 1902).

Guillarmou, Angélina, *Kinésithérapie gynécologique: Valeur hémostatique de certains mouvements musculaires contre les méno et métrorrhagies chroniques (système de Brandt). Etude pratique*. Thèse (Paris: Steinheil, 1896).

Guillaume, Émile, *Le Myome utérin à la ménopause*. Thèse (Lyon: J. Prudhomme, 1910).

Guillit de Chatellus, Thomas, *Recherches physiologique et médicales sur l'influence et les modifications qu'apportent dans l'économie de la femme et la première apparition et la cessation absolue des règles*. Thèse (Montpellier: Auguste Ricard, 1807).

Guimbail, Henri, *De la folie à la ménopause*. Thèse (Paris: A. Delahaye, 1884).

Guyétant, Sébastien, *Le Médecin de l'âge de retour et la vieillesse: conseils aux gens du monde, qui ont passé l'âge de quarante-cinq ans* (Paris: Dufey, 1836).

Guyétant, Sébastien, *Conseils aux femmes, ou Moyens de se préserver et de se guérir de la leucorrhée* (Paris, chez l'auteur, 1836).

Guyétant, Sébastien, *Notice historique et biographique sur M. Noel des Questonnières, ancien Commissaire-général des Armées Françaises, agé de 116 ans* (par l'auteur du Médecin de l'âge du retour et de la vielliesse) (Paris: chez l'auteur, 1844).

Guyétant, Sébastien, *Nouvelles Considérations sur la longévité humaine* (Paris: Chez l'auteur, 1863).

Guyétant, Sébastien, *L'Âge de retour et la vieillesse: Conseils au gens du monde* (Paris: L. Brunet, 1870).

Guyon, Jean Casimir Félix, *Étude sur les cavités de l'utérus à l'état de vacuité* (Paris: Rignoux, 1858).

Guyon, Jean Casimir Félix, *Des tumeurs fibreuses de l'utérus* (Paris: Adrien Delahaye, 1860).

Guyot, Gilbert Joseph Magdeleine, *Quelques propositions sur la femme considérée dans les différentes périodes de la vie.* Thèse (Montpellier: Jean Martel, 1817).

Haime, Auguste, *Réflexions sur les différents âges de la vie de l'homme* (Tours: Ladevèze, 1857).

Halford, H., 'On the Climacteric Disease', *Medical Transactions*, 4 (1813): 316–328.

Hallé, Jean-Noël, 'Âge', *Encyclopédie méthodique, Médecine*, vol. 1 (Paris: Panckoucke, 1787), 358–361.

Haller, Albrecht von, *Elementa physiologiae corporis humani*, vol. 8, Part II (Berne: Sumptibus Sumptibus Societatis Typographicae, 1766).

Halley, Edmond, 'An Estimate of the Degrees of the Mortality of Mankind, drawn from the curious tables of the births and funerals of the city of Breslaw, with an attempt to ascertain the price of annuities upon lives', *Philosophical Transactions*, 17 (1693): 596–610

Hardy, A. & J. Béhier, *Traité élémentaire de pathologie interne* (Paris: Labé, 1850–1858).

Harreaux, Charles-Victor, *Essai sur une variété d'hypocondrie particulière aux femmes de l'âge critique.* Thèse (Paris: Rignoux et Ce, 1837).

Hart, David Berry & Alexander Hugh Freeland Barbour, *Manual of Gynecology* [1882], 2nd ed. (Edinburgh: W. & A. K. Johnston, 1883).

Hayès, Dr, *Hygiène de l'âge critique* (Paris: Librairie des publications modernes, 1891).

Hébert, Etienne-Léandre, *Dissertation sur la cessation des règles, les accidens auxquels la femme est alors exposée, et les précautions qu'elle doit prendre pour les éviter* (Paris: Didot Jeune, 1817).

Hecquet, Philippe, *De purgandâ medicinâ a curarum sordibus* (Paris: Chavelier, 1714).

Hecquet, Philippe, *Lettre sur la convulsionnaire en extase, ou la vaporeuse en rêve* (unpublished, 1736).

Hegar, Alfred, 'Zur Ovariotomie, die intraperitoneale Versorgung des Stiels der Ovarientumoren; Schicksale und Effecte versenkter Ligaturen, abgeschnürter Gewebsstücke, Brandschorfe, vollständig getrennte Massen oder zurückgelassener Flüssigkeiten in der Bauchhöhle', *Gynäkologie*, 36, *Klinische Vorträge* 109 (1877): 811–830.

Helmont, Jan Baptista van, *Ortus medicinæ* (London: Elzevirium, 1652).

Helvétius, Claude-Adrien, *Œuvres complètes*, 4 vols (London: No publisher named, 1777).

Herpain, Jacques, *Essai sur la nymphomanie ou fureur utérine.* Thèse (Paris: Didot Jeune, 1812).

Heumann, Christoph-Augustus-Francis, *Dissertatio Medica Solemnis De Cessante, Ob Aetatem, Mensium Fluxu Et Morbis Inde Oriundis* (Helmstadt: Schnorrii, 1776).

Hippocrates, *The Genuine Works of Hippocrates*, trans. Francis Adams, 2 vols (London: Sydenham Society, 1849).

Hippocrates, *Œuvres complètes d'Hippocrate*, trans. Adolf M. Hakkert (Amsterdam: A. Littre, 1961).

Hirsch, Madeleine, *Douleurs cellulitiques et ménopause.* Thèse (Paris: Amédée Legrand, 1928).

Hoffmann, Friedrich, *De annorum climactericorum rationali & medica explicatione. Opera Omnia Physico, Tomus Quintus* (Geneva: Fratres de Tournes, 1704).

Hoffmann, Friedrich, *Opera omnia physica-medica*, 6 vols (Geneva: Fratres de Tournes, 1748).

Hooghe, Dr, 'De l'influence des maladies zygomatiques sur la grossesse, la parturition et ses suites', *Annales de la Société de Médecine d'Anvers*, 36 (1874), 70 [70–86].

Houlès, Joseph-Hortense, *De la ménopause considérée au point de vue de l'hygiène.* Thèse (Montpellier: Isadore Tournel, 1843).

Houzé de L'Aulnoit, Alfred, *Hygiène industrielle: Des avantages de la création de caisses de secours en faveur des femmes nouvellement accouchées... et étude sur la statistique et les causes de la mortalité des enfants* (Lille: L. Danel, 1874).

Hufeland, Christoph Wilhelm, *Die Kunst das menschliche Leben zu verlängern*, 2 vols (Jena: Franz Haas, 1797).

Hufeland, Christoph Wilhelm, *Enchiridion medicum oder Anleitung zur medizinischen Praxis: Vermächtniss einer fünfzigjährigen Erfahrung* (Berlin: Jonas, 1836).

Hufeland, Christoph Wilhelm, *La Macrobiotique, ou L'Art de prolonger la vie de l'homme, suivi de Conseils sur l'éducation physique des enfants*, trans. A.-J.-L. Jourdan (Paris: J.-B. Baillière, 1836).

Hufeland, Christoph Wilhlem, *Hufeland's Art of Prolonging Life*, ed. Erasmus Wilson (London: J. Churchill, 1853).

Hunauld, Pierre, *Dissertation sur les vapeurs et les pertes de sang* (Paris: Jean-Noel Leloup, 1756).

Hurtaut, Pierre-Thomas-Nicolas, *Essais de médecine sur le flux menstruel et la curation des maladies de la tête, ou Par rapport à la première partie on donne une théorie nouvelle sur le flux périodique des femmes: & par rapport à la seconde, on propose un remède nouveau contre les maladies céphaliques*, trans. Robert Emett (Paris: J. B. Despilly, Jac. Ch. Chardon. & S. Severin, 1754).

Hyvert, Roger, *Description, emploi et valeur en clientèle des traitements nouveaux: Médicaments, médications et formules, spécialités pharmaceutiques* (Paris: Maloine, 1912).

Icard, Séverin, *La Femme pendant la période menstruelle: Psychologie morbide* (Paris: Alcan, 1890).

Irish, J. C., *Treatment of Uterine Fibro-Myomata by Abdominal Hysterectomy.* Boston: Damrell & Upham, 1890).

Jacob, P. F. T., *Essai sur la doctrine des crises.* Thèse (Paris: Didot Jeune, 1817).

Jacobs, C., 'Fibrome utérin: Quelques Observations cliniques tirées de 633 opérations abdominales', *Bulletin de la Société Belge de Gynécologie et Obstétrique*, 8 (1905–1906): 73–79.

Jacquemart, P., *Contribution à l'étude du rôle étiologique de la ménopause.* Thèse (Paris: Olliet-Henry, 1884).

Jallon, L. J. S., *Essai sur l'âge critique des femmes.* Thèse (Paris: Didot Jeune, 1805).

Jaumes, Jean-Antoine-Placide, *Aperçu sur diverses maladies qui peuvent affecter les femmes à l'âge du retour* (Montpellier: Jean Martel aîné, 1816).

Jayle, Félix Léon, *Septicémie péritonéale aiguë post-opératoire.* Thèse (Paris: Carré, 1895).

Jayle, Félix Léon, *Opothérapie ovarienne dans la ménopause artificielle post-opératoire et la ménopause naturelle* (Paris: Masson, 1898).

Jayle, Félix Léon, 'Opothérapie ovarienne dans la ménopause artificielle post-opératoire et la ménopause naturelle', *Revue de gynécologie et chirurgie abdominale* 2 (April 1898): 239–272.

Jayle, Félix Léon, 'Résultats éloignés de la castration chez la femme', *Bulletin de l'Académie de médecine* (1896): 196–197.

Jayle, Félix Léon, 'Effets physiologiques de la castration chez la femme', *Revue de gynécologie et de chirurgie abdominale*, 3 (May–June 1897): 403–436.

Jayle, Félix Léon, *La Gynécologie* (Paris: Masson, 1918).

Jeannet des Longrois, Jean-Baptiste-Claude, *Conseils aux femmes de quarante ans* (Paris: Méquignon, 1787).

Jeannin, Louis-Marie-André, *Considérations physiologiques, pathologiques et hygiéniques sur l'âge de retour des femmes*. Thèse (Strasbourg: F.G. Levrault, 1830).

Jolanda (Maria Plattis), *Talismans de jeunesse (les raffinements de la femme): conseils et règles de la vie féminine contemporaine, mondanité, éducation, maternité, hygiène* (Paris: A. Méricant, *c.*1910).

Joliet, Charles, *Le Médecin des dames, scènes parisiennes* (Paris: Calmann Lévy, 1885).

Jones, Emma K., Janelle R. Jurgenson, Judith M. Katzenellenbogen, & Sandra C. Thompson, 'Menopause and the Influence of Culture: Another Gap for Indigenous Australian Women?' *BMC Women's Health* 12/43 (2012): 12–43. Doi: 10.1186/1472-6874-12-43.

Jordan, Claude, *Voyages historiques de l'Europe*, 8 vols, vol. 8 (Paris: Nicolas Le Gras, 1693).

Jouard, Gabriel, *Essai sur quelques points de l'histoire naturelle médicale de la femme, considérés sous les rapports physique, anatomique, physiologique, avec des applications à la pathologie*. Thèse (Paris: S. A. Huguelet, 1803).

Jouard, Gabriel, *Nouvel Essai sur la femme considérée comparativement à l'homme principalement sous les rapports moral, physique, philosophique* (Paris: Chez Crochard, 1804).

Joulin, Désiré-Joseph, *Étude bibliographique sur les maladies des femmes* (Paris: P. Asselin, 1861).

Jozan, Antoine Émile, *Traité pratique complet des maladies des femmes* (Paris: Garnier Frères, 1894).

Jund, Léon-Paul-Louis, *Contribution à l'étude des génesthopathies, états mélancoliques cenesthopathiques de l'âge critique*. Thèse (Nancy: A. Crepin-Leblond, 1909).

Jungfleisch, Émile-Clément, 'Sur la constitution des aloïnes de l'Aloès du Natal', *Comptes rendus hebdomadaires des séances de l'Académie des Sciences*, 155 (Paris: Gauthiers-Villard, 1912), 172–175.

Junod, C. L., *De l'époque critique chez les femmes et des précautions à prendre pour en prévenir et combattre quelques accidens ou maladies*. Thèse (Paris: Didot Jeune, 1822).

Keiffer, J. H., 'La Menstruation dans ses rapports avec la pathologie générale', *Journal obstétrique*, 4 (1897): 289–300.

Keller, Raymond, *A propos des métrorragies chez la femme au delà de la ménopause* (Lille: A. Taffin-Lefort, 1926).

Kennedy, Henri, 'Observations on Climacteric Disease', *Dublin Journal* of *Medical Science*, 25/74 (1844): 245.

Kersseboom, Willem, *Proeven van politique rekenkunde, vervat in drie verhandelingen over de meenigte des volks in de provintie van Hollandt en Westvrieslandt; de probable leeftyt der weduwen, de duurzaamheid der huwelyken, de relatie van de meenigte des volks tegen het getal der geborene, en dat der gehuwde paaren &c. als meede over de waardye van lyfrente in proportie van losrente: waarby gevoegt zyn eenige aanmerkingen op de gissingen over den staat van het menschelyk geslacht & begrepen in zeekere inleiding tot de algemeene geographie* (Gravenhage: Jan van den Bergh, 1738).

Kersseboom, Willem, *Observatien, waar in voornamentlyk getoont word wat is gelyktydigheid, dewelke vereischt word in alle calculatien, die tot voorwerp hebben de probable leevenskracht van persoonen van eenigen voorgestelden ouderdom. Hier is bygeveen proeve van de constante ondervinding, dat die van de vrouwelijke sexe doorgaans maar eenige weinige jaaren doormalkander langer leven, dan die van de mannelyke* (The Hague: Jan van den Bergh, 1740).

Kisch, Enoch Heinrich, *Das klimaterische Alter der Frauen: Physiologischer und pathologischer Beziehung* (Erlangen: Ferdinand Enke, 1874).

Kisch, Enoch Heinrich, *Die Sterilität des Weibes: Ihre Urscahen und ihre Behandlung* (Wein & Leipzig: Urban & Schwarzenberg, 1886).

Kisch, Enoch Heinrich, *Causes et traitement de la stérilité chez la femme*, trans. Dr Frédéric Weiss (Paris: G. Steinheil, 1888).

Kisch, Enoch Heinrich, *The Sexual Life of Woman in Its Physiological, Pathological and Hygienic Aspects*, trans. M. Eden Paul (New York: Rebman, 1923).

Kœberlé, Eugène, *Documents pour servir à l'histoire de l'extirpation des tumeurs fibreuses de la matrice par la méthode sus-pubienne* (Paris: J.-B. Baillière et fils, 1864).

Kœberlé, Eugène, *De l'ovariotomie* (Paris: Baillière et fils, 1865).

Kracauer, Siegfried, *Die Melancholie der Frauen nach dem Climacterium*. Dissertation (Breslau: F. Jungfer, 1882).

Krafft-Ebing, Richard von, *Lehrbuch der Psychiatrie: Auf Klinischer Grundlage für Praktische Arzte und Studirende* [1879], 5th ed. (Stuttgart: F. Enke, 1893).

Krafft-Ebing, Richard von, *Psychopathia Sexualis mit besonderer Berücksichtung der conträren Sexualempfindung, eine medicinisch-gerichtliche Studie für Ärzte und Juristen* [1886], 12th ed. (Stuttgart: Verlag von Ferdinand Enke, 1903).

Krauβ, P. 'Uber psychische Storungen bei Frauen nach der Kastration', *Zeitschrift für die gesamte Neurologie und Psychiatrie*, 12/141 (1932): 750–765.

Labarraque, Jacques-Philippe, *Aperçu physiologico-pathologique sur la menstruation en général, et quelques conseils d'hygiène pour l'âge critique en particulier*. Thèse (Montpellier: Jean Martel aîné, 1827).

Laborde, Jacques, *Quelques Considérations sur la puberté chez la femme et sur la ménopause*. Thèse (Paris: Rignoux, 1860).

Labretoigne-Lavalette, I. A., *Réfléxions sur les maladies qui surviennent aux femmes à l'époque de la cessation des règles*. Thèse (Montpellier: Imprimerie Auguste Ricard, 1805).

Lacassagne, Alexandre, *Précis d'hygiène privé et sociale* (Paris: G. Masson, 1874).

Lacassagne, Alexandre, *La Verte vieillesse* (Paris: A. Rey, 1920).

Lachaise, Claude, *Topographie médicale de Paris ou Examen général des causes qui peuvent avoir une influence marquée sur la santé des habitans de cette ville, le caractère de leurs maladies, et le choix des précautions hygiéniques qui leur sont applicables* (Paris: J. B. Baillère, 1822).

Lachaise, Claude, *Hygiène physiologique de la femme ou de la femme considérée dans son système physique et moral* (Paris: Mequignon Marvis, 1825).

Lachaise, Claude, *Les Médecins de Paris jugés par leurs œuvres, ou Statistique scientifique et morale des médecins de Paris* (Paris: Chez l'auteur, 1845).

Laffitte, Guillaume, *Contribution à l'étude de l'eczema rubrum facial dans ses rapports avec la puberté et la ménopause*. Thèse (Montpellier: Boehm & Fils, 1875).

Lafontaine-Margariteau, Louis-Marie, *Conseils hygiéniques aux femmes depuis leur naissance jusqu'à l'âge critique, ayant pour but principal de les préserver de la leucorrhée (fleurs blanches), ou de la diminuer si elle existe*. Thèse (Paris: Didot le Jeune, 1835).

Lagneau, Gustave, *Recherches comparatives sur la menstruation en France* (Paris: Victor Masson, 1866).

Lamaze, Henri, *Essai sur la cessation du flux menstruel et sur les moyens propres à prévenir les accidents et les maladies qui peuvent affecter les femmes à cette époque* (Paris: Didot Jeune, 1805).

Lambert, Madame de (Anne-Thérèse de Marguenat de Courcelles), *De l'amitié, suivi de Traité de la vieillesse* [1736] (Paris: Payot, 2018).

La Molinière, Adrien Claude le Fort de, *Les Vapeurs* (Paris: Prault, 1753).

Lamothe, Bernard, *Dissertation sur l'hystéricie ou vapeurs hystériques en general* (Montpellier: Jean Martel aîné, 1802).

Landouzy, Hector, *Traité complet de l'hystérie* (Paris: J. B. Baillière, 1846).

Landouzy, Louis, *Les Sérothérapies: Leçons de thérapeutique et matière médicale* (Paris: Georges Carré et C. Naud, 1898).

Landouzy, Louis, *Glossaire médical: 9500 mots, noms, ou expressions, 426 figures et 5 carte* (Paris: C. Naud, 1902).

Lange, Martin, *Traité des vapeurs où leur origine, leurs effets, et leur remèdes sont mécaniquement expliqués* (Paris: Veuve Denis Nion, 1689).

Lanique, Gaston, *De l'hystérectomie vaginale totale appliquée au traitement du prolapsus utérin complet* (Nancy: Imprimerie Coopérative de l'Est, 1894).

Lapasse, Louis-Charles-Edouard, *Hygiène de longévité, guérison des migraines, maux d'estomac, maux de nerfs et vapeurs* (Paris: Victor Masson/Garnier Frères, 1861).

Larcher, Louis-Julien, *La Femme jugée par les grands écrivains des deux sexes; ou, La Femme devant Dieu, devant la nature, devant la loi et devant la société: riche et précieuse mosaïque de toutes les opinions émises sur la femme* [1846], 3rd ed. (Paris: Garnier Frères, 1854).

Larcher, Oscar, *Contributions à l'histoire des polypes fibreux intra-utérins à apparitions intermittentes* (Paris: Asselin, 1867).

Lasègue, Charles, *Études médicales*, 2 vols (Paris: Asselin, 1884).

Lasmoles, Albert Léonce Henri, *De la ménopause postopératoire.* Thèse (Bordeaux: Y. Cadoret, 1927).

Latzko, W. & J. Schnitzler, 'Ein Beitrag zur Organotherapie bei Osteomalacie', *Deutsche medizinische Wochenschrift*, 23/37 (1897): 587–592.

Laugier, Jacques, *De la ménopause: (âge critique).* Thèse (Montpellier: Jean Martel aîné, 1861).

Laumonier, Jean-Baptiste Philippe René, 'Observations sur un dêpot de la trompe et sur l'extirpation des ovaires', *Histoire de la Société Royale de Médecine*, 5 (1787): 296–299.

Laumonier, Jean-Baptiste Philippe René, *Discours sur l'anatomie, prononcé à l'ouverture du cours de 1791* (Rouen: Imprimerie de P. Seyer & Behourt, 1791).

Laurens, André du, *Discours de la conservation de la veue: Des maladies mélancoliques des catarrhes, & de la vieillesse*, 3rd ed. [1594] (Rouen: Claude le Villain, 1600).

Laurent, Émile, *Fétichistes et érotomanes* (Paris: Vigot Frères, 1905).

Laville, Jean-Charles Auguste, *Considérations générales sur les causes et les moyens préservatifs des maladies des femmes à l'époque de la cessation des menstrues.* Thèse (Paris: Didot Jeune, 1816).

Lavirotte, Jean-Claude, *De la femme à l'état physiologique, et des névroses qui peuvent l'atteindre aux différentes époques de sa vie.* Thèse (Paris: Rignoux, 1844).

Laynard, Boyd, *Secret de beauté santé et longévité* (Paris: B. Grasset, 1909).

Leake, John, *Medical Instructions Towards the Prevention, and Cure of Chronic Diseases Peculiar to Women* [1779], 2 vols (London: R. Baldwin, 1780–1781).

Le Barzic, Hyacinthe, *Contribution à l'étude du traitement des troubles de la ménopause naturelle par l'opothérapie ovarienne.* Thèse (Paris: Jouve & Boyer, 1899).

Leblanc, C., *Essai sur la métrite aiguë de la matrice ou inflammation* (Paris: Didot le Jeune, 1823).

Lebout, F. J., *La Vrai Médecine aux prises avec le charlatanisme, ou Examen critique de plusieurs doctrines médicales très dangereuses pour le peuple, et particulièrement*, dite curative de M. Leroy (Paris: Béthune et Plon, 1837).

Le Cat, Claude-Nicolas, *Nouveau Système, sur la cause de l'évacuation périodique du sexe. Lettre à l'auteur du Journal de médecine, suivie d'une réponse à des objections faites contre ce système, par laquelle il devient encore plus solidement établi, & l'hypothèse oposée radicalement détruite* (Amsterdam: no publisher named, 1765).

Leclerc, Claude-Bartholomé-Jean, *An morborum, cessante mensium fluxu, therapeia, quae difficillema, rationali medicina duce, felicior?* Thèse (Paris: Quillau, 1786).

Leclercq, Arthur, *L'Âge critique, goutte, affections paragoutteuses, obésité*, 2nd ed. (Paris: Octave Doin, 1922).

Le Dran, Henri François, 'Du cancer des mammelles', in Fortuné Barthélemy de Félice, ed., *Encyclopédie ou dictionnaire universel raisonné des connoisances humaines*, 57 vols (Yverdon: 1770–1780), vol. 27, 314–316.

Leduc, Violette, *La Bâtarde* (Paris: Gallimard, 1964).

Lefevre, Joseph-Paul, *Considérations générales sur la ménopausie, ou cessation naturelle des menstrues*. Thèse (Paris: Didot Jeune, 1826).

Legrain, Paul Maurice, *Du délire chez les dégénérés: Observations prises à l'asile Sainte-Anne, 1885–1886* (Paris: A. Delahaye et E. Lecrosnier, 1886).

Legrand, Maximillien-Albert, *La Longévité à travers les âges* (Paris: Flammarion, 1911).

Le Moniet, Sébastien, *Hystérectomie abdominale totale et hystérectomie abdomino-vaginale pour fibromes de l'utérus* (Paris: G. Steinheil, 1894).

Lemoyne, N. N. Firmin, *Considérations générales sur les phénomènes qui se manifestent à la cessation du flux menstruel et sur le régime que doivent adopter les femmes pour franchir heureusement cette époque*. Thèse (Paris: Didot Jeune, 1824).

Leroy, Louis, *La Médecine naturelle et curative, ou la Purgation dirigée contre la cause des maladies*, 4e édition (Paris: chez l'auteur, 1817).

Léry, Jean de, *Histoire d'un voyage fait en Brésil, autrement dite Amérique* (Geneva: Pour Antoine Chuppin, 1578).

Lestrade, Jean-Nicolas, *Considérations générales sur l'époque critique des femmes, et sur les maladies qui sont attachées à cet âge*. Thèse (Paris: Didot Jeune, 1815).

Létu, J. B. D., *Essai sur la doctrine des crises et des jours critiques dans les maladies aiguës*. Thèse (Montpellier: Jean Martel aîné, 1816).

Le Vacher, Gilles, *Dissertation sur le cancer des mammelles* (Besançon: J.-B. Charmet, 1740).

Lévy, Édouard, *Les Bouffées de chaleur de la ménopause opératoire* (Paris: Georges Carré & C. Naud, 1900).

Lévy, Michel, *Traité d'hygiène publique et privée*, 2 vols (Paris: J.-B. Baillière et fils, 1844–1845).

Leynseele, Charles Van, *Hygiène de la femme, ou l'art de conserver la santé et de prolonger la vie, depuis la naissance jusqu'à l'extrême vieillesse*, 2 vols (Gand: H. Hoste, 1860).

Leyral, Antoine, *Essai sur la prophylactique des femmes parvenues à l'époque de la cessation des règles*. Thèse (Montpellier: Imprimerie Auguste Ricard, 1806).

L'Héritier, Sébastien-Didier, *Traité complet des maladies de la femme, étudiées sous les rapports physiologique, nosographique et thérapeutique* (Paris: Bulletin du Bureau Clinique, 1838).

Liaubet, Joseph-Damien, *Dissertation sur la névropathie ou vapeurs*. Thèse (Montpellier: Imprimerie de Coucourdan, 1801).

Liébault, Jean, *Les Trois Livres de la santé, fœcondité, et maladies de femmes* [1582] (Lyon: J. Veyrat, 1598).

Liébault, Jean, *Trésor des remèdes secrets pour les maladies des femmes*. Pris du Latin, fait français par Jean Liébault (Paris: Jacques du Puys à la Samaritaine, 1585).

Liébeaux, F. A. Hippolyte, *Dissertation sur la ménaphanie: La Non-apparition des menstrues chez les filles pubères*. Thèse (Paris: Didot le Jeune, 1830).

Linguet, Simon Nicolas Henri, *Annales politiques, civiles et littéraires du dix-huitième siècle* (London: Spilsbury, 1783).

Lipinska, Mélanie, *Histoire des femmes médecins depuis l'antiquité jusqu'à nos jours.* Thèse (Paris: Librairie G. Jacques & Cie, 1900).

Lissac, Maurice, *Traitement des troubles consécutifs à la castration chez la femme: Opothérapie ovarienne.* Thèse (Paris: Georges Carré, 1896).

Lombroso, Cesare & Guglielmo Ferrero, *La donna delinquente: la prostituta e la donna normale* (Tur: L. Roux, 1893).

Londe, Charles, *Gymnastique médicale, ou L'Exercice appliqué aux organes de l'homme, d'après les lois de la physiologie, de l'hygiène et de la thérapeutique* (Paris: Crouillebois, 1821).

Long, George, ed., *The Standard Library Cyclopædia of Political, Constitutional, Statistical, and Forensic Knowledge: Forming a Work of Universal Reference on Subjects of Civil Administration, Political Economy, Finance, Commerce, Laws and Social Relations*, 4 vols, vol. 1 (London: Henry G. Bohn, 1848).

Longrois, M. Jeannet des, *Conseils aux femmes de quarante ans; dans l'ordre social, les femmes ont à souffir de mille dépendances; comme dans l'univers physique, de mille infirmités* (Paris: Méquignon, 1787).

Lorenz, Otto Henri, *Catalogue général de la librairie française: 1840–1865*, 4 vols (Paris: O. Lorenz, 1869).

Loua, Toussaint, *La France sociale et économique d'après les documents officiels les plus récents* (Paris: Berger-Levrault, 1888).

Louyer-Villermay, Jean-Baptiste, *Recherches historiques et médicales sur l'hypocondrie isolée, par l'observation et l'analyse, de l'hystérie et de la mélancolie* (Paris: Mequignon, 1802).

Lucas, Prosper, *Traité philosophique et physiologique de l'hérédité naturelle dans les états de santé et de maladie*, 2 vols (Paris: J. B. Baillière, 1850).

Lugol, J. G. A., *Recherches et observations sur les causes des maladies scrofuleuses* (Paris: Fortin & Masson, 1844).

Lund, Léon-Paul-Louis, *Contribution à l'étude des génesthopathies; États mélancholiques cénesthopathies de l'âge critique.* Thèse (Nancy: A. Crepin-Leblond, 1909).

Luscan, Gabriel, *Goître exophtalmique et ménopause* (Montpellier: Firmin et Montane, 1923).

Lutaud, Auguste Joseph, *Consultations sur les maladies des femmes* (Paris: Rueff, 1895).

Lutaud, Auguste Joseph, *Manuel complet de gynécologie médicale et chirurgicale* (Paris: A. Maloine, 1900).

Lutaud, Auguste Joseph, *Études sur la rage et la méthode Pasteur* [1887], 2nd ed. (Paris: Journal de médecine de Paris, 1891).

Luys, Jules-Bernard, *Des maladies héréditaires* (Paris: Baillière, 1863).

Luys, Jules-Bernard, *Traité clinique et pratique des maladies mentales* (Paris: A. Delahaye & E. Lecrosnier, 1881).

Luys, Jules-Bernard, *Hôpital de la Charité: Leçons cliniques sur les principaux phénomènes de l'hypnotisme, dans leurs rapports avec la pathologie mentale* (Paris: G. Carré, 1890).

Luys, Jules-Bernard, *Le Traitement de la folie* (Paris: Rueff, 1893).

Macé, J. A., *Essai sur les hémorrhagies utérines après la délivrance.* Thèse (Paris: Didot le Jeune, 1814).

Magnan, Valentin, *Des anomalies, des aberrations et des perversions sexuelles* (Paris: A. Delahaye & E. Lecrosnier, 1885).

Magnan, Valentin and Paul Maurice Legrain, *Les Dégénérés: État et syndrômes épisodiques* (Paris: Rueff, 1895).

Maladière-Montécot, Georges-Michel, *Considérations générales sur la ménespausie, ou cessation des menstrues et sur les moyens à employer pour prévenir les accidents et les maladies qui peuvent l'accompagner.* Thèse (Paris: Didot Jeune, 1818).

Malthus, Thomas Robert, *An Essay on the Principle of Population* [1823] (New York: Cosimo Classics, 2010).

Manditch, Lioubicha, *Cécité partielle à la suite de cessation brusque des règles*. Thèse (Strasbourg: Éditions Universitatires de Strasbourg, 1924).

Manelphi, Ioannis, *Hippocratis Aphorismi Nicolao Leoniceno Vincentino interprete, una cum annotationibus* (self-published, 1640).

Marañon, Gregorio, *L'Âge critique (étude pathogénique et clinique)*. Trans. J. Sanjuro D'Arella/édition entièrement revue par l'auteur (Paris: Librarie Félix Alcan: 1934).

Marañon, Gregorio, *The Evolution of Sex and Intersexual Conditions*, trans. Warren Bradley Wells (London: Allen & Unwin, 1932).

Marcé, Victor, *Traité pratique des maladies mentales* (Paris: Baillière, 1862).

Marchal, Eugène, *Étude sur la mortalité des femmes en couches dans la ville de Metz* (Metz: J. Verronnais, 1867).

Marie, Pierre, 'L'Hystérie à la consultation du Bureau Central des Hôpitaux de Paris—Étude statistique', *Progrès médical*, 10 (27 July 1889), 69.

Martin, Dr, 'L'Enseignement de l'hygiène dans les établissements d'enseignement supérieur', *Revue internationale de l'enseignement* 16 (1888), 1–22.

Martin, Franklin H., *Lectures on the Treatment of Fibroid Tumours of the Uterus: Medical Electrical and Surgical* (Chicago: W. T. Keener, 1897).

Martin, Laurent, *Les Dangers de l'amour, de la luxure et du libertinage pour l'homme, pour la femme, pendant la jeunesse, pendant l'âge mûr, pendant la vieillesse* (Paris: Lebigre-Duquesne Frères, 1865).

Marvaud, Guy-François, *Considérations générales sur la cessation des règles et sur l'âge faussement appelé critique*. Thèse (Paris: Didot Jeune, 1829).

Massia, Edouard de, *Âge critique chez la femme*. Thèse (Montpellier: Boehm, 1851).

Mathieu, André, *Quelques Propositions sur l'hygiène en général*. Thèse (Montpellier: Publisher not identified, 1807).

Maurice, P. *De la ménespausie*. Thèse (Paris: Didot Jeune, 1832).

Mauriceau, François, *Des maladies des femmes grosses et accouchées, avec la véritable et bonne méthode de les bien aider dans leurs accouchements naturels, et les moyens de remédier à tous ceux qui sont contre nature, et aux indispositions des enfans nouveau-nés* (Paris: J. Hénault, 1668).

Mauriceau, François, *Aphorismes touchant la grossesse, l'accouchement, les maladies, et autres dispositions des femmes* (Paris: L. d'Houry, 1694).

Mauriceau, François, *Observations sur la grossesse et l'accouchement des femmes, et sur leurs maladies & celles des enfans nouveau-nez: En chacune desquelles les causes & les raisons des principaux évenemens sont décrites & expliquées* (Paris: Chez l'auteur, 1695).

Mayer, Dr Alex, *Conseils aux femmes sur l'âge de retour; médecine et hygiène* (Paris: J. B. Baillière et Fils, 1875).

Maygrier, Charles, *Étude sur l'opération de Porro: Opération césarienne suivie de l'amputation de l'utérus et des ovaires* (Paris: A. Delahaye et L. Lecrosnier, 1880).

Meige, Pierre Ulysse, *Dissertation sur la métrite, considérée dans son état aigu et chronique*. Thèse (Paris: Didot Jeune, 1827).

Ménissier, E. D., *Considérations générales sur quelques maladies qui affectent les femmes à l'âge critique*. Thèse (Paris: Didot Jeune, 1808).

Menville, Charles, *Conseils aux femmes à l'époque de l'âge de retour, ou de l'âge critique, et de moyens de combattre et prévenir les maladies qui peuvent survenir à cette époque de la vie* (Paris: Germer Baillière, 1839).

Menville, Charles, *De l'âge critique chez les femmes, des maladies qui peuvent survenir à cette époque de la vie et des moyens de les combattre et de les prévenir* (Paris: Imprimerie de Bourgogne et Martinet, 1840).

Menville, Charles, *Histoire médicale et philosophique de la femme, considérée dans toutes les époques principales de sa vie, avec tous les changements qui surviennent dans son physique et son moral, avec l'hygiène applicable à son sexe et toutes les maladies qui peuvent l'atteindre aux différents âges* (Paris: Aymot & Labé, 1845).

Mercy, François Christophe Florimond de Chevalier de, *Traduction des oeuvres médicales d'Hippocrate, sur le texte grec, d'après l'édition de Foës*, 4 vols (Toulouse: Fagès, Meilhace et Comp., 1801).

Mercy, François Christophe Florimond de Chevalier de, *Nouvelle Traduction des aphorismes d'Hippocrate, conférés sur l'édition grecque publiée en 1811, ou l'on trouve les variantes des manuscrits de la Bibliothèque du Roi et des commentaires spécialement applicables à l'étude de la médecine pratique*, 6 vols (Paris: Adrien Égron, 1817).

Messager, Virginie, *Traité pratique des maladies des femmes* (Paris: Chez l'auteur, 1851).

Messager, Virginie, *Traité pratique des fleurs blanches et des ulcérations de la matrice* (Paris: Chez l'auteur, 1851).

Messager, Virginie, *Manuel de la jeune mère, ou Conseils aux jeunes femmes sur les soins que demandent… leur santé et celle de leurs enfants en bas âge; suivi d'Une instruction sur les soins de la toilette, ou Moyens de conserver et de rendre aux diverses parties du corps leur fraîcheur et leur état naturel* (Paris: Chez l'auteur, 1852).

Messager, Virginie, *Guide pratique de l'âge critique, ou Conseils aux femmes sur les maladies qui peuvent les attaquer à cette époque de leur vie; suivis de Réflexions et d'observations sur les maladies laiteuses* (Paris: chez l'auteur, 1843).

Meurisse, Bernard, *Syndrome utérin et manifestations hystériques* (Lille: L. Quarré, 1895).

Michaux, Émile, *De l'influence menstruelle sur la production d'accidents rhumatismaux*. Thèse (Paris: A. Parent, 1876).

Michelet, Jules, *La Femme* [1860] (Paris: Calmann Lévy, 1879).

Migalli, Bouchra Youachim, *De la ménopause retardée dans les myomes utérins*. Thèse (Lyon: Bosc Frères & Riou, 1925).

Millot, Jacques-André, *De Uteri prolapsus. Theses anatomicae et chirurgicae* (Paris: P. A. le Prieur, 1771).

Millot, Jacques-André, *L'Art d'améliorer et perfectionner les générations humaines*, 2 vols (Paris: Imprimerie de Migneret, 1801).

Millot, Jacques-André, *La Gérocomanie ou code physiologique et philosophique pour conduire les individus des deux sexes à une longue vie, en les dérobant à la douleur et aux infirmités* (Paris: F. Buisson, 1807).

Molk, Marcel, *Kritik der vaginalen und abdominalen totalen Hysterektomie in Fällen von Fybromyomen*. Dissertation (Strassburg: J. Singer, 1901).

Mond, Richard, 'Kurze Mittheilungen über die Behandlung der Beschwerden bei natürlicher oder durch operation veranlasster Amenorrhee mit Eierstocksconserven (Ovariin Merck)', *Münchener medizinische Wochenschrift*, 14 (1896): 314–316.

Monin, Ernest, *Les Troubles nerveux de cause sexuelle* (Paris: O. Doin, 1890).

Monin, Ernest, *L'Hygiène des riches* (Paris: A. Silvestre. 1891).

Monin, Ernest, *La Vulgarisation médicale* (Paris: Réunion amicale de la presse scientifique, 1893).

Monnet, L. J. F., *Dissertation sur l'hystérie, appelée vulgairement vapeurs* (Paris: Didot Jeune, 1808).

Monod, Charles & Félix Jayle, *Cancer du sein* (Paris: Rueff & Cie, 1894).

Montmort, Pierre Rémond, *Essay d'analyse sur les jeux de hazard* (Paris: Quillau, 1708).

Moreau (de la Sarthe), Jacques Louis, *Histoire naturelle de la femme, suivie d'un traité d'hygiène appliqué à son régime physiques et moral aux différentes époques de la vie*, 3 vols (Paris: Duprat, 1803).

Morel, Bénédicte-Augustin, *Traité des dégénérescences* (Paris: J. B. Balliere, 1857).
Morel, Bénédicte-Auguste, *Traité des maladies mentales* (Paris: Victor Masson, 1860).
Morély, Paul, *Essai sur l'ouverture des collections annexielles par la voie vaginale* (Paris: G. Steinheil, 1899).
Moride, *Accidents du retour d'âge et maladies du système veineux: Varices et ulcères variqueux, hémorroîdes, varicocèles, phlebites, oedèmes chronique, congestions, hémorragies, etc. leur traitement par l'exilir de Virginie* (Paris: Pharmacie Moride, *c.*1897).
Mossé, Prosper, *État actuel de l'opothérapie ovarienne: Étude expérimentale et clinique* (Paris: J.-B. Baillière et fils, 1899).
Mouton, Auguste, *Influence de l'utérus sur le système physique et moral de la femme.* Thèse (Paris: Didot le Jeune, 1834).
Müller, Peter & Ernst Börner, *Sterility: Developmental Anomalies of the Uterus and the Menopause* (New York: William Wood, 1887).
Muret, Henri, *Essai sur le traitement des principaux dérangements des menstrues, considérées dans les différents âges de la femme* (Paris: Didot Jeune, 1826).
Muret, Jean-Louis, *Mémoire sur l'état de la population dans le pays de Vaud* (Yverdon: F.-B. de Félice, 1766).
Muret, Maurice, *De l'organothérapie par l'ovaire? Communication faite à la reunion de la Société vaudoise de médecine à Lavey le 18 juin 1896* (Lausanne: Georg, 1896).
Muret, Théodore, *Comment on dégénère.* Feuilleton de l'Union Monarchique (Paris: Imprimerie de E. Proux, 1847).
Navet, Stanislas-Victor-Amédée, *Propositions sur le tempérament de la femme, sur sa menstruation et sur son âge critique.* Thèse (Paris: Didot Jeune, 1830).
Necker, Suzanne, *Réflexions sur la divorce* (Lausanne: Durand Ravanel, 1794).
Négrier, Charles N., *Recherches anatomiques et physiologiques sur les ovaires dans l'espèce humaine, considérés spécialement sous le rapport de leur influence dans la menstruation* (Paris: Béchet Je. et Labé, 1840).
Netzel, William, *Opération césarienne rendue nécessaire par un myome incarcéré dans le petit bassin*, trans. H. Cazin (Paris: V. A. Delahaye, 1876).
Nicaise, Auguste, *Essai sur l'âge de retour chez la femme.* Thèse (Paris: Rignoux, 1838).
Nicolau, Pierre, *Contribution à l'étude des métrorragies de la ménopause (métrorragies d'origine ovarienne).* Thèse (Montpellier: Firmin & Montane, 1912).
Nicolon, J.-J., *Observations sur la ménorrhagie qui survient à l'approche de l'âge critique, et sur l'aménorrhée par vice de conformation.* Thèse (Strasbourg: Levrault, 1808).
Niemeyer, Ludwig Heinrich Christian, *De menstruationis fine et usu.* Dissertation (Göttingen: Dieterich, 1796).
Noé, J., *La Nicine Rol dans le traitement des hémorroïdes, varices, phlébites, artériosclérose, emphysème, asthme, bronchites, métrites, accidents de l'âge critique, cirrhoses, affections cardiaques et vasculaires, etc.* (Paris: Nicine Rol, 1908).
Noirot, Louis, *Études statistiques sur la mortalité et la durée de la vie dans la ville et l'arrondissement de Dijon depuis le 19e siècle jusqu'à nos jours* (Paris: J. Baillière, 1850).
Nordau, Max, *Entartung* [1892], 3rd ed. (Berlin: Carl Dunder, 1896).
Nosely, Jean-Baptiste, *Dissertation sur l'âge critique.* Thèse (Paris: Rignoux, 1848).
Novak, Emil, *Menstruation and Its Disorders* (New York & London: D. Appleton & Co., 1928).
Nye, Robert A., *Masculinity and Male Codes of Honor in Modern France* (New York/ Oxford: Oxford University Press, 1993).
Nye, Robert A., 'The Evolution of the Concept of Medicalization in the Late Twentieth Century', *Journal of the History of the Behavioural Sciences*, 39/2 (2003): 115–129. Doi: 10.1002/jhbs.10108.

Obici G., 'Le psicosi in rapporto alle fasi fisiologiche dell'organismo', *Rivista sperimentale di freniatria*, 31 (1903): 154.

Odier, Louis, 'Extrait mortuaire de Genève pour les années 1778 & 1779', *Société établie à Genève pour l'encouragement des arts et de l'agriculture. Mémoires*, 1–2 (1780): 144–156.

Olive, Antoine-Alexandre, *Dissertation inaugurale sur la première menstruation, l'âge critique et les soins hygiéniques que réclament les femmes à ces deux époques*. Thèse (Paris: Didot Jeune, 1819).

Oliver, James, 'Sudden and Complete Inversion of the Uterus and Cervix after the Menopause; Very Small Fibroid Nodule in the Fundus; Gangrene, Operation; Recovery', *The Lancet*, 152/3921 (1898): 1057–1058 Doi: 10.1016/S0140-6736(01)82896-8.

Ottosson, Anders, 'The Age of Scientific Gynaecological Masseurs. "Non-Instrusive" Male Hands, Female Intimacy, and Women's Health Around 1900', *Social History of Medicine*, 29/4 (2016): 802–828. Doi: 10.1093/shm/hkw013.

Pagès, Louis-Antoine, *De la ménopause et de son influence dans la production de l'aliénation mentale*. Thèse (Nancy: A. Parent, 1876).

Paré, Ambroise, *De la génération de l'homme, recveilli des anciens et modernes* [1573], in *Œuvres complètes d'Ambroise Paré*, ed. J. F. Malgaigne, vol. 2 (Paris: J. B. Baillière, 1840).

Pascal, Jean-Albert, *La Ménopause prématurée par la castration ovarienne: Contribution à l'étude du traitement des fibromes utérins*. Thèse (Bordeaux: Veuve Cadoret, 1887).

Pauchet, Victor, *L'Automne de la vie; l'homme et la femme à l'âge critique*, préface de M. Brieux de l'Académie Française (Paris: Editions J. Oliven, 1932).

Paumerelle, Claude, *La Philosophie des vapeurs* (Lausanne: J. Fr. Bastien, 1774).

Paumerelle, Claude, *La Philosophie des vapeurs*, 2nd ed. (Paphos: Royez, 1784).

Paumerelle, Claude, *La Philosophie des vapeurs*, ed. Sabine Arnaud (Paris: Mercure de France, 2009).

Péan, Jules, 'De la prétendue bénignité des fibromes utérins', *Annales de gynécologie et d'obstétrique*, 39/1 (1893): 460–466.

Péan, Jules & Léopold Urdy, *Hystérotomie: De l'ablation partielle ou totale de l'utérus par la gastrotomie: Étude sur les tumeurs qui peuvent nécessiter cette opération* (Paris: Adrien Delahaye, 1873).

Peloux, C. A. M., *Essai sur l'époque critique et sur les moyens propres à prévenir les accidents et les maladies qui en dépendent*. Thèse (Paris: Didot Jeune, 1812).

Perkins, Anne E., 'Dangers of the Menopause', *American Journal of Nursing*, 10/12 (1910): 945–948.

Perrier, Charles, *Anatomie et physiologie de l'ovaire*. Thèse (Paris: P. Asselin, 1866).

Perrin, George, *Du Traitement des troubles de la ménopause par les bains carbo-gazeux et l'eau Velléda* (Clermont-Ferrand: Bussac, 1924).

Perrin, Georgette, *L'Hypertension de la ménopause, son traitement à Royat*. Thèse (Paris: Jouve, 1926).

Perthuisot, Ernest, *De la crise médicale: Pléthore, discrédit, concurrence, imposition* (Lyon: A. Storck & Cie, 1898).

Peteghem, Émile van, *Des endométrites de la ménopause*. Thèse (Paris: Ollier-Henry, 1893).

Pétrequin, Joseph-Pierre-Éléonor, *Recherches sur la menstruation*. Thèse (Paris: Didot le Jeune, 1836).

Phelippeaux, Adrien, *Histoire clinique d'un fibrome utérin du poids de 150 grammes, opération et guérison. Considérations sur quelques faits de gynécologie. Discussion. Commentaires* (Paris: V. Adrien Delahaye, 1878).

Pichot, F. L., *Étude clinique sur le cancer du corps et de la cavité de l'utérus* (Paris: Henri Rey, 1876).

Pigeonnat, Jules-Henri, *Gros Fibromes utérins (Hystérectomie abdominale, méthode-péritonéale)* (Paris: Henri Jouve, 1896).

Pignod, Jean, *Des troubles oculaires de la femme non diathésiques coïncidant avec les troubles de la menstruation et la ménopause.* Thèse (Lyon: Imprimerie Paul Legendre, 1900).

Pinel, Philippe, *Nosographie philosophique, ou la méthode de l'analyse appliquée à la médecine*, 2 vols (Paris: Maradon, 1797).

Pinel, Philippe, *Traité medico-philosophique sur l'aliénation mentale* (Paris: Richard, 1800).

Pinel, Philippe, *La Médecine clinique rendue plus précise et plus exacte par l'application de l'analyse, ou Recueil et résultat d'observations sur les maladies aiguës, faites à la Salpêtrière* (Paris: Brosson, Gabon et Cie, 1802).

Pinel, Philippe, *Traité médico-philosophique sur l'aliénation mentale*, 2nd ed. (Paris: J. A. Brosson, 1809).

Pinel, Philippe, *Nosographie philosophique, ou la méthode de l'analyse appliquée à la médecine*, 3 vols (Paris: J. A. Brosson, 1810).

Pingault, Jérémie-André, *De la cessation des règles.* Thèse (Montpellier: Tournel, 1799).

Plihon, Gustave-Adolphe, *De la ménopause (âge critique).* Thèse (Paris: Rignoux, 1859).

Poirson, Hubert Quirin Franklin, *Dissertation sur la ménespausie.* Thèse (Strasbourg: F. G. Levrault, 1827).

Poquillon, Jean-Baptiste-Louis, *De la ménopause, ou de l'âge dit critique chez la femme.* Thèse (Paris: Rignoux, 1846).

Potocki, Julien, *De l'opération césarienne, et, en particulier, de l'opération césarienne avec double suture de l'utérus, par la méthode de Saenger* (Paris: G. Steinheil, 1886).

Pouchet, Félix-Archimède, *Théorie positive de l'ovulation spontanée et de la fécondation des mammifères et de l'espèce humaine, basée sur l'observation de toute la série animale* (Paris: J. B. Baillière, 1847).

Pouchet, Georges, *Précis d'histologie humaine d'après les travaux de l'école française* (Paris: Masson, 1864).

Poullet, Dr, *La Gynécologie à l'étranger* (Lyon: Riotor, 1879).

Poupinel, Gaston Ferdinand, *Des tumeurs mixtes de l'ovaire* (Paris: Masson, 1887).

Poussié, Jean-Antoine, *Réflexions sur l'hygiène qui convient aux femmes arrivées à l'âge de retour.* Thèse (Montpellier: Jean Martel aîné, 1813).

Poussié, Julien, *Essai sur les crises et leur existence dans les maladies* (Montpellier: Ricard, 1840).

Pozzi, Samuel, *Étude sur les fistules de l'espace pelvi-rectal supérieur, ou fistules pelvi-rectales supérieures.* Thèse (Paris: G. Masson, 1873).

Pozzi, Samuel, *De la valeur de l'hystérotomie dans le traitement des tumeurs fibreuses de l'utérus.* Thèse (Paris: G. Masson, 1875).

Pozzi, Samuel, *Relevé statistique des opérations pratiquées dans le service de gynécologie de l'hôpital Broca* (Paris: Masson, 1899).

Pozzi, Samuel & Félix Jayle, *Traité de gynécologie clinique et opératoire* [1890], 4th ed., 2 vols (Paris: Masson et Cie, 1905–1907).

Pozzi, Samuel, *Notice sur les travaux scientifiques du Dr. S. Pozzi* (Paris: G. Masson, 1912).

Pozzi, Samuel, *Notes d'un voyage chirurgical en Argentine et au Brésil* (Mâcon: Protat frères, 1912).

Pressavin, Jean-Baptiste, *Nouveau Traité des vapeurs, ou traité des maladies des nerfs, dans lequel on développe les crais principes des vapeurs* (Paris: La Veuve Reguilliat, 1770).

Prévost, Marcel, *Les Demi-vierges* (Paris: Alphonse Lemerre, 1894).

Privat, J. Léon, *Notice statistique et médicale sur la Malou-lès-Bains (Hérault), suivies de l'application des eaux alcalino-ferrugineuses et arsénicales de la Malou-l'Ancien au traitement du rhumatisme, de la névropathie, de la paraplégie et de la chloro-anémie* (Paris: Baillière, 1858).

Proust, Jean-Eugène, *Influence de la ménopause sur le cancer du sein et castration ovarienne thérapeutique par les rayons X*. Thèse (Bordeaux: Impr. de l'Académie et des Facultés, 1929).

Prus, C. R. 'Recherches sur les maladies de la vieillesse', *Mémoires de l'Académie Royale de Médecine*, 8 (1840): 1–27.

Ptolémée, Claude, *L'Uranie de Messire Nicolas Bourdin, seigneur de Villennes, ou La Traduction des quatre livres des jugemens des astres de Claude Ptolémée* (Paris: Cardin Besongne, 1640).

Ptolemy, Claudius, *Tetrabiblos*, trans. & ed. F. E. Robbins, Book IV, Chapter X (Cambridge, Mass.: Harvard University Press, 1940).

Puyo, Bernard-Grégoire Emile, *De la ménopause*. Thèse (Paris: A Parent, 1865).

Quicherat, L. & A. Daveluy, *Dictionnaire latin-français: Contenant tous les mots employés par les auteurs latins et les principales inscriptions latines jusqu'au VIe siècle de notre ère avec renvois aux sources des mots rares*, 46th ed. (Paris: Librairie Hachette, 1910).

Raciborski, Adam, *Dissertation sur les tumeurs stercorales*. Thèse (Paris: Didot Jeune, 1834).

Raciborski, Adam, *De la puberté et de l'âge critique chez la femme, au point de vue physiologique, hygiénique et médical* (Paris: J. B. Baillière, 1844).

Raciborski, Adam, *Du rôle de la menstruation dans la pathologie et la thérapeutique* [1844] (Paris: J.-B. Baillière, 1856).

Raciborski, Adam, *Traité de la menstruation, ses rapports avec l'ovulation, la fécondation, l'hygiène de la puberté et de l'âge critique* (Paris: J. B. Baillière, 1868).

Ramon, Albert, *Hystérectomie abdomino-vaginale: Méthode péan dans les cas de gros fibromes utérins* (Paris: G. Steinheil, 1893).

Ramondenc, Sucrion, *Considérations sur l'état de la femme à l'époque de la cessation des règles*. Thèse (Montpellier: Jean Martel, 1820).

Rastoul, Philémon, *Fragments d'hygiène prophylactique (fonctions génératrices, fonctions de mouvement)*. Thèse (Montpellier: Pierre Grollier, 1862).

Raulin, Joseph, *Traité des affections vaporeuses du sexe, avec l'exposition de leurs symptômes, de leurs différentes causes, et la méthode de les guérir* (Paris: Jean-Thomas Hérissant, 1758).

Ravarit, Dr, 'Remèdes de commères au XXe siècle', *La Chronique médicale*, 16 (1908): 239–240.

Raymond, Dominique, *Traité des maladies qu'il est dangereux de guérir*, 2 vols (Avignon: F. B. Merande, 1757).

Raymond, Dominique, *Traité des maladies qu'il est dangereux de guérir* [1757], new ed. (Paris: Brunot-Labbé, 1816).

Raynal, Guillaume-Thomas, *Histoire philosophique et politique des établissemens et du commerce des Européens dans les deux Indes*, 6 vols (Geneva: Jean-Leonard Pellet, 1780).

Regemann, Johann L., *De morbis ex menstruis per aetatem cessantibus* (Leiden: Lugdunum Batavorum, 1737).

Régis, Émmanuel, *Manuel pratique de la médecine mentale* (Paris: Octave Doin, 1885).

Régis, Émmanuel, 'Cas de folie consécutive à une ovarosalpingectomie', *Journal de médecine de Bordeaux*, 37 (10 September 1893), 413–417.

Régis, Émmanuel, *A Practical Manual of Mental Medicine* (Philadelphia: Blakiston, 1898).

Régis, Émmanuel, *Précis de psychiatrie* [1904], 3rd ed. (Paris: Octave Doin, 1906).

Rémond, Antoine & Paul Voivenel, 'Essai sur le rôle de la ménopause en pathologie mentale', *L'Encéphale: Revue de psychiatrie clinique, biologique et thérapeutique*, 6/2 (1911): 113–126.

Renou, Jean de, *Œuvres pharmaceutiques* [1626], 2nd ed. (Lyon: Nicholas Gay, 1637).

Retz, Noël, *Nouvelles ou Annales de médecine, chirurgie et pharmacie*, vol. 5 (Paris: Méquignon, 1789).

Reveillé-Parise, J. H., *Traité de la vieillesse, hygiénique, médicale et philosophiques* (Paris: J. B. Baillère, 1853).

Rhazis, Le Docteur, *La Menstruation et l'âge critique; causes des règles—complications. La ménopause. Début et caractère* (Paris: De Porter, 1909).

Ribes, François, *Discours sur la vie de la femme*. Thèse (Montpellier: Sevalle-Castel, 1836).

Ricard, Henri, *Étude sur les troubles de la sensibilité génésique à l'époque de la ménopause*. Thèse (Paris: A. Derenne, 1879).

Richelot, Gustave Antoine, *La Femme-médecin* (Paris: E. Dentu, 1875).

Richerand, Anthelme Balhasar Baron, *Nouveaux Eléments de physiologie*, 4 vols (Paris: Richard, Caille & Ravier, 1801–1825).

Richerand, Anthelme Balhasar Baron, *Des erreurs populaires relatives à la médecine* (Paris: Caille & Ravier, 1812).

Ripeault, Ch.-Aug.-Dés, *De la ménopause*. Thèse (Paris: Rignoux, 1848).

Robert, L. J. M., *Manuel de santé ou Nouveaux Elémens de médecine pratique*, 2 vols (Paris: Imprimerie de Crapelet, 1805).

Rocque, Henri-Eugène, *Essai sur la physiologie et la pathologie de la ménopause*. Thèse (Paris: Rignoux, 1858).

Rocques, Joseph, *Nouveau Traité des plantes usuelles, spécialement appliqué à la médecine domestique, et au régime alimentaire de l'homme sain ou malade*, 2 vols (Paris: P. Dufart, 1837).

Roederer, Johann Georg, *Icones uteri humani observationibus illustratae* (Göttingen: Vandenhoeck, 1758).

Roeser, Pierre-Henry, *Vieillesse et longévité* (Paris: A. Maloine, 1910).

Roussel, Pierre, *Système physique et moral de la femme* (Paris: Chez Vincent, 1775).

Routh, Charles Henry F., *On Some Points Connected with the Pathology, Diagnosis and Treatment of Fibrous Tumours of the Womb: Lettsomian Lectures on Midwifery and Diseases of Women* (London: T. Richards, 1864).

Roux de Brignolles, Gabriel, *Sclérose utéro-annexielle en dehors de la ménopause* (Paris: Vigot Frères, 1909).

Royer-Collard, Antoine-Athanase, *Essai sur l'aménorrhée, ou Suppression du flux menstruel* (Paris: Gabon, 1802).

Rozier, Charles du, *Notice historique sur Maugras* (Paris: Brunueax, 1843).

Rudbeck, Olaus, *Atlantica Atland Eller Manheim* (Uppsala: Henricus Curio, 1679).

Rudbeck, Olaus, *Olaus Rudbeck's Atlantica* [1684], ed. Axel Nelson, 5 vols (Stockholm: Almqvist & Wiksell, 1937–1950).

Ruf, Jakob, *De conceptu et generatione hominis, de matrice et ejus partibus, nec non de conditione infantis in utero et gravidarum cura et officio* (Frankfurt: Tiguri, 1554).

Rüff, Jakob, *The Expert Midwife, or An excellent and most necessary treatise of the generation and birth of man Wherein is contained many very notable and necessary particulars requisite to be knovvne and practised* (London: S. Burton, 1637).

Sahuqué Adrienne, *Les Dogmes sexuels* (Paris : Félix Alcan, 1932).

Sarwey, Otto, *Über die Kastration der Fraue*. Dissertation (Tübingen: Heinrich Laupp Jr, 1890).

Saucerotte, Constant, *Nouveaux Conseils aux femmes sur l'âge prétendu critique, ou conduite à tenir lors de la cessation des règles* (Paris: Madame Auger-Méquinon, 1828).

Saury, Honoré, *Étude clinique su la folie héréditaire* (Paris: Delahaye, 1886).

Sauvé, Prosper-Louis, *Réflexions sur l'âge critique, et particulièrement sur le régime le plus convenable pour préserver les femmes des accidens qui ont coutume de survenir cette époque de leur vie*. Thèse (Strasbourg: F. G. Levrault, 1826).

Scanzoni, Friedrich Wilhelm (von Lichtenfels), *Lehrbuch der Krankheiten der weiblichen Sexualorgane* (Vienna: Wilhelm Braumüller, 1857).

Scanzoni, Friedrich Wilhelm (von Lichtenfels), *Traité pratique des maladies des organes sexuels de la femme*, trans. M. Dor & A. Socin (Paris : J. B. Baillière et fils, 1858).

Scherer, Else, *Über das Verhalten des Blutdruckes im Klimakterium und der Menopause*. Dissertation (Göttingen : Fritz Scherer, 1925).

Schultz, Dr Marie & Dr Alfred Auvard, *Hygiène génitale de la femme, menstruation, fécondation, stérilité, grossesse, accouchement, suites de couches* (Paris: Octave Doin, 1902).

Schultz, Marie, *Hygiène générale de la femme, alimentation, vêtements, soins corporels, d'après l'enseignement et la pratique du Dr Auvard* (Paris: O. Doin, 1903).

Schultz, Marie, *La Philosophie indoue, rapport adressé à M. le ministre de l'Instruction publique en France, à la suite d'une mission confiée à l'auteur pour étudier, aux Indes, la nature, la valeur et l'enseignement de cette philosophie* (Paris: Comité de publications théosophiques, 1909).

Schultz, Marie & Alfred Auvard, *L'Évoluisme* (Paris: A. Maloine, 1914).

Schweighaeuser, Jacques Frédéric, *Archives de l'art des accouchemens, considéré sous ses rapports anatomiques, physiologique et pathologique*, 2 vols (Strasbourg: Louis Eck, 1802).

Schwob, Aimé, *Contribution à l'étude des psychoses menstruelles considérées surtout au point de vue médico-légal*. Thèse (Lyon: Storck, 1893).

Scialom, D., *Associations névroso-organiques (hystérie et neurasthénie)* (Montpellier: G. Firmin, Montane et Sicardi, 1902).

Selvy, Jean-André, *Dissertation sur la métrorrhagie, ou hémorragie utérine qui a lieu dans l'âge critique*. Thèse (Montpellier: Jean Martel aîné, 1814).

Seré, Louis de, *La Virilité et l'âge critique chez l'homme et chez la femme* (Paris: A. Delahaye et Lecrosnier, 1885).

Serge-Paul, Dr, *Physiologie de la vie sexuelle chez l'homme et chez la femme, suivie d'une étude sur la procréation des sexes à volonté* (Paris: Bibliothèque populaire des sciences médicales, 1910).

Serres, Louis de, *Discours de la nature, causes, signes et curation des empeschemens de la conception et de la stérilité des femmes* (Paris: Antoine Chard, 1625).

Seville, Isidore of, *Etymologies*, [*c*.625] trans. Stephen A. Barney, W. J. Lewis, J. A. Beach, and Oliver Berghof (Cambridge: Cambridge University Press, 2006).

Simon, François, *Essai sur les crises*. Thèse (Paris: Didot le Jeune, 1831).

Simonnet, Henri, *Contribution à l'étude de la sécrétion interne de l'ovaire, les propriétés du liquide folliculaire* (Paris: Doin, 1927).

Simonnet, Henri, 'Concentration, propriétés da la folliculine', *Annales de physiologie et de physicochimie biologique*, 1/3 (1927): 586–609.

Simonnet, Henri, 'Contribution à l'étude de la sécrétion interne de l'ovaire, les propriétés du liquide folliculaire', *Annales de physiologie et de physicochimie biologique*, 1/3 (1927): 610–662.

Sinéty, Louis de, *Sur quelques points d'anatomie et de physiologie de l'ovaire et de l'utérus* (Paris: Association française pour l'avancement des sciences, 1875).

Sinéty, Louis de, *Anatomie pathologique de la métrite chronique* (Paris: A. Parent, 1878).

Sinéty, Louis de, *Manuel pratique de gynécologie et des maladies des femmes* (Paris: O. Doin, 1879).

Sinéty, Louis de, *Des inflammations qui se développent au voisinage de l'utérus: Considérées surtout dans leurs formes bénignes* (Paris: A. Delahaye et E. Lecrosnier, 1882).

Siracoff, Georges, *Brachialgie de la ménopause.* Thèse (Lausanne: Imprimerie G. Varney-Burnier, 1902).

Solier, Jean-Louis, *Essai sur les crises.* Thèse (Montpellier: Boehm, 1857).

Sollier, Paul, *Guide pratique des maladies mentales: Séméiologie, pronostic, indications* (Paris: G. Masson, 1893).

Sorbait, Paul de, *Insitutionum medicarum et anatomicarum, methodus medendi, cum controversiis, annexa sylva medica. Diende sequuntur: Curationes Omnium morborum, virorum, mulierum et puerorum. A capite ad calcem, nec non cura morbi venerei, et tractatus de febribus, peste et venenis* (Nuremberg: Michael & Johan Friderici, 1672).

Sornay, F., *L'Âge critique et la crise religieuse chez les jeunes gens: Lettre aux jeunes gens des cercles d'études de la région des bords de Saône* (Belley: L. Chaduc, 1907).

Sorokina, M., *Über die Psychosen des Climacteriums.* Thèse (Bern: Gottfried Iseli, 1910).

Souleyre, Charles, *Neurasthénie et génitopathies féminines, Etude des formes utérines secondaires de la névrose* (Paris: Bailliere, 1898).

Stahl, Georg Ernst, *Theoria medica vera: Physiologiam & pathologiam* (Halle: Literis Orphanotrophei, 1707).

Stahl, Georg Ernst, *Œvres médico philosophiques et pratiques de G.E. Stahl*, 6 vols. Trans. T. Blondin (Paris: J. B. Baillière, 1859–1864).

Stahl, Georg Ernst, & Gottfried Wilhelm Leibniz, *La Controverse entre Stahl et Leibniz sur la vie, l'organisme et le mixte*, ed. and trans. Sarah Carvallo (Paris: J. Vrin, 2004).

Stapfer, M., 'La Kinésithérapie gynécologique: Traitement des maladies des femmes par le massage', *Annales de gynécologie* (1892): 81–118.

Stopin, Raoul, *Essai sur les métrorrhagies de la ménopause* (Paris: Henri Jouve, 1898).

Storer, Horatio Robinson, *Successful Removal of the Uterus and Both Ovaries by Abdominal Section; The Tumor, Fibro-Cystic, Weighing Thirty-Seven Pounds* (Boston: David Clapp & Sons, 1866).

Süßmilch, Johan Peter, *Die göttliche Ordnung in den Veränderungen des menschlichen Geschlechts, aus der Geburt, dem Tode und der Fortpflanzung desselben erwiesen: Worin die Regeln der Ordnung bewiesen werden, welche Gottes Weisheit und Güte in dem Lauf der Natur zur Erhaltung, Vermehrung und Verdoppelung des menschlichen geschlechts, vestgesetzet hat, woraus denn die wahren Grundsätze einer vernünftigen Bevölkerung hergeleitet werden* [1741], 2nd ed., vol. 2 (Berlin: Verlag des Buchhandens der Realschule, 1761).

Swieten, Gerard van, *Commentaires sur les aphorismes d'H. Boerhaave, de la connaissance et de la cure des maladies*, trans. M. Moublet, 6 vols (Lyon: Frères Perisse, 1775).

Tardieu, Ambroise, *Étude médico-légale sur l'avortement, suivie d'observations et de recherches pour servir à l'histoire médico-légale des grossesses fausses et simulées* (Paris: J. B. Baillière, 1864).

Tessier, Madeleine, *Établissement de la ménopause.* Thèse (Paris: Ollier-Henry, 1911).

Teysset, François-Hyacinthe, *Quelques Généralités sur l'hygiène des vieillards.* Thèse (Montpellier: Jean Martel, 1825).

Thierry, Alexandre, 'Statistiques compare de la mortalité des femmes en couches dans les hôpitaux de Paris et dans ceux d'Allemagne et d'Angleterre', *Extrait du Moniteur des Hôpitaux*, 1856: 1–3.

Thilo, Marie de, *L'Hygiène de la femme, I. Hygiène générale. II. L'enfance. III. La jeune fille. IV. La femme mariée. V. L'âge critique. VI. La vieillesse* (Paris: Fischbacher, 1891).

Thilo, Marie de, *L'Hygiène intime: Conseils aux femmes pour tous les âges de la vie* (Paris: Fischbacher, 1892).

Thomas, Antoine-Léonard, *Essai sur le caractère, les mœurs et l'esprit des femmes dans les différens siècles* (Paris: Moutard, 1772).

Thomas, François de Troisvèvre, *Physiologie des tempéramens ou Constitutions; nouvelle doctrine applicable à la médecine pratique, à l'hygiène, à l'histoire naturelle et à la philosophie* (Paris: J. B. Baillière, 1826).

Thyssen, Eduard, *Contribution à l'étude de l'hystérie traumatique* (Paris: A. Davy, 1888).

Tillionbois de Valleuil, T. M., *Essai sur l'hygiène des femmes considérées pendant la grossesse, l'accouchement et les couches* (Paris: Didot Jeune, 1818).

Tilt, Edward John, *On Diseases of Menstruation and Ovarian Inflammation, in Connection with Sterility, Pelvic Tumours, and Affections of the Womb* (London: John Churchill, 1850).

Tilt, Edward John, *The Change of Life in Health and Disease: A Practical Treatise on the Nervous and Other Affections Incidental to Women at the Decline of Life* [1857], 3rd ed. (London: J. Churchill, 1870).

Tilt, Edward John, *Elements of Health, and Principles of Female Hygiene* (London: Henry G. Bohn, 1852).

Tissot, Samuel-Auguste, *Traité des nerfs et de leurs maladies*, 2 vols (Paris: Théophile Barrois le jeune, 1779).

Tissot, Samuel-Auguste, 'Avis pour les femmes', in *Œuvres choisies de Tissot*, ed. J. N. Hallé, 11 vols, vol. 1 (Paris: Allut, 1810).

Titius, David, *De fine mensium initiis morborum variorum opportu: Dissertatio inauguralis medica* (Halle: Henckelii, 1710).

Tourtelle, Étienne, *Theses medicae. Ex theoria. De naturâ, diversitate & viribus mineralium aquarum, medicatarum vocitatarum. Ex Praxi* (Montpellier: Jacques François Couché, 1782).

Tourtelle, Étienne, *Elémens d'hygiène, ou De l'influence des choses physiques et morales sur l'homme, et des moyens de conserver la santé*, 2 vols. (Strasbourg: F. G. Levrault, 1797).

Tourtelle, Étienne & George Williamson, *Elements of Hygiene (Principles of Health) or, A treatise on the influence of physical and moral causes on man, and on the means of preserving health* (Baltimore: J. Robinson, 1809).

Tourtelle, Étienne & Jean Noël Hallé, *Encyclopédie des sciences médicales*, VII: *Hygiène*, ed. M. Bricheteau (Paris: Bureau de l'Encyclopédie, 1837).

Tramar, Comtesse de (Marie-Fanny de Lamarque de Lagarrigue), *Règles du savoir-vivre dans la société moderne* (Paris: Havard, 1905).

Tramar, Comtesse de (Marie-Fanny de Lamarque de Lagarrigue), *Que veut la femme? Être jolie, être aimée et dominer* (Paris: Malet, 1911).

Tramar, Comtesse de (la Marquise Isarn de Villafort), *L'Amour obligatoire: Les Etapes de la vie d'une femme; la carrière de l'homme* [1900], 3rd ed. (Paris: Librairie Universelle, 1913).

Transtour, J. A., *Considérations générales sur quelques maladies qui affectent les femmes à l'âge critique*. Thèse (Paris: Didot Jeune, 1812).

Trécul, Jean-Hyacinthe, *La Catarrhe utérin*. Thèse (Paris: Didot Jeune, 1819).

Trifet, Alexandre, *Maladies des femmes* (Paris: Chez l'auteur, 1875).

Vacher, Gilles, *Dissertation sur le cancer des mamelles, ou Sans recourir à aucune hippothèse, on donne une véritable idée de la nature* (Besançon: Jean-Baptiste Charmet, 1740).

Valenc, Pierre, *Dissertation sur l'aménorrhée ou suppression des règles*. Thèse (Paris: Didot jeune, 1816).

Vallès, Jules, *Jacques Vingtras: Le Bachelier*, 2nd ed. [1881] (Paris: G. Charpentier, 1885).

Valleteau de Moulliac, Emile-Joseph-Amédée, *Contribution à l'étude de l'âge critique chez l'homme (Troubles nerveux et psychiques)* (Bordeaux: A. Destout ainé & Cie, 1907).

Vandenesse, 'Âge se prend, en médecine', in Denis Diderot & Jean le Rond d'Alembert, *Encyclopédie*, vol. 1 (1751), 170a–171a.

Varanda, Jean de, *Traité des maladies des femmes* (Paris: Robert de Ninville, 1666).

Variot, Gaston, 'Trois Expériences sur l'action physiologique du suc testiculaire injecté sous la peau, suivant la méthode de M. Brown-Séquard', *Comptes rendus des séances de la Société de Biologie et de ses filiales*, 41 (1889): 451–454.

Velpeau, Alfred Armand Louis Marie, *Traité complet de l'art des accouchemens, ou tocologie théorique et pratique: avec un abrégé des maladies qui compliquent la grossesse, le travail et les couches, et de celles qui affectent les enfans nouveau-nés* (Brussels: Dumont, 1836).

Verdé de Lisle, N. M., *Dissertation sur la métrite aiguë, ou inflammation aiguë de la matrice*. Thèse (Paris: Didot Jeune, 1827).

Vermorel, E., *De l'origine thyroïdienne de certaines tachycardies ou palpitations, dites nerveuses, de la puberté et de la ménopause*. Thèse (Paris: Alfred Leclerc, 1907).

Verne, Honoré-Jean, *Essai sur la cessation des menstrues et sur quelques maladies qui attaquent les femmes à cette époque critique*. Thèse (Paris: Didot Jeune, 1809).

Vernière, François-Pierre-Prosper, *Aperçu des dangers de l'âge critique*. Thèse (Montpellier: Jean Martel aîné, 1811).

Vialenc, Pierre, *Dissertation sur l'aménorrhée, ou suppression des règles*. Thèse (Paris: Didot Jeune, 1816).

Viault, François Gilbert & Félix Jolyet, *Traité élémentaire de physiologie humaine*, 2nd ed. corrigée et très augmentée (Paris: Octave Doin, 1894).

Vigarous, Joseph-Marie-Joachim, *Cours élémentaire de maladies des femmes, ou Essai sur une nouvelle méthode pour étudier et pour classer les maladies de ce sexe*, 2 vols (Paris: Deterville, 1801).

Villeneuve, Louis André Félix, *Quelques Faits pour servir à l'histoire des injections sous-cutanées de suc de tissu testiculaire et ovarien par la méthode Brown-Séquard. Observations recueillies par MM. Vaudey et Lachaud* (Marseille: Barlatier & Barthelet, 1889).

Vinay, Charles, *La Ménopause* (Paris: Masson, 1908).

Virey, Julien-Joseph, *Hygiène philosophique, ou De la santé dans le régime physique, moral et politique de la civilisation moderne*, 2 vols (Paris: Crochard, 1828).

Virey, Julien-Joseph, *Histoire naturelle du genre humain* (Paris: Crochard, 1834).

Viridet, Jean, *Dissertation sur les vapeurs qui nous arrivent* (Yverdon: J. Jacques Guenath, 1726).

Voisin, Auguste-Félix, *De l'hématocèle rétro-utérine et des épanchements sanguins non enkystés de la cavité péritonéale du petit bassin: Considérés comme accidents de la menstruation* (Paris: J.-B. Baillière et fils, 1860).

Walshe, Walter Hayle, *The Nature and Treatment of Cancer* (London: Taylor & Walton, 1846).

Wargentin, Pehr Wilhelm, 'Mortalitaten i Sverige, i anledning af Tabell-Verket', *Kongl. Vetenskaps-academiens Handlingar*, 27 (1766): 1–25.

Wargentin, Pehr Wilhelm, *Wargentin: Naissance des sciences de la population*, trans. Nathalie Le Bouteillec & Jean-Marie Rohrbasser (Paris: Ined, 2017).

Wells, Thomas Spencer, *Diseases of the Ovaries* (London: John Churchill, 1865).

Wells, Thomas Spencer, *Du traitement des kystes et des tumeurs ovariques* (Paris: Leclerc, 1867).

Wells, Thomas Spencer, *Des tumeurs de l'ovaire et de l'utérus, leur diagnostic et leur traitement* (Paris: G. Masson, 1883).

Whytt, Robert, *Observations on the Nature, Causes and Cure of those Disorders, which have been commonly called Nervous, Hypochondriac or Hysteric; to which are prefixed some remarks on the sympathy of nerves* (Edinburgh: T. Becket & P. A. De Hondt, 1765).

Whytt, Robert, *Les Vapeurs et maladies nerveuses, hypocondriaques ou hystériques reconnues & traitées dans les deux sexes* [1765], 2 vols (Paris: Vincent, 1767).

Willette, Théodore, *Étude sur les accidents nerveux de la ménopause.* Thèse (Paris: A. Parent, 1877).
Windrif, Louis-Joseph, *Essai sur les phénomènes de l'âge critique chez la femme; sur les principaux accidens que l'on remarque à cette époque, et sur les moyens de les prévenir.* Thèse (Strasbourg: Levrault, 1811).
Wion Pigalle, Amélie, *Le Conseiller secret des femmes, ou Conseils sur les moyens de se préserver des maladies qui atteignent spécialement les femmes* (Paris: Georges Kugelmann, 1861).
Wion (Vion) Pigalle, Amélie, *De la peur du choléra et de l'influence pernicieuse que ce sentiment exerce sur la santé* (Paris: Chez l'auteur, 1865).
Zacherl, Hans, *Die Wechseljahre der Frau* (Vienna: Julius Springer, 1928).
Zalzal, N., *Troubles cardiaques de la ménopause.* Thèse (Lyon: Imprimerie Nouvelle, 1885).

Archives

Ms. Joly de Fleury-284, fol. 51, Bibliothèque Nationale de France (site Richelieu).
Remèdes et recettes à l'usage de la famille de Gramont et particulièrement de Marie-Gabrielle de Sinety, duchesse de Gramont (s.d., XVIIIe s-vers 1850): *Archives du duché de Caderousse (1008–XIXe siècle),* Papiers personnels et familiaux Maison de Gramont: 2 E 9/165.
AD Bas-Rhin 5 M22, no. 6

Secondary Reading

Achenbaum, W. Andrew, *Crossing Frontiers: Gerontology Emerges as a Science* (Cambridge: Cambridge University Press, 1995).
Ackernecht, Erwin H., 'Hygiene in France, 1815–1848', *Bulletin of the History of Medicine,* 22/2 (1948): 117–155.
Aiello, E. J., Y. Yutaka, S. S. Tworoger, C. M. Ulrich, M. L. Irwin, D. Bowen, R. S. Schwartz, C. Kumai, J. D. Potter, & A. McTiernan, 'Effect of a Yearlong, Moderate-Intensity Exercise Intervention on the Occurrence and Severity of Menopause Symptoms in Postmenopausal Women', *Menopause,* 11 (2004): 283–288.
Albury, W. R., 'Heart of Darkness: J. N. Corvisart and the Medicalization of Life', in Jean-Pierre Goubert, ed., *La Médicalisation de la société française, 1770–1830* (Waterloo: Historical Reflections Press, 1982), 17–31.
Altman, Daniel, Li Yin, & Henrik Falconer, 'Long-Term Cancer Risk After Hysterectomy on Benign Indications: Population-Based Cohort Study', *International Journal of Cancer,* 138 (2016): 2631–2638. Doi: 10.1002/ijc.30011.
Aprile, Sylvie & Fabrice Bensimon, eds, *La France et l'Angleterre au XIXe siècle* (Paris: Créaphis, 2006).
Archambault, Paul, 'The Ages of Man and the Ages of the World: A Study of Two Traditions', *Revue d'études augustiniennes et patristiques,* 12/3–4 (1966): 193–228.
Ariès, Philippe, *L'Enfant et la vie familiale sous l'ancien régime* (Paris: Le Seuil, 1973).
Arnaud, Robert, *La Ménopause à travers l'histoire* (Lausanne: Laboratoires Ciba-Geigy, 1995).
Arnaud, Sabine, *On Hysteria: The Invention of a Medical Category Between 1670 and 1820* (Chicago: University of Chicago Press, 2015).
Aronson, Jeffrey K. & Manoj Ramachandran, 'The Diagnosis of Art: Dr. Péan's Operation', *Journal of the Royal Society of Medicine* (2008): 423–424. Doi: 0.1258/jrsm.2008.08k001.

Ashley, Susan A., *'Misfits' of Fin-de-Siècle France and Italy: Anatomies of Difference* (London: Bloomsbury, 2017).

Banner, Lois W., *In Full Flower: Aging Women, Power, and Sexuality* (New York: Vintage Books, 1993).

Barton, Tamsyn, *Ancient Astrology* (London: Routledge, 2002).

Baskett, Thomas F., *Pages of History in Canadian Obstetrics and Gynecology* (Toronto: Rogers Media, 2003).

Bauer, Thomas, *La Sportive dans la littérature française des Années folles* (Lille: Presses Universitaires de Septentrion, 2011).

Begert, Lucie, Izel Demirbas, & Aude Fauvel, 'Terre promise ou terre interdite? La Suisse: l'Eldorado ambigu des premières femmes médecins, 1867–1939 [Promised land or forbidden land? Switzerland, the ambiguous El Dorado of the first women doctors, 1867–1939]', *Revue d'histoire des sciences humaines*, 35 (2019): 59–96.

Behar, Cem, 'Le Pasteur Jean-Louis Muret (1715–1796): De la controverse sur la dépopulation à l'analyse démographique', *Population*, 3 (1996): 609–644.

Behar, C. & Y. Ducel, 'L'Arithmétique politique d'Antoine Deparcieux', in Thierry Martin, ed., *Arithmétique politique dans la France du XVIIe siècle* (Paris: Institut National d'Études Démographiques, 2003), 147–194.

Beizer, Janet L., *Ventriloquized Bodies: Narratives of Hysteria in Nineteenth-Century France* (New York: Cornell University Press, 1994).

Berriot-Salvadore, Evelyne, *Un corps, un destin: La Femme dans la médecine de la Renaissance* (Paris: Champion, 1993).

Benoit, Claude, 'L'Art de "bien vieillir" chez deux grandes femmes de lettres: George Sand et Colette', *Gérontologie et société*, 28/114 (2005): 167–193. Doi: 10.3917/gs.114.0167.

Blell, Mwenza, 'Menopausal Symptoms Among British Pakistani Women: A Critique of the Standard Checklist Approach', *Menopause*, 22/1 (2015): 79–87.

Bois, Jean-Pierre, *Histoire de la vieillesse* (Paris: Presses Universitaire de France, 1994).

Bonnet-Cadilhac, Christine, 'Les Aménorrhées dans le "Corpus hippocratique": La Vision du médecin actuel', in Antoine Thivel & Arnaud Zucker, eds, *Le Normal et le pathologique dans la collection hippocratique.* Actes du xe colloque international hippocratique (Nice: Publications de la Faculté des Lettres, Arts et Sciences humaines, 2002), 575–589.

Bordelais, Patrice, *Le Nouvel Age de la vieillesse* (Paris: Odile Jacob, 1993).

Borell, Merriley, 'Brown-Séquard's Organotherapy and Its Appearance in America at the End of the Nineteenth Century', *Bulletin of the History of Medicine*, 50 (1976): 309–320.

Borell, Merriley, 'Organotherapy and the Emergence of Reproductive Endocrinology', *Journal of the History of Biology*, 18 (1985): 1–30. Doi: 10.1007/BF00127955.

Bove, Riley, Elizabeth Secor, Lori B. Chibnik, Lisa L. Barnes, Julie A. Schneider, David A. Bennett, & Philip L. De Jager, 'Age at Surgical Menopause Influences Cognitive Decline and Alzheimer Pathology in Older Women', *Neurology*, 82 (2014): 222–229. Doi: 10.1212/WNL.0000000000000033.

Bozon, Michel & Juliette Rennes, 'The History of Sexual Norms: The Hold of Age and Gender', trans. Siân Reynolds, *CLIO: Women, Gender, History*, 42/2 (2015): 7–23.

Brad-Chopard, Armelle, 'Le Vieillissement au féminin et au masculin chez Simone de Beauvoir', *Recherches féministes*, 26/2 (2013): 37–50. Doi: 10.7202/1022770ar.

Braun, Saori I., Youngdeok Kim, Amy E. Jetton, Minsoo Kang, & Don W. Morgan, 'Sedentary Behavior, Physical Activity, and Bone Health in Postmenopausal Women', *Journal of Aging and Physical Activity*, 25/2 (2017): 173–181. Doi: 10.1123/japa.2016-0046.

Brenner, Thomas, 'Toward the Cultural History of Alcohol in France', *Journal of Social History*, 23/1 (1989): 71–92.

Brockliss, L. W. B., 'Before the Clinic: French Medical Teaching in the Eighteenth Century', in Caroline Hannaway & Ann la Berge, eds, *Constructing Paris Medicine* (Amsterdam: Rodopi, 1998), 71–115.

Brockliss, Lawrence & Colin Jones, *The Medical World of Early Modern France* (Oxford: Oxford University Press, 2004).

Brończyk-Puzoń, Anna, Dariusz Piecha, Justyna Nowak, Aneta Koszowska, Karolina KulikKupka, Anne Dittfield, & Barbarakk Zubelewicz-Szodzińska, 'Guidelines for Dietary Management of Menopausal Women with Simple Obesity', *Przeglad Menopauzalny*, 14/1 (2015): 48–52. Doi: 10.5114/pm.2015.48678.

Brown, Jeannette S., 'Hysterectomy and Urinary Incontinence: A Systematic Review', *The Lancet*, 356/9229 (2000): 535–539. Doi: 0.1016/S0140-6736(00)02577-0.

Buckley, Thomas C. T. & Alma Gottlieb, eds, *Blood Magic: The Anthropology of Menstruation* (Berkeley: University of California Press, 1988).

Burton, June K., *Napoleon and the Woman Question: Discourses of the Other Sex in French Education, Medicine, and Medical Law 1799–1815* (Lubbock: Texas Tech University Press, 2007).

Cantor, David, ed., *Reinventing Hippocrates* (Abingdon: Palgrave, 2016).

Caprais, Annabelle, *La Place et le rôle des femmes dans la gouvernance des fédérations sportives françaises.* Thèse, Education, Université de Bordeaux (2020). HAL Archives ouvertes, Id: tel-03114344. <https://hal.archives-ouvertes.fr/tel-03114344v2>.

Capron, Alexander Morgan, 'Where Did Informed Consent for Research Come From?', *The Journal of Law, Medicine & Ethics*, 46/1 (2018): 12–29. Doi:10.1177/1073110518766004.

Carlino, Carla, 'Écrire la catastrophe du vieillir: Le Cas de Colette', in A. Soncini Fratti, ed., *Horizons de recherche/Research Horizons* (Bologna: Emil, 2014), 173–182.

Censer, Jack R. & Lynn Hunt, *Liberty, Equality, Fraternity: Exploring the French Revolution* (University Park, Pa: Pennsylvania State University Press, 2001).

Chaperon, Sylvie, *La Médecine du sexe et les femmes: Anthologies des perversions féminines au XIXe siècle* (Paris: La Musardine, 2008).

Chaperon, Sylvie, 'Simone de Beauvoir, la promesse faite aux femmes', *L'Humanité* (9 January 2008): 1–4. <https://www.humanite.fr/node/384540> (viewed 11 May 2020).

Charland, Louis C., 'Benevolent Theory: Moral Treatment at the York Retreat', *History of Psychiatry*, 18/1 (2007): 61–80.

Charlap, Cécile, *La Fabrique de la ménopause.* Thèse de sociologie (Strasbourg: Université de Strasbourg, 2015).

Charlap, Cécile, *La Fabrique de la ménopause* (Paris: CNRS, 2019).

Chazal, Gérard, *Les Lumières et l'idée de nature* (Dijon: Éditions universitaires de Dijon, 2011).

Cherici, Céline, 'Serge Voronoff (1866–1951): Savant maudit ou génie de son époque?' *Bulletin d'histoire et d'épistémologie des sciences de la vie*, 21/1 (2014): 57–69. Doi:10.3917/bhesv.211.0057.

Chevalier, Jim, 'The Queen's Coffee and Casanova's Chocolate: The Early Modern Breakfast in France', in Tamara S. Wagner & Narin Hassan, eds, *Consuming Culture in the Long Nineteenth Century: Narratives of Consumption, 1700–1900* (Lanham, Md: Lexington Books, 2007), 191–208.

Chevron, Audrey, François Margueritte, Xavier Fritel, Aniie Serfaty, Cyrille Huchon, & Arnaud Fauconnier, 'Hystérectomie: Évolution des pratiques entre 2009 et 2019 en France', *Gynécologie obstétrique fertilité & sénologie*, 49 (2021): 816–822. Doi: 10.1016/j.gofs.2021.07.002.

Class, Monika, 'Medical Case Histories as Genre: New Approaches', *Literature and Medicine*, 32/1 (2014): 12–26.

Coddens, Michel, 'La Théorie de l'hérédité-dégénéréscence. Morel, Lombroso, Magnan et les autres', *L'En-je lacanien*, 27/2 (2016): 123–149. Doi: 10.3917/enje.027.0123.

Coffin, Jean-Christophe, *La Transmission de la folie* (Paris: Harmattan, 2003).

Conrad, Peter, *The Medicalization of Society: On the Transformation of Human Conditions into Treatable Disorders* (Baltimore: Johns Hopkins University Press, 2007).

Conti, F. F., J. D. E. Brito, N. Bernardes, S. Dias Dda, C. Malfitano, M. Morris, S. F. Llesuy, M. C. Irigoyen, & K. De Angelis, 'Positive Effect of Combined Exercise Training in a Model of Metabolic Syndrome and Menopause', *American Journal of Physiology. Regulatory, Integrative and Comparative Physiology*, 309/12 (2015). R1532-9. Doi: 10.1152/ajpregu.00076.

Cooper Owens, Deirdre, *Medical Bondage: Race, Gender, and the Origins of American Gynecology* (Atlanta, Ga: University of Georgia Press, 2017).

Coquillard, Isabelle, 'Les Docteurs régents de la faculté de médecine de Paris et la fourniture de soins aux "bons pauvres malades" dans les paroisses parisiennes (1644–1791)', *Revue Historique*, 4/668 (2013): 875–904. Doi: 10.3917/rhis.134.0875.

Cosnier, Colette, *Le Silence des filles: De l'aguille à la plume* (Paris: Fayard, 2001).

Coury, Charles, 'The Teaching of Medicine in France from the Beginning of the Seventeenth Century', in Charles Donald O'Malley, ed., *The History of Medical Education* (Berkeley: University of California Press, 1970), 121–172.

Crawford, Patricia, 'Printed Advertisements for Women Medical Practitioners in London, 1670–1710', *Journal for the Social History of Medicine Bulletin*, 35 (1984): 66–70.

Creese, Mary R. S. & Thomas M. Creese, *Ladies in the Laboratory II: West European Science, 1800–1900: A Survey of Their Contributions to Research* (Lanham, Md/Oxford: Scarecrow Press, 2004).

Crozier, Ivan, 'Philosophy in the English Boudoir: Contextualising Havelock Ellis's Discourses about Sexuality, with Particular Reference to His Writing on Algolagnia', *Journal of the History of Sexuality*, 13 (2004): 275–305.

Cryle, Peter, '*Les Choses et les mots*: Missing Words and Blurry Things in the History of Sexuality', *Sexualities*, 12 (2009): 439–452.

Cryle, Peter & Alison Moore, *Frigidity: An Intellectual History* (Basingstoke: Palgrave Macmillan, 2011).

Cryle, Peter & Elizabeth Stephens, *Normality: A Critical Genealogy* (Chicago: University of Chicago Press, 2017).

Davidson, Arnold, *The Emergence of Sexuality; Historical Epistemology and the Formation of Concepts* (Cambridge, Mass.: Harvard University Press, 2004).

Davis, Oliver, *Age Rage and Going Gently: Stories of the Senescent Subject in Twentieth-Century French Writing* (Amsterdam/New York: Rodopi, 2006).

Dean-Jones, L., *Women's Bodies in Classical Greek Science* (Oxford: Oxford University Press, 1996).

Delanoë, Daniel, 'Les Troubles psychique attribués à la ménopause et le regard des hommes', in Pascale Bélot-Foucarde & Diane Winaver, eds, *La Ménopause: Regards croisés entre gynécologues et psychanalystes* (Toulouse: Érès, 2004), 151–170.

Delanoë, Daniel, *Sexe, croyances et ménopause* (Paris: Hachette Littératures, 2007).

Démier, Francis & Claire Barillé, *Les Maux et les soins: Médecins et malades dans les hôpitaux parisiens au XIXe siècle* (Paris: Éditions de la Maison des sciences de l'homme, 2007).

De Moulin, Daniel, *A Short History of Breast Cancer* (Leiden: Martinus Nijhoff, 1983).

Deutscher, Penelope, 'Beauvoir's Old Age', in Claudia Card, ed., *Cambridge Companion to Beauvoir* (Cambridge: Cambridge University Press, 2003), 286–304.

Diasio, Nicoletta, '"Habillée de temps": La Femme à l'âge critique dans le discours médical au tournant du XIXe siècle', in Virginie Vinel, ed., *Féminin/masculin: Approches anthropologiques des catégories et des pratiques médicales* (Strasbourg: Cahiers du portiQue, 2007), 101–129.

Diasio, Nicoletta, 'Maillage des temps et gouvernement des corps dans la construction des rapports d'âge et de genre', *SociologieS: Dossiers, genre et vieillissement*, 5 November 2012 <http://journals.openedition.org/sociologies/4118>.

Ding, D.-C., I.-J. Tsai, C. Y. Hsu, J.-H. Wang, S.-Z. Lin, & F.-C. Sung, 'Risk of Hypertension After Hysterectomy: A Population-Based Study', *BJOG: International Journal of Obstetrics & Gynaecology* (2018): 1–8. Doi: 0.1111/1471-0528.15389.

Dinges, Martin, Kay Peter Jankrift, Sabine Schlegelmilch, & Michael Stohlberg, *Medical Practice 1600–1900*, trans. Margot Saar (Leiden/Boston: Brill/Rodopi, 2016).

Dirlewanger, Dominique, *Les Couleurs de la vieillesse: Histoire culturelle des représentations de la vieillesse en Suisse et en France* (1940–1990) (Neuchâtel: Éditions Alphil-Presses universitaires suisses, 2018).

Doig, Ann Kathleen & Felicia B. Sturzer, eds, *Women, Gender and Disease in Eighteenth-Century England and France* (Cambridge: Cambridge Scholars, 2014).

Dorlin, Elsa, *La Matrice de la race: Généologie sexuelle et coloniale de la nation française* [2006] 2nd ed. (Paris: La Découverte/Poche, 2009).

Dormire, Sharon & Chularat Howharn, 'The Effect of Dietary Intake on Hot Flashes', *Journal of Obstetrics, Gynecology and Neonatal Nursing*, 36/3 (2007): 255–262.

Douville, Olivier, 'Folie hystérique et hystérie virile', *Figures de la psychanalyse*, 1/27 (2014) : 25–33. Doi:10.3917/fp.027.0025.

Dowbiggin, Ian, *Inheriting Madness, Professionalization and Psychiatric Knowledge in Nineteenth-Century France* (Berkeley: University of California Press, 1991).

Duchet, Claude, *Mythes et représentations de la femme au dix-neuvième siècle* (Paris: Champion, 1977).

Duffy, Larry & Catherine Emerson, eds, *La Nature dévoilée: French Literary Responses to Science* (Hull: Hull University Press, 2000).

Dugast-Portes, Francine, 'Colette: Écrire le vieillir', in Alain Montandon (dir.), *Écrire le vieillir* (Clermont-Ferrand: Presses Universitaires Blaise Pascal, 2005), 159–170.

Dulieu, Louis, *La Médecine à Montpellier*, 4 vols (Avignon: Presses Universelles, 1971–1988).

Dumasy-Queffélec, Lise & Hélène Spengler, eds, *Médecine, sciences de la vie et littérature en France et en Europe de la Révolutioin à nos jours: Le Médecin entre savoirs et pouvoirs*, vol. 3 (Geneva : Librairie Droz, 2014).

Dupâquier, Jacques, *L'Invention de la table de mortalité, de Graunt à Wargentin* (Paris: Presses Universitaires de France, 1996).

Dutt, Carsten & Reinhard Laube, eds, *Zwischen Sprache und Geschichte: Zum Werk Reinhart Kosellecks* (Göttingen: Wallstein, 2013).

Edelman, Nicole, *Les Métamorphoses de l'hystérique: Du début du XIXe siècle à la Grande Guerre* (Paris: La Découverte, 2013).

Edwardson, C. L., T. Gorely, M. J. Davies, L. J. Gray, K. Khunti, E. G. Wilmot, T. Yates, & S. J. Biddle, 'Association of Sedentary Behaviour with Metabolic Syndrome: A Metananalysis', *PLos One*, 7/4 (2012): e34916. Doi: 10.1371/journal.pone.0034916.

Eghihan, Greg, *The Routledge History of Madness and Mental Health* (London/New York: Routledge, 2017).

Elden, Stuart, *Mapping the Present: Heidegger, Foucault and Project of a Spatial History* (London: Continuum, 2001).

Engammare, Max, *Soixante-trois: La Peur de la grande année climactérique à la Renaissance* (Geneva: Droz, 2013).

Engelhardt, Dietrich von, 'Krankheit und Heilung bei Thomas Mann', *Praxis* 95/1 (2006): 13–21.

Erekson, Elisabeth A., Deanna K. Martin, MPH, & Elena S. Ratner, 'Oophorectomy: The Debate Between Ovarian Conservation and Elective Oophorectomy', *Menopause*, 20/1 (2013): 110–114. Doi: 10.1097/gme.0b013e31825a27ab.

Evans, Martha, *Fits and Starts: A Genealogy of Hysteria in Modern France* (Ithaca, NY/ London: Cornell University Press, 1991).

Faure, Olivier, 'La Médecine gratuite au XIXe siècle: De la charité à l'assistance', *Histoire, économie & société*, 3–4 (1984): 593–608.

Fausto-Sterling, Anne, *Sexing the Body: Gender Politics and the Construction of Sexuality* (New York: Basic Books, 2000).

Fauvel, Aude, 'Cerveaux fous et sexes faibles (Grande-Bretagne, 1860–1900)', [Crazy Brains and the Weaker Sex: The British Case (1860–1900)], *CLIO: Femmes, genre, histoire*, 37 (2013): 41–64. Doi: 10.4000/cliowgh.352.

Fauvel, Aude, 'Women and Psychiatric Institutionalisation in France', in P. Bourdelais and J. Chircop, eds, *Vulnerabilities, Social Inequalities and Health in Perspective* (Lisbon: Edições Colibri, 2010), 61–72.

Feinson, Marjorie Chary, 'Where are the Women in the History of Aging?,' *Social Science History*, 9/4 (1985): 429–452. Doi: 10.1017/S0145553200015170.

Feller, Elise, 'Les Femmes et le vieillissement dans la France du premier XXe siècle', *CLIO: Femmes, genre, histoire*, 7 (1998). Doi: 10.4000/clio.353.

Ferenczi, Sandor, 'Die psychiatrische Schule von Bordeaux über die Psychoanalyse', in Sandor Ferenczi, *Bausteine zur Psychoanalyse* (Bern: Hans Huber, 1939), 12–24.

Fisher, Kate & Rebecca Langlands, eds, *Sex, Knowledge and Receptions of the Past* (Oxford: Oxford University Press, 2015).

Fischer, Kate & Jana Funke, 'The Age of Attraction: Age, Gender and the History of Modern Male Homosexuality', *Gender & History*, 31/2 (2019): 266–283.

Flatt, Thomas & Linda Partridge, 'Horizons in the Evolution of Aging', *BMC Biology*, 16/93 (2018):1–13. Doi: 10.1186/s12915-018-0562-z.

Flint, F., 'Sociology and Anthropology of the Menopause', in P. A. van Keep, D. M. Serr, and R. B. Greenblatt, eds, *Female and Male Climacteric: Current Opinion 1978* (Lancaster: MIT Press, 1979), 1–9.

Foley, Susan, *Women in France Since 1789: The Meanings of Difference* (Basingstoke: Palgrave, 2004).

Fontaine, Jacqueline, *Les Étudiantes en médecine à la faculté de Montpellier au cours de la Troisième République* (Paris: L'Harmattan, 2016).

Formanek, Ruth, ed., *The Meanings of Menopause: Historical, Medical and Clinical Perspectives* (Hillsdale, NJ: The Analytic Press, 1990).

Formanek, Ruth, 'Menopause: Two Views', *Annals of the New York Academy of Sciences*, 592/1 (1990): 418. Doi: 10.1111/j.1749-6632.1990.tb30357.x.

Formanek, Ruth & Valerie Ann McKeon, 'Dispelling Menopause Myths', *Journal of Gerontological Nursing*, 14/8 (1988): 26–29.

Forsgren, Catharina & Daniel Altman, 'Long-Term Effects of Hysterectomy: A Focus on the Aging Patient', *Aging Health*, 9/2 (2013): 179–187. Doi: 10.2217/ahe.13.7.

Foucault, Michel, *Les Mots et les choses: Une archéologie des sciences humaines* (Paris: Editions Gallimard, 1966).

Foucault, Michel, *Histoire de la sexualité*, 4 vols (Paris: Gallimard, 1984–2018).

Foucault, Michel, *'Il faut défendre la société': Cours au Collège de France (1975–1976)*, ed. François Ewald & Alessandro Fontana (Paris: l'Association pour le Centre Michel Foucault, 2012).

Foucault, Michel, *La Naissance de la clinique* [1963] (Paris: Presses Universitaires de France, 2015).

Foucault, Michel, *La Sexualité: Cours donné à l'université de Clermont-Ferrand (1964), Suivi de Le Discours de la sexualité: Cours donné à l'université de Vincennes (1969)*, ed. Claude-Olivier Doron (Paris: Gallimard/Seuil, 2018).

Foxcroft, Louise, *Hot Flushes, Cold Science: A History of the Modern Menopause* (London: Granta Books, 2011).

Frampton, Sally, *Belly-Rippers, Surgical Innovation and the Ovariotomy Controversy* (London: Palgrave, 2018).

Frampton, Sally & Roger L. Kneebone, 'John Wickham's New Surgery: "Minimally Invasive Therapy", Innovation, and Approaches to Medical Practice in Twentieth-Century Britain', *Social History of Medicine*, 30/3 (2017): 544–566. Doi: 10.1093/shm/hkw074.

Frank, Rosalyn M., *The Hidden Face of a Midwifery Treatise from 17th Century England: The Chamberlen Family, Dr. Peter Chamberlen and the Contributionsof Huarte de San Juan to The Compleat Midwife's Practice Enlarged* (Creative Common: Roslyn M. Frank: 2016).

Franzel, Sean & Stefan-Ludwig Hoffman, *Sediments of Time: On Possible Histories*, ed. Hent de Vries (Stanford, Calif.: Stanford University Press, 2018).

Freckelton, Ian, 'Sterilization of Intellectually Disabled Minors', *Journal of Law & Medicine*, 14/3 (2007): 299–305.

Füzéki, E., L. Vogt, & W. Banzer, 'Sedentary Behaviour and Health', *Gesundheitswesen*, 77/3 (2015): 148–160. Doi: 10.1055/s-0034-1370951.

Gambaudo, Sylvie, 'The Regulation of Gender in Menopause Theory', *Topoi*, 36/3 (2017): 549–559. Doi: 10.1007/s11245-015-9351-2.

Garcia Rodríguez, Miguel Emilio, & Miguel Javier García Basulto, 'Vaginal Hysterectomy: Historical Notes', *Gaceta Médica Espirituana*, 21/1 (2019): 59–69.

Garg, Suneela, Nandini Sharma, & Ragini Sahay, 'Socio-Cultural Aspect of Menstruation in an Urban Slum in Delhi, India', *Reproductive Health Matters*, 9/17 (2001): 16–25.

Garrabé, Jean, 'Les Chaires de clinique des maladies mentales et des maladies nerveuses à Paris', *L'Information psychiatrique*, 88/7 (2012): 549–557. Doi: 10.3917/inpsy.8807.0549.

Gayet-Ageron, Angèle, Nassira Amamra, Virginie Ringa, Valérie Tainturier, Claudine Berr, Françoise Clavel-Chapelon, Cécile Delcourt, Pierre D. Delmas, Pierre Ducimetière, & Anne-Marie Schott, 'Estimated Numbers of Postmenopausal Women Treated by Hormone Therapy in France', *Maturitas*, 52/2–3 (2005): 269–305. Doi: 10.1016/j.maturitas.2005.05.002.

Georgakis, Marios K., Theano Beskou-Kontou, Ioannis Theodoridis, Alkistis Skalkidou, & Eleni Th. Petridou, 'Surgical Menopause in Association with Cognitive Function and Risk of Dementia: A Systematic Review and Meta-analysis', *Psychoneuroendocrinology*, 106 (2019): 9–19. Doi: 10.1016/j.psyneuen.2019.03.013.

Gerhard, Rudolf, 'Santé publique et éducation: Notions d'hygiène sociale au XVIIIe et au XIXe siècle: Étienne Tourtelle (1756–1800), Jules Levy (1805–1872), Jules Rochard (1819–1896)', *Histoire des sciences médicales*, 17/A1 (1982): 146–150.

Gibert, Bertrand, 'Des Avatars littéraires: Le Cas du Docteur Pozzi', *Poétique*, 2/190 (2021): 171–202.

Godfrey, Jessica E., *Attitudes to Post-Menopausal Women in the High and Late Middle Ages, 1100–1400* (Jessica E. Godfrey, 2011).

Goetz, Rose, 'Les Âges de la vie dans les *Rapports du physique et du moral de l'homme* de Pierre-Jean-Georges Cabanis', *Le PortiQue: Revue de philosophie et de sciences humaines*, 21 (2008). Doi:10.4000/leportique.1713.

Goldstein, Jan, 'The Uses of Male Hysteria: Medical and Literary Discourses in Nineteenth-Century France', in Ann La Berge & Mordechai Feingold, eds, *French Medical Culture in the Nineteenth Century* (Amsterdam: Rodopi, 1994), 210–247.

Goodfellow, Sarah, *'The Sexual Hush': Representations of Late-Life Sexuality in Western Europe and America, 1870–1930*. Ph.D. thesis (Pennsylvania State University, College of Liberal Arts, 2004).

Goubert, Jean-Pierre, ed., *La Médicalisation de la société française, 1770–1830* (Waterloo: Historical Reflections Press, 1982).

Grassi, Marie-Claire, 'L'Art épistolaire français (XVIIIe et XIXe siècles)', dans Alain Montadon, ed., *Pour une histoire des traités de savoir-faire en Europe* (Clermont-Ferrand: Association des publications de la Faculté des Lettres et Sciences humaines de Clermont-Ferrand, 1994), 301–331.

Greer, Germaine, *The Change: Women, Ageing and the Menopause* (London: Bloomsbury, 2018).

Grob, Gerald N., *Aging Bones: A Short History of Osteoporosis* (Baltimore: Johns Hopkins University Press, 2014).

Gueslin, André & Dominique Kalifa, eds, *Les Exclus en Europe, 1830–1930* (Paris: Les Éditions de l'Ateler, 1999).

Guincêtre, Pierre & Pierre Julien, 'La Publicité médico-pharmaceutique de l'Astrologue Normand en 1904', *Revue d'histoire de la pharmacie*, 78 (1990): 390–397.

Haber, Carole, *Beyond Sixty-Five: The Dilemna of Old Age in America's Past* (Cambridge: Cambridge University Press, 1983).

Hacking, Ian, *The Social Construction of What?* (Cambridge, Mass.: Harvard University Press, 1999).

Hällström, T. & S. Samuelsson, 'Mental Health in the Climacteric: The Longitudinal Study of Women in Gothenburg', *Acta Obstetricia Gynecologica Scandinavica Supplement*, 130 (1985): 13–18. Doi: 10.3109/00016348509157141.

Hamilton, M. T., D. G. Hamilton, & T. W. Zderic, 'Sedentary Behaviour as a Mediator of Type 2 Diabetes', *Medicine and Sports Science*, 60 (2014): 11–26. Doi: 10.1159/000357332.

Harnacke, Caroline, 'The Ashley Treatment: Improving Quality of Life or Infringing Dignity and Rights?', *Bioethics*, 30/3 (2016): 141–150.

Hartun, Heike, ed., *Alter und Geschlecht: Repräsentationen, Geschichten und Theorien des Alter(n)s* (Beilefeld: Transcript Verlag, 2005).

Harvey, Graham, *Eternal Eve: The History of Gynecology & Obstetrics* (New York: Doubleday, 1951).

Hassan, Narin, *Diagnosing Empire: Women, Medical Knowledge and Colonial Mobility* (London & New York: Routledge, 2016).

Hauger, Christian, *Le Professeur Eugène Kœberlé, précurseur de la chirurgie abdominale moderne, (1828–1915), l'homme et son œuvre*. Thèse (Université Louis Pasteur (Strasbourg 1): Faculté de médecine, 1986).

Hewitt, Jessie, *Institutionalizing Gender: Madness, the Family, and Psychiatric Power in Nineteenth-Century France* (Ithaca, NY/London: Cornell University Press, 2020).

Hickey, Martha & Gita D. Mishra, 'Timing and Type of Menopause and Risk of Cardiovascular Disease', *Menopause: The Journal of the North American Menopause Society*, 28/5 (2021): 477–479. Doi: 10.1097/GME.0000000000001747.

Hoberman, John, *Testosterone Dreams: Rejuvenation, Aphrodisia, Doping* (Berkeley: University of California Press, 2005).

Hoffmann, Paul, *La Femme dans la pensée des lumières*, 2nd ed. (Geneva: Slatkine Reprints, 1977/1995).

Holmes, Diana, 'Colette, Beauvoir and the Change of Life', *French Studies*, 53/4 (1999): 430–443. Doi: 10.1093/fs/53.4.430.

Hörder, Helena, Lena Johansson, & Xin Xin Guo, 'Midlife Cardiovascular Fitness and Dementia: A 44-Year Longitudinal Population Study in Women', *Neurology*, 90/15 (2018): e1298–e1305; Doi: 10.1212/WNL.0000000000005290.

Horstmanshoff, Manfred, Helen King, & Claus Zittel, *Blood, Sweat and Tears: The Changing Concepts of Physiology from Antiquity into Early Modern Europe* (Leiden: Brill, 2012).

Houck, Judith A., *Hot and Bothered: Women, Medicine, and Menopause in Modern America* (Cambridge, Mass.: Harvard University Press, 2008).

Hu, F. B., M. J. Stampfer, G. A. Colditz, A. Ascherio, K. M. Rexrode, W. C. Willett, & J. E. Manson, 'Physical Activity and Risk Stroke in Women', *Journal of the American Medical Association*, 283/22 (2000): 2961–2967.

Huebner, Marianne, David Meltzer, Wenjuan Ma, & Holly Arrow, 'The Masters Athlete in Olympic Weightlifting: Training, Lifestyle, Health Challenges, and Gender Differences', *PLoS One*, 15/12 (2020): Article e0243652. Doi: 10.1371/journal.pone.0243652.

Hugon, Anne, ed., *Histoire des femmes en situation coloniale: Afrique et Asie, XXe siècle* (Paris: Karthala, 2004).

Huguet, Françoise, *Les Professeurs de la faculté de médecine de Paris: Dictionnaire biographique 1794–1939* (Paris: Éditions du CNRS, 1991).

Illich, Ivan, *Medical Nemesis* (London: Calder & Boyars, 1974).

Ingelsson, Erik, Cecilia Lundholm, Anna L. V. Johansson, & Daniel Altman, 'Hysterectomy and Risk of Cardiovascular Disease: A Population-Based Cohort Study', *European Heart Journal*, 32 (2011): 745–750. Doi: 10.1093/eurheartj/ehq477.

Izquierdo, Mikel, R. A. Merchant, J. E. Morley, S. D. Anker, I. Aprahamian, H. Arai, M. Aubertin-Leheudre, R. Bernabei, E. L. Cadore, M. Cesari, L.-K. Chen, P. de Souto Barreto, G. Duque, L. Ferrucci, R. A. Fielding, A. García-Hermoso, L. M. Gutiérrez-Robledo, S. D. R. Harridge, B. Kirk, S. Kritchevsky, F. Landi, N. Lazarus, F. C. Martin, E. Marzetti, M. Pahor, R. Ramírez-Vélez, L. Rodriguez-Mañas, Y. Rolland, J. G. Ruiz, O. Theou, D. T. Villareal, D. L. Waters, C. Won Won, J. Woo, B. Vellas, & M. Fiatarone Singh, 'International Exercise Recommendations in Older Adults (ICFSR): Expert Consensus Guidelines', *Journal of Nutrition, Health & Aging*, 25/7 (2021): 824–853. Doi: 10.1007/s12603-021-1665-8.

Jablonka, Eva & Marion J. Lamb, *Evolution in Four Dimensions: Genetic, Epigenetic, Behavioral, and Symbolic Variation in the History of Life*, rev. ed. (Cambridge, Mass.: MIT Press, 2014).

Jackson, Mark, *A Global History of Medicine* (Oxford: Oxford University Press, 2018).

Jasienska, Grazyna, *The Fragile Wisdom: An Evolutionary View on Women's Biology and Health* (Cambridge, Mass.: Harvard University Press, 2013).

Jones, Colin, 'Montpellier Medical Students and the "Medicalisation" of Eighteenth-Century France', in R. Porter & A. Wear, eds, *Problems and Methods in the History of Medicine* (London: Croom Helm, 1987), 57–80.

Jones, Colin & Roy Porter, 'Introduction', in Colin Jones & Roy Porter, eds, *Reassessing Foucault: Power, Medicine and the Body* (London: Routledge, 1994), 1–16.

Katz, Stephen, 'Simon de Beauvoir's The Coming of Age: The Humanities and Gerontology's Diagram of Science', *Age, Culture, Humanities: An Interdisciplinary Journal*, 3 (2016): 1–10.

Katzmarzyk, P. T., T. S. Church, C. L. Craig, & C. Bouchard, 'Sitting Time and Mortality from All Causes, Cardiovascular Disease, and Cancer', *Medicine and Science in Sports and Exercise*, 41/5 (2009): 998–1005. Doi: 10.1249/MSS.0b013e3181930355.

Kendall, Kristina L. & Ciaran M. Fairman, 'Women and Exercise in Aging', *Journal of Sport and Health Science*, 3/3 (2014): 170–178. Doi: 10.1016/j.jshs.2014.02.001.

Kern-Coquillat, Françoise, 'Les Femmes médecins dans le service de santé (1914–1918)', *Deportate, esuli, profughe (DEP): Rivista telematica de studi sulla memoria femminile*, 24 (2014): 48–75.

Kerr, John Martin Munro, Robert William Johnstone, & Miles H. Phillips, *Historical Review of British Obstetrics and Gynecology, 1800–1950* (Edinburgh/London: E. & S. Livingstone, 1954).

Kertzer, David I. & Peter Laslett, eds, *Aging in the Past: Demography, Society and Old Age* (Berkeley: University of California Press, 1995).

Khan, Aamir, Manjeet Shehmar, & Janesh K. Gupta, 'Uterine Fibroids: Current Perspectives', *International Journal of Women's Health*, 6 (2014): 95–114.

King, Helen, *Hippocrates' Woman: Reading the Female Body in Ancient Greece* (London/New York: Routledge, 1998).

King, Helen, *Midwifery, Obstetrics and the Rise of Gynaecology* (London: Routledge, 2007).

King, Helen, *The One-Sex Body on Trial: The Classical and Early-Modern Evidence* (London: Routledge, 2013).

King, Jeannette, *Discourses of Ageing in Fiction and Feminism: The Invisible Woman* (London: Palgrave, 2013).

Kohn, Grace E., Katherine M. Rodriguez, & Alexander W. Pastuszuk, 'The History of Estrogen Therapy', *Sexual Medicine Review*, 7/3 (2019): 416–421. Doi: 10.1016/j.sxmr.2019.03.006.

Kolip, Petra, ed., *Weiblichkeit ist keine Krankheit: Die Medikalisierung körperlicher Umbruchphasen im Leben von Frauen* (Weinheim/Munich, 2000).

Komesaroff, Paul, Philipa Rothfield, & Jeanne Daly, eds, *Reinterpreting the Menopause: Cultural and Philosophical Issues* (New York: Routledge, 1997).

Köninger, Angela & Rainer Kimmig, 'Geschichte der operativen Gynäkologie am Beispiel der Hysterektomie—eine Zeitreise', in Rolf Kreienberg & Hans Ludwig, eds, *125 Jahre Deutsche Gesellschaft für Gynäkologie und Geburtshilfe* (Berlin/Heidelberg: Springer-Verlag, 2011), 93–140.

Koselleck, Reinhart, '"Neuzeit": Zur Semantik moderner Bewegungsbegriffe', *Vergangene Zukunft: Zur Semantik geschichtlicher Zeiten* (Frankfurt am Main: Suhrkamp, 1979), 260–277.

Koselleck, Rheinhart, 'Wie neu is die Neuzeit?' *Historische Zeitschrift*, 251 (1990): 539–554.

Koselleck, Reinhart, *The Practice of Conceptual History: Timing History, Spacing Concepts*, trans. Todd Presner (Stanford, Calif.: Stanford University Press, 2002).

La Berge, Ann, 'Dichotomy or Integration? Medical Microscopy and the Paris Clinical Tradition', in Caroline Hannaway & Ann Le Berge, eds, *Constructing Paris Medicine* (Amsterdam: Rodopi, 1998), 275–312.

La Berge, Ann and Caroline Hannaway, 'Paris Medicine: Perspectives Past and Present', in Caroline Hannaway and Ann La Berge, *Constructing Paris Medicine* (Amsterdam: Rodopi, 1998), 1–70.

La Berge, Ann & Mordechai Feingold, eds, *French Medical Culture in the Nineteenth Century* (Amsterdam: Rodopi, 1994).

Ladimer, Bethany, *Colette, Beauvoir and Duras: Age and Women Writers* (Gainsville, Fla: University of Florida Press, 1999).

Laqueur, Thomas W., *Making Sex from the Greeks to Freud* (Cambridge, Mass.: Harvard University Press, 1990).

Laqueur, Thomas W., *Solitary Sex: A Cultural History of Masturbation* (New York: Zone Books, 2003).

Laughlin-Tommaso, Shannon K., Anisha Satish, Zaraq Khan, Carin Y. Smith, Walter A. Rocca, & Elizabeth A. Stewart, 'Long-Term Risk of De Novo Mental Health Conditions After Hysterectomy With Ovarian Conservation: A Cohort Study', *Menopause: The Journal of the North American Menopause Society*, 27/1 (2020): 33–42. Doi: 10.1097/GME.0000000000001415.

Laughlin-Tommaso, Shannon K., Zaraq Khan, Amy L. Weaver, Carin Y. Smith, Walter A. Rocca, & Elizabeth A. Stewart, 'Cardiovascular and Metabolic Morbidity after Hysterectomy with Ovarian Conservation: A Cohort Study', *Menopause: Journal of the North American Menopause Society*, 25/5 (2017): 483–492. Doi: 10.1097/GME.0000000000001043.

Le Bouteillec, Nathalie & Jean-Marie Rohrbasser, eds, *Wargentin: Naissance des sciences de la population* (Paris: Institut National d'Études Démographiques, 2017), 122–124.

Le Bras, Hervé, *Naissance de la mortalité: L'Origine politique de la statistique et de la démographie* (Paris: Gallimard, 2000).

Lebrun, Caroline, 'Adolescence et ménopause: L'Angoisse des grands passages', *Dialogue*, 204 (2014): 63–77.

Le Dœuff, Michèle, *Le Sexe du savoir* (Paris: Aubier, 1998).

Le Naour, Jean-Yves & Catherine Valenti, 'Du sang et des femmes: Histoire médicale de la menstruation à la Belle Époque', *CLIO: Histoire, femmes et sociétés*, 14 (2001): 207–229. Doi:10.4000/clio.114.

Léonard, Jacques, *La Médecine entre les pouvoirs et les savoirs: Histoire intellectuelle et politique de la médecine française au XIXième siècle* (Paris: Editions Aubier, 1992).

Leproult, Rachel & Eve Cauter, 'Role of Sleep Loss in Hormonal Release and Metabolism', *Endocrine Development*, 17 (2017): 11–21. Doi: 10.1159/000262524.

Leridon, Henri, 'Théories de la fécondité: Des démographes sous influence?' *Population*, 70/2 (2015): 331–373. Doi: 10.3917/popu.1502.0331.

Lesch, John E., *Science and Medicine in France: The Emergence of Experimental Physiology, 1790–1855* (Cambridge, Mass.: Harvard University Press, 1984).

Li, Pei-Chen, I.-Ju Tsai, Chung Y. Hsu, Jen-Hung Wang, Shinn-Zong Lin, Dah-Ching Ding, & Fung-Chang Sung, 'Risk of Hyperlipidemia in Women with Hysterectomy: A Retrospective Cohort Study in Taiwan', *Nature Scientific Reports*, 8 (2018): 1–9. Article 12956. Doi: 0.1038/s41598-018-31347-z.

Liotard-Schneider, Frédérique, *Les Experts de l'intime et les femmes, médecins et démographes en France de 1945 à 1975*. Thèse d'histoire (Paris: Ouest-Nanterre, 2010).

Livi, Jocelyne, *Vapeurs de femmes: Essai historique sur quelques fantasmes médicaux et philosophiques* (Paris: Navarin, 1984).

Lock, Margaret M., *Encounters with Aging: Mythologies of Menopause in Japan and North America* (Berkeley: University of California Press, 1993).

Logan, Cheryl A., *Hormones, Heredity and Race: Spectacular Failure in Interwar Vienna* (New Brunswick, NJ: Rutgers University Press, 2013).

Löwy, Ilana, 'Le Genre du cancer' [The gender of cancer], trans. Geneviève Knibiehler, *CLIO: Femmes, genre, histoire*, 37 (2013): 65–83.

Löwy, Ilana, *Preventive Strikes: Women, Precancer, and Prophylactic Surgery* (Baltimore: Johns Hopkins University Press, 2010).

Löwy, Ilana & Jean-Paul Gaudillière, 'Médicalisation de la ménopause, mouvements pour la santé des femmes et controverses sur les thérapies hormonales', *Nouvelles Questions féministes*, 25/2 (2006): 48–65.

Lupton, Deborah, 'Foucault and the Medicalisation Critique', in Alan Peterson and Alan Bunton, eds, *Foucault, Health and Medicine* (London/New York: Routledge, 1997), 94–110.

McClive, Cathy, *Menstruation and Procreation in Early-Modern France* (London/New York: Routledge, 2015).

McClive, Cathy & Nicole Pellegrin, eds, *Femmes en fleurs, femmes en corps: Sang, santé, sexualité du moyen âge aux Lumières* (Saint-Étienne: L'École du genre, 2010).

McGregor, Deborah Kuhn, *From Midwives to Medicine: The Birth of American Gynecology* (New Brunswick, NJ: Rutgers University Press, 1998).

McLean, Ian, *The Renaissance Notion of Woman: A Study in the Fortunes of Scholasticism* (Cambridge: Cambridge University Press, 1980).

Macmillan, James F., *France and Women 1789–1914: Gender, Society and Politics* (London/New York: Routledge, 2000).

Malenfant, Émilie, 'Vieillir sans laisser de trace: Où sont les femmes âgées dans l'histoire?' *HistoireEngagee.ca* (19 December 2016): <http://histoireengagee.ca/?p=6123>.

Marchand, André, *Opothérapie: Émergence et développement d'une technique thérapeutique (France, 1889–1940). Histoire, Philosophie et Sociologie des sciences.* Thèse (Paris: Conservatoire national des arts et métiers, 2015).

Marchand, Suzanne, 'Cachez ce sang que je ne saurais voir. Les Menstruations au Québec (1900–1950)', *Rabaska: Revue d'ethnologie de l'Amérique française*, 10 (2012): 69–80. Doi: 10.7202/1013541ar.

Martin-Fugier, Anne, *La Bourgeoise* (Paris: Grassset, 1983).

Matterns, Susan P., *The Slow Moon Climbs: The Science, History and Meaning of Menopause* (Princeton: Princeton University Press, 2019).

Mayer, Ernst, *The Growth of Biological Thought: Diversity, Evolution, and Inheritance* (Cambridge, Mass.: Harvard University Press, 1982).

Mbarga, Josiane Marie Pascaline, *L'Expérience de la ménopause: Étude ethnographique en Suisse Romande et au Centre-Cameroun.* Thèse (Lausanne: Institut des Sciences Sociales, 2012).

Medvei, Victor C., *A History of Endocrinology* (Lancaster: MTP Press, 1982).

Micale, Mark, *Approaching Hysteria: Disease and Its Interpretations* (Princeton: Princeton University Press, 1995).

Micale, Mark, *Hysterical Men: The Hidden History of Male Nervous Illness* (Cambridge, Mass.: Harvard University Press, 2008).

Minois, George, *Histoire de la vieillesse: De l'antiquité à la Renaissance* (Paris: Fayard, 1987).

Mitchinson, Wendy, *The Nature of Their Bodies: Women and Their Doctors in Victorian Canada* (Toronto: University of Toronto Press, 1991).

Moilanen, J., A. M. Aalto, E. Hemminki, A. R. Aro, J. Raitanen, & R. Luoto, 'Prevalence of Menopause Symptoms and Their Association with Lifestyle Among Finnish Middle-Aged Women', *Maturitas*, 67/4 (2010): 368–374. Doi: 10.1016/j.maturitas.2010.08.007.

Monteleone, P., G. Mascagni, A. Gianni, A. R. Genazzani, & T. Simoncini, 'Symptoms of Menopause: Global Prevalence, Physiology and Implications', *Nature Reviews. Endocrinology*, 14/4 (2017). Doi: 10.1038/nrendo.2017.180.

Montesi, Élide, *Les Filles d'Hippocrate* (Tilly: Éditions Acrodacrolivres, 2015).

Moore, Alison M. Downham, 'Foucault's Scholarly Virtues and Sexuality Historiography', *History: The Journal of the Historical Association*, 105/366 (2020): 446–469. Doi: 10.1111/1468-229X.13015.

Moore, Alison M. Downham, 'The Historicity of Sexuality: Knowledge of the Past in the Emergence of Modern Sexual Science', *Modern Intellectual History*, 18/2 (2021): 1–24. Doi: 10.1017/S147924431900026X.

Moore, Alison M. Downham & Stuart Elden, 'Foucault's 1960s Lectures on Sexuality', *Theory, Culture and Society*, Special Issue on Foucault Before the Collège de France (2021): 1–15.

Moore, Alison M. Downham & Rashmi Pithavadian, 'Aphrodisiacs in the Global History of Medical Thought', *Journal of Global History*, 16/1 (2021): 24–43. Doi: 10.1017/S1740022820000108.

Moore, Alison Downham, Fouzieyha Towghi, Holly Ashford, Tinashe Dune, & Rashmi Pithavadian, 'The Global Proliferation of Radical Gynaecological Surgeries: A History of the Present', *History & Anthropology*, 32/4 (2021): 1–25. Doi: 10.1080/02757206.2021.1987232.

Moore, Alison M., '*L'Amour morbide*: How a Transient Mental Illness Became Defunct', *Intellectual History Review*, 29/2 (2019): 291–312. Doi: 10.1080/17496977.2017.1374078.

Moore, Alison M., 'Conceptual Layers in the Invention of Menopause in Nineteenth-Century France', *French History*, 32/2 (2018): 226–248. Doi: 10.1093/fh/cry006.

Moore, Alison M., *Sexual Myths of Modernity: Sadism, Masochism and Historical Teleology* (New York: Lexington, 2015).

Moore, Alison M., ed., *Sexing Political Culture in the History of France* (New York: Cambria, 2012).

Morel, Marie-France, 'Nathalie Sage-Pranchère, mettre au monde: Sages Femmes et accouchées en Corrèze au XIXe siècle', *CLIO: Femmes, genre, histoire*, 29 (2009). <http://journals.openedition.org/clio/9339>.

Mosconi, Nicole, 'Aux sources du sexisme contemporain: Cabanis et la faiblesse des femmes', *Le Télémaque*, 39 (2011): 115–130.

Moscucci, Ornella, *The Science of Woman: Gynaecology and Gender in England, 1800–1929* (Cambridge: Cambridge University Press, 1993).

Moscucci, Ornella, 'Medicine, Age and Gender: The Menopause in History', *British Menopause Society*, 5/4 (1999): 149–153.

Moulinié, Véronique, 'Andropause et ménopause: La Sexualité sur ordonnance', [The Andropause and the Menopause: Sexuality by Prescription] *CLIO: Histoire, femmes et sociétés*, 37 (2013): 105–121. Doi: 10.4000/clio.11016.

Moulinié, Véronique, *La Chirurgie des âges: Corps, sexualité et représentations du sang* (Paris: Éditions de la Maison des sciences de l'homme, 2016).

Muir, Kate, 'Women have struggled to get help with the menopause for decades but it's about to change', *The Guardian*, 6 October 2021. <https://www.theguardian.com/commentisfree/2021/oct/06/women-menopause-change-hormone-replacement-therapy>.

Muir, Kate, 'Mission Menopause: My hormones went off a cliff—and I'm not going to be ashamed', *The Guardian*, 9 May 2021. <https://www.theguardian.com/society/2021/may/09/mission-menopause-my-hormones-went-off-a-cliff-and-im-not-going-to-be-ashamed>.

Müller, Jan-Werner, 'On Conceptual History', in Darrin M. McMahon and Samuel Moyn, eds, *Rethinking Modern European Intellectual History* (New York: Oxford University Press, 2014), 74–92.

Nicol-Smith, Louise, 'Causality, Menopause, and Depression: A Critical Review of Literature', *BMJ* 313 (1996), article 1229. <https://doi.org/10.1136/bmj.313.7067.1229>.

Nussbaum, Martha & Saul Levmore, *Aging Thoughtfully: Conversations About Retirement, Romance, Wrinkles and Regret* (Oxford: Oxford University Press, 2017).

Nye, Robert A., 'The Evolution of the Concept of Medicalization in the Late Twentieth Century', *Journal of the History of the Behavioural Sciences*, 39/2 (2003): 115–129.

O'Dowd, Michael J. & Elliot E. Philipp, *The History of Obstetrics & Gynecology* (New York: Parthenon, 1994).

Offen, Karen, *The Woman Question in France, 1400–1870* (Cambridge: Cambridge University Press, 2017).

Offen, Karen, 'Depopulation, Nationalism and Feminism in Fin-de-Siècle France', *American Historical Review*, 89/3 (1984): 648–676. Doi: 10.2307/1856120.

Ogilvie, Marilyn Bailey, *Women in Science: Antiquity Through the Nineteenth Century. A Biographical Dictionary with Annotated Bibliography* (Cambridge, Mass.: MIT Press, 1986).

Oliveira, Juliana S., Marina B. Pinheiro, Nicola Fairhall, et al., 'Evidence on Physical Activity and the Prevention of Frailty and Sarcopenia Among Older People: A Systematic Review to Inform the World Health Organization Physical Activity Guidelines', *Journal of Physical Activity and Health*, 17/12 (2020): 1247–1258. Doi: 10.1123/jpah.2020-0323.

Olsen, Niklas, *History in the Plural: An Introduction to the Work of Reinhart Koselleck* (New York: Berghahn, 2012).

Orrells, Daniel, *Sex: Antiquity and Its Legacy* (London: Bloomsbury, 2015).

Ottaway, Susannah R., *The Decline of Life: Old Age in Eighteenth-Century England* (Cambridge: Cambridge University Press, 2004).

Ottaway, Susannah R., Lynn A. Botehlo, & Katherin Kittredge, eds, *Power and Poverty: Old Age in the Pre-Industrial Past* (Westport, Conn.: Greenwood Press, 2002).

Oudshoorn, Nellie, *Beyond the Natural Body: An Archeology of Sex Hormones* (London & New York: Routledge, 1994).

Palluaut, Florent, *Medical Students in England and France, 1815–1858, A Comparative Study.* Thesis (University of Oxford: Trinity College, 2003).

Panke-Kochinke, Birgit, *Die Wechseljahre der Frau: Aktualität und Geschichte 1772–1996* (Opladen: Leske & Budrich, 1998).

Parkin, T. G., *Old Age in the Roman World: A Cultural and Social History* (Baltimore: Johns Hopkins University Press, 2003).

Power, Geraldine, 'Yvette Guilbert: A Career of Public Applause and Personal Disappointment', *Context*, 27 and 28 (2004): 31–41.

Pearsall, Chad, 'Biography of Emma F. Angell Drake, 1849–1934', in National Woman Suffrage Association, *Biographical Database of NAWSA Suffragists, 1890–1920.* <https://documents.alexanderstreet.com/d/1009656460>.

Pernau, Margrit & Dominic Sachsenmaier, eds, *Global Conceptual History: A Reader* (London: Bloomsbury, 2016).

Phung, T. K. T., Berit Lindum Waltoft, Thomas Munk Laursen, Annette Settnes, Lars Vedel Kessing, Preben Bo Mortensen, & Gunhild Waldemar, 'Hysterectomy, Oophorectomy and Risk of Dementia: A Nationwide Historical Cohort Study', *Dementia and Geriatric Cognitive Disorders*, 30/1 (2010): 43–50. Doi: 0.1159/000314681.

Pick, Daniel, *Faces of Degeneration: A European Disorder, c.1848–c.1918* (Cambridge: Cambridge University Press, 1993).

Pierron, Agnès, *Les Nuits blanches du Grand-Guignol* (Paris: Seuil, 2002).

Pitts-Taylor, Victoria, ed., *Cultural Encyclopedia of the Body* (Westport, Conn.: Greenwood Press, 2008).

Planiol, Thérèse, *Herbes folles hier, femmes médecins aujourd'hui* (Anjou: Editions Cheminements, 2000).

Power, Geraldine, 'Yvette Guilbert: A Career of Public Applause and Personal Disappointment', *Context*, 27 and 28 (2004): 31–41.

Quinlan, Sean M., *Morbid Undercurrents: Medical Subcultures in Postrevolutionary France* (Ithaca, NY: Cornell University Press, 2021).

Quinlan, Sean M., *Medicine and the Social Body in France: From Individual Self to Social Theory in Learned Medical Practice, 1750–1850* (Bloomington, Ind.: Indiana University Press, 2000).

Quinlan, Sean M., *The Great Nation in Decline: Sex, Modernity and Health Crises in Revolutionary France, c.1750–1850* (Aldershot: Ashgate, 2007).

Rahman, Sabbir T., Nirmala Pandeya, Rachel E Neale, Donald S. A. McLeod, Peter D. Baade, Philippa H. Youl, Roger Allison, Susan Leonard, & Susan J. Jordan, 'Risk of Thyroid Cancer Following Hysterectomy', *Cancer Epidemiology*, 72 (2021): 1–8. Article 101931. Doi: 10.1016/j.canep.2021.101931.

Ramsey, Matthew, *Professional and Popular Medicine in France, 1779–1830* (Cambridge: Cambridge University Press, 1988).

Ramsey, Matthew, 'Academic Medicine and Medical Industrialism: The Regulation of Secret Remedies in Nineteenth-Century France', in Ann La Berge and Mordechai Feingold, eds, *French Medical Culture in the Nineteenth Century* (Amsterdam: Rodopi, 1994), 25–78.

Riddle, John M., *Contraception and Abortion from the Ancient World to the Renaissance* (Cambridge, Mass./London: Harvard University Press, 1992).

Ringa, Virginie, Noëlle Varnoux, Stéphanie Paiult, & Gérard Bréart, 'Hormone Therapy Use among Postmenopausal French Women before the Publication of the Women's Health Initiative Study: Duration of Use and Factors Associated with Discontinuation', *Reproductive Endocrinology*, 83/6 (2005): 1771–1779. Doi: 10.1016/j.fertnstert.2004.12.040.

Rizk, Botros, Mostafa I. Abuzeid, Ibrahim Alkatout, & Liselotte Mettler, eds, *Advances in Minimally Invasive Gynecologic Reproductive Surgery* (Boca Raton, Fla/London: CRC Press, 2021).

Roberts, Celia, *Messengers of Sex: Hormones, Biomedicine and Feminism* (Cambridge: Cambridge University Press, 2007).

Robin, D. M., A. R. Larsen, & C. Levin, *Encyclopedia of Women in the Renaissance: Italy, France, and England* (Santa Barbara, Calif.: ABC-CLIO, 2007).

Rocca, Walter A., Liliana Gazzuola-Rocca, Carin Y. Smith, Brandon R. Grossardt, Stephanie S. Faubion, Lynne T. Shuster, James L. Kirkland, Elizabeth A. Stewart, & Virginia M. Miller, 'Accelerated Accumulation of Multimorbidity After Bilateral Oophorectomy: A Population-Based Cohort Study', *Mayo Clinic Proceedings*, 91/11 (2016): 1577–1589. Doi: 10.1016/j.mayocp.2016.08.002.

Rochebrochard, Elise de la, 'One in Thirty Children in France Conceived through Assisted Reproductive Technology', *Population et Sociétés*, 556 (2018): Hal-01990070. https://hal.archives-ouvertes.fr/hal-01990070/document.

Rose, Nikolas, 'Medicine, History and the Present', in Colin Jones & Roy Porter, eds, *Reassessing Foucault: Power, Medicine and the Body* (London: Routledge, 1994), 48–72.

Rouche, Hélène, 'La Différence des sexes chez Adrienne Sahuqué et Simone de Beauvoir: Leur Lecture des discours biologiques et médicaux', *Cahiers du genre*, 1/34 (2003): 105–125. Doi: 10.3917/cdge.034.0105.

Rozenbaum, Henri & Jean-Jacques Peumery, *Histoire illustré de la ménopause* (Paris: Dacosta, 1990).

Rusnock, Andrea A., *Vital Accounts: Quantifying Health and Population in Eighteenth-Century England and France* (Cambridge: Cambridge University Press, 2002).

Rutkin, H. Darrel, 'The Use and Abuse of Ptolemy's *Tetrabiblos* in Renaissance and Early-Modern Europe: Two Case Studies (Giovanni Pico Mirandola and Filippo Fantoni)', in Alexander Jones, ed., *Ptolemy in Perspective: Use and Criticism of His Work from Antiquity to the Nineteenth Century* (New York: Springer, 2010), 135–150.

Sage Pranchère, Nathalie, *L'École des sages-femmes: Naissance d'un corps professionnel 1786–1917* (Tours: Presses Universitaires, 2017).

Salkin Sbiroli, Lynn, 'Generation and Regeneration: Reflections on the Biological and Ideological Role of Women in France (1786–96)', in M. M. Roberts & Roy Porter, eds, *Literature and Medicine during the Eighteenth Century* (London: Routledge, 1993), 266–285.

Sanchez, Jean-Christophe, 'Observations des météores et médecine aux temps modernes', *Histoire, médecine et santé*, 1 (2012): 95–113. Doi:10.4000/hms.224.

Sarde, Michèle, *Françoise et la cinquantaine* (Paris: Seuil, 2003).

Scalenger, Sara, 'Menstruation and Menopause', in Bonny G. Smith, ed., *The Oxford Encyclopedia of Women in World History*, vol. 1 (Oxford: Oxford University Press, 2008), 264–266.

Schäfer, Daniel, *Old Age and Disease in Early Modern Medicine*, trans. Patrick Baker (London: Routledge, 2015).

Schäfer, Daniel, 'Die alternde Frau in der frühneuzeitlichen Medizin—eine "vergessene" Gruppe alter Menschen', [The Aging Woman in Early Modern Medicine—A 'Forgotten' Group of the Elderly] *Sudhoffs Archiv*, 87 (2003): 90–108.

Schiebinger, Londa, *Nature's Body: Gender in the Making of Modern Science* (Boston: Beacon, 1993).

Schlumbohm, Jürgen, 'Comment l'obstétrique est devenue une science: La Maternité de l'université de Gôttingen, 1751–1830', *Actes de la recherche en sciences sociales*, 143 (2002): 18–30. Doi: 10.3406/arss.2002.2851.

Schmidt, Susanne, *Midlife Crisis: The Feminist Origins of a Chauvinist Cliché* (Chicago: University of Chicago Press, 2020).

Scully, Diana, *Men Who Control Woman's Health: The Miseducation of Obstetrician-Gynecologists* (Boston: Houghton Mifflin, 1980).

Seignan, Gérard, 'L'Hygiène sociale au XIXe siècle: Une physiologie morale', *Revue d'histoire du XIXe siècle*, 40 (2010) : 113–130. Doi: 10.4000/rh19.3996.

Sengoopta, Chandak, *The Most Secret Quintessence of Life: Sex, Glands and Hormones, 1850–1950* (Chicago: University of Chicago Press, 2006).

Shackelford, Jole, 'The Chemical Hippocrates: Paracelsian and Hippocratic Theory in Petrus Severinus' Medical Philosophy', in David Cantor, ed., *Reinventing Hippocrates* (Abingdon: Routledge, 2016), 59–88.

Shackelford, Jole, *A Philosophical Path for Paracelsian Medicine: The Ideas, Intellectual Context, and Influence of Petrus Severinus (1540–1602)* (Copenhagen: Museum Tusculanum Press, 2004).

Sievert, Lynette Leidy, 'Menopause Across Cultures: Clinical Considerations', *Menopause*, 21/4 (2014): 421–423. Doi: 10.1097/GME.0000000000000099.

Sionneau, Sylvain, *Les Hors-la-loi de la médecine au xixe siècle en Maine-et-Loire* (La Crèche: Geste, 2015).

Smith, Bonnie G., ed., *The Oxford Encyclopaedia of Women in World History* (Oxford: Oxford University Press, 2008).

Soumaya, Naamane Gessous, *Printemps et automne sexuels: puberté, ménopause, andro-pause au Maroc* (Marseille: Autre Temps, 2000).

Sournia, Jean-Charles, *Histoire de la médecine* (Paris: Éditions la Découverte, 1992).

Speert, Harold, *Obstetric and Gynecologic Milestones: Essays in Eponymy* (New York: Macmillan, 1958).

Speert, Harold, *Obstetrics and Gynecology in America: A History* (Chicago: American College of Obstetricians and Gynecologists, 1980).

Squier, Susan, 'The Traffic Between Technologies of Reproduction and Age-Extension', in Kathleen Woodwood, ed., *Figuring Age, Women, Bodies, Generations* (Bloomington and Indianapolis: Indiana University Press, 1999), 86–99.

Staum, Martin, *Cabanis: Enlightenment and Medical Philosophy in the French Revolution* (Princeton: Princeton University Press, 1980).

Stead, Evanghélia, 'Musa medicinalis: Variation sur la médecine et les lettres au tournant du siècle', *Romantisme*, 94 (1996): 111–124. Doi: 10.3406/roman.1996.3162.

Stearns, Peter, *Fat History: Bodies and Beauty in the Modern West* (New York: New York University Press, 1997).

Steele, Valerie, *Paris Fashion: A Cultural History* (Oxford: Oxford University Press, 1988).

Stewart, Elizabeth A., Stacey A. Missmer, & Walter A. Rocca, 'Moving Beyond Reflexive and Gynecologic Prophylactic Surgery', *Mayo Clinic Proceedings*. 96/2 (2021): 291–294. Doi: 10.1016/j.mayocp.2020.05.012.

Stewart, Joan Hinde, *The Enlightenment Age: Women, Letters and Growing Old in Eighteenth-Century France* (Oxford: Voltaire Foundation, 2010).

Stewart, Mary Lynn, *For Health and Beauty: Physical Culture for Frenchwomen 1880s–1930* (Baltimore: Johns Hopkins University Press, 2000).

Stoff, Heiko, *Ewige Jugend: Konzepte der Verjungung vom spaten 19. Jahrhundert bis ins Dritte Reich* (Cologne: Bohlau, 2004).

Stolberg, Michael, 'A Woman's Hell? Medical Perceptions of Menopause in Preindustrial Europe', *Bulletin of the History of Medicine*, 73/3 (1999): 404–428.

Stolberg, Michael 'A Woman Down to Her Bones: The Anatomy of Sexual Difference in the Sixteenth and Early Seventeenth Centuries', *Isis*, 94/2 (2003): 274–299.

Stolberg, Michael, 'Von den 'Stufenjahren' zur 'Menopause': Das Klimakterium im Wandel der Zeit [From 'anni climacterici' to 'menopause': The historical roots of the concept of climacteric]. *Wurzburger Medizinhistorische Mitteilungen*, 24 (2005): 41–50.

Stolberg, Michael, 'Menstruation and Sexual Difference in Early Modern Medicine', in Andrew Shail & Gillian Howie, eds, *Menstruation, A Cultural History* (New York: Palgrave, 2005), 90–101.

Stoller, Silvia, ed., *Simone de Beauvoir's Philosophy of Age: Gender, Ethics, Time* (Berlin: De Gruyter, 2014).

Strasser, Anne, 'Simone de Beauvoir, du *Deuxième sexe* à *La Vieillesse*: Quand l'intime gagne le politique', *Itinéraires*, 2 (2012): 93–103. Doi: 10.4000/itineraires.1135.

Strassmann, Beverly I., 'The Biology of Menstruation in Homo Sapiens: Total Lifetime Menses, Fecundity, and Nonsynchrony in a Natural-Fertility Population', *Current Anthropology*, 38/1 (1997): 123–129.

Sturm, Jules, *Bodies We Fail: Productive Embodiments of Imperfection* (Bielefeld: Transcript Verlag, 2014).

Sullivan-Fowler, Micaela, 'Doubtful Theories, Drastic Therapies: Autointoxication and Faddism in the Late Nineteenth Century and Early Twentieth Centuries', *Journal of the History of Medicine and Allied Sciences*, 50 (1995): 364–390.

Sussman, George D., 'The Glut of Doctors in Mid-Nineteenth-Century France', *Comparative Studies in Society and History*, 19/3 (1977): 287–304.

Taunton, Nina, *Fictions of Old Age in Early Modern Literature and Culture* (New York: Routledge, 2007).

Tazzioli, Martina, Sophie Fuggle, & Yari Lanic, 'Introduction', in Sophie Fuggle, Yari Lanic, & Martina Tazzioli, eds, *Foucault and the History of Our Present* (Basingstoke: Palgrave, 2015), 1–12.

Thane, Pat, *Old Age in English History* (Oxford: Oxford University Press, 2000).

Thébaud, Françoise, *Écrire l'histoire des femmes et du genre* (Paris: ENS Éditions, 2017).

Thénard-Duvivier, Franck, ed., *Hygiène, santé et protection sociale de la fin du XVIIIe siècle à nos jours* (Paris: Ellipses, 2012).

Théré, Christine, 'Âge de retour et retour d'âge: L'Asymétrie entre les sexes dans les discours médicaux en France (1770–1836)', [Life Change and Change of Life: Asymmetrical Attitudes towards the Sexes in Medical Discourse in France (1770–1836)] *CLIO: Femmes, genre, histoire*, 42 (2015): 54–75.

Theriot, Nancy M., 'Women's Voices in Nineteenth-Century Medical Discourse: A Step Toward Deconstructing Science', *Signs*, 19/1 (1993): 1–31.

Tiersten, Lisa, *Marianne in the Market: Envisioning Consumer Society in Fin-de-Siècle France* (Berkeley: University of California Press, 2001).

Tillier, Annick, 'Un Âge critique. La Ménopause sous le regard des médecins des XVIIIe et XIXe siècles', *CLIO: Femmes, genre, histoire*, 21 (2005): 269–280. Doi: 10.4000/clio.1471.

Tomkins, Alannah, 'Case Notes and Madness', in Mark Jackson, ed., *The Routledge History of Disease* (London: Routledge, 2016), 529–546.

Tomlinson, Maria Kathryn, *From Menstruation to Menopause: The Female Fertility Cycle in Contemporary Women's Writing in French* (Liverpool: Liverpool University Press, 2021).

Toulalan, Sarah, '"Elderly Years Cause a Total Dispaire of Conception": Old Age, Sex, and Infertility in Early Modern England', *Social History of Medicine*, 29/2 (2016): 333–359.

Troyansky, David, *Old Age in the Old Regimes: Image and Experience in Eighteenth-Century France* (Ithaca, NY/London: Cornell University Press, 1989).

Troyansky, David, *Aging in World History* (New York: Routledge, 2016).

Ulijaszek, S. J., M. Mann, & S. Elton, *Evolving Human Nutrition: Implications for Public Health* (Cambridge: Cambridge University Press, 2012).

Ulin, Mara, Mohamed Ali, Zunir Tayyeb Chaudhry, Ayman Al-Hendy, & Qiwiei Yang, 'Uterine Fibroids in Menopause and Perimenopause', *Menopause*, 27/2 (2020): 238–242. Doi: 10.1097/GME.0000000000001438.

Vanderpooten, Claude, Samuel Pozzi, chirurgien et ami des femmes (Ozoire-la-Ferrière: Éditions La Fine, 1992).

Vergès, Françoise, *Le Ventre des femmes: Capitalisme, racialisation, féminisme* (Paris: Albin Michel 2017).

Vernus, Michel, *Médecine populaire en Franche-Comté: Petites et grandes histoires des faiseurs de secrets et autres rebouteux* (Pontarlier: Éditions du Belvédère, 2013).

Vial, Robert, *Histoire de l'enseignement des Hôpitaux de Paris: Les Blouses blanches en formation initiale et continue* (Paris: L'Harmattan, 1999).

Viala, Alain, *La Galanterie, une mythologie française* (Paris: Éditions du Seuil, 2019).

Vila, Anne C., 'Sex and Sensibility: Pierre Rousseau's *Système physique et moral de la femme*', *Représentations*, 52 (1995): 76–93.

Vinel, Virginie, 'Ménopause et andropause à la lumière du 'dispositif de sexualité', *Le PortiQue*, 13–14 (2004). Doi: 10.4000/leportique.628.

Waisse, Silvia, Maria Amaral, & Thereza Cer Galvão, 'Roots of French Vitalism: Bordeu and Barthez, between Paris and Montepellier', in Ana M. Alfonso-Goldfarb, ed., *História, Ciências, Saúde—Manguinhos*, 18/3 (2011). http://scielo.br.

Wang, Y., W. Shan, Q. Li, & W. Shan, 'Tai Chi Exercise for Quality of Life in a Perimenopausal Women Organization', *Worldviews Evidence Based Nursing*, 14/4 (2017): 294–305. Doi: 10.1111/wvn.12234.

Warman, Carolyn, 'From Lamarck to Aberration: Nature, Hierarchies, and Gender', *Journal of the History of Sexuality*, 18/1 (2009): 8–25.

Watkins, Elizabeth Siegel, *The Estrogen Elixir: A History of Hormone Replacement Therapy in America* (Baltimore: Johns Hopkins University Press, 2009).

Weber, Eugen, *Peasants into Frenchmen: The Modernization of Rural France, 1870–1914* (Stanford, Calif.: Stanford University Press 1976).

Weiner, Dora B., '"Le Geste de Pinel": The History of a Psychiatric Myth', in Mark S. Micale & Roy Porter, eds, *Discovering the History of Psychiatry* (New York: Oxford University Press, 1994), 232–242.

Weisz, George, 'The Emergence of Specialism in the Nineteenth Century', *Bulletin of the History of Medicine*, 77 (2003): 536–575.

Wellman, Kathleen Anne, 'Physicians and Philosophes: Physiology and Sexual Morality in the French Enlightenment', *Eighteenth-Century Studies*, 35/2 (2002): 267–277.

Weston, Robert, *A Country Doctor in the French Revolution: Marie-François-Bernardin Ramel* (New York: Routledge, 2020).

Wilbush, Joel, '*La Ménespausie*: The Birth of a Syndrome', *Maturitas*, 1 (1979): 145–151.

Wilbush, Joel, 'What's in a Name? Some Linguistic Aspects of the Climacteric', *Maturitas*, 3 (1981): 1–9.

Wilbush, Joel, 'Menorrhagia and Menopause: A Historical Review', *Maturitas*, 10 (1988): 5–26.

Williams, Elizabeth A., *A Cultural History of Medical Vitalism in Enlightenment Montpellier* (London: Routledge, 2003).

Williams, Elizabeth A., *The Physical and the Moral: Anthropology, Physiology, and Philosophical Medicine in France, 1750–1850* (Cambridge: Cambridge University Press, 1994).

Williams, Elizabeth A., 'Eating after the Climacteric: Food, Gender and Aging in the Long Eighteenth Century', chapter 4 in James Kennaway and Rina Knoeff, eds, *Lifestyle and Medicine in the Enlightenment: The Six Non-Naturals in the Long Eighteenth Century* (London: Routledge, 2020), unpaginated.

Williams, Elizabeth A., 'Hysteria and the Court Physician in Enlightenment France', *Eighteenth-Century Studies*, 35/2 (2002): 247–255. Doi: 10.1353/ecs.2002.0021.

Williams, Elizabeth A., 'Physicians, Vitalism, and Gender in the Salon', *Studies in Eighteenth-Century Culture*, 29 (Baltimore: Johns Hopkins University Press, 2000), 1–21.

Wolfe, Charles T., 'Introduction: Vitalism without Metaphysics? Medical Vitalism in the Enlightenment', *Science in Context*, 21/4 (2008): 461–463. Doi: 10.1017/S0269889708001919.

Wolfe, Charles T., 'The Animal Economy as Object and Program in Montpellier Vitalism', *Science in Context*, 21/4 (2008): 537–579. Doi: 10.1017/S0269889708001956.

Wolfe, Charles T., 'Models of Organic Organization in Montpellier Vitalism', *Early Science & Medicine*, 22 (2017): 1–24. Doi: 10.1163/15733823-02223p07.

Index

Note: Figures are indicated by an italic '*f*' following the page numbers.

For the benefit of digital users, indexed terms that span two pages (e.g., 52–53) may, on occasion, appear on only one of those pages.